Advances in Pattern Recognition

Springer

London
Berlin
Heidelberg
New York
Barcelona
Hong Kong
Milan
Paris
Singapore
Tokyo

Advances in Pattern Recognition is a series of books which brings together current developments in all areas of this multi-disciplinary topic. It covers both theoretical and applied aspects of pattern recognition, and provides texts for students and senior researchers.

Springer also publishes a related journal, **Pattern Analysis and Applications**. For more details see: http://link.springer.de

The book series and journal are both edited by Professor Sameer Singh of Exeter University, UK.

Also in this series:

Principles of Visual Information Retrieval
Michael S. Lew (Ed.)
1-85233-381-2

Statistical and Neural Classifiers: An Integrated Approach to Design
Šarūnas Raudys
1-85233-297-2

NETLAB: Algorithms for Pattern Recognition
Ian T. Nabney
1-85233-440-1

Object Recognition: Fundamentals and Case Studies
M. Bennamoun and G.J. Mamic
1-85233-398-7

Jasjit S. Suri, S. Kamaledin Setarehdan
and Sameer Singh (Eds)

Advanced Algorithmic Approaches to Medical Image Segmentation

State-of-the-Art Applications in Cardiology, Neurology, Mammography and Pathology

With 239 Figures

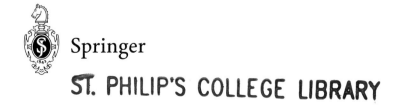

Springer

Jasjit S. Suri, PhD
Clinical Research Division, Magnetic Resonance Division,
Marconi Medical Systems Inc., 595 Minor Road, Cleveland, OH 44143, USA

S. Kamaledin Setarehdan, PhD
Department of Electrical, Electronic and Computer Engineering,
Faculty of Engineering, PO Box 14395/515, University of Tehran, Tehran, Iran

Sameer Singh, PhD
Department of Computer Science, University of Exeter, Exeter, EX4 4PT, UK

Series editor
Professor Sameer Singh, PhD
Department of Computer Science, University of Exeter, Exeter, EX4 4PT, UK

British Library Cataloguing in Publication Data
Advanced algorithmic approaches to medical image
    segmentation : state-of-the-art applications in cardiology,
    neurology, mammography and pathology. - (Advances in
    pattern recognition)
    1.Diagnostic imaging 2. Algorithms
    I.Suri, Jasjit S. II.Setarehdan, S. Kamaledin III. Singh,
    Sameer, 1970-
    616'.0754
    ISBN 1852333898

Library of Congress Cataloging-in-Publication Data
A catalog record for this book is available from the Library of Congress

Advances in Pattern Recognition ISSN 1617-7916

ISBN 1-85233-389-8 Springer-Verlag London Berlin Heidelberg
a member of BertelsmannSpringer Science+Business Media GmbH
http://www.springer.co.uk

Typesetting: Editors and Ian Kingston Editorial Services, Nottingham, UK
Printed and bound at The Cromwell Press, Trowbridge, Wiltshire
34/3830-543210 Printed on acid-free paper SPIN 10783286

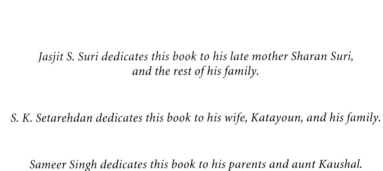

Jasjit S. Suri dedicates this book to his late mother Sharan Suri, and the rest of his family.

S. K. Setarehdan dedicates this book to his wife, Katayoun, and his family.

Sameer Singh dedicates this book to his parents and aunt Kaushal.

The Editors

Dr. Jasjit Suri was born in India in 1964, received his high school diploma from *Sainik School Rewa* (one of only 21 schools of its kind in India), in the state of Madhya Pradesh (MP), a Bachelor's degree in Electronics and Computer Engineering from *Maulana Azad College of Technology* (a Regional Engineering College, and number one in the state of MP), Bhopal, a Master's degree in Computer Science from the *University of Illinois*, Chicago (with a specialization in Neuro Imaging), and a Doctorate in Electrical Engineering from the *University of Washington*, Seattle, with a specialization in Cardiac Imaging. Dr. Suri has been working in the area of Medical Image Segmentation for more than 12 years and has published more than 75 publications in the areas of Cardiac Imaging, Brain Magnetic Resonance, Abdomen Computed Tomography, Dental X-rays, Ultrasound and Pathology Imaging. Dr. Suri has given more than 25 presentations/seminars at several international conferences in Europe, Australia and the United States. He has worked with the IBM Scientific Center (Computer Graphics Division), performing surface rendering of blood vessels using MRA on RISC 6000 (using Open GL), and with Siemens in the CT Research Division performing treatment planning system design (performing surface rendering) on DEC alpha. He has also spent time as a Research Scientist at the *University of Wisconsin*, Madison, designing an Ultrasound Lesion Detection System based on surfaces. He was a faculty member at MACT, Bhopal, India, teaching Computer Arch. Design/Imaging. Dr. Suri has worked in the areas of MR image-guided thermal ablation for prostate imaging using high frequency ultrasound (HIFU), and in image-guided neuro-surgery, orthopedics, and perfusion imaging systems for the breast and human brain. He was honored with the Indian President's Gold Medal in 1980. He is on the review/editorial boards of several international imaging science journals, including: *Journal of Real Time Imaging, Journal of Engineering Medicine and Biology, Journal of Pattern Analysis and Applications, Journal of Computer Assisted Tomography, Journal of Radiology*, and *IEEE Transactions of Information Technology and Biomedicine*. Dr. Suri has also served as a board member of the program committees of the following conferences: "Image Processing of International Association of Science and Technology for Development (IASTED)", "IEEE Computerized-Based Medical Systems" hosted by the National Institutes of Health, "International Conference on Visualization, Imaging and Image Processing" hosted by IASTED and has peer reviewed several international conferences/journal papers in the areas of Medical Imaging and Mathematical Imaging. During his career, Dr. Suri has received more than 45 scholarly, scientific extra-curricular awards and holds the honor of an outstanding award (by the State Ministry of Defense, India) of "managing and allroundership" for managing 600 college level students for one full year. Dr. Suri is a *Senior IEEE member* and life member of: Tau-Beta-Pi, Engineering Honor Society, Eta-Kappa-Nu, Engineering Honor Society, and a member of: the New York Academy of Sciences, Sigma Xi Research Honor Society, Engineering in Medicine and Biology Society, ACM, The International Society for Optical Engineering, and Cleveland Engineering. Dr. Suri received the *"Who's Who in the World"* award for the year 2000 and is listed in *Marquis Who's Who* – 18th edition. Dr. Suri is also a recipient of the *"International Executive Who's Who"* award for the year 2000 and is listed in the 2001 edition of the International *Who's Who of Information Technology*. Dr. Suri also received the prestigious "One Thousand Great Americans Award" from the International Biographic Center, Cambridge, England for 2001. His major interests are in Computer Vision, Graphics, Image Processing, Medical Imaging, User interfaces and applications of mathematical imaging for human body organs. Dr. Suri wishes to continue building health care diagnostic medical imaging systems based on his 18 years of extensive computer science and engineering experience.

Dr. S. Kamaledin Setarehdan was born in Iran in 1965. He graduated from the *College of Alborz*, Tehran, Iran and ranked in the top 0.1% in the national conquers for a B.Sc. place in Engineering in 1983. He received a B.Sc. degree in Electronic Engineering from *Tehran University*, Tehran, Iran and an M.Sc. degree in Biomedical Engineering from *Sharif University of Technology*, Tehran, Iran. He was awarded the MCHE bursary by the Ministry of Culture and Higher Education of Iran to pursue his studies towards a Ph.D. degree. He received his Ph.D. degree in Electronic Engineering from the *University of Strathclyde*, Glasgow, UK, with a specialization in Medical Imaging and Signal Processing. Dr. Setarehdan has published many regular and invited journal and conference papers in the areas of Biomedical Engineering and Medical Image Processing, with some of his papers having won awards at international conferences in Europe and the United States.

Professor Sameer Singh was born in New Delhi, India, and graduated from *Birla Institute of Technology*, India with a Bachelor of Engineering degree with a distinction in Computer Engineering. He received his Master of Science degree in Information Technology for Manufacturing from the *University of Warwick*, UK, and a Ph.D. in speech and language analysis of stroke patients from the *University of the West of England*, UK. His main research interests are in Image Processing, Medical Imaging, Neural Networks and Pattern Recognition. He is the Director of the Pattern Analysis and Neural Networks group at Exeter University, UK. He serves as the Editor-in-Chief of the *Pattern Analysis and Applications Journal* published by Springer, Editor-in-Chief of the Springer book series on "Advances in Pattern Recognition", Chairman of the British Computer Society Specialist Group on Pattern Analysis and Robotics, Editorial Board member of the *Neural Computing and Applications Journal*, and Editorial Board member of the "Perspectives in Neural Computing" book series published by Springer. He is a Fellow of the Royal Statistical Society, a Chartered Engineer, and a member of IAPR, IEE and IEEE.

Preface

The field of medical imaging has experienced an explosive growth in recent years due to several imaging modalities, such as X-ray, computed tomography (CT), magnetic resonance (MR) imaging, positron emission tomography (PET), single positron emission computer tomography (SPECT), ultrasound and its fusion. The digital revolution and the computer's processing power in combination with these imaging modalities have helped humans to better understand the complex human anatomy and its behavior to a certain extent. Computer power and medical scanner data alone are not enough; we need the art to extract the necessary boundaries, surfaces, and segmented volumes of these organs in the spatial and temporal domains. This art of organ extraction is segmentation. Image segmentation is essentially a process of pixel classification, wherein the image pixels are segmented into subsets by assigning the individual pixels to classes. These segmented organs and their boundaries are very critical in the quantification process for physicians and medical surgeons, in any branch of medicine which deals with imaging.

This book primarily focuses on state-of-the-art model-based segmentation techniques applied to CT imaging, MR imaging, ultrasound imaging, X-ray imaging and pathology imaging. These modalities are applied to different body parts such as the brain, heart, breast and at the cellular level. Different applications are covered, such as the human brain in magnetic resonance, cardiovascular imaging in ultrasound and X-rays, breast cancer lesion detection in mammograms and cytology imaging. Readers will find the following new items in this book: (1) A collection of principles of image generation for ultrasound, MR, CT, X-ray and PET. (2) A collection of algorithms for brain segmentation applied to MR. (3) A collection of algorithms for neuro-applications using MR such as in functional Magnetic Resonance Imaging (fMRI), spectroscopy, mixture modeling and Multiple Sclerosis (MS). (4) A collection of algorithms for parametric and geometric deformable models for brain segmentation. (5) A collection of algorithms for left ventricle segmentation and analysis using least squares and constrained least squares models for cardiac X-rays. (6) A collection of algorithms for left ventricle analysis in echocardioangiograms. (7) A collection of algorithms for breast lesion detection in digital mammograms. (8) A collection of algorithms for the detection of cells in cell images. (9) Discussions on the future of segmentation techniques. And finally, (10) a collection of state-of-the-art references in segmentation. Since this book is an algorithmic approach to segmentation, it is meant for dedicated researchers who would like to reach a certain level of understanding of model-based segmentation techniques.

The book is organized into 4 sections. The first section of the book focuses on the principles of image generation and cardiac image segmentation algorithms. Section 2 focuses on neuro applications. Section 3 focuses on mammography imaging and Section 4 on cytology imaging.

Section 1 consists of three chapters. Chapter 1 discusses the principles of image generation, and Chapter 2 and Chapter 3 discuss left ventricle (LV) segmentation in ultrasound and X-ray images. We will now discuss the details of each chapter in Section 1.

Chapter 1 discusses the basic principles of image generation for ultrasound, X-rays, MR, CT and PET. In MR, we discuss the process of acquiring 2-D/3-D MR image data, how magnetic resonance images use three orthogonal magnetic field gradients in addition to the static main magnetic field and the radio frequency transmitter and receiver, to encode the three-dimensional position information into, or localize, the Nuclear Magnetic Resonance (NMR) signals received. We also discuss some of the latest techniques in MR imaging. In ultrasound image generation, we discuss how a piezoelectric transducer generates a short burst of ultrasound in response to an electrical stimulus which is then transmitted into the body. We also discuss how cross-sectional images of body tissues are generated. In X-rays, we discuss the cardiac X-ray image generation process. We also discuss the principles of image generation for CT and PET. The chapter concludes by comparing different standard medical imaging modalities.

Chapters 2 and 3 concentrate on the model-based segmentation techniques applied to cardiac analysis. In Chapter 2, we present novel contributions towards the automatic identification of cardiac left ventricular central point and epicardial and endocardial boundaries from standard echocardiographic image sequences, which are the basis for the quantification of cardiac function and wall motion visualization. The techniques, which are based on fuzzy logic and the wavelet transform, focus on simulating a human expert's ability to integrate the scattered local and global intensity and motion information in the sequences of echocardiographic frames through the eye-brain fuzzy reasoning process to come up with closed cardiac boundaries. The left ventricular center point approximation in both short axis and long axis echo images is presented in a fuzzy reasoning approach. This identifies a pixel in the image using the most descriptive local and regional left ventricular center point features, which are acquired from the interpretations of a human expert. The key problem of edge detection in echocardiographic images is alleviated through the development of a new technique, based on the definition of the global maximum point of the wavelet transform. This wavelet transform-based multiscale edge detection technique is shown to produce less root mean square error when compared to other conventional edge operators on a variety of noisy edge profiles. Finally, a complete cardiac left ventricular boundary extraction, left ventricular wall motion visualization and cardiac functional assessment system is presented. This is based on the ability of the fuzzy reasoning techniques to carry out automatic left ventricular central point identification and "radial search-based" left ventricular boundary edge detection using the new edge detection technique of the global maximum of the wavelet transform.

In Chapter 3, we present a review of model-based segmentation techniques applied to different types of cardiac imaging. The major part of this chapter is on left ventricle (LV) analysis using X-rays. This chapter first discusses the problems associated with the LV X-ray images. It then presents a pixel-based Bayesian approach to LV chamber boundary estimation which uses spatial and temporal information, where the gray scale values of the location throughout the cardiac cycle were taken as a vector. The distribution of this vector was assumed to be bi-variate normal. For each observed vector, one class was assigned according to the ground truth, which was available by filling the left ventricle region surrounded by the ground truth left ventricle boundary. The pixels were then classified using a Bayesian classifier. The above methods do produce boundaries but, due to the reasons stated above, the boundaries fall short, have jaggedness, over-estimation, under-estimation, irregularities and are not close to the ground truth boundaries, thereby making the system incomplete and unreliable. In the inferior wall region, the papillary muscles have a non-uniform structure, unlike the anterior wall region. This non-uniformity causes further variation in the apparent boundary during the cardiac cycle. Because of this, the initial boundary position of the inferior walls is sometimes over-estimated. In an attempt to correct the initial image processing boundaries, we present two linear calibration algorithms to estimate the LV boundaries without taking the LV apex information. This approach uses a training-based optimization procedure over the initial boundaries to correct its bias. This bias correction can be thought of as a calibration procedure, where the boundaries produced by the image processing techniques are corrected using the global shape information gathered from the ideal database.

For further improving upon the left ventricle boundary error, we present a greedy left ventricle boundary estimation algorithm, which fuses the boundaries coming from two different techniques. To reduce further error in the apex zone, we developed an apex estimation technique using the end diastole apex, the so-called temporal dependence approach. This estimated the end systole apex and was then used in the end systole boundary estimation process. Using the weighted least squares algorithm, this developed the apex estimation using the ruled surface model. Though the apex error was reduced, the inferior wall zone could not be controlled in many subjects due to the large classifier error, which was due to the overlap of the left ventricle and the diaphragm. This was validated by using a training-based system which utilized the LV gray scale images and the estimated boundaries. The surface fitting approach was used along with mathematical morphology to identify the diaphragm edges and separate the LV from the diaphragm. Then, the classifier boundaries were merged with edge-based left ventricle boundaries, and the better of the two was taken for calibration. By penalizing the apex vertex in the linear calibration, this forced the estimated curve to pass through the LV apex, this convex hull approach drastically reducing the apex error. Linear calibration was further improved upon in the quadratic calibration scheme for left ventricle boundary quantification yielding the segmentation accuracy to 2.5 millimeters, the target set by cardiologists. This chapter concludes by discussing LV boundary quantification techniques.

Section 2 of this book consists of Chapters 4, 5, 6, 7 and 8. These chapters cover a wide variety of applications of segmentation in neuro-imaging.

In Chapter 4, we present an extensive cortical segmentation review. The extensive growth in functional brain imaging, perfusion-weighted imaging, diffusion-weighted imaging, and brain scanning techniques has led to a tremendous increase in the importance of brain segmentation both in 2-D and 3-D data sets. Also, recent growth in active contour brain segmentation techniques in 2-D has brought the engineering community, such as those in computer vision, image processing and graphics, closer to the medical community, such as to neuro-surgeons, psychiatrists, oncologists, radiologists and internists. This chapter is an attempt to review the state-of-the-art brain segmentation of 2-D and 3-D techniques using Magnetic Resonance Imaging. Particular emphasis is placed on the fusion of classification algorithms with deformation models to robustly segment the brain data sets. The chapter concludes by discussing the state-of-the-art method of fMRI.

Chapter 5 covers illustrative descriptions of the use of various segmentation methods focusing on the automatic quantification of MS lesions in a clinical set-up. This part of the book will be useful as an advanced level reference to neurologists. For image processing scientists, it covers introductory issues in brain tissue segmentation and various brain tissue artifacts like partial volume averaging, and poor contrast-to-noise ratio deteriorating the demarcation of tissue edges. Improved pulse sequences are given as good examples for MR physicists who are interested in software developments for better lesion-to-tissue contrast, robust automation in MS lesion volume measurement and quantification of brain tissue components. The success of segmentation is evidenced as well in illustrated color-coded tissue composition information and better visualization of White Matter (WM), Gray Matter (GM), Cerebrospinal Fluid (CSF) and MS lesions as distinct, well-defined Multiple Sclerosis features interesting to neurologists.

In Chapter 6, we focus on finite mixture modeling and its application to MR brain images. For neurological image segmentation, we show how the brain magnetic resonance images are used in the segmentation process. The pixel classification problem is posed by assigning numeric labels to each pixel. Given a known or estimated number of classes, each class can be associated with a numeric label. One widely used model is the mixture model, wherein the pixels constituting a discrete image are assumed to arise from a density function which in itself is composed of several underlying densities. For instance, in the simple case, we could have a set of three Gaussian densities, each of which is characterized by unique mean and variance values. Each of these individual components is weighted by a scale factor. The assumption of such a model for an image transforms the image segmentation problem into a parameter estimation problem. Upon estimating the parameters (means and variances in this simple example) of the underlying component densities of the mixture, a suitable labeling rule can be applied to assign labels to the pixels in the image and segment it into various regions. We can also incorporate other appropriate models for phenomena such as the partial volume effect in this framework for optimal image segmentation. Various statistical models which have been applied for segmenting medical images are presented, and their advantages and disadvantages are outlined. We then focus on some of the more recent advances in the application of mixture models for image segmentation. It has been shown that a spatially-variant mixture model has been formulated for pixel labeling. This model eliminates a severe limitation of the classical mixture model when applied for Bayesian pixel labeling. Based on this model, a generalized expectation-maximization algorithm has been proposed for Bayesian image segmentation. This algorithm incorporates Markov Random Fields (MRFs) within the mixture model framework. MRFs have been widely applied for obtaining visually appealing image segments in cases where the data is extremely noisy. However, an intrinsic drawback in most of these techniques is the extreme computational requirements. Most of the algorithms using MRFs involve complex searches for global minima of some energy functions. To facilitate easy computation, sub-optimal approaches which terminate algorithms in local minima have been adopted. In this part of the book, an attractive alternative to these former approaches is the use of mixture models which result in both visually appealing segmentation as well as less computationally intensive algorithms when using MRFs. These algorithms are applicable to images which suffer from high statistical noise where pixel misclassification is a common occurrence. The use of these algorithms has been shown to result in a significant reduction in the percentage of mis-classified pixels in the image. We also discuss the segmentation accuracies of these techniques. The results of applying these techniques to Computed Tomography (CT) and Magnetic Resonance Images (MRI) are presented to better understand the use of mixture models for medical image segmentation.

Chapter 7 is a quick reference for imaging scientists, neurologists and brain-spectroscopists. The author discusses the purpose, need and technical aspects of an automated program for Magnetic Resonance Spectroscopic Imaging (MRSI), interesting to beginners and advanced level Multiple Sclerosis-biochemists, physicists and neurologists devoted to research or a clinical setup. Additional information on spectroscopic image post-processing shows the applications of MRI brain tissue segmentation, using the co-registration of MRI data sets with Multiple Sclerosis plaque and Alzheimer's Disease. This is very beneficial to neuroscientists. In this direction, the application of a simple MR spectra processing method – the Automated Proton Spectroscopic Image Processing algorithm – is defined as robust, efficient clinical routine imaging software with less operater bias. In the last part of this chapter, the main emphasis is on well resolved spectral peaks and their clinical profiles in serial longitudinal scan examinations in Multiple Sclerosis and patients with Alzheimer's Disease. In the brain that has MS, NAA, Creatine, Choline, Myo-inositol, lipids and amino acids in MR visible spectral peaks are stimulations to advanced level clinical neurologists, imaging-spectroscopists and biochemists. Less common metabolites such as lactate, alanine, acetate, glutamate, glutamine and taurine are illustrated as examples of protein regulation and energy deficiency in Multiple Sclerosis, and as surrogate metabolic markers which are associated with neuronal loss, gliosis and demyelination. This chapter requires the clinical neurologist to have read up on the importance of in-vivo MR spectroscopic markers in decision making and to understand the disease process during clinical trials or routine examination. This chapter is a good example of the application of an automated Chemical Shift Imaging application in metabolite quantification, characterization and screening.

Finally, Section 2 concludes with Chapter 8, where we present a fast region-based level set approach for the extraction of White Matter (WM), Gray Matter (GM), and Cerebrospinal Fluid (CSF) boundaries from two dimensional magnetic resonance slices of the human brain. The raw contour was placed inside the images, which was later pushed or pulled towards the convoluted brain topology. The forces applied in the level set approach utilized four kinds of speed control functions based on shape, region, edge and curvature. Regional and shape speed functions were determined based on a fuzzy membership function computation using the fuzzy clustering technique, while the edge and curvature speed functions were based on gradient and signed distance transform functions, respectively. The level set algorithm was implemented to run in the "narrow band" using a "fast marching method". The system was tested on synthetic convoluted shapes and real magnetic resonance images of the human head. The entire system took approximately one minute to estimate the WM/GM boundaries on an XP1000 running with the Linux Operating System when the raw contour was placed half way from the goal, and took only a few seconds if the raw contour was placed close to the goal boundary with one hundred percent accuracy.

Section 3 discusses segmentation techniques in mammography. A large number of standard techniques have been applied in this area, and several new methods suited specifically to mammography have been developed. In Chapter 9, we investigate some of the important issues related to the segmentation and analysis of digital mammograms. This chapter presents a seamless view of analyzing mammograms from their acquisition to the classification of pathology as being benign or malignant. We consider various approaches suited to the detection of microcalcifications and masses. We detail issues surrounding image acquisition, enhancement, segmentation, feature extraction and performance assessment on classification. This chapter does not cover classification techniques in detail, as fairly standard techniques including statistical and neural classifiers have been used in mammography studies across the board. In particular, this chapter provides an algorithmic approach to a range of image and data analysis operations. It is outside the scope of this chapter to present a large group of image segmentation algorithms, however, we have made an attempt to present the majority of algorithms that have been popularly used in the last decade. The studies proposing them are discussed in brief where necessary, to give an overall view that forms the basis of the suggested algorithms. These algorithms cover enhancement, image segmentation and feature extraction in mammography.

Section 4 of this book focuses on segmentation application in pathology and cytology imaging. The focus is on the robust color segmenter based on non-parametric analysis of the L*u*v* vectors derived from the input image. The segmenter is one of the main modules of the image guided decision support system which integrates components for both remote microscope control and decision support. The task of the image guided decision support system is to locate, retrieve and display cases which exhibit morphological profiles consistent to the case in question, and to suggest the most likely diagnosis according to majority logic. The segmentation algorithm detects color clusters and delineates their borders by employing the gradient ascent mean shift procedure. It randomly tessellates the color space with search windows and moves the windows until convergence to the nearest mode of the underlying probability distribution is achieved. The nonparameteric analysis of the color space is suitable for cell images, typically characterized by only a few, non-Gaussian clusters. As a result, the segmentation module is capable of fast, accurate, and stable recovery of the main homogeneous regions in the input image.

The book concludes with Chapter 11, discussing the pros and cons of the state-of-the-art segmentation techniques and the future of image segmentation techniques.

Jasjit S. Suri
S. Kamaledin Setarehdan
Sameer Singh

Acknowledgements

This book is not the result of one individual's endeavours. Rather, it represents the work of several noted engineering and computer scientists, professors, physicists, and radiologists. In a way, they are the real authors of this book, and the editors are indeed indebted to all of them. In particular, the editors' appreciation and gratefulness go to Springer-Verlag London Ltd. for helping create this *invitational book*. From Springer-Verlag, London, UK, we are very thankful to Rosie Kemp and Karen Barker for their excellent coordination of this book at every stage.

Dr. Suri would like to thank Marconi Medical Systems, Inc., for the MR data sets and encouragements during his experiments and research. Thanks are due to Dr. Elaine Keeler and Dr. John Patrick from Marconi Medical Systems, Inc., for their support and motivation. Thanks are also due to my past Ph.D. committee research professors, particularly Professors Linda Shapiro, Robert M. Haralick, Dean Lytle and Arun Somani for their encouragement. Thanks are due to Dr. George Thoma, Chief Imaging Science Division from the National Institute of Health, and Dr. Ajit Singh, Siemens, for their motivations.

The editors would also like to extend thanks to all the contributing authors: Dr. Rakesh Sharma, Dr. Dorin Comaniciu, Dr. Peter Meer, Dr. John J. Soraghan, Dr. S. Sanjay Gopal, Dr. P. A. Narayana, Dr. Xiaolan Zeng, Keir Bovis and Laura Reden.

Thanks go to Anthony Goreham, Queen's College, Oxford, UK, on the issues related to LaTeX. Thanks go to Rick Hedrick for helping us to sort out the missing volume numbers and issue numbers of several articles listed in the bibliography of this book. The editors would also like to thank everyone who directly or indirectly participated in making this book an excellent research and educative tool.

Lastly, Dr. Suri would like to thank his lovely wife Malvika, a special person in my life, who gave strong support and love during this undertaking. Thanks go to my little baby, Harman Suri, who gave me his love all the time. Thanks go to my father, a mathematician and a General Manager, who inspired me all the time. Thanks go to my late mother, who passed away a few days before my Ph.D. graduation, and who wanted to see me write this book. I love you, Mom. I also would like to thank my mother-in-law and father-in-law and their family for their love and support. Dr. Setarehdan would also like to thank his wife, Katayoun, for her love and support. Finally, Professor Singh would like to thank his parents and aunt Kaushal.

Contents

The Contributors

Jasjit S. Suri, Ph.D.
Marconi Medical Systems, Inc.
Cleveland, OH, USA

Sameer Singh, Ph.D.
University of Exeter
Exeter, UK

S. K. Setarehdan, Ph.D.
University of Tehran
Tehran, Iran

John J. Soraghan, Ph.D.
University of Strathclyde
Glasgow, UK

Dorin Comaniciu, Ph.D.
Rutgers University
Piscataway, NJ, USA

Peter Meer, Ph.D.
Rutgers University
Piscataway, NJ, USA

Rakesh Sharma, Ph.D.
University of Texas Medical School
Houston, TX, USA

P. A. Narayana, Ph.D.
University of Texas Medical School
Houston, TX, USA

Yansun Xu, Ph.D.
Marconi Medical Systems, Inc.
Cleveland, OH, USA

Sanjay S. Gopal, Ph.D.
Marconi Medical Systems, Inc.
Cleveland, OH, USA

Xiaolan Zeng, Ph.D.
R2 Technology, Inc.
Los Altos, CA, USA

Keir Bovis, M.Sc.
University of Exeter
Exeter, UK

Laura Reden, B.S.
Marconi Medical Systems, Inc.
Cleveland, OH, USA

Chapter 1

Basic Principles of Image Generation for Ultrasound, X-Rays, Magnetic Resonance, Computed Tomography and Positron Emission Tomography

Jasjit S. Suri, S. K. Setarehdan, Rakesh Sharma, Sameer Singh, Yansun Xu, Laura Reden

1.1   Introduction

The usual aim in generating any kind of image in a body organ is to decide whether or not an abnormality is present and/or to follow the temporal variations of the abnormality during the course of a therapeutic treatment. Therefore, the two main goals of a human expert observer are: to detect the abnormality and to recognize it as such. Logically, the detection must occur prior to any useful recognition, however both procedures can be aided by improving the quality of the image by means of any post-processing techniques.

Since most medical images are traditionally viewed by a human observer, most research in medical imaging instrumentation has been directed so as to facilitate the detection process by human experts. However, due to technical or health limitations – for example, the limited dose of radiation that can be given to the patient – it is often the case that a feature of interest in a medical image cannot be seen or detected as clearly as the observer would wish. This also brings up the issues of subjectivity and intra-observer and inter-observer variability, which cannot be avoided due to the different knowledge levels or the way the observers have been trained.

The question that arises here is: how we can process a given image with its limited quality in order to produce one with higher visually appreciated quality? The processing of medical images is a rapidly evolving technique and with the advancement in digital technology and the computing power of processors, the production of good quality two-dimensional (2-D) or three-dimensional (3-D) anatomical data is now possible. These images are generated using different imaging modalities such as magnetic resonance, computed tomography, X-ray, ultrasound and positron emission tomography. Understanding the principles behind these image generation modalities plays an important role in the development of a useful sequence of post-processing steps. For example, this will help us to decide how to image an organ for its best quantitative analysis. For the best diagnostic utility, the imaging of organs and the principles involved in imaging them play an important role in post-processing and segmentation.

The post-processing discussed in this book uses modalities such as X-rays, magnetic resonance (MR), computer tomography (CT), positron emission tomography (PET) and ultrasound. This chapter will concentrate on using these modalities in cardiology, neurology, radiology and pathology.

The layout of this chapter is as follows: Sub-section 1.2 discusses in depth the principles of ultrasound imaging and the echocardiogram image generation process. Sub-section 1.3 discusses the X-ray image generation applied to cardiac image analysis. These images are called cardio-angiograms or ventriculograms. Sub-section 1.4 presents the MRI image generation process. Sub-section 1.5 discusses briefly the principles of Computer Tomography. Sub-section 1.6 highlights PET imaging principles and its image generation process. The chapter concludes by comparing the standard medical imaging modalities in Sub-section 1.7.

1.2   Ultrasound Image Generation

Ultrasound is the term used to describe the generation and transmission of longitudinal mechanical vibrations through matter when the frequency of oscillations is greater than the highest audible frequency, almost 20 kHz. For diagnostic ultrasound, the frequency is usually in the range of 1 to 10 MHz (see Carr [4]). Medical applications of ultrasound include surgery and therapy. However, in this book we are concerned only with diagnostic ultrasound and, in particular, pulse-echo imaging techniques.

Pulse-echo systems are able to produce cross-sectional images of soft tissue organs by transmitting a short duration ultrasound wave (pulse) into the body and detecting the reflections at tissue boundaries (echo). Ultrasound imaging of the body organs has several desirable properties when compared to the other medical imaging modalities. It is believed to be relatively safe (see Dunn [2]). There is no ionizing radiation in ultrasound, and most examinations are non-invasive and do not affect the patient (see McDicken [3]), so consequently examinations may be readily repeated. In comparison to MRI and CT, ultrasound involves less complicated instruments and is easily portable. Ultrasound allows soft tissues, which are difficult to detect by conventional X-ray techniques, to be imaged in detail. Unlike other medical imaging techniques, ultrasound offers interactive visualization of the underlying anatomy in real-time and has the ability to image dynamic structures within the body.

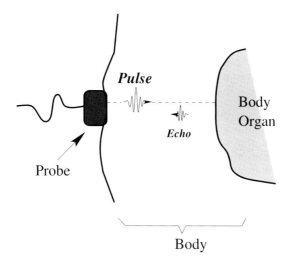

Figure 1.1: The principle of pulse-echo ultrasonic imaging.

1.2.1 The Principle of Pulse-Echo Ultrasound Imaging

In pulse-echo ultrasound imaging, a short burst of ultrasound is generated and transmitted into the body by a piezoelectric transducer. The piezoelectric transducer generates short length mechanical vibrations in response to an electrical stimulus. The reverse effect is also possible in piezoelectric materials, that is, they can convert mechanical vibrations to electrical currents. Therefore, the same device can be operated as a pressure transducer. In most systems, the tasks of transmitting and receiving are implemented by the same transducer and the transducer is housed in a hand-held probe. After transmitting a short burst of ultrasound oscillations into the body through physical contact with the probe, the transducer operates in the receive mode. The reflected signals from the different tissue boundaries and also the scatters resulting from the inhomogeneities in the media[1] are recorded by the transducer (see Figure 1.1).

Following a relatively long period of time, sufficient for the returning echoes to die out, another burst of ultrasound is emitted and the cycle is repeated. Because there are only small differences in the speeds of ultrasound in different tissues, the distance traveled by a pulse of ultrasound is proportional to time. The traveling time for the received echoes is then used to calculate the position of acoustic interfaces. The received echo and the computed information can be displayed in a number of ways. Commonly used display methods are the A-scan, M-scan and B-scan, which will be described in later sub-sections of this chapter.

---

[1] Media is plural and medium is singular.

1.2.1.1   Propagation of Ultrasound in Body Tissues

When a burst of an ultrasound wave passes through the different body layers, it has to deal with the effect of a non-homogeneous and imperfect transmission medium. An ultrasound wave is described by its frequency f and its amplitude A, and when it propagates in a medium we can talk about its velocity v and its wavelength λ in that medium. Since the frequency of oscillation of the ultrasound wave is almost fixed by the material and the structural shape and sizes of the piezoelectric crystal, its wavelength varies directly with the propagation velocity of the medium according to the relationship:

$$v = f \times \lambda. \tag{1.1}$$

1.2.1.2   Attenuation and Penetration Depth

The imperfections of the body tissues result in the attenuation of the ultrasound wave due to several phenomena including absorption, scattering, reflection, mode conversion and beam divergence. Despite the complexity of the phenomena, the attenuation property of soft tissue increases approximately linearly with frequency over the frequency range used by diagnostic ultrasound (see Carr [4]). Thus, a given power and frequency establish a maximum depth of penetration beyond which echoes are too weak to be detected. The ultrasound wave amplitude A along the path of propagation may be expressed as:

$$A(z) = A_0 e^{-\alpha z}, \tag{1.2}$$

where α is the attenuation coefficient, A_0 is the incident intensity, and z is the distance traversed. Simple automatic systems are designed to compensate for the attenuation of echoes from dipper layers in homogeneous tissue. Since in this compensator the gain is purely a function of depth (time), it is called the Time Gain Compensator (TGC).

1.2.1.3   Reflection, Refraction and Scattering

There are two known phenomena for echo back of the transmitted waves, namely reflection and scattering. Reflection occurs at the specular (mirror-like) interfaces of two different tissues, which are reflectors whose size is greater than the wavelength of the incident ultrasonic wave and whose irregularities are much smaller than the wavelength of the incident wave. Specular reflection is only a portion of the transmitted wave and the remainder propagates into the second medium. The amount that is reflected and the amount that continues depend on the difference in the characteristic impedances of the two tissues. The characteristic impedance of the medium is defined as (see Feigenbaum [6]):

$$Z = \rho \times v, \tag{1.3}$$

which determines how sound travels through a medium, where ρ is the density of the material and v is the velocity of sound waves in it. At a specular interface,

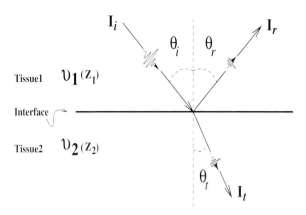

Figure 1.2: Reflection and refraction of the ultrasound beam.

the intensity of the reflected wave, I_r, is given by (see Geiser [11]):

$$I_r = I_i \left(\frac{Z_2 - Z_1}{Z_2 + Z_1} \right)^2 . \tag{1.4}$$

When ultrasound is reflected from a specular interface, the angle of reflection, θ_r, is equal to the angle of incidence, θ_i. There is also a change in the direction of the continuing portion of ultrasound in the second medium, which is referred to as refraction. These are illustrated in Figure 1.2. The relationship between the angle of incidence θ_i and the angle of refraction θ_t is dependent on the speed of sound in the two tissues:

$$\frac{sin\theta_i}{sin\theta_t} = \frac{v_1}{v_2}, \tag{1.5}$$

where v_1 and v_2 refer to the velocity of sound in tissue 1 and tissue 2, respectively.

Specular reflection only accounts for part of the returning waves. When the propagating ultrasound coincides with the cellular structures which are much smaller in size than the wavelength of the ultrasound wave, a very different kind of reflection occurs which is known as scattering. In scattering, each small particle acts as a point source producing spherical wavelets (Huygen's principle). The intensity I_s of the scattered wave is inversely proportional to the fourth power of the wavelength and directly proportional to the sixth power of the radius, i.e.:

$$I_s \propto \frac{r^6}{\lambda^4} . \tag{1.6}$$

1.2.1.4 Echo Display: A-Scan

In the A-scan display or A-mode (Amplitude-mode), the echoes detected by the transducer are first rectified and the envelope detected. The resulting

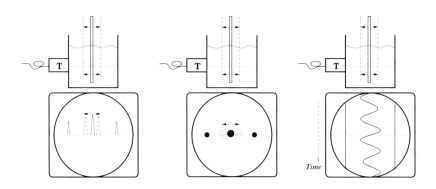

Figure 1.3: Commonly used display methods for ultrasound data. **Left**: A-Scan; **Middle**: B-Scan; **Right**: M-Scan.

signal is then displayed along the horizontal trace in the position which is calculated by the Time-Of-Flight of the ultrasound, given the sound speed in the medium. When the reflecting object moves forward or backward relative to the transducer, the displayed signal exhibits similar movements (see Figure 1.3, Left). A-scans are useful for accurate measurement of dimensions (see Feigenbaum [6]).

1.2.1.5   Echo Display: B-Scan

The idea in B-scan or B-mode (Brightness-mode) is to convert the amplitude of the displayed signal in the A-scan to a proportional intensity. In other words, the received echoes are plotted as brightness-modulated lines along the ultrasound beam path using an oscilloscope, like a display system (see Figure 1.3, Middle).

1.2.1.6   Echo Display: M-Scan

In M-scan or M-mode (Motion-mode), the brightness-modulated lines of the B-scan are plotted against time and the lines from successive pulses are plotted side by side to display how the positions of the objects vary with time (see Figure 1.3, Right). M-scans are useful in studying the movements of moving objects (see Feigenbaum [6]).

1.2.1.7   Two-Dimensional Real-Time B-Scan

A two-dimensional (2-D) B-scan is formed from multiple B-scan lines scanned across the desired scan-plane. This can be done mechanically using a set of rotating or oscillating crystals or electronically using a phased array transducer. Each 2-D B-scan image consists of an ensemble of equi-angularly spaced B-scan lines relative to the probe position. Interpolation and compounding of

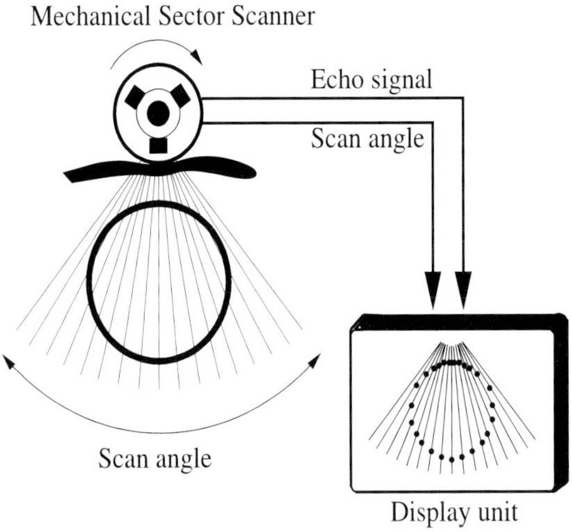

Figure 1.4: 2-D B-scan image creation principle. The principle of creation of a 2-D B-scan image using a mechanical sector scanner probe.

successive sweeps are usually used to fill in gaps between adjacent lines in the image, which is known as the "digital scan conversion" process. The term "real-time" refers to the capability to generate 2-D B-scan images at frame rates greater than 5/s (see McDicken [3]). Due to the high velocity of sound in soft tissue, it is possible to image at frame rates up to 40/s with an appropriate probe. The principle of creation of a 2-D B-scan image using a mechanical sector scanner with a set of rotating crystals is shown in Figure 1.4. As each crystal passes over the heart, it transmits pulses and receives echoes. The next element then takes over. The echo signal and the scan angle are both used in the display system. Each echo signal is displayed in B-scan form with the same angle as the ultrasound beam. The result is a tomographic image of the heart.

In the phased array transducers beam, steering is carried out electronically using a large number of small tranducers (typically 32), which are fired in a very rapid, precisely controlled sequence. Figure 1.5 schematically shows the principle of this method. The top element is pulsed first, and since it is very small, the ultrasound wave it generates is circular. Very soon afterwards the second element is pulsed, and so on. The individual small ultrasound waves combine to make one compound wave which, because of the pulsing sequence, travels at an angle to the axis of the transducer array. Continuously changing the pulsing sequence scans the ultrasound beam in a manner similar to a mechanical scanner.

Figure 1.6 demonstrates examples of real standard two-dimensional B-scan ultrasonic images driven from the human heart.

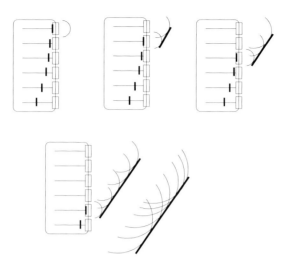

Figure 1.5: 2-D B-scan image creation principle. The principle of creation of a 2-D B-scan image using a phased array transducer.

1.2.2 B-Scan Quality and the Ultimate Limits

There are various artifacts, error sources and ultimate limitations in the generation of ultrasound images which affect their quality and accuracy. Some of them are characteristic of how the system is implemented and some are inherent to the nature of pulse-echo imaging. The following review gives an intuitive feel for the types of problems which arise in 2-D B-scan image formation. It also reflects the difficulty of the subsequent processing of these images. Despite these errors, diagnostically useful images are still obtainable by careful selection of imaging parameters. More description of the different kinds of artifacts can be found in Harris [13] and McDicken [3].

1.2.3 Propagation-Related Artifacts and Resolution Limits

This group of artifacts is related to the spatial wave property, ultrasound beam size, direction and speed in the body tissue.

1.2.3.1 Side Lobes

One of the error sources in 2-D images is that not all of the acoustic energy is propagated in the direction perpendicular to the transducer face. This phenomenon, which is a characteristic of the ultrasound probe, generates "side lobes". A side lobe refers to a minor ultrasound beam which is created within the main beam traveling in a different direction (see Kremkau [14]). Side lobes with large enough intensities could produce echoes from objects off the main beam path, producing artifacts in the B-scans. This phenomenon is shown

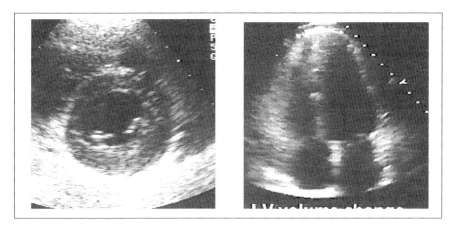

Figure 1.6: Examples of standard echocardiographic views of the heart. **Left**: Parasternal mid-papillary muscle level short-axis view. **Right**: Apical long-axis four-chamber view (Courtesy of S. K. Setarehdan, University of Strathclyde, Glasgow, UK).

in Figure 1.7 in which object C has produced an artifact on the line of sight of object A. Side lobes exist in all types of transducers, and their energy and direction with regard to the main beam are determined by the frequency of the transducer and its active area. The angle between the side lobes and the central axis of the main lobe is given by:

$$\sin\theta = \frac{m\lambda}{D}, \tag{1.7}$$

where λ is the wavelength, θ is the angle of the side lobe, m is the side lobe number (1, 2, 3, ...) and D is the diameter of the transducer face.

1.2.3.2 Speckle

The characteristic granular appearance of ultrasound images, commonly referred to as "speckle", is the result of a complex superposition of many factors, most importantly the constructive-destructive interference of the ultrasound pulses back-scattered from the tiny multiple reflectors which constitute the body tissues and which was discussed earlier in this sub-section. Speckle typically has the unfortunate aspect of falling into the high-sensitivity region of human vision to spatial frequency and can severely degrade the clinical information content of the images. Consequently, speckle reduction and filtering, or development of techniques that are less sensitive to the speckle noise, are important aspects in ultrasonic image processing.

1.2.3.3 Refraction

Refraction changes the beam direction at oblique interfaces. This phenomenon results in improper positioning of an object in the image (see Fish [10] and

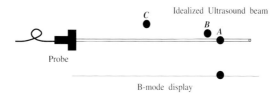

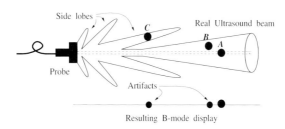

Figure 1.7: An ideal ultrasound beam and its B-scan display (top), and the real ultrasound beam (notice the side lobes and low lateral resolution) and its B-scan display (bottom).

Kremkau [14]), as illustrated in Figure 1.8.

1.2.3.4   Speed Errors

The speed of sound in soft tissue is not constant as assumed by pulse-echo systems. Excluding air and bone, the speed of sound ranges between 1450 m/s in fat to 1750 m/s in tendon and is on average 1540 m/s (see McDicken [3]). It also varies with temperature and tissue condition. Variation in the speed of sound results in incorrect placement of the interfaces in the image. This also distorts the shape of the objects within the image.

1.2.3.5   Range Ambiguity

The maximum depth that can be imaged unambiguously is determined by the pulse repetition frequency (see Kremkau [14]). In other words, a second pulse should be transmitted only after all echoes are received from the first one. Otherwise, echoes from the first pulse will appear as artifacts in the second image. A trade-off should be made between the range ambiguity and the frame rate.

1.2.3.6   Axial Resolution

Axial resolution is defined as the minimum distance between two objects positioned axially that can be imaged as two separate objects. It is defined by the length of the ultrasound burst which is used for imaging. Axial resolution improves with shorter pulse lengths which need higher ultrasound frequencies.

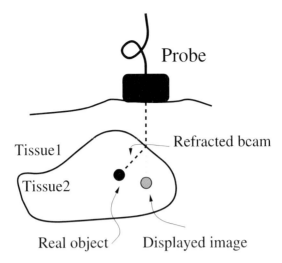

Figure 1.8: Imaging error due to refraction.

1.2.3.7 Lateral and Elevational Resolutions

These resolutions are defined by the minimum distance between two objects positioned laterally or elevationally that can be imaged individually. Because the ultrasound beam is not a fine, laser-like line, objects which lie laterally or elevationally close together are displayed on the same line of sight. This is shown diagrammatically in Figure 1.7 for object B which produces an artifact on the line of sight of object A. Reduction of the beam width by focusing techniques is usually done to make the beam as narrow as possible. The highest resolution (smallest beam size) occurs at the focal spot. Modern multi-element transducers improve lateral resolution through dynamic focusing. Dynamic focusing involves rapidly sweeping the focus along the beam axis to coincide with the range of received echoes for a given instant in time. In general, axial resolution is much finer than lateral resolution (see Skorton *et al.* [7]).

1.2.4 Attenuation-Related Artifacts

Artifacts due to attenuation are related to the amplitude properties of the ultrasound pulses, echoes and electrical signals. When a pulse of ultrasound passes through a highly absorbing layer, it is greatly attenuated and only produces weak echoes at deeper interfaces.

1.2.4.1 Contrast Resolution

Contrast resolution is defined as the smallest detectable difference in echo intensity. The echo contrast dynamic range is usually much more than the dynamic range of human perception of gray levels (approximately 100 dB to 20 dB) (see Kremkau [14]) and it is therefore necessary to compress the echo contrast dynamic range to the range most sensitive to the human eye. Some image processing techniques consider contrast resolution enhancement during the early processing steps.

1.2.4.2   Shadowing

Shadowing occurs when ultrasound pulses are greatly attenuated behind strong reflectors like bone or lung (see Fish [10] and Kremkau [14]). The only way to image the shadowing region is to change the "look direction" of the ultrasound probe.

1.2.4.3   Enhancement

Enhancement is the opposite of shadowing. Some tissues or fluids are weakly echogenic. Regions below these tissues or fluids return echoes of greater than expected amplitude (see Kremkau [14] and Fish [10]), which makes a very bright region in the image. Time-Gain Compensator is also partly responsible for this phenomenon.

One of the main applications of diagnostic ultrasound is the study of cardiac anatomy and function, known as Echocardiography. It was originated by the work of Edler and Hertz in the 1950's (see Feigenbaum [6]). It was they who first demonstrated the relationship between ultrasonic echoes and the structure and function of the heart. From the time of their pioneering research, remarkable progress has been made, beginning with the widespread acceptance of M-mode studies, followed by real-time imaging, Doppler and duplex techniques, and color-coded Doppler imaging (see Wells [8], [9]). In Chapter 2 we will cover the Echocardiography issue and discuss the different image processing approaches for automatic quantification of echocardiographic images.

1.3   X-Ray Cardiac Image Generation

Cardiac catheterization (CC) involves inserting a pigtail catheter into the left ventricle (LV) chamber of the heart (see the 3-D structure of the heart showing the LV chamber in Figure 3.2 and also the color plates at the end of this book), through one of the arteries passing through the groin in a human. In 1940, this procedure was introduced to the medical field of cardiovascular research for the purpose of heart treatment and its diagnosis (for details, see Hood *et al.* [16] and Zisserman *et al.* [17]). During this procedure, a contrast agent or dye is inserted through the catheter, which causes it to mix with the blood in the LV chamber of the heart. During the bolus injection of this contrast agent, the X-ray source is turned on and the dosage is passed through the human chest (from posterior to inferior) covering the LV chamber in a right anterior oblique (RAO) view of 30 degrees to yield the projection images called ventriculograms (LVgrams). The RAO projection is recommended and used by most investigators to correct foreshortening of the projected long axis[2] of the chamber and to visualize the

---

[2]The segment joining the mid of the aortic valve plane and the apex.

plane of the mitral valve in order to grossly detect the presence of mitral valve regurgitation[3]. Since this procedure is invasive, there must be an awareness of its risks and complications. Details of these risks are given in Conti *et al.* [18], but here we very briefly present some of the most common risks CC can cause: (**1**) death, (**2**) arrhythmia (irregular heart beat), (**3**) profound hypotension (low blood pressure), (**4**) complications involving the arterial system, (**5**) accidental perforations of the heart, (**6**) catheter problems, (**7**) embolism (plaque dislodging from one place and blocking another artery/vein), (**8**) bleeding and (**9**) ventricular fibrillation (rapid irregular beating of ventricle).

1.3.1   LV Data Acquisition System Using X-Rays

A cardiac imaging X-ray cine film acquisition system is shown in Figure 1.9. The major components of the system are an X-ray source, an image intensifier, a cine or video camera, and an analog-to-digital converter (ADC) (a detailed version can be seen in Shung *et al.* [19]). A high enough voltage is applied to the X-ray source, which produces the X-ray beam. The beam is made to pass through the chest of the human patient and is received by the detector. Note that the X-ray beam source and the detector axis are aligned along the same common line, called the axis of the tube. The LV is made to lie in the center of the X-ray beam. The image intensifier converts the X-ray beam into an optical image. For a clear delineation of the LV to be imaged from its neighboring tissue, a radio opaque contrast agent, such as an iodine compound, is injected into the organ to absorb part of the X-ray beam energy. This brings out a relatively high or brighter region compared to the surrounding background in the image produced by the image intensifier. The function of the silvered mirror is to focus the incoming X-ray beam into the cine camera, which is placed transversely to the direction of the incoming X-ray beam. The remainder of the light comprising the image is partially transmitted through the silvered mirror along the axis of the detector (image intensifier) and into the lens of a video camera. Usually, the video camera produces an analog signal resulting from scanning the image produced by the image intensifier. Alternatively, the images produced by the image intensifier can be projected from a video camera. The analog signal is nothing but a voltage level which corresponds to the pixel value in the image. The analog-to-digital converter converts this voltage, which represents the gray scale of a pixel as a digital value. Examples of X-ray images are shown in Figure 1.10. Typical X-ray ventriculograms for end diastole (ED[4]) and end systole (ES[5]) frames are shown in Figure 1.11.

1.3.2   Drawbacks of Cardiac Catheterization

Though CC provides definitive anatomical information not obtainable from other imaging modalities and is relatively economical and effective for studying

---

[3]Backwards motion.

[4]This is the last time frame of the expansion stage or diastole cycle.

[5]This is the last frame of the contraction stage or systole cycle.

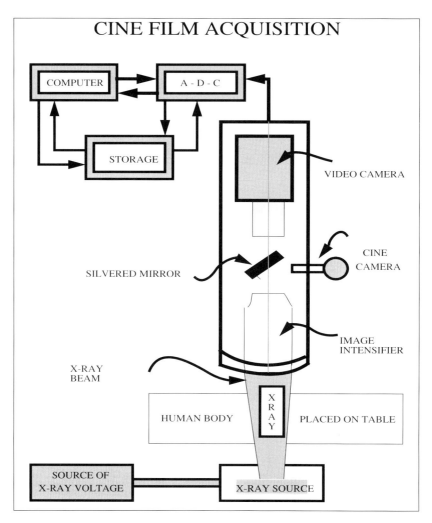

Figure 1.9: Digital cine film data acquisition system: overall system for gray scale cine film acquisition. The optical system consists of the image intensifier, silvered mirror, cine camera and video camera. A video camera outputs the analog signal obtained by scanning the image produced by the image intensifier. A computer and data storage are accessories for processing of the digital data.

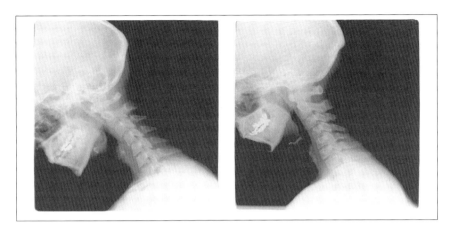

Figure 1.10: Sample X-ray images of cervical and lumbar spine (Courtesy of George Thoma, National Library of Medicine, NIH, Bethesda, MD).

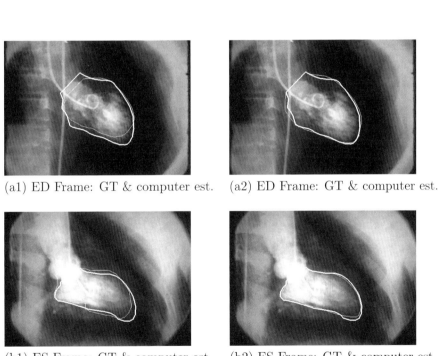

(a1) ED Frame: GT & computer est.   (a2) ED Frame: GT & computer est.

(b1) ES Frame: GT & computer est.   (b2) ES Frame: GT & computer est.

Figure 1.11: Examples of cardiac X-ray images (ventriculograms). **Top**: ED frames, **Bottom**: ES frames. GT stands for ground truth boundary, shown with a thick boundary. Thick boundaries are computer-estimated techniques [28].

cardiac disorders, it has a weakness which controls the dynamics of the dye flow in the LV chamber. These dynamics have put an extra burden on post-processing of LV gray scale data. As a result, it has led CVPR[6] researchers to model the LV modeling process in a special way. The most critical drawback in CC is its low quality, especially in the apical,[7] anterior wall and inferior wall zones (see Figure 3.11 for the labeling of the LV in projection ventriculograms). There are several reasons for poor quality in the LV apex: first, the contrast agent is unable to reach the apex zone of the LV due to the curling of the catheter, which is necessary to avoid irritation to the patient, as shown in Figure 3.11 (for details on catheter design, we refer the reader to the excellent US patent by Rickerd [20] and Stephen *et al.* [21]); second, the contrast agent is unable to reach the apex if the LV is extremely large in size; third, the abnormality of the LV shape causes an irregularity that contributes to the poor propagation of the contrast agent towards the apex (see MacCallum [22] and Mall [23]); fourth, the dynamics of the blood mixing with the contrast agent is not homogeneous in the LV chamber. This is because of the muscle resistivity. Some boundary muscle tissues are thick and resist the contrast agent penetrating towards the LV apex. In addition to the LV apex, the LV anterior and interior wall zones do not receive the dye well enough. The inferior wall of the LV chamber is of particularly poor quality because of the superposition of the diaphragm over the LV. (Later, Suri *et al.* [246] will show how to separate the diaphragm from the LV in LVgrams.) The projection of the ribs over the LV in the LVgrams is another cause of poor contrast. Motion artifacts and noise due to the scattering of the X-ray radiation by tissue volumes not related to the LV also contribute to the low quality of LVgrams. All of these above factors pose a great challenge in LV segmentation and modeling.

1.4   Magnetic Resonance Image Generation

The layout of this section is as follows: physical principles of NMR are discussed in Sub-section 1.4.1. The basics of MRI are covered in Sub-section 1.4.2. Sub-section 1.4.3 discusses the gradient echo imaging. Some of the latest techniques in MR image generation are discussed in Sub-section 1.4.4. The 3-D Turbo FLASH technique is discussed in Sub-section 1.4.5. Spiral MRI is discussed in Sub-section 1.4.6. Fat suppression is discussed in Sub-section 1.4.7. Perfusion-weighted imaging is discussed in Sub-section 1.4.8. Sub-section 1.4.9 discusses Time of Flight MR angiography. Fast spectroscopic imaging is discussed in Sub-section 1.4.10 and finally, the MRI section concludes with Sub-section 1.4.11, which presents some recent fast MR imaging techniques.

---

[6]Computer Vision and Pattern Recognition.
[7]Bottom one third of the LV.

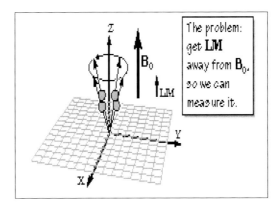

Figure 1.12: The precession of protons is represented around the z-axis like a spinning top to generate linear magnetization (Courtesy of Marconi Medical Systems, Inc.).

1.4.1   Physical Principles of Nuclear Magnetic Resonance

For Magnetic Resonance, RF pulses are applied to spinning nuclei as 90° excitation pulses. These create the magnetic field B_1 for the precessing nuclei at the Larmor frequency to flip them into the transverse plane with B_0 (see Figure 1.12). As seen in this figure, around two-thirds of all nuclei exhibit motion like a "spinning top" in different axes. This creates a magnetic moment due to nuclear angular momentum (linear magnetization M_z) in the high magnetic field B_0 direction at different axes. This motion is known as "Larmor precession". The Larmor (angular) precessing frequency is the product of the magnetic field strength and a specific constant Gyromagnetic ratio, where the angular frequency per unit magnetic field B_0 is known as the Gyromagnetic ratio, a constant for each type of nuclei. For example, for 1-H=42.58 MHz, 31-P=17.24 MHz and 23-Na=11.26 MHz at a magnetic field strength equal to 1.0 Tesla. The physical basis of precession is described in detail in Chapter 5. The resultant coherent transverse magnetization precesses at the Larmor frequency of hydrogen in the transverse plane. It creates a voltage, or stated another way, the NMR signal is induced in the receiver coil in the transverse plane. The signal can be located in three dimensions, so the system can position each signal at the correct point in the image. First, it locates the slice and then the signal is encoded along both axes of the image by all the gradients.

In this section we will briefly discuss the principles of Nuclear Magnetic Resonance (NMR). For more details, interested readers can refer to any standard textbook on the principles of NMR (for example, see Stark *et al.* [29]).

Magnetic Resonance Imaging (MRI) is based on the physical phenomenon called Nuclear Magnetic Resonance (NMR). In NMR, nuclei precess in the presence of a static magnetic field B_0. These spinning nuclei are exposed to 90° and 180° radio frequency (RF) pulses. These RF pulses are produced from

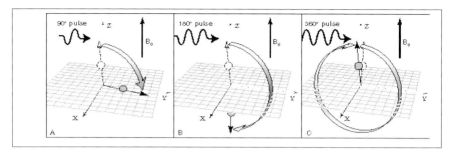

Figure 1.13: Events of magnetization vector flipping during the RF pulse application. The flipping event of magnetization is shown as a ribbon. **Left**: 90° pulse. **Middle**: 180° pulse. **Right**: 360° pulse, returning magnetization to the original position (Courtesy of Marconi Medical Systems, Inc.).

an RF source at a certain frequency proportional to the static magnetic field. The sequence of the pre-defined 90°–180° RF pulse train generates a spin echo as a result of the RF 180° pulse-induced flipping of the magnetization into the transverse plane. This spin echo emits RF specific NMR signals. These different events are shown in Figures 1.13–1.17 at different stages and are described very briefly here.

Figure 1.13 shows the events of the net magnetization starting in parallel with the z-direction aligned with B_0 magnetic field with the low energy state. This also shows how the linear magnetization M_z can be flipped to various directions, depending on the RF pulse used. At equilibrium, the magnetization vector only has a linear component M_z, with no transverse M_{xy} component. In other words, some population of nuclei are aligned with the magnetic field B_0 in a low energy state: this is shown as linear magnetization M_z in equilibrium and as a net magnetization **M**. The other population of nuclei are non-aligned with B_0. If a "90° electromagnetic RF energy pulse" is introduced to the nuclei, the excess of the aligned linear magnetization M_z component (shown as a ribbon in Figure 1.13) is flipped by 90° and generates transverse magnetization M_{xy} in the $x - y$ plane, perpendicular to the z-direction (see Figure 1.13 (left)). At this point, the 90° RF pulse can be called the "excitation pulse". If a "180° electromagnetic RF energy pulse" is introduced to the nuclei in the equilibrium state, the majority of the nuclei are inverted through 180° (see Figure 1.13 (middle)). So, the net magnetization **M** now becomes $-M_z$ and is seen in the opposite direction to z of the main field B_0, resulting in $-M_z$ buildup (see Figure 1.13 (middle)). This follows with the subsequent decay in $-M_z$ amplitude or buildup of M_z towards equilibrium. If a "360° electromagnetic RF energy" is introduced to the nuclei, the majority of these nuclei in the equilibrium state participate and their net magnetization **M** is flipped through 360° so that their net magnetization **M** also returns to M_z direction without any effect (see Figure 1.13 (right)).

After flipping the protons to 90°, the linear magnetization M_z component disappears and the transverse magnetization M_{xy} component appears as net

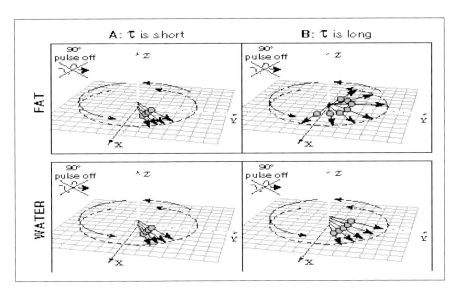

Figure 1.14: Various events are represented after a 90° pulse at **Left Column**: Short τ. **Right Column**: Long τ. Note the difference in the water and fat proton behavior at short τ and long τ during echo generation and dephasing. Note that τ is the interval between the 90° and 180° pulses (Courtesy of Marconi Medical Systems, Inc.).

magnetization **M** (see Figure 1.14). The same figure shows the various events after applying the 90° excitation pulse and transverse magnetization M_{xy} generation represented for the application of 90° pulse at short τ (left side panels) and long τ, respectively (right side panels), where τ is the interval between the 90° and 180° pulses. The time interval τ depends upon the molecule's environment or the bond interactions of the nuclei in the molecule. It is important to use a suitable τ interval time, as it proportionately determines the rate of decay of transverse magnetization M_{xy} or the rate of incoherence over time, shown as straight arrows. It also determines the induced field B_1, shown as circular arrows.

Similarly, Figure 1.15 shows the events after applying 90° RF pulse and different dephasing rates for water and fat protons at short τ and long τ intervals. In the left and middle columns of this figure, we see the difference in behavior of the water and fat protons as a source of T_2 contrast due to different free induction decay rates of incoherence or dephasing at a short and a long τ. The right-hand figure shows the 180° flipping behavior after the 180° pulse is applied at a long τ. It shows faster dephasing of nuclei in fat than in water at long τ. This flipping event after the 180° inversion of dephased M_{xy} magnetization components in the reverse direction generates spin echo in the reverse direction as NMR signal energy.

Figure 1.15 shows the late events of the 90° and 180° pulse-induced changes in magnetization **M**, which are introduced for their excitation phases and sub-

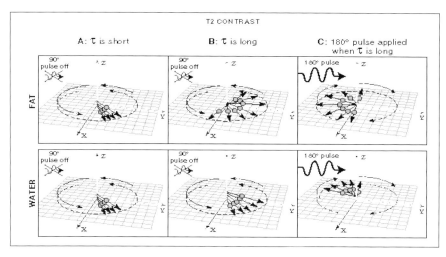

Figure 1.15: Various events after applying a 90° pulse of dephasing are shown for water and fat protons. **Left Column**: at short τ. **Middle Column** and **Right Column**: long τ. Note the difference in behavior of the water and fat protons as a source of T_2 contrast. Also note the behavior of the 180° pulse applied at long τ showing slower dephasing of water. Note that τ is the interval between the 90° and 180° pulses (Courtesy of Marconi Medical Systems, Inc.).

sequent dephasing events leading to "spin echo" generation. The rate of 90° excitation is nuclei specific for different molecules. Faster rates are seen in fat molecules than in water molecules, resulting in different dephasing rates of transverse magnetization M_{xy} magnitudes (see Figure 1.15, middle and right columns) at longer τ interval after the 180° RF pulse is applied. The advantage of long τ intervals is that it allows sufficient build up time of magnetization M_{xy} and the NMR signal, before the new RF pulse is applied. Interestingly, the 180° RF pulse application introduces perfect 180° flip with "spin echo formation" in the opposite direction to all those dephased transverse magnetization components generated after the 90° RF pulse terminated, without changing the rate of rephasing or transverse magnetization M_{xy} recovery (see Figure 1.15, right column). In this process of recovery and rephasing, characteristic electromagnetic energy is emitted as a "spin echo", which is received by the RF receiver coil as an NMR signal. This NMR signal has its temporal or spatial frequency components with individual amplitudes and phases varying with time and space.

The characteristic behavior of the larger number of fat protons and the lower number of free protons in fat molecules results in strong transverse magnetization M_{xy} or strong T_2 signals of fat. Figure 1.16 shows the different rates of linear magnetization recovery of fat protons and water protons in the z-direction. This characteristic of different proton behavior is affected by "spin-spin" interactions. This creates the T_2-weighted images. A detailed description of the NMR signal, relaxation time and contrast relationship can be seen in

Stark *et al.* [29].

One obvious question can be raised here, namely, how is the NMR signal generated? The answer lies with the "spin echo" generation. Initially, the spins or both their magnetization components M_z and M_{xy} may be perturbed by absorption of electromagnetic RF energy at the precessional frequency or "Larmor frequency". The intensity and duration of the RF pulse determines the rotation or perturbation of both of the magnetization components. As a result, precessing nuclei are changing the magnitudes of M_z and M_{xy} in the z- and xy-directions, which later return to the equilibrium M_z with the release of energy at the same Larmor precessional frequency. This excitation and subsequent release of energy at the condition of released RF energy frequency equals the Larmor precessional frequency, known as the "Nuclear Magnetic Resonance (NMR)" effect due to "spin echo". As a result, this NMR effect, an electromagnetic signal, is induced in the RF coil after termination of the RF $90°$ excitation pulse as the nuclei re-align with the magnetic field B_0, giving up energy in the form of weak NMR electromagnetic current signals at their Larmor frequencies or "free induction decay" (FID). The FID decays in amplitude with time, so-called FID. Its initial amplitude depends upon the number of nuclei and the rate of decay depends upon the coherence of the precessional motions of the nuclei. In MRI, the signal is represented as the signal-to-noise ratio. Thus the strength and magnitude of this NMR signal depends upon the number of nuclei and the spin environment. Interestingly, the $180°$ pulse produces no NMR signal but produces the spin-echo effect for the NMR signal. So, a sequence of a $90°$-$180°$ RF pulse with the set interval "τ" produces the magnetization and relaxation time properties needed.

These NMR signals are encoded with the characteristics of the protons, interactions among themselves (Transverse Relaxation Time or T_2) and their interactions with their surrounding materials (Longitudinal Relaxation Time or T_1). These relaxation times represent the NMR characteristic of protons and contrast (see Figure 1.17 for T_2 contrast and signal differentiation). In the next sub-section, we will focus on the MRI image generation process in detail.

1.4.2   Basics of Magnetic Resonance Imaging

The layout of this sub-section is as follows: Sub-section 1.4.2.1 introduces a brief history of MRI. Sub-section 1.4.2.2 discusses the three gradients. Spatial encoding and slice thickness control are discussed in Sub-section 1.4.2.3. Frequency encoding is discussed in Sub-section 1.4.2.4. Back-projection is discussed in Sub-section 1.4.2.5. The two-dimensional Fourier Transform is presented in Sub-section 1.4.2.6. A discussion on k-space is presented in Sub-section 1.4.2.7. Sub-section 1.4.2.8 discusses the Nyquist Theorem. Data collection and image formation are discussed in Sub-section 1.4.2.9. Fast Fourier Transform and image matrix generation are discussed in Sub-section 1.4.2.10. The last three sub-sections cover scan time, signal amplitude and spatial resolution in k-space, respectively.

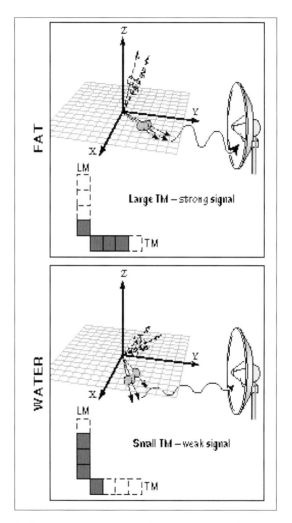

Figure 1.16: This figure represents the different rates of longitudinal magneti-zation recovery of fat protons and water protons in the resultant z-direction. **Top**: strong fat signal at large transverse magnetization. **Bottom**: weaker water signal at small transverse magnetization (Courtesy of Marconi Medical Systems, Inc.).

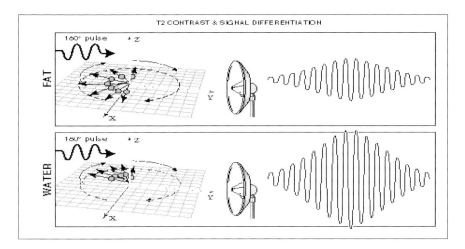

Figure 1.17: RF $180°$ pulse is applied, resulting in different dephasing rates for fat and water protons. Note the difference between dephasing rates and the echo produced. The resultant NMR signal is received by an RF coil. **Top**: fat protons. **Bottom**: water protons with different T_2 contrast and signal intensity (Courtesy of Marconi Medical Systems, Inc.).

1.4.2.1 Brief History of MRI

Magnetic Resonance images are acquired using a technique called Nuclear Magnetic Resonance (NMR). This has been used extensively as a powerful analytical tool for biological studies as well as for physical and chemical investigations at the molecular level since its inception in the mid-1940s. The first imaging technique based on NMR was developed by Paul C. Lauterbur in 1972 at SUNY Stony Brook in New York [30]. He was able to generate the first set of two-dimensional cross-sectional NMR images with the contrast of proton density and spin lattice relaxation time. He used a radio frequency (RF) magnetic field and spatially defining magnetic field gradients as well as a main static magnetic field. The main magnetic field was used to make the spins resonate at the targeted radio frequency. The RF magnetic field was generated by an RF transmitter which was used to induce interactions among the spins in the imaging object. An RF receiver was employed to collect the RF signals emitted from the imaging object. The two-dimensional images were formed (reconstructed) from the collected RF signals due to the application of the magnetic field gradients in three orthogonal directions during the NMR data acquisition. Lauterbur termed his technique "NMR Zeugmatography", which is now known as NMR in the world of physics and Magnetic Resonance Imaging (MRI) in the medical world. The term NMR will be used to indicate the physics of Nuclear Magnetic Resonance which will be discussed in this section. The term MRI means the use of the NMR technique to produce medically diagnostic images, or as a diagnostic imaging modality. The physical principles of MR will be explained in the next sub-section. Figure 1.18 shows a typical MRI system layout.

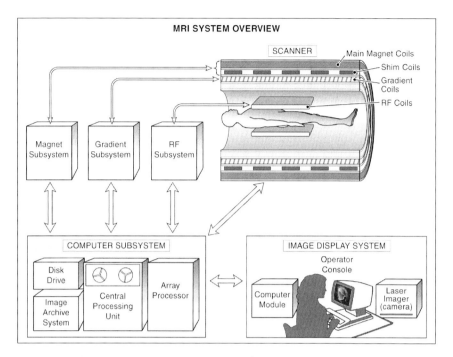

Figure 1.18: A typical MRI system layout (Courtesy of Marconi Medical Systems, Inc.).

1.4.2.2   Three Gradients

The passage of current through the gradient coils (see Figure 1.19, right) induce a magnetic gradient field around it. This alters the static magnetic field strength B_0 in a linear fashion by the gradient coils. In a clinical MRI scanner, the x-gradient alters the magnetic field along the magnetic horizontal axis, the y-gradient alters along the vertical axis and the z-gradient alters the magnetic field along the long axis (see Figure 1.19, left). Based on the magnetic field strength, the precessional frequency experienced by the nuclei situated along the axis of the gradient can be predicted or spatially-encoded.

1.4.2.3   Spatial-Encoding and Slice Thickness Control

This permits in-plane discrimination of the position within the slice. Slice selection is a prerequisite for this process. A slice is selectively excited by transmitting an RF pulse with a band of frequencies. These frequencies coincide with the different specific Larmor frequencies of different spins. For a particular slice, the slice select gradient is defined by:

$$B(r) = \omega(r)\,, \tag{1.8}$$

where $B(r)$ is the linear gradient and $\omega(r)$ is the frequency at the position r. At this slice select gradient, the gradient amplitude G_r is related to the magnetic

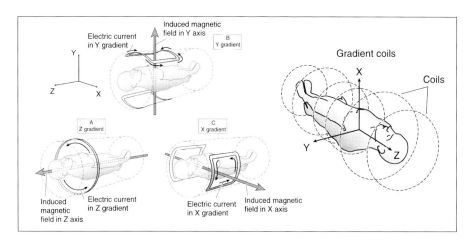

Figure 1.19: **Left**: Events of changing the static magnetic field with the gradient coils. **Right**: Gradient coils (Courtesy of Marconi Medical Systems, Inc.).

field B_0 with the following relationship:

$$B = B_0 + G_r, \qquad (1.9)$$

where B is the magnetic field. This leads to the resonance of nuclei within this slice, and only the RF corresponding to the slice position is received (because the other slice nuclei precessional frequencies differ along the gradient). This is based on the scan plane selection by any gradient out of the x-, y-, or z-gradients during the pulse sequence: axial slices are selected by the altered z-magnet axis (by the z-gradient), sagittal slices are selected by the altered x-magnet axis (by the x-gradient), coronal slices are selected by the altered y-magnet axis (by the y-gradient), and oblique slices are selected by using a combination of any of these three. Figures 1.20, 1.21, and 1.22 represent brain MR images in the axial directions using T_1-weighted, T_2-weighted, and PD-weighted scanning, respectively. Sample images for MR angiography are shown in Figure 1.23.

Equation (1.10) shows how the slices are selected:

$$\delta w = \gamma \, G_z \left(Z_{max} - Z_{min} \right) = \gamma \, G_z \, \Delta Z \qquad (1.10)$$

where δw is the frequency spread within a slice, $Z_{max} - Z_{min}$ is the slice dimension, G_z is the z-gradient and γ is the Gyromagnetic ratio. The slice thickness is selected by a band of nuclei excited by the excitation pulse. The slope of the slice-select gradient (bandwidth or range of frequencies) determines the difference in the precessional frequency between two points on the gradient. For the sake of argument, at a known RF, a steep slope or narrow bandwidth will achieve a thin slice and a shallow slope or broad bandwidth will achieve a thick slice. The gradient slope also determines the gap between slices.

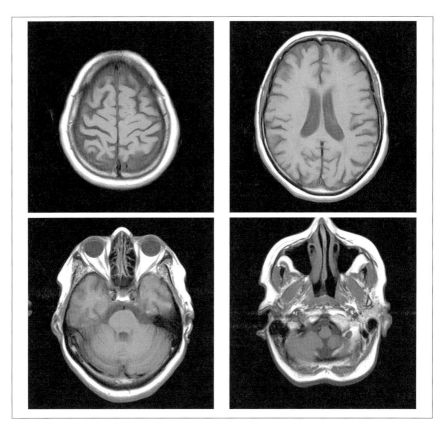

Figure 1.20: MR T_1-weighted axial brain images with the following imaging parameters: T_E=16 ms, T_R=400 ms, FOV=24 cm, Matrix Size=220 × 256, Flip Angle=90°, NSA=2, Slice Thickness=5 mm, Gap=1 mm (Courtesy of Marconi Medical Systems, Inc.).

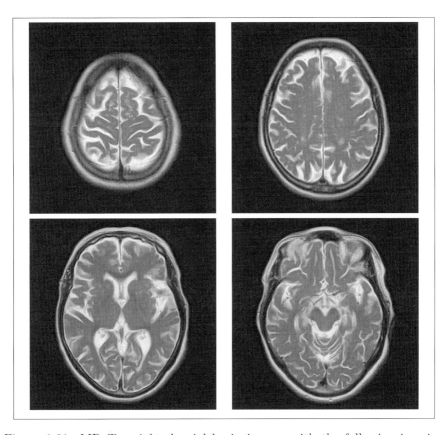

Figure 1.21: MR T_2-weighted axial brain images with the following imaging parameters: T_E=105 ms, T_R=3600 ms, FOV=22 cm, Matrix Size=220 × 256, Flip Angle=90°, NSA=2, Slice Thickness=5 mm, Gap=2 mm (Courtesy of Marconi Medical Systems, Inc.).

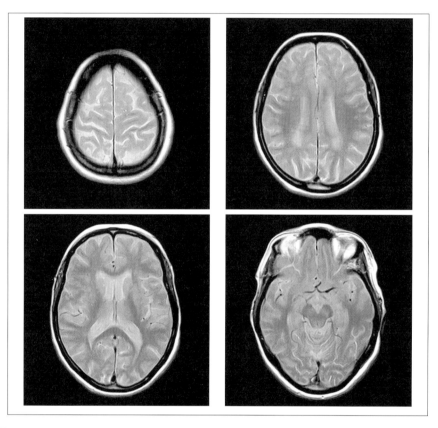

Figure 1.22: MR *PD*-weighted axial brain images with the following imaging parameters: T_E=21 ms, T_R=3600 ms, FOV=22 cm, Matrix Size=220 × 256, Flip Angle=90°, NSA=2, Slice Thickness=5 mm, Gap=2 mm (Courtesy of Marconi Medical Systems, Inc.).

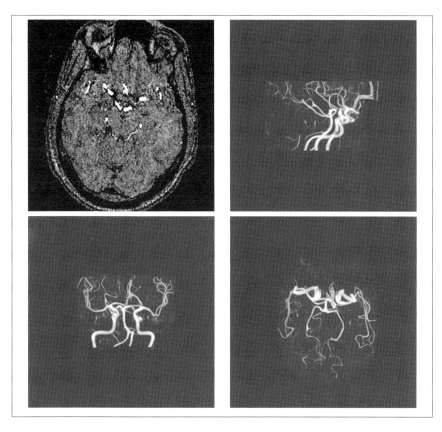

Figure 1.23: Magnetic resonance angiographic data set (volume Time of Flight (ToF) technique) with the following imaging parameters: T_E=6.7 ms, T_R=27 ms, FOV=20 cm, Matrix Size=220 × 256, Flip Angle=30°, NSA=1, Slice Thickness=1 mm, Gap=0 mm. **Top Left**: Transverse raw image. **Top Right**: Sagittal MIP. **Bottom Left**: Coronal MIP. **Bottom Right**: Transverse MIP. For details on MIP, see Suri *et al.* [369] (Courtesy of Marconi Medical Systems, Inc.).

1.4.2.4   Frequency Encoding

Using the frequency-encoding scheme, one can obtain information about the individual pixels within the slice. Once the slice is selected using the selective 90° pulse, the G_z (slice selective gradient) is turned on during the 90° pulse and turned off after the next 90° pulse over the individual pixels within that slice. A selective 180° RF refocusing pulse is applied and the G_z gradient is turned on during this pulse. The echo is received after a time T_E. This echo is a signal from the entire slice in one dimension, as shown in Equation (1.11):

$$s(t) = \int_{-\frac{L}{2}}^{\frac{L}{2}} f(x)\ e^{\gamma\,G_x\,xt}\ e^{-\frac{t}{T_2}}\ dx\,, \qquad (1.11)$$

where $s(t)$ is the rate of complex free induction decay (FID), L is the field of view (FOV), $f(x)$ is the spin density, γ is gyro-magnetic ratio. $G_x\ x\ t$ is the frequency distribution introduced by the gradients. This depends on the gyro-magnetic ratio (γ), the gradient in the transverse x-direction (G_x) and the time of decay (t) in the x-direction. To get spatial information in the x-direction of the slice, another gradient G_x (frequency encoding gradient or read out gradient) is applied in the x-direction during the maximum sampling time and the echo is received (read out).

   The slice pixels experience a different gradient magnitude. For example, in the magnetic gradient from left to right, the center of this slice volume will not experience the gradient in the x-direction, but pixels on the right side of the slice will experience a higher net magnetic field and pixels on the left side will experience a lower net magnetic field. The number of pixels and specific location correspond to a re-created MRI image. Initially, all the protons experience the same frequency of precession (E). Suppose each pixel has its frequency at a specific point in time prior to turning on the G_x gradient. These pixels have the same frequency consisting of different magnitudes at each pixel. The received signal is a complicated sinc wave. Each individual pixel will have the same precessional frequency E but a different magnitude. The signal will be the sum of all the signals from each pixel, i.e., the sum of the amplitudes $= 0 + 1 + (-2) + 1 + 2 + 0 + 1 + 0 + 1 = 4$. The frequency E of each pixel, and the shape of the signal will be the same, i.e., $4\cos(Et)$. The signal is a decaying complex sinc wave. Imagine that an RF pulse is transmitted with reasonable frequencies for a particular slice, then all the protons in the slice start to precess in phase at the Larmor frequency $= E$. Each pixel contains a different number of protons corresponding to the amplitude of the signal. These are designated as a cosine wave for simplicity, because precessing protons in the pixel oscillate. In other words, pixels of the entire slice produce a signal without spatial discrimination and spatial information. For encoding pixels, the summed signal has to be separated into its components, pixel by pixel. Suppose the frequency-encoding gradient in the x-direction is applied, these pixels experience different frequencies. Pixels in the center will not feel the gradient. They will remain at the same frequency, E_0 resulting in a constant amplitude of each pixel as the number of protons remains the same. Pixels on

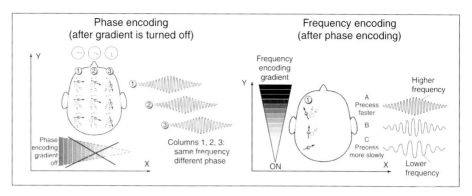

Figure 1.24: **Left**: Phase encoding steps. **Right**: Frequency encoding steps (Courtesy of Marconi Medical Systems, Inc.).

the right (an assumption) experience a slightly higher frequency, $E+$ because they are at a higher magnetic field strength. The protons oscillate at a high frequency but, on the contrary, pixels on the left will experience a slightly lower field strength and thus have a precessional frequency a little lower than other pixels, $E-$. The summed signal of all the individual signals in each column of pixels has a different frequency. So, the same frequency signals may be added up arithmetically column-wise as shown below in Equations (1.12), (1.13), (1.14), and the summation in Equation (1.15).

$$0 + \cos\left(E - t\right) + -2\cos\left(E - t\right) = -\cos\left(E - t\right) \tag{1.12}$$

$$\cos\left(Et\right) + 2\cos\left(Et\right) + 0 = 3\cos(Et) \tag{1.13}$$

$$\cos\left(E + t\right) + 0 + \cos\left(E + t\right) = 2\cos\left(E + t\right). \tag{1.14}$$

Total sum of the signals:

$$-\cos\left(E - t\right) + 3\cos(Et) + 2\cos\left(E + t\right). \tag{1.15}$$

Figure 1.24 shows the phase encoding and frequency encoding where phase and frequency increase in a gradual manner.

The Fourier transformed MR signal before the application of the G_x gradient will be different from the signal after the application of the G_x gradient. For a cosine wave, Fourier transformation is a symmetric pair of spikes at the cosine frequency with an amplitude equal to the magnitude of the signal. In practice, a band of frequencies or the bandwidth of a signal is its characteristic. For simplicity, three different frequencies are Fourier transformed. This can be observed from the center, and the center frequency comes with the frequency spike amplitude as the sum of the amplitudes of the pixels in the center, i.e. $3\cos Et$. Suppose a high frequency comes from the right. The amplitude of that frequency spike represents the sum of the amplitude of the right side pixels, i.e., $2\cos(E + t)$. Naturally then, the lower frequency comes from the left. The amplitude of that frequency spike represents the sum of the amplitude of the left side pixels i.e., $\cos(E - t)$ (in spatial direction). It is clear that the frequency and position have a one-to-one relationship. This provides some spatial encoding information from the slice, as can be seen from the above example (see Figure 1.24) of the slice matrix decomposed into three different pixel groups in the x-directions, or we get three different gray shades corresponding to these pixel groups. These pixel groups may be further decomposed into their three individual pixels in the y-direction in one of two ways: back-projection or two dimensional Fourier Transform.

1.4.2.5 Back-Projection

An area is assigned to an image and the gradient is applied over it. The gradient may be rotated by an angle, reapplied by the same angle and so on, to complete a 360° rotation with a set of different equations. These equations can be solved for pixel values in the matrix (the back-projection approach by rotation of the frequency gradient). This approach picks up a smaller field of view (FOV), but it is very sensitive to external magnetic field inhomogeneities B_0' and magnetic field gradients.

1.4.2.6 Two-Dimensional (2-D) Fourier Transform (FT)

The Fourier Transform method is not sensitive to either external magnetic field inhomogeneities or gradient field inhomogeneities and phase-encoding is performed. In the 2-D Fourier Transform method, the slice selection gradient (G_z) (assuming an axial slice), the gradient for frequency-encoding in the x-direction (G_x) and the phase-encoding gradient (G_y) in the y-direction are applied. The G_y gradient is turned on followed by the read-out gradient G_x applied right after the RF pulse or before the G_x gradient, or anywhere in between. In other words, G_y is usually applied between the 90° and 180° RF pulses or between the 180° pulse and the echo. Suppose a slice has 9 pixels before the G_y (phase-encoding) or G_x (frequency-encoding) gradient is applied. Each pixel shows the same phase and designated frequencies. This phase may be represented as precessional positions at a given point in time. After the 90° RF pulse, all the protons in the selected slice precess at the same frequency. At any point in time, protons in all pixels are oriented in the same direction without any phase difference. This is because they all oscillate at the same frequency.

Suppose the G_y gradient – a magnetic field gradient in the y-direction – is applied over the slice. The pixels in the upper right, center and left side of the matrix experience a higher net magnetic field; pixels in the middle right, center and left side of the matrix experience no change in the magnetic field (no phase change). Pixels in the lower right, center and left side of the matrix experience a lower net magnetic field. In other words, the top row protons will be out of phase with the middle row protons (precessing faster in a stronger field), while the bottom row protons also will be out of phase with the middle row protons (precessing slower in a weaker field) and the top row protons. Thus, the phase-encoding gradient G_y application has caused a difference in the rows of pixels, based on phase values. Such differences in the spatial position up and down in phase are termed phase-encoding. This is expressed in Equations (1.16) and (1.17) as:

$$\theta = \gamma G_y \, y \, \delta \, t_y \, , \tag{1.16}$$

where θ is the phase angle, γ is the Gyromagnetic ratio, G_y the gradient in the y-direction, δt_y the duration of the phase-encoding gradient, and:

$$v(t, G_y) = \int \int e^{-\frac{t}{T_2}} f(x, y) \, e^{i\gamma \, G_x \, xt} \, e^{-i\gamma \, G_y \, y \, \delta t_y} \, , \tag{1.17}$$

where G_y is the phase-encoding gradient, $i\gamma \, G_x \, xt$ is the frequency distribution, and x, y are the dimensions in the slice direction. The signal is read out by turning on G_y (the phase-encoding gradient) and G_x (the frequency-encoding gradient). Note, the integral has limits from 0 to t. This shows that the middle column protons do not experience any change of precessional frequency or the frequency remains the same, but the pixels in the middle column will have different phase shifts. Suppose protons in the right side column experience a greater magnetic field. These protons will have a faster precessional frequency and, in each pixel, these protons will have the same phase shift. They will shift from their different, unique phase positions. These protons have the same increased frequency with different phases.

Similarly, protons in the left column will experience a lower precessional frequency when the G_x gradient is on. These protons in the middle column are all out of phase with the other pixels in the column due to the phase shift (caused by applying the G_y gradient). In other words, protons in each pixel have a distinct frequency and a distinct phase, which are unique and encoded for the x and y coordinates of that pixel. Let us consider the signal received during several repetition T_R cycles, where the phase shift changes, such as $-3, -2, -1, 0, +1, +2, +3$ and so on. Similarly, the frequency changes as $E - 3, E - 2, E - 1, 0, E + 1, E + 2, E + 3$ and so on. The same may be written as $(Et - 3), (Et - 2), (Et - 1), 0, (Et + 1), (Et + 2), (Et + 3)$. The variation in phase or frequency depends upon the strength of the gradients applied (the steeper the gradients, the greater are the phase shifts and the more the precessional frequencies change). For example, in the middle row, there will be no phase shift. In the upper row, suppose the phase shift will be negative and in the lower row, the phase shift will be positive. Each column has its own unique frequency, $E-$ for top row, E_0 for the middle row and $E+$ for the bottom row, caused by the G_x gradient. If both phase and frequency are combined during the readout signal, each pixel has its own unique phase shift and frequency. In general, phase-encoding takes a longer time because each step of the phase-encoding is completed in one independent repetition time (T_R). For example, to distinguish 128 rows, taking 128 phase-encoding steps with a different gradient G_y, this needs time T_R x 128 with $\frac{360^\circ}{128} = 2.90$ phase shift difference between the rows, i.e. 0, 2.90, 2(2.90), 3(2.90) and so on. Each time the phase-encoding step is followed by frequency-encoding, it generates the MR signal for each row, i.e. the first $T_R=1$ signal with no phase shift, the second T_R=2 produces a signal with some phase shift, the third T_R=3 produces a signal with more phase shift, and so on.

1.4.2.7 k-space

Each of the signals fills one line of the row of data space (a presentation of received signals in the time domain). The digital information for signals of these rows is conventionally known as k-space. In appearance, various k-space data look like trajectories. Each signal has information about the entire picture and it goes into each row of data space as the sum of all the signals from the individual pixels in the slice. Digitized information of the signal is true k-space in a spatial frequency domain. The incremented T_R values with increased phase shifts and simultaneous frequency-encoding steps provide specific signals.

This signal information in a digitized form is a series of parallel rows. These are received and placed into rows of data space (top three, middle and bottom rows) for a number of times like 32, 64, 128, 256, depending upon the matrix size. So the phase shift is added after each T_R. The frequency-encoding step is applied to get a new signal which is different from the previous ones. This new signal is put into another row in the data space. Each row is placed at an interval equal to T_R in msec. This is completed through a cycle from one 90° pulse to the next 90° pulse. Digitization for all of the signal information is done by sampling. The signal in the data space is phase-encoded and frequency-encoded. It can be represented by a matrix size such as 128 × 256. This means 256 frequency-encoding steps and 128 phase-encoding steps. For each phase-encoding step, 256 different frequencies are used in one signal generation. Thus the phase- and frequency-encoding steps are independent. Data space is converted to a specific image by the Fourier transformation of the signal. They are Fourier transformed signal shapes as 3-D space with a set of spikes.

1.4.2.8   Sampling Time, bandwidth and the Nyquist Theorem

The frequency-encoding gradient is switched on during the collection of the signal, and is therefore often called the readout gradient. The duration of the frequency-encoding gradient during the readout time is called the sampling time. During the sampling time, the system samples up to 1024 different frequencies. The sampling rate is the rate at which the samples are taken during readout. The number of samples taken determines the number of frequencies sampled. During the sampling time, the system must be able to receive and sample a range of frequencies. The signal is received at the point and this range of frequencies is called the receive bandwidth or simply bandwidth. Each frequency is allocated a frequency column that is mapped on the FOV along the frequency axis. The sampling time, sampling rate and receive bandwidth are all linked by a mathematical principle called the Nyquist theorem.

The Nyquist theorem states that any signal must be sampled at least twice per cycle in order to represent, or reproduce, it accurately. In addition, enough cycles must occur during the sampling time to achieve enough frequency samples. For example, if 256 samples are to be taken, at least 128 cycles must occur during the sampling. The number of cycles occurring per second is determined by the receive bandwidth, which is proportional to the sampling time if each cycle is sampled twice. If ω_{max} is the maximum frequency in the signal, $\triangle T_s$ being the sampling interval, then the sampling rate ω_s is given by:

$$\omega_s = \frac{1}{\triangle T_s} \, 2\,\omega_{max}\,. \tag{1.18}$$

Mathematically, the Nyquist theorem states:

$$\triangle t_{sampling} = \frac{1}{f_{max}} = \frac{2\pi}{\gamma G_x \, L_x}\,, \tag{1.19}$$

where L_x is the maximum bandwidth and G_x is the x-gradient. The ratio $\frac{L_x}{N_x}$ is known as resolution. This represents the ratio of the maximum bandwidth to the number of sampled points (NX). So, from Equation (1.18), we obtain the sampling interval, given as:

$$\triangle T_s = 2 \, \frac{\omega_{max}}{\omega_s}\,, \tag{1.20}$$

where the symbols have the same meaning as stated above. The number of cycles occurring per second is determined by the receive bandwidth. Bandwidth is proportional to the sampling rate, i.e., if the sampling rate increases, the bandwidth also increases. In addition, the sampling time is inversely proportional to the sampling rate or the receive bandwidth. The receive bandwidth is, therefore, inversely proportional to the sampling time (as shown in Equation (1.20)).

1.4.2.9 Data Collection and Image Formation

When all three gradients, G_x, G_y and G_z, are applied over the body slice determined by applying slice selection, these gradients produce a frequency shift on one axis and a phase shift on the other axis. In fact, the system can locate the individual signal within the image by measuring the number of times the magnetic moments cross the receiver coil. The frequency of the position of the event around the precessional path (phase) and other information about individual signals are stored as k-space (a rectangular shape with two axes) in the spatial frequency domain. The question arises as to how the data is collected? During each T_R signal, each slice is phase-encoded and frequency-encoded. A certain value of frequency shift is obtained according to the slope of the frequency-encoding gradient, which is determined by the size of the field of view (FOV). The FOV remains unchanged during the scan, so the frequency shift value remains the same. A certain value of the pulse shift is also obtained according to the slope of the phase-encoding gradient. The slope of the phase-encoding gradient determines the line of k-space based on the data of that frequency-encoding and phase-encoding gradient.

In order to fill out different lines of k-space, the slope of the phase-encoding gradient must be altered after each T_R. The number of different phase-encoding slopes applied determines the number of k-space lines filled. If 128 different phase-encoding slopes are selected, 128 lines of k-spaces are filled to complete the scan. If 256 different phase-encoding slopes are selected, 256 lines of k-space are filled to complete the scan. The slope of the phase-encoding gradient determines the magnitude of the phase shift between two points in a patient. In order to fill the different lines of k-space, a different phase shift must be obtained. This is done by switching the phase-encoding gradient to a different amplitude or slope (sine waves).

1.4.2.10   Fast Fourier Transform and Image Matrix Generation

The Fast Fourier Transform (FFT) process offers calculation of the amplitude of individual frequencies. In FFT, the signal intensity (in the time domain) is converted into signal intensity (in the frequency domain). The FOV is divided into pixels, depending upon the frequency samples and the phase-encoding performed. This can be represented as pixels depending on frequency-encoding or phase-encoding. To create an image, each pixel is allocated a signal intensity. It corresponds to the amplitude of the signal originating from the anatomy at the position of each pixel in the matrix. The matrix represents a signal amplitude with a distinct frequency and phase shift. Once the whole k-space is filled, the data acquisition is over. The number of times the signal is filled is called the number of signal averages (NSA) or the number of excitations (NEX).

1.4.2.11   Scan Time

For every T_R, each slice is slice-selected, phase-encoded and frequency-encoded. The maximum number of slices that can be selected and encoded depends upon the length of the T_R, i.e. a longer T_R allows more slices to be selected than a shorter T_R. The phase-encoding gradient slope is altered in every T_R. This is applied to each selected slice in order to phase-encode it. At each phase-encode, a different line of k-space is filled. The number of phase-encoding steps therefore affects the length of the scan. The scan time is also affected by the number of times the signal is phase-encoded with the same phase-encoding gradient slope or number of excitations. For example, each signal is phase-encoded twice with the same amplitude as the phase-encoding gradient slope. For this, T_R must be repeated twice for each slope and for each line of k-space. Therefore: Scan Time $= T_R \times$ number of phase-encoding $\times$ NEX.

1.4.2.12   Signal Amplitude

k-space is drawn as a rectangle with two axes (phase on the horizontal axis and frequency on the vertical axis). Above the center, all phases are positive and below the center, all phases are negative. The steepness of the slope of the phase-encoding gradient depends on how much current is driven through the gradient coil. For a 256 phase-encoding, 128 positive gradient lines fill in the positive half of k-space, and 128 negative gradient lines fill in the negative half of the k-space soon after the central lines are filled first. The central lines of k-space are filled using the shallow phase-encoding slopes, and the outer lines are filled using the steep phase-encoding slopes. Shallow phase-encoding slopes do not produce large phase shifts along their axis, so the resultant signal has a large amplitude. Similarly, steep phase-encoding slopes produce large phase shifts along their axis with small amplitude. The vertical axis of k-space corresponds to the frequency-encoding axis. The center of the echo represents the maximum signal amplitude as all the magnetic moments are in-phase.

The magnetic moments are either rephasing or dephasing on either side of the echo peak, so the signal amplitude will be less toward these sides. The amplitude of the frequencies sampled is mapped relative to the frequency axis. The rephasing and dephasing portions of the echo are mapped to the left and the right of the frequency axis. To sum this up, the center of the k-space has data with the highest signal amplitude along both the phase and frequency axes. The outer portions of k-space contain data with lower signal amplitude along both the phase and frequency axes.

1.4.2.13 Spatial Resolution in k-space

The number of phase-encodings steps performed determines the number of pixels in the FOV along the phase-encoding axis. This indicates that there are more pixels in the FOV along the phase axis and each pixel is a smaller unit. If the FOV is fixed, voxels of smaller dimensions result in an image with a higher spatial resolution. Spatial resolution means that two points within the image are easily distinguishable when the pixels are smaller. When the amplitude of the phase-encoding gradient slope increases, the degree of phase shift along the gradient also increases. Two points adjacent to each other have a different phase value and can therefore be differentiated from each other. Therefore, data collected after the steep phase-encoding gradient slopes produce greater spatial resolution in the image. In other words, the central lines of k-space contain data with low spatial resolution. The center lines are filled by shallow phase-encoding gradient slopes (high signal amplitude). The outer lines of k-space contain data with high spatial resolution. The outer lines are filled by steep phase-encoding gradient slopes (low signal amplitude). The k-space filling and image propagation depend on a combination of the polarity and amplitude of both the frequency and the phase-encoding gradients. The amplitude of the frequency-encoding gradient determines the left and right sides of the k-space points traversed. It also determines the size of the FOV in the frequency direction of the image. The amplitude of the phase-encoding gradient determines how far up and down a line of k-space is filled. It determines the size of the FOV in the phase direction of the image. The polarity of each gradient defines the direction traveled through k-space. This may be explained as follows: if the frequency-encoding gradient is positive, k-space traversed is from left to right. If the frequency-encoding gradient is negative, k-space is traversed from right to left. The phase-encoding gradient on the positive side fills the top half of the k-space. The phase-encoding gradient on the negative side fills the bottom half of k-space.

1.4.3   Gradient-Echo (GRE)

The layout of this sub-section is as follows: Sub-section 1.4.3.1 discusses partial or fractional echo imaging. Partial averaging is discussed in Sub-section 1.4.3.2. Pre-scanning is discussed in Sub-section 1.4.3.3. Data acquisition is discussed in Sub-section 1.4.3.4.

In a gradient echo sequence, the frequency-encoding switches negatively to dephase the FID and then positively to rephase it. After rephasing, a gradient echo is produced. When the frequency-encoding gradient is negative, k-space is traversed from right to left. The starting point of k-space filling is towards the center. So, k-space is initially traversed from the center to the left for a distance, which depends on the amplitude of the negative lobe of the frequency-encoding gradient. It can be observed that the phase-encode will be positive, so a line in the top half of k-space is filled. The sample of this gradient determines the distance traveled. It means that the data line is filled up in k-space if the amplitude of the phase gradient is higher. Therefore, the combination of the phase gradient and the negative lobe of the frequency gradient determines the point in k-space for the beginning of data storage. The frequency-encoding gradient is switched on positively. During its application, data is read from the echo. As the frequency-encoding gradient is positive, data is placed in a line of k-space from left to right. The distance traveled depends on the amplitude of the positive lobe of the gradient. This distance determines the size of the FOV. If the phase gradient is negative, then a line in the bottom half of k-space is filled in exactly the same manner as above. The manner in which k-space is filled depends on the data acquisition. k-space filling can be modified using the following methods: (**1**) rectangular FOV, (**2**) anti-aliasing, (**3**) using ultra fast pulse sequences, (**4**) using respiratory compensation, (**5**) Echo Planar Imaging, (**6**) using partial echo imaging and (**7**) partial averaging. Only partial echo imaging and partial averaging will be discussed here.

1.4.3.1   Partial or Fractional Echo Imaging

This is performed when the signal or echo is partially read during the application of the frequency-encoding gradient. The system samples the first half of the echo to fill half of the k-space frequency area. Later, the system calculates the other half of the original image as its mirror image. Filling half of the k-space area along the frequency axis is known as partial or fractional echo. In partial echo imaging, the sampling window is shifted during readout. Only the peak and the dephasing part of the echo are sampled. The peak of the echo occurs closer to the RF excitation pulse. T_E is reduced and partial echo imaging is performed. It allows for maximum T_1 and proton density weighting with more slices for a given T_R.

1.4.3.2   Partial Averaging

The negative and positive halves of k-space on each side of the phase axis are symmetrical and mirror images of each other. Approximately half of the lines of k-space are selected and filled during the acquisition. The system has enough data to produce an image, i.e., if 70% of the k-space is filled, only 70% of phase-encoding is selected to complete the scan and the remaining lines are filled with zeros. In this manner, the scan time is reduced at the cost of lengthy image acquisition time where the "scan time" is the product of phase-encoding, NEX and T_R scan parameters.

1.4.3.3   Pre-scan

Pre-scanning is carried out for calibration before the data acquisition. Its main tasks are to find the central frequency, find the exact magnitude of the RF and adjust the magnitude of the received signal. The central frequency is normally chosen on the water protons' resonant frequency within the area of the examination. The exact magnitude of the transmitted radio frequency (the maximum signal in the coil) is chosen. This RF magnitude should be equal to the energy needed for magnetization vector 90° flipping. This is measured as transmit gain or power spectrum. The magnitude of the received signal is always chosen above the background noise without distortion. All these pre-scan calculations are specific to the pulse sequence used, based on the patient and scan parameters chosen.

1.4.3.4   Data Acquisition

Data can be acquired in one of the following ways: (**1**) sequential; (**2**) interleaved; (**3**) three-dimensional volumetric. Sequential acquisitions acquire all the data from the lines of k-space (slice 1) and then go on to acquire all the data from the lines of k-space (slice 2). The slices are displayed as they are acquired. Two-dimensional acquisition in interleaved manner fills one line of k-space for slice 1 and then fills the same line of k-space for slices 2, 3, etc. Once this line is filled for all slices, the next line of k-space is filled for other slices 1, 2, 3, etc. Three-dimensional acquisition fills these different k-space lines in the third dimension as slice thickness in the volume of interest. The interleaved slices are subsequently imaged in different directions at variable flip angles. This results in data acquisition for oblique[8] imaging.

1.4.4   The Latest Techniques for MR Image Generation

The following are the latest developments in image generation techniques: (**1**) increasing speed by use of fractional NEX, FSE, fast gradient echo methods. (**2**) reducing echo time (T_E) by using fractional echo and fractional RF. (**3**) increasing resolution by using asymmetric FOV. (**4**) reducing aliasing by using no phase wrap or frequency wrap methods. (**5**) increasing coverage by using

---

[8]Diagonal.

phase offset RF pulses. (**6**) achieving contiguous slices by 3-D acquisition. (**7**) achieving spatial (saturation (SAT) pulses) or spectral (chemical presaturation) saturation. (**8**) increasing signal to noise ratio (SNR) by use of narrow bandwidth (variable BW). (**9**) tissue suppression by using inversion recovery (IR) or short inversion time (TI) inversion recovery (STIR) and Fluid Attenuation (FLAIR) with Magnetization Transfer (M_T). (**10**) flow correction by use of flow-related enhancement (FRE), MR Angiography(2-D/3-D TOF- or Phase Contrast-MRA), Maximum Intensity Projection (MIP), cardiac gating, spatial presaturation pulses, gradient moment nulling, better gradient with rise time, low flip angle by Tilted Optimized Non-saturating Excitation (TONE), multiple overlapping thin slice acquisition (MOTSA), even or odd echo numbers and echo dephasing-rephasing. The physical principles of a few commonly-used techniques are described next from the point of view of modifying parameters and their user-friendliness.

1.4.4.1   Fast Spin Echo (FSE) Imaging

This is done by a train of multiple spin echoes (echo train length (ETL)) generated from closely resembling multiple 180° RF pulses with a small inter-echo spacing. This provides multiple views from a single 90° RF excitation multiple Spin-Echo pulse sequence (see Figure 1.25). In other words, instead of many k-spaces for echoes, only one k-space is generated with information from all the echoes. A large number of echoes in the train shortens the imaging time from the central portion of k-space (low spatial frequencies). The number of slices acquired also decreases. In the k-space center, the least phase-encoding step enhances a large signal. In a multi-echo FSE, every single echo is used several times to fill in the single line in k-space. In dual echo imaging, we need twice the number of lines to fill in k-space. So, this will increase the scan time or will scan half the number of echoes per ETL. This problem is best solved by a shared-echo approach where the first and last echoes in the train are emphasized for TE1 and TE2, respectively.

Fast Spin Echo (FSE) image resolution depends upon its early echo and late echo T_2-weighted characteristics. At short $TE_{effective}$, the first echo of the train will be centered around the k-space center. This will give good tissue resolution; otherwise a longer $TE_{effective}$ produces poor resolution. The first half of the echoes in the train fill k-space for the early echo (PD-weighted) and the second half of the echoes in the train fill k-space for the late echo. This technique minimizes scan time, provides good SNR, increases speed, provides high image resolution, and minimizes image artifacts. It has several disadvantages, such as false multiple sclerosis (MS) lesion, Magnetization Transfer Contrast effects, magnetic susceptibility effects, and brighter lipids which appear on T_2-weighted images. However, it also has certain merits such as: less acquisition time, minimization of MS lesions and generation of high resolution images (for example in 3-D FSE).

In this area of research, MS lesion delineation is done by incorporating both FLAIR and MTC into FSE Attenuated Fluid by Fast Inversion Recovery with Magnetization Transfer Imaging (AFFIRMATIVE) with a variable echoes pulse sequence (see Figures 1.26 and 1.27).

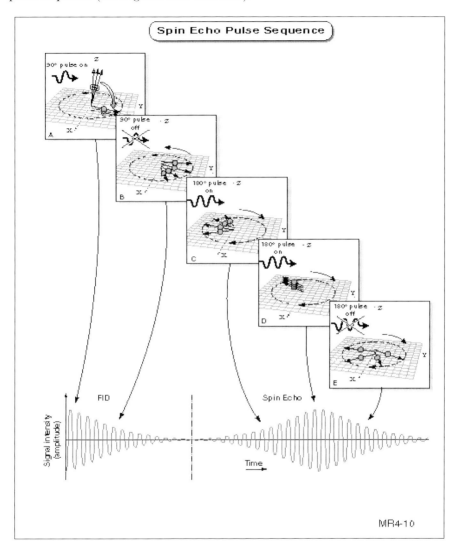

Figure 1.25: Spin Echo pulse sequence (Courtesy of Marconi Medical Systems, Inc.).

This pulse sequence uses an inversion pulse of $180°$, each preceded by a magnetization transfer pulse for equilibrium. This is followed by a flow-compensated, multi-slice, dual echo FSE sequence. Each $90°$ pulse is preceded by an M_T pulse for the acquisition of FLAIR/MTC images. After a variable delay for magnetization recovery, a second imaging sequence is played out to acquire FSE images. These three repeated scans use effective T_E=17/102 ms, ETL=8 (4 per echo), Inversion Time =2500 ms, T_R=10 sec, NEX=1, FOV=24

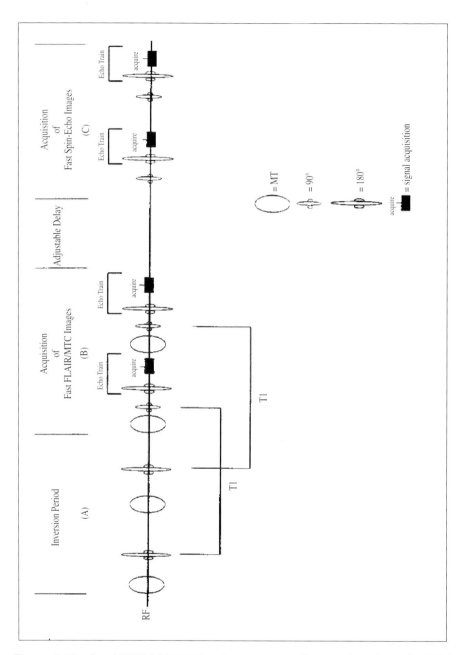

Figure 1.26: An AFFIRMATIVE pulse sequence diagram based on the FSE scheme showing events during early and late echo FLAIR/MTC images (Courtesy of Ponnada A. Narayana, Texas School of Medicine, Houston, TX).

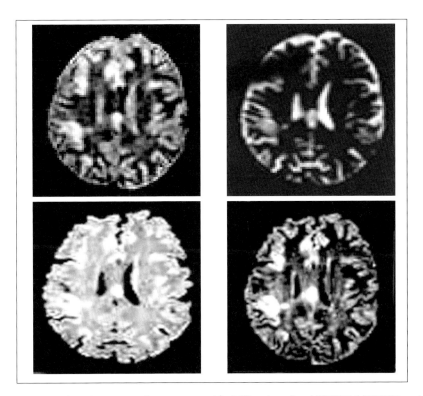

Figure 1.27: Axial images of a patient with MS using the AFFIRMATIVE pulse sequence based on: **Top Left**: early echo FSE image. **Top Right**: late echo FSE image. **Bottom Left**: early echo FLAIR/MTC image. **Bottom Right**: late echo FLAIR/MTC echo image, showing clear MS lesions.

cm, acquisition matrix=256 × 256 (see Bedell *et al.* [31]).

1.4.4.2 Quadruple Contrast Imaging

In most of the FSE images, the main problem is partial volume averaging (PVA) which reduces the chances of tissue fraction analysis and the visibility of lesion pathology, like MS lesions in the white matter area. PVA minimization by CSF signal suppression in fluid-attenuated inversion recovery (FLAIR) is used to visualize MS lesions in darker white matter. Fractional analysis of tissue volumes is done using the Quadruple Contrast pulse sequence based upon the time-multiplexing concept. Four types of images are acquired: WM/CSF-suppressed (GM-visible); GM/CSF-suppressed (WM-visible); CSF-suppressed(FLAIR); and PD-weighted images. The physical principle of this pulse sequence is the same as the FSE scheme. Four sets of slice-selective inversion pulses are applied followed by four FSE acquisition trains (the first to null CSF, the second after a TI_1=3000 ms GM-visible inversion pulse, the third inversion pulse after TI_2 to suppress WM and CSF, and the fourth inversion pulse to visualize the rest of the tissue) in the FLAIR image acquisition as shown in Figures 1.28 and 1.29 (see Bedell *et al.* [32]). This method uses an image matrix of 256 × 128 with zero fill to 256 × 256; FOV=240 mm; slice thickness=3 mm; ETL=12; NEX=1; receiver bandwidth=31.25 MHz; effective echo time=10 ms.

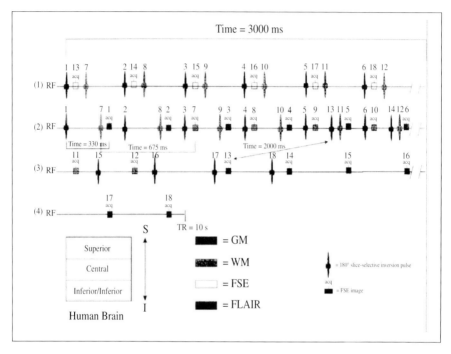

Figure 1.28: A Quadruple Contrast pulse sequence diagram consisting of four sets of slice-selective inversion pulses and FSE (*PD*-weighted) acquisition trains for GM-visible, WM-visible, FLAIR and FSE images acquired in an interleaved manner. The slice numbers are shown for the inversion recovery acquisition (Courtesy of Ponnada A. Narayana, Texas School of Medicine, Houston, TX).

1.4.4.3   Gradient-Echo (GRE) Imaging

A single excitation RF pulse is used with reversed polarity on the frequency-encoding gradient. This rephases the gradient-dependent dephasing at the center of the signal acquisition period (giving rise to a GRE). The gradient-echo amplitude depends on T_2^* and the flip angle. The idea is to acquire incomplete longitudinal relaxation (T_1-based steady-state magnetization) within a short T_R. This also introduces T_2 weighting into the generated images. Spoiled or crushed residual magnetization and refocusing of the transverse phase coherence are the best ways of tackling the said residual magnetization. The gradient-spoiled methods use killer pulses placed at the end of each T_R period

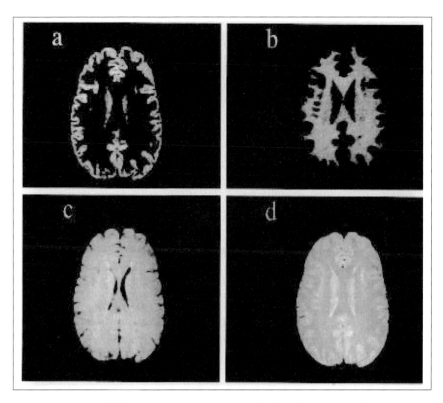

Figure 1.29: Axial MR images acquired with the Quadruple Contrast pulse sequence from the ventricular region of a normal volunteer. The images shown are: (a) GM-visible, (b) WM-visible, (c) FLAIR, and (d) PD-weighted FSE (Courtesy of Ponnada A. Narayana, Texas School of Medicine, Houston, TX).

on the slice-selection axis. These allow for image contrast weighted towards T_1 differences through T_R and flip angle (without T_2 differences). Recently, several fast GRE sequences have been used, such as: MP-FISP, FMP-SPGR, MP-SPGR[9], spoiled MP-Fast-Low-Angled Shot (Turbo MP-FLASH), FAST, RF-spoiled FAST, CE-FAST, RAM-FAST. The signal intensity can be represented as:

$$s = \frac{sin(\alpha)}{1 + \frac{T_1}{T_2} + cos(\alpha)\left(\frac{T_1}{T_2} - 1\right)}, \quad (1.21)$$

where T_1 and T_2 are relaxation times and α is the flip angle (see Figure 1.30). In non-spoiled steady-state GRE methods, residual magnetization is rephased at the end of each T_R period. It is done by the use of a rewinder gradient pulse. This is applied with a second phase-encoding gradient pulse applied after each frequency-encoding pulse. The rewinder pulse has an amplitude equal to, but opposite in sign to, the first phase-encoding pulse. The image

---

[9]Multi-planar spoiled Gradient-Recalled Acquisition in the steady-state GRASS.

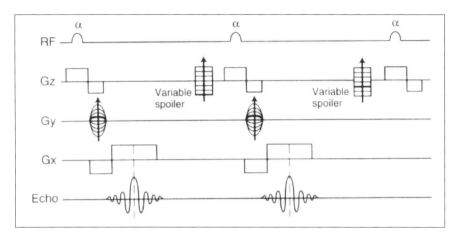

Figure 1.30: A representative SPGR (Multi-planar spoiled Gradient-Recalled Acquisition in the steady-state GRASS) pulse sequence diagram showing the physical events during image generation.

contrast depends on the ratio T_2/T_1, PD flow and magnetic susceptibility. This may be also called RF phase-offset spoiling.

1.4.4.4   Echo Planar Imaging (EPI)

The goal of EPI is to acquire all the k-space data from a single excitation (single-shot EPI) or segments of k-space (multi-shot EPI). This generates images with high resolution at the expense of time with better contrast. The acquisition window depends upon inhomogeneity $(T_2{}^*)$ for specific tissues to minimize tissue saturation or signal loss (1 ms/line sampling time for a single planar image in 100 ms). The oscillating gradient G_x criss-crosses k-space up and along the frequency-encoding or read direction k_x up to 128 times during a single 128 x 128 sequence. Incremental phase-encoding is provided at the end of each crossing k_x in the form of a brief pulsed (blipped) phase-altering gradient. After the short phase-encoding pulse, the blip increments G_y and the sign of G_x is reversed. Later, G_x traverses a second line in k-space. This process is continued for as long as there is enough transverse magnetization (T_2* or T_2) to support the repeated gradient echo. Multi-shot or interleaved (IEPI) sequences can cover only a portion of k-space at a time. The trajectories can be interleaved based on the available gradient power. These trajectories control the sensitivity of the pulse sequence to off-resonance effects. For example, the Siemens Vision 25 mt/m at a 300 rise time with the commercial GOD package uses a 400 micro seconds sample, 300 micro sec (rate of gradient fall = 1 ms per line) with the help of a gradient booster. Figure 1.31 illustrates the diffusion-weighted images.

The physical principle of this technique is to acquire three series of images with diffusion gradients.

These gradients are oriented along three orthogonal directions with pro-

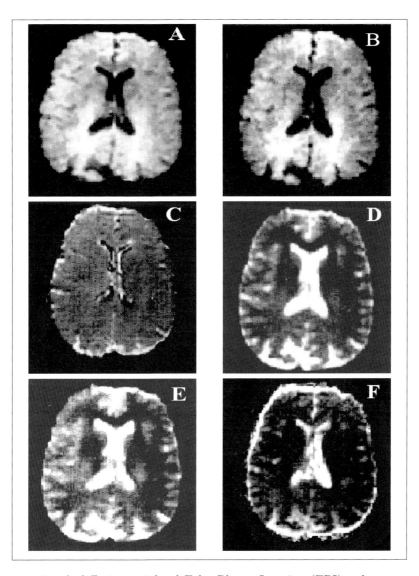

Figure 1.31: A diffusion-weighted Echo Planar Imaging (EPI) pulse sequence diagram and images. **Top Left**: CSF-suppressed multi-shot. **Top Right**: multi-slice selection. **Middle Left**: dephasing gradient. **Middle Right**, **Bottom Left** and **Bottom Right** are: spin-echo diffusion-weighted EPI acquisitions (Courtesy of Ponnada A. Narayana, Texas School of Medicine, Houston, TX).

gressive adjustments in diffusion sensitivity. For apparent diffusion coefficients (ADC) measurement, the following parameters can be used with CSF suppression: T_E=130 ms, slice thickness= 5 mm, FOV=40 cm, effective T_R 7000 ms, inversion time TI=1600 ms. The trapezoidal diffusion gradients are calculated as:

$$b \quad = \quad \gamma^2 \, G^2 \, [\delta^2 \, (\frac{1}{3\delta}) + \frac{1}{30} \, \epsilon^3 - \frac{1}{6} \, \delta \, \epsilon^2] \, , \qquad (1.22)$$

where γ is the Gyromagnetic ratio, G is the gradient strength for diffusion, δ is the gradient duration, and ϵ is the gradient ramp time. In the orthogonal directions, diffusion sensitivity is enhanced by combining the X-, Y-, Z-gradients. Two data sets of 128×128 from overlapping regions of k-space are acquired for each diffusion-weighted image. These data sets are combined with averaging of overlapping regions after the zero and first order phase correction. Finally, the data yields 256×128 data sets. The zero order and first order corrections are made by setting k-space center phase (kx=0 and ky=0) and time shifting. This shifting sets one data set relative to the other in k-space until full overlap is achieved. Later, the data set performs zero-filling and 2-D Fourier transform is applied to generate diffusion-weighted images.

1.4.5   3-D Turbo FLASH (MP-RAGE) Technique

These images are suitable for T_1-weighted 3-D measurements, i.e. in cardiac perfusion, liver diagnostics and abdominal imaging. These images are generated using specific optimal parametric settings at: short T_E, narrow bandwidth to yield high SNR, good contrast ($T_R = 3.5$–11 ms; $T_E = 1.7$–4.5 ms; slice thickness $= 500$–800 mm; FOV $= 200$–500 mm) chosen as appropriate for different applications. For example, an inversion pulse with a non-selective RF pulse, narrow bandwidth with reordered phase-encoding pulse applications is used in a neuro-imaging technique.

1.4.6   Non-Rectilinear k-Space Trajectory: Spiral MRI

In spiral MRI sequences, the read and phase gradients are rapidly switched or oscillated along an expanding sine wave in a sinusoidal pattern. k-space is covered with a series of spiral trajectories. The number of spiral trajectories per image acquisition depends on the spatial resolution generated and is the scan time required. This requires nonlinear data sampling and a special 2-D FT reconstruction algorithm. For image generation, a train of 180° RF pulses is combined with spiral trajectories of k-space or a hybrid of FSE. These generate a "RARE spirals" sequence at continuous transverse magnetization. This provides a short spiral of repeated gradient echoes between the 180° RF pulses. In this case, k-space is not covered with annular rings. Hence, it is called "spiral imaging". The longer T_2 decay permits k-space to be filled in one shot.

1.4.7 Fat Suppression

The bright fat signal on a short T_R Spin Echo sequence mimics the bright T_2-weighted FSE or T_1-weighted signal. For example, the bright T_2-weighted FSE or T_1-weighted signal from the Gd-DTPA-enhanced MS lesion mimics the fat signal. To avoid the signal from the fat, the chemical saturation method uses a frequency-selective RF excitation pulse. This allows a narrow-bandwidth excitation profile centered over the lipid resonance before the 90° pulse or a partial flip angle pulse. After excitation of the lipid protons, crusher gradients are applied. These gradients dephase transverse magnetization from the lipids longer than the acquisition time. The entire acquisition period leaves the slice lipids saturated and the lipids appear hypointense.

1.4.8 High Speed MRI: Perfusion-Weighted MRI

Perfusion-weighted MRI allows the early detection of an organ in a perfusion-rich region. This is done by the use of T_1- and T_2^*-weighted shortening-induced magnetic susceptibility changes. This distinguishes between blood-filled volumes and the capillary surface area effect by using long-range T_2^* shortening.

1.4.9 Time of Flight (TOF) MR Angiography

Based on 2-D or 3-D Fourier transformation, magnetic resonance angiography (MRA) uses 2-D FSE or 3-D GRE techniques. In 2-D TOF-MRA, a presat (presaturation) pulse is applied above or below each slice to eliminate the signal from the vessels flowing in the opposite direction. For this technique, scan parameters are set with a short T_R=20 msec, a flip angle of 45-60° and a short T_E of 10-30 msec. In the case of 3-D TOF-MRA, a slab of 5 cm containing 50 slices can be used to generate the images. A typical example of the 2-D TOF technique is shown Figure 1.32, with the carotid bifurcation separating at the external or internal atherosclerotic lesion location.

1.4.10 Fast Spectroscopic Imaging

The Spectroscopic Imaging (SI) experiment provides data for one frequency axis, and one to three spatial axes ($A_x \times B_y \times N$). These data points go through k-space in columns by acquiring N data points per excitation. It needs $A_x \times B_y$ excitations with their chemical shift information. The chemical shift information is encoded by incrementing the evolution period t between each excitation. The spectral bandwidth is the reciprocal of t but independent of the imaging filter bandwidth. Such an approach reduces the measuring time at condition $N.A_x.B_y$. For example, a bandwidth (8 Hz) at 4 ppm is covered by fewer frequency domain points at a longer T_2 with suppressed water. This allows SI measurement for lipid bleeds free in a VOI (water suppression-excitation-evolution-volume selection imaging).

In this direction, several approaches are in use: (1) a hard pulse for excitation; (2) a binominal pulse for water suppression; (3) a selective VOI in less

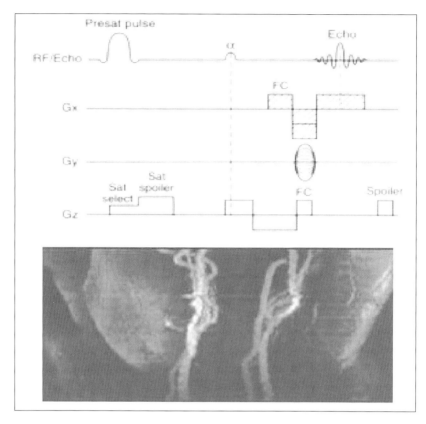

Figure 1.32: 2-D Time of Flight MR Angiography pulse sequence diagram and image projection showing bilateral carotid artery bifurcation with bilateral Atherosclerotic plaque (Courtesy of Rakesh Sharma, Texas School of Medicine and Methodist Hospital, Houston, TX).

scan time by using PRESS[10] or STEAM[11]; (4) the use of longitudinal magnetization manipulation before the readout pulse by FLAIR or EPI are good practices to use. Good global shimming is a pre-requisite for volume selective Chemical Shift Imaging (CSI). Good shimming is achieved by: using a slice thickness of 1–2 cm; field of view (FOV) = 16–24 cm; data matrix = 16 × 16; in-plane resolution 1–1.5 cm in each direction; individual voxels are 1.0–4.5 cc; phase-encoding matrix 16 × 16; T_R 1500 ms; scan time acquired 7 minutes (while a matrix of 32 × 32 requires a scan time of 26 minutes). How are different chemical shift images for different voxels produced? This is done with a FID in the presence of a constant gradient, which samples the spatial FT for the distribution of the metabolite proton frequencies at a fixed point in the k-space line. In general, the combination of two methods (constant gra-

---

[10]Point Resolved Spectroscopy.
[11]Stimulated T_E acquisition mode.

dient in one direction and pulse in the other) is used for 2-D chemical shift imaging to acquire one line in k-space. For CSI image generation, multiple FIDs with different strength gradient pulses in different directions are repeated multiple times in k-space. 2-D/3-D CSI needs phase-encoding in two or three dimensions. This provides an estimate of spatial and frequency distributions by discrete Fourier Transformations (DFT) in time and space. The reconstructed image (spatial distribution of spins at a particular location) is judged by a point spread function (PSF). In the brain, this is used for routine multiple sclerosis lesion characterization (multi-section Spin-Echo MRSI). This method uses Chemical Shift Spectroscopy (CHESS) water saturation pulse, octagonal outer volume saturation (OVS) pulse for scalp water/lipid suppression. This imaging spin-echo pulse sequence is detailed in Chapter 5. The OVS sequence has eight sinc-gauss section-selective pulses, which excite eight sections outside the skull outline. Their orientation and position are calculated from coordinates (four in the superior plane and four in the inferior plane) measured by a gradient-recalled acquisition in the steady-state (GRASS) sequence.

For image formation, RF pulses are applied in four pairs, each pair followed by an 8 msec crusher gradient pulse of 14mT/m. The pulse diagonal pairs look at opposite octagonal arrangements at an adjusted flip angle with RF pulses in the spin-echo sequence. The following parameter settings can be used: slice section thickness is 15 mm; 180° pulse flanked by 4-msec gradient crushers in three directions; a result slew rate is 16 mT/m at 90° pulse band at spectral width of 1 kHz; TE 270 msec to acquire a 256 msec echo. So, sequential parallel slice sections are excited by adjusting the transmitter for $90^\circ/180^\circ$ RF pulses. Soon after the last gradient crusher pulse, a 2-D phase-encoding (32×32) is used for 240 mm (FOV) data acquisition by k-space sampling scheme. Another important aspect is the normalization of the metabolite images. This is a spatially-dependent signal amplitude correction within the transverse plane for NAA, creatine, choline, acetate, lactate, water and myo-inositol. Chemical artifacts are also dependent on the Larmor frequency of the metabolite, relative metabolite: water chemical shift (cross correlation), position and field gradient relationship. The shape of the VOI and heterogeneity of the metabolite distribution in the image depends on T_1 relaxivities, and flip angles across the VOI (see Wild *et al.* [33]). Emphasis was given to recent ultrafast imaging methods. A concise text on this topic is reproduced partially in Chapter 5. Interested readers can refer to this chapter for further details.

1.4.11 Recent MR Imaging Techniques

Other fast imaging methods include: dynamic contrast-enhanced breast MRI done using two- and three-dimensional variable flip angle fast low-angle shot T_1 measurement (see Brookes *et al.* [35]); dynamic-breathing MRI (see Suga *et al.* [36]); ultrafast MRI (see Outwater [37]); hepatic lesion fat suppressed T_2-weighted MR imaging pulse sequence (see Kanematsu *et al.* [38]); coronary MR angiography (see Duerinckx [39]); fast-FLAIR MTC pulse sequence (see Filippi [40]); Single Shot Fast Spin Echo (SSFSE) pulse sequence (see Kadoya *et al.* [41]); Fast Spin Echo Diffusion Coefficient Mapping MRI (see Brockstedt *et al.* [42]); adiabatic multiple Spin Echo pulse sequence (see Zweckstetter *et al.* [43]); half-Fourier Turbo Spin Echo MRI (HASTE[12]) (see Coates *et al.* [44]); 3-D Time of Flight MR angiography by Ultrafast MP-RAGE sequence (see Yamashita *et al.* [45]); Coherent and Incoherent steady-state spin-echo (COSESS[13] and INSESS[14]) sequences (see Werthner *et al.* [46]); phase-modulated binominal RF pulses for spectrally selective imaging (see Thomasson *et al.* [47]); Dual Echo Steady-State Free Precession (DESS-FP) pulse sequence (see Hardy *et al.* [48]); optimized ultra-Fast Imaging Sequence (OUFIS) (see Zha *et al.* [49]); fast three - dimensional Inversion-Recovery GRE pulse sequence (see Foo *et al.* [50]); diffusion-weighted EPI pulse sequences for glioma (see Tien *et al.* [51]); Time of Flight carotid vascular contrast MRA pulse sequences (see Tkach *et al.* [52]); incremental Flip Angle Snapshot FLASH MRI pulse sequence (see Urhahn *et al.* [53]); Steady-State Free Precession Rapid 2-DFT MRI: FAST and CE-FAST sequences (see Gyngell [54]).

In conclusion, the following are among the new developments in image generation: (**1**) the need to increase speed; (**2**) to reduce TE; (**3**) to increase resolution; (**4**) to reduce aliasing; (**5**) to increase tissue coverage; (**6**) to achieve contiguous slices; (**7**) to increase SNR; (**8**) to apply tissue suppression, flow correction, cardiac gating; (**9**) spatial presaturation; (**10**) gradient moment nulling; (**11**) better gradients with rise time; (**12**) low flip angle; (**13**) multiple overlapping thin slices; (**14**) even or odd spin echo numbers; and (**15**) metabolite characterization.

1.5   Computer Tomography Image Generation

X-ray Computer Tomography (CT) provides cross-sectional images of body organs. While the resulting images from CT are more clearly visualized when compared to conventional X-ray images, the radiation doses in CT are significantly higher. CT is therefore not used as an examination technique unless additional clinical information indicates its need. In CT, an X-ray beam, which is initially generated as a point source, is collimated to form a single slice of a flat fan-shaped X-ray beam. The X-ray source and the detector are rotated around the patient and the two-dimensional or three-dimensional distribution of the X-ray radiation densities within the structure being imaged are recorded as projections from many angles of view. The information is then used to reconstruct the cross-sectional images of the body organs using mathematical reconstruction techniques including filtered back-projection or Fourier reconstruction. In recent generation CT equipment, a true "fan-beam" of X-ray is generated and directed towards a circular array of detectors passing through the patient (see Figure 1.33). Next, we will explain how CT scanners combine the projection data to form a cross-sectional image. In this explanation,

---

[12]Half-Fourier acquisition single-shot turbo spin echo.
[13]Coherent Spin Echo in the Steady State as fast imaging pulse sequence.
[14]Incoherence steady-state spin echo.

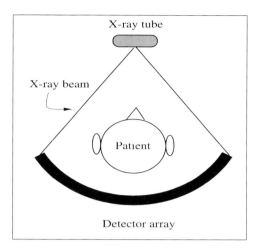

Figure 1.33: CT scanner configuration with a true "fan beam" of X-ray.

for simplicity, we will only describe the Fourier transform-based reconstruction technique for the scanner, which uses a single collimated X-ray beam. In practical and modern scanners which use true "fan beam" geometries, different assumptions are required. Interested readers may refer to the book by Seeram [55].

1.5.1   Fourier Reconstruction Method

As explained earlier, information which is obtained in CT scanners is in the form of a series of samples of the absorption summed through the thickness of the body. The absorption can be modelled as a two-dimensional function $f(x, y)$ and its projection $g_\rho(R)$ is:

$$g_\theta(R) = \int \int f(x, y)\, \delta\, (x cos(\theta) + y\, sin(\theta) - R)\, dx\, dy\,, \qquad (1.23)$$

where the delta function selects the projection of interest at an angle θ from the x-axis and R is the line $R = x\, cos(\rho) + y\, sin(\rho)$ (see Figure 1.34). Consider the two-dimensional Fourier transform of the cross-section absorption function $f(x, y)$ that we wish to reconstruct as:

$$F(u, v) = \int \int f(x, y)\, exp\, (-2\pi i\rho\, (ux + vy))\, dx\, dy\,. \qquad (1.24)$$

For convenience, we may write the Fourier transform of $f(x, y)$ in polar coordinates as:

$$F(\rho, \beta) = \int \int f(x, y)\, exp\, (-2\pi i\rho\, (x cos(\beta) + y sin(\beta)))\, dx\, dy\,, \qquad (1.25)$$

where $u = r\, cos(\beta)$ and $v = r\, sin(\beta)$. An important theorem in Fourier theory, the Central Slice Theorem, establishes the connection between the slice and its

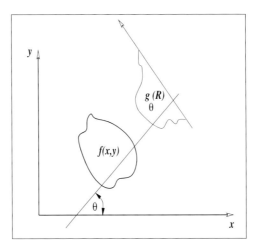

Figure 1.34: Projection of a shape in CT.

projections. According to this theorem, the one-dimensional Fourier transform of the projection is equivalent to the values of the two-dimensional Fourier transform of the image, measured on lines through the origin of the Fourier transform space at the same angles as the original projections were acquired (Figure 1.35) [56]. This it can be written as:

$$F(\rho, \beta) = F\{g_\beta(R)\}. \tag{1.26}$$

This means, in principle, that the two-dimensional Fourier transform of the image can be reconstructed by interpolating the projections onto a two-dimensional Fourier transform. Then by calculating the inverse two-dimensional Fourier transform, the cross-sectional image may be computed (see Figure 1.35) [56]. Some sample CT images of the heart and a CT scanner are shown in Figure 1.36.

1.6   Positron-Emission Tomography Image Generation

Positron-emission tomography is a non-invasive medical imaging technique that measures the metabolic activity of the human body cells. Unlike the other medical imaging techniques described previously, PET produces images of the body's basic biochemistry or function. Hence it is extremely valuable for assessing changes in organ performance that precede structural changes and which are usually imaged by traditional diagnostic techniques. Unlike conventional anatomical-based imaging tools like CT, MR and ultrasound, PET provides functional imaging. This ability to give a direct measure of the body's metabolic functions gives PET many advantages over other diagnostic imaging techniques; it can detect early metabolic changes which may be precursors to

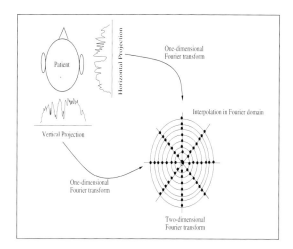

Figure 1.35: Demonstration of the Central Slice Theorem and its application to image reconstruction in CT scanners.

disease, it can monitor response to treatment, and it can eliminate the need for costly redundant testing or invasive surgical procedures. PET is clinically useful in the diagnosis and monitoring of certain types of cancers, some kinds of brain disorders and cardiac diseases [57], [58], [59]. Even in diseases, such as Alzheimer's disease, where there is no gross structural abnormality, PET is able to show a biochemical change. A PET scan is a simple procedure. It is based on the use of a small amount of a radioactive material, known as a radio-tracer, similar to that which is used in other nuclear medicine procedures. The radioactivity, which includes common elements (oxygen, carbon, nitrogen, fluorine), is attached to a compound that is familiar to the human body. Compounds like glucose, water, ammonia, and certain drugs may be used. Replacing the naturally occurring atoms in a compound with a labeled atom leaves one with a compound that is chemically and biologically identical to the original, so it will behave in a manner which is identical to its unlabeled versions and is also traceable. For example, glucose labeled with positron-emitting fluorine (18F) is a PET radio-tracer commonly used to measure energy metabolism. Radio-labeling of drugs can reveal both the location of action ("receptor site") and the efficacy of the interaction ("binding capacity"). The range of available PET tracers - and thus the number of bodily processes that can be imaged with PET - is currently quite broad, with still more in development. The radioactive drug is usually injected into the patient and a specially designed PET scanner images how the body processes the drug. Chemical compounds we would like to follow through the body are labeled with radioactive atoms that decay very rapidly by emitting positrons or positive-electrons. It is identical to an electron in mass and electrical charge but has an opposite charge. In fact, the PET camera detects the position of these positrons in the body.

A PET camera makes tens of thousands of measurements each second. Each

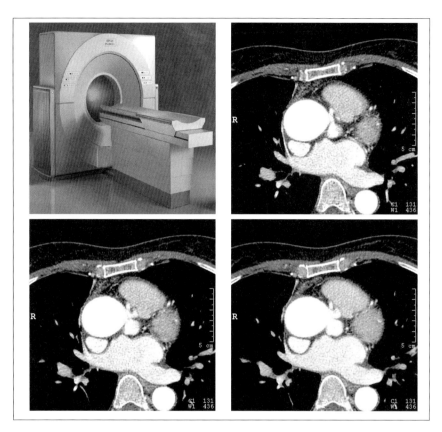

Figure 1.36: Sample cardiac CT images and a CT scanner (Courtesy of Marconi Medical Systems, Inc.).

measurement looks at a very small volume of tissue, only about 2 mm^3. Taken together, these tens of thousands of highly precise measurements create a 3-D measurement of an entire organ. Such 3-D measurements can be viewed as images or analyzed in detail by sophisticated computer programs. PET has been in clinical use since the early 1990s.

1.6.1   Underlying Principles of PET

A positron is a positive electron which is identical to an electron in mass, but has an opposite charge of $+1$ if the electron is defined as having a charge of -1. In PET, positrons are all produced by nuclear decay. Basically, unstable nuclei are generated in a cyclotron by bombarding a certain target material with protons. In a typical reaction, a bombarding proton enters the nucleus of the target material and releases a neutron in the process. For example, bombarding 18-O, which is an isotope of oxygen that has two extra neutrons, results in the proton being captured and a neutron being released from the target nucleus. Changing the number of protons in a nucleus is important and changes the atomic species. In this case, the atom changes from oxygen to fluorine. In chemical language, this can be represented as [18-O + proton = 18-F + neutron]. In another similar reaction, nitrogen changes to carbon with the participants being [14-N + proton = 11-C + alpha], where an alpha is a particle that is composed of two protons and two neutrons. The new nucleus created in this manner is unstable and eventually decays into a more stable form. The time needed for this decay depends on the particular species created, and ranges in time from almost nothing to thousands of years for different species. In addition to other conditions, the target material in PET is chosen so that the product of the bombardment decays to a more stable state isotope by emitting a positron. Considering the 18-F example above, there are too many protons in its nucleus. In order to remain stable, one of these protons decays into a neutron and emits a positron and a neutrino, which can be represented as [proton (+1 charge) = neutron (0 charge) + positron (+1 charge) + neutrino (0 charge)]. The result is one 18-O again (the original target material), a positron, and a neutrino. The neutrino is an odd little particle which has no mass, no charge, and travels at a rate near the speed of light so, once created, in practice it is out of the picture. The positron, on the other hand, being the positive electron that is needed in PET, is still available. The energy left over from the nuclear decay process is shared between the positron and the departing neutrino. This energy is in the form of kinetic energy and, because of the fundamental conservation laws, the positron collides with other particles and loses kinetic energy through scattering until it almost comes to rest. Once the positron has lost most of its kinetic energy, it is ready to participate in the annihilation reaction. The positron will encounter an electron and the two will completely annihilate each other, converting all their mass into energy. The result of the annihilation process is two photons. The conservation law for energy expresses that the energy of the system before annihilation, which includes positron rest mass energy, electron rest mass energy and the small bit of remaining kinetic energy, must be the same as the energy of the system after annihilation. Similarly, the conservation law for momentum dictates that the momentum of the system before annihilation, which is basically zero since both the positron and electron are almost at rest, must be the same as the momentum of the system after annihilation. The only final possible state for the system under these conditions is one in which the two photons travel apart in opposite directions at approximately 180° (see Figure 1.37), so that the net momentum of the system is zero and each has an energy corresponding to half the energy of the initial system. Since the rest mass of the positron and electron are identical (511keV), each photon has 511 keV of energy. The slight deviation from 180° is due into the residual kinetic energy of the positron.

Having two 511 keV photons flying off at 180° from each other, the next step in PET is to detect these photons with a PET camera. This allows us to determine the site of the annihilation that is within approximately 2 mm of the nucleus which released the positron initially. Therefore, we can spatially locate the site of the tracer, effectively finding out where this nucleus goes in the body,

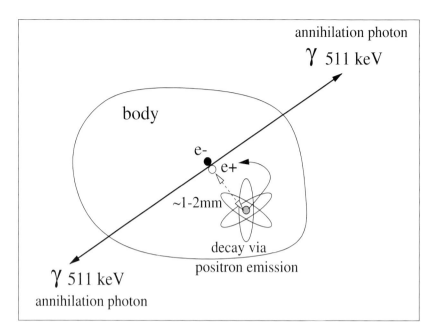

Figure 1.37: Positron emission and annihilation.

and that is the goal in PET. The annihilation photons are usually detected by interaction with an inorganic scintillator, such as bismuth germinate or thallium doped. The 511 keV photons are absorbed and the energy re-radiated as a shower of ultraviolet secondary photons. The secondary photons are detected by an optically-coupled array of photomultiplier tubes (see Figure 1.38), and the resulting signals are passed to processing electronics. The detection procedure is shown schematically in Figure 1.39.

1.6.2 Usage of PET in Diagnosis

How is PET used? Since the compounds that can be labeled in PET are limited only by the imagination of the investigators and the physical half-life of the positron emitting radio-tracer, the range of PET applications is limited only by the imagination of the user. PET has been used to study normal organ function and disease states. For example, PET research triggered a revolution in our understanding of energy metabolism during normal brain work. Current concepts of the neural systems of human cognition are being strongly influenced by PET. Even cell-to-cell communication systems are being explored by radio-labeling drugs that mimic the body's own hormones and neurotransmitters. In disease-related research, PET has many applications including diagnosis, outcome prediction, treatment assessment, and post-recovery. PET is not limited to any one organ and has already been applied to the brain, heart, lung, liver and bone. PET can be applied to the study of many types of disorder including congenital, developmental, infectious, neoplastic, traumatic, and degenerative

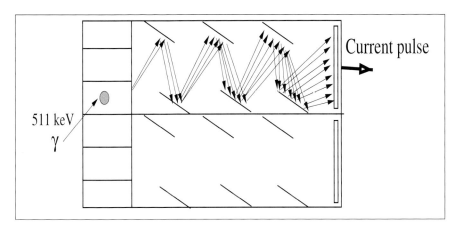

Figure 1.38: Schematics of the photomultiplier tube in PET.

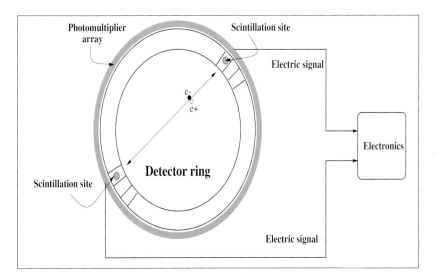

Figure 1.39: Schematics of the site locating procedure in PET.

diseases.

1.6.2.1   PET in Cardiac and Neurological Applications

Well-accepted clinical uses for PET include the diagnosis of Alzheimer's Disease, Huntington's Disease, Parkinsonism (and other movement disorders), the presurgical evaluation of focal epilepsy and cardiac ischemia, and post-treatment evaluation of brain tumors. New clinical applications being developed at several centers include the diagnosis of depressive disorders, head trauma, liver and bone cancer. PET explores the brain's organization for perception, action, language, attention, and emotion. Other areas are in neurosurgery, depression, epilepsy, head trauma, stuttering and deafness. Samples of PET images applied to the brain can be seen in the color section in Plate 1.

1.6.3   Fourier Slice Theorem

One of the useful tools for visualizing the data acquisition and reconstruction process is the Fourier transform of a projection of a 1-D sample. For a one dimensional Fourier transform, we have:

$$P(v_{xr}, \phi) = \int dx_r \, p(x_r, \phi) \, \exp(-2\pi I \, x_r \, v_{xr}). \tag{1.27}$$

For the two dimensional Fourier transform, we have:

$$F(v_x, v_y) = \int dx \int dy \, f(x, y) \, p(x_r, \phi) \, \exp(-2\pi i (xv_x + yv_y)). \tag{1.28}$$

The Central-Section theorem is a special case of the more general projection theorem, which can be stated as:

$$dx_r \, p(x_r, \phi) w(x_r) = \int dx \int dy \, f(x, y) \, w(x \, cos\phi + y \, sin\phi), \tag{1.29}$$

where $w(.)$ is any function.

1.6.4   The Reconstruction Algorithm in PET

Given the PET scanner projection data, the goal is to estimate the original tracer distribution $f(x, y)$. This can be mathematically given as the inverse of the 2-D Fourier transform as:

$$f(x, y) = \int dv_x \int dv_y \, \exp(2\pi i (xv_x + yv_y x))) \, F(v_x, y_y). \tag{1.30}$$

Changing to polar coordinates, where $F(\rho, \phi)$ is $F(v_x, v_y)$, and using the relationship $F(\rho, \phi) = F(-\rho, \phi + \pi)$, we get:

$$f(x, y) = \int_{-\infty}^{\infty} d\phi \int d\rho \, \rho \, \exp(2\pi i \rho (x cos\phi + y sin\phi))) \, F(\rho, \phi). \tag{1.31}$$

Splitting the above equation into polar coordinates and then integrating, we get:

$$f(x,y) = \int_{-\infty}^{\infty} d\phi \int d\rho \, |\rho| \, \exp(2\pi i\rho(x cos\phi + y sin\phi))) \, F(\rho, \phi) \,. \qquad (1.32)$$

1.6.5 Image Reconstruction Using Filtered Back-Projection

If $P(\rho, \phi)$ is the Fourier transform of the projection data and $\rho = v_{xr}$ and $x_r = x\,cos(\phi) + y\,sin(\phi)$, then the function $f(x,y)$ can be given as:

$$f(x,y) = \int_{-\infty}^{\infty} d\phi \int dv_{xr} \, |v_{xr}| \, \exp(2\pi i v_{xr} x_r) P(v_{xr}, \phi) \,. \qquad (1.33)$$

We can split this into filtering and back-projection operations as follows:

1. Let W be the apodizing window, thus the filtering we get is:

$$p^*(x,y) = \int dv_{xr} \, \exp(2\pi i v_{xr} x_r) \, |v_{xr}| \, W(v_{xr}) \, P(v_{xr}, \phi) \,. \qquad (1.34)$$

2. Now, taking the back-projection of the filtered projection p^*, we get:

$$f(x,y) = \int d\phi \, p^*(x_r, \phi) \,. \qquad (1.35)$$

1.7 Comparison of Imaging Modalities: A Summary

Here, we briefly present a comparison of the different medical imaging modalities.

1. *Image Generation*: An MR image is produced when an RF-pulse excites the hydrogen nuclei of the atoms in the body in static and changing magnetic fields. A CT or X-ray image is produced when X-rays penetrate the organ being imaged and exposes a film. An ultrasound image is produced by collecting the reflected signals from the different tissue boundaries resulting from the inhomogeneities in the medium, when a signal is excited using a piezoelectric transducer.

2. *Image Acquisition Type*: One can acquire MR images using multiplanar and oblique techniques, but one can only obtain cross-sectional anatomy in CT. An X-ray is a flat planar imaging technique. One can acquire both multiplanar and oblique views in ultrasound imaging.

3. *Image Resolution and Image Acquisition Timing*: MR requires long data acquisition times, however with the advancement of faster pulse sequence

generation, we have started to see faster image acquisition times. MR image resolution is typically around 1.0 mm, while for CT the image resolution is typically around 0.5 mm.

4. *Clinical Usage*: The MR imaging technique is used in neuro-imaging (brain and spine), mammography imaging, angiography (MRA), metastatic disease examination, lesion determination, many non-invasive diseases and whole body imaging, such as in the abdomen, etc. MR can be used as a diagnostic tool in many scenarios, such as: (a) If the anatomical area is subject to artifact by X-rays or ultrasound cannot penetrate the area, such as in the posterior fossa, brain stem and abdominal areas. (b) When deep vascular imaging is needed. (c) In certain neurological disorders such as demyelination, nutritional or metabolic disorders or diffuse infection. Clinical usages of CT exams are in bone diseases and bone injury, such as in the head, neck and spine. It is also used in vascular diagnosis such as in aneurysm examinations. An X-ray has its clinical usage in bone imaging, such as for fractures and any degenerative diseases. It is also used in mammography (breast screening), in Gastrointestinal examinations such as esophageal studies. An ultrasound scan is clinically very useful in gynecological exams and lesion detection in the abdomen. A PET imaging scan is clinically useful in studying and understanding energy metabolism during normal activities in the brain, heart, lung, liver, and bone studies. PET can be applied to the study of disorders such as congenital, developmental, infectious, neoplastic, traumatic, and degenerative diseases.

5. *Parameters Affecting Image Contrast*: A variety of imaging parameters affect tissue characteristics and pulse sequences affect the image contrast seen in an MR image. In a CT image, high-density tissues block X-rays, producing bright areas on the image, while low-density tissues block X-rays, producing dark regions in the image. An ultrasound image is also affected by the imaging parameters used for tissue characteristics.

6. *Image Visualization*: An MR image shows excellent tissue contrast, while a CT image shows excellent bone detail. An X-ray image also shows bone detail. An ultrasound image shows good boundaries inside the body.

7. *Body Composition Reflection*: An MR image reflects the physical and chemical composition of tissues, while a CT image reflects the density of the tissues. An X-ray reflects superimposition of bone over soft tissue. A PET image reflects functional information, such as metabolic changes, in the body. An ultrasound image reflects the amount of attenuation by the organ being imaged.

8. *Expense of Exam*: MR is a more expensive exam than CT and X-ray, while a CT exam is more expensive than an X-ray exam. An ultrasound exam costs almost the same as an X-ray exam.

9. *Radiation Exposure*: A patient is exposed to ionizing radiation in CT imaging, while there is no radiation exposure in MR; however, RF deposited into the body, as well as any metal and/or implanted devices in the patient's body, may pose a safety issue. There is no danger of radiation exposure or the effects of a magnetic field and RF exposure in ultrasound, hence it poses the least risk to the patient.

10. *Claustrophobia Issue*: There is no claustrophobia issue for the patient in X-ray, but there may be some in CT and, to a greater degree, in MR. There is absolutely no risk of claustrophobia in ultrasound imaging, as the patient is not at all enclosed during the examination.

11. *Patient Scanning*: A grossly obese patient cannot be scanned using an MR, CT or PET system. Obesity does not matter in X-ray and ultrasound scanning; however, the quality of images is affected if the person being scanned is highly obese.

12. *Popularity and Applications*: Though it is somewhat subjective looking at the trend, one can say that MRI is the most popular exam these days and has the largest number of applications in patient care and management. Both invasive and non-invasive techniques exist in the market today, which use MRI systems much more than CT and X-ray systems. The popularity of ultrasound is equally high in certain applications. However, we have also started to see an extensive usage of the fusion of MR, CT, X-ray, PET, SPECT and ultrasound for better visualization of pathology understanding and aiding in patient treatments.

1.7.1 Acknowledgements

The authors would like to thank Marconi Medical Systems, Inc., for the MR data sets. Jasjit Suri would also like to thank Dr. Larry Kasuboski and Dr. Elaine Keeler, both from Marconi Medical Systems, for encouraging him to attend internal MR Physics workshops. Thanks go to Dr. Kecheng Liu and Dr. Agus Priatna, from Marconi Medical Systems, for their valuable suggestions on the MR section of this chapter. The authors would also like to thank Professor Narayana, University of Texas Medical School, Houston, TX, for contributing some of the MR images.

Chapter 2

Segmentation in Echocardiographic Images

S. K. Setarehdan, John J. Soraghan

2.1 Introduction

Echocardiography, ultrasonography of the living heart, has become an important basic tool of diagnosis, treatment evaluation, and research in cardiology. It has achieved a prominent place among the other cardiac imaging modalities for many practical and safety reasons. Since it is basically a pulse-echo imaging system it has all the advantages of the ultrasonic imaging techniques which were described in Chapter 1. Another important reason for its success is that the information it provides is helpful in understanding the mechanisms and evaluating the status and causes of cardiovascular disease in patients. It also provides anatomical information in terms of the heart chambers and their sizes.

Echocardiographical data was initially studied in a qualitative fashion by visually considering some particular alterations of cardiac shape, size, and motion. These were used to identify specific abnormalities of cardiac structure and function. Recently, however, research has been directed towards the effective use of the extensive amount of diagnostic information of echo data, and particularly 2-D echocardiographic (2-DE) images by performing quantitative measurements on 2-DEs using image processing techniques. Quantitative analysis of echo data, in general, is a wide research area which covers such topics as the acoustic properties of the myocardium and myocardial tissue characterization. In this chapter, we are concerned only with the quantitative analysis of global and regional cardiac LV function and morphology.

A physiological and anatomical overview of the human heart, the most common echocardiographic views and the recommended standard models and methods [60] for quantitative analysis of cardiac performance using 2-DE images are given in Section 2.2. This review shows that the recommended methods are commonly based upon the segmentation of the LV cavity and its centroid from end-systolic and end-diastolic frames or from the frames recorded in a complete cardiac cycle. In fact, as a routine clinical test, echocardiography has been used in a vast number of studies for quantification of cardiac function and LV wall motion analysis. However, each of them has required expert clinicians to view a sequence of echocardiographic frames in real time, slow motion, and stop frame modes for segmentation of the LV cavity by manual tracing of the cardiac muscle borders. The tedious nature of manual tracing of the LV boundaries, as well as significant intra-observer and inter-observer variability in measurements, encouraged many researchers in computer vision and image processing to investigate automatic or semi-automatic techniques for boundary detection in standard 2-DE images.

In Section 2.3, we review the state of the art in LV boundary extraction algorithms that were applied to 2-DE images and in particular we identify three distinctive common strategies. Among these strategies the center-based (also known as radial search-based) strategy, which comprises the separate stages of LV centroid approximation and LV boundary edge detection, has gained more attention because of a number of advantages. The review shows that previous algorithms mostly had little success outside the research environment due to the many noisy effects which plague 2-DE data (the most important being the granular appearance known as "speckle noise") and which make conventional segmentation and edge detection techniques inappropriate for contour estimation in 2-DE images.

These algorithms mostly tend to treat all the areas in a 2-DE image equally and in a *crisp* way; however, not only are the actual contrast and noise level by no means constant, but also, as a grey tone image, a 2-DE possesses a different kind of ambiguity and is *fuzzy* in nature. When the regions or object boundaries in an image are ill-defined (fuzzy), the use of traditional image processing methods like segmentation and thresholding which involve hard decisions will produce less satisfactory results. In comparison, a human expert can estimate these boundary locations with minimal effort. Although the overall image is fuzzy, a dark hole in the center indicates the relative location of the ventricular chamber. Knowing the position of the center of the chamber, an experienced human operator is able to estimate the intensity changes at the epicardial and endocardial borders through an eye–brain fuzzy reasoning process and piece together the scattered evidence from these border points to come up with closed contours. He/she uses the extracted edges in some confident areas of the image to guide a search in those areas where intensity changes are less obvious and help identify a rough area where border points are likely to appear. As to the dropouts in the image, human operators seem to be capable of making use of the identified boundary pixels to interpolate the missing ones.

In Section 2.4 we present a novel fuzzy reasoning-based Left Ventricular Center Point (LVCP) estimation algorithm applicable to the standard Short Axis (SA) and Long Axis (LA) echocardiographic images. The algorithm uses the most descriptive features of the pixel coincident with the LVCP in the fuzzy domain. This section comprises a major part of the chapter since accurate LVCP estimation is an important initial step in most of the existing LV boundary segmentation algorithms which was usually done manually in the past. Moreover, an accurate LVCP reference point is important for the quantitative analysis of LV wall motion using 2-DE images.

To solve the edge detection problem, we initially explain the idea behind the development of the multiresolution edge detection techniques in Section 2.5. This is then followed by a description of the relationship between the Wavelet Transform and multiresolution edge detection. Next, we develop the concept of Global Maximum of Wavelet Transform (GMWT) based edge detection.

Finally, Section 2.6 combines the fuzzy-based LVCP extraction algorithm with the multiscale edge detection technique of GMWT to develop a fully automatic 'center-based' LV cavity segmentation in 2-DE images. Examples of the application of the complete algorithm to frames of a complete cardiac cycle are presented.

2.2   Heart Physiology and Anatomy

The heart functions as a pump and is responsible for the circulation of the blood through the blood vessels and the body's circulatory system. The heart actually comprises two pumps in one. The right side of the heart pumps blood through the *pulmonary circulation*, which carries blood to the lungs, where carbon dioxide is exchanged for oxygen. The left side of the heart pumps blood through the *systemic circulation*, which carries oxygenated blood to all remaining tissues of the body and returns the deoxygenated blood to the heart [61]. Each pump consists of a relatively thin walled primer pump, the atrium, and a thick walled power pump, the ventricle. Both atria contract at about the same time to fill the ventricles with blood, and both ventricular power pumps contract at about the same time to produce the major force that causes blood to flow through the high resistance circuits. The term *cardiac cycle* refers to this repetitive pumping process that begins with the onset of cardiac muscle contraction and ends with the beginning of the next contraction [61]. As the chamber which pumps blood at high pressure into the systemic circuit the Left Ventricle (LV) is the most critical component of the heart, and its performance is commonly studied to examine cardiac condition.

The general anatomy of the heart is shown in Figure 2.1. The information provided by the echocardiography of the heart chambers was traditionally studied by specialists in a qualitative fashion by visually considering some particular alterations of the chamber shape, size, and wall motion. These were used to identify specific abnormalities of cardiac structure and function. Recently, however, research has been directed towards the effective use of the extensive amount of diagnostic information of echo data by performing quantitative measurements on 2-DEs using image processing techniques in order to quantify cardiac function and pumping performance.

2.2.1   Cardiac Function

Quantitative measurement of cardiac function is a critical step in the evaluation and management of almost all patients with suspected or clinically evident heart failure. As it is the main power pump of the heart, cardiac function

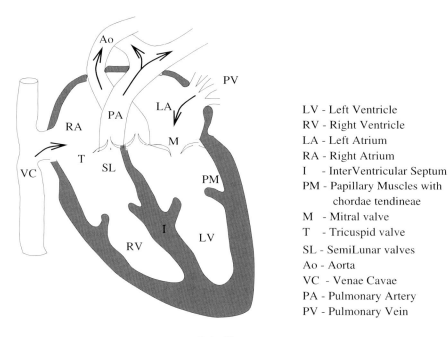

LV - Left Ventricle
RV - Right Ventricle
LA - Left Atrium
RA - Right Atrium
I   - InterVentricular Septum
PM - Papillary Muscles with
        chordae tendineae
M   - Mitral valve
T   - Tricuspid valve
SL - SemiLunar valves
Ao - Aorta
VC - Venae Cavae
PA - Pulmonary Artery
PV - Pulmonary Vein

Figure 2.1: Heart anatomy.

is closely related to the left ventricular function and shape attributes such
as the thickness of the wall, the enclosed area, end-diastolic volume (EDV),
end-systolic volume (ESV), ejection fraction, wall motion and pressure–volume
ratio. Virtually all indices of left ventricular pump performance have been
derived from the measurement of volume and pressure [62]. The indices derived
from volume measurements, such as the left ventricular EDV, ESV, stroke
volume (SV) and *Ejection Fraction* (EF), have proved to be of greatest clinical
value [62]. EDV is useful for evaluating and following the course of patients
with left ventricular volume overloading lesions or myocardial disease. In both
of these conditions, effective stroke volume delivered to the systemic circulation
may be initially reduced [62]. When both EDV and ESV are measured, the
left ventricular stroke volume can be estimated:

$$SV = EDV - ESV \qquad (2.1)$$

In the absence of valvular regurgitation, *Cardiac Output* (CO) can be estimated
as the product of stroke volume and Heart Rate (HR):

$$CO = HR \times SV \qquad (2.2)$$

When ESV and EDV are known, the ejection fraction can be calculated as the
ratio of stroke volume to EDV:

$$EF = \frac{SV}{EDV} \qquad (2.3)$$

Ejection fraction is a widely used index of left ventricular function and is generally considered to be the best single predictor of prognosis in both coronary and valvular heart disease [62]. *Regional LV wall motion* analysis is of particular importance in the assessment of coronary artery and ischemic heart disease. Normal subjects show a posterior systolic movement of the left side of the septum between 3–8 mm and an anterior systolic motion of 8–12 mm. A coronary artery disease, however, may cause reduced or absent regional LV wall motion. The assessment of the *local LV wall thickness* is also an important factor which should be considered when studying endocardial motion, since this is less affected by overall motion of the heart in space. Traditionally, the only clinically useful approach to calculating some of the above parameters and also to examining LV morphology and wall motion, involved angiographic procedures that required direct injection of contrast media into the heart during cardiac catheterization. At present, however, diagnostic information of this type can often be obtained with less or non invasive procedures such as echocardiography.

2.2.2   Standard LV Views in 2-DEs

Most of the heart is covered by bony structures or by lung tissue which are both virtually impenetrable to ultrasound. The left lung does not, however, cover the heart completely and thus opens an ultrasound window in the third, fourth and fifth intercostal spaces (Figure 2.2). This region, which is termed the left parasternal area, provides the best access for echocardiography. Additional important access can usually be obtained from the cardiac apex, by subcostal and suprasternal routes (Figure 2.2).

Even with this limited access to the heart it is possible to direct an ultrasound beam at most cardiac structures to make an almost infinite variety of cross-sectional images of the heart.

In practice, however, only a few common views and slices are used for diagnostic purposes. The standard views include parasternal Short Axis (SA) (Figure 2.3(a)), parasternal Long Axis (LA) (Figure 2.3(b)), apical 2-chamber LA (Figure 2.3(c)), and apical 4-chamber LA (Figure 2.3(d)). Furthermore, in the parasternal SA view there are three slices which are commonly used: at the level of the mitral valve, at the level of the papillary muscles (Figure 2.3(a)), and at the apex between the papillary muscles and apical tip. All these standard views are usually used for qualitative assessment of the structural, anatomical, and functional performances of the heart or to discover and study abnormalities due to heart disease [63]. However, each view has special features which make it appropriate for some special purpose studies. For example, the apical 4-chamber view, Figure 2.3(d), is particularly used to evaluate LV wall motion in those regions most liable to suffer from scarring due to coronary artery disease and myocardial infarction [64]. The epicardium is best seen with the SA view which is important in the evaluation of LV wall thickening. In the following sub-section we will also see that the SA mid-papillary muscle level and 2-chamber and 4-chamber LA views are commonly used for quantitative

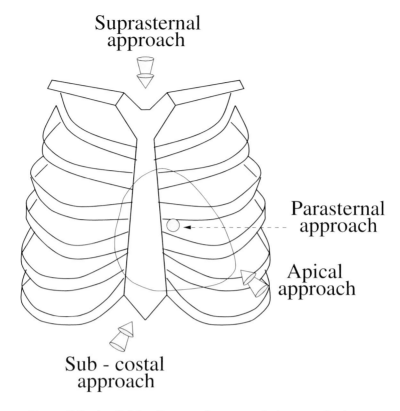

Figure 2.2: Available ultrasound access windows to the heart.

measurement of LV volumes, systolic and diastolic functions and LV mass.

2.2.3 LV Function Assessment Using 2-DEs

Different cardiac imaging modalities including MRI, CT scanners, Radio-nuclide Ventriculography, Positron Emitted Tomography (PET), and Echocardiography have been extensively used to measure the LV systolic and diastolic functions and also in regional wall motion analysis. It is reported, however, that LV volumes are best measured using 2-DE images [65]. In fact, one of the major applications of 2-DE images is in the assessment of LV systolic function [65]. In a comparative study, Stamm *et al.* found that real-time EF estimation by echocardiography was the most accurate of several algorithms tested [66] [67]. Considering the results of these and other similar studies in addition to the advantages of ultrasonic imaging in general (the absence of ionizing radiation, non-invasivity, portability, reproducibility, real-time processing, low cost), standard echocardiography is a very useful and attractive technique for quantitative analysis of cardiac function compared to other modalities.

Various methods and models with different degrees of accuracy have been proposed and used for the quantitative measurement of LV volumes from 2-DEs

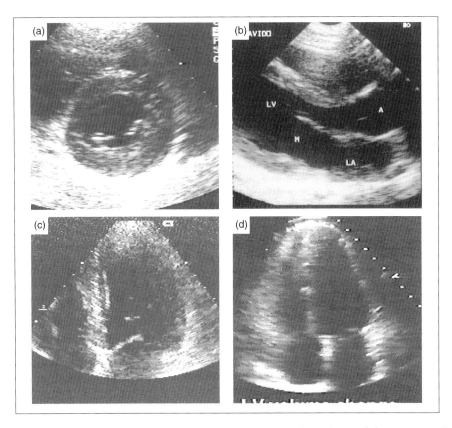

Figure 2.3: The standard echocardiographic views of the heart (a) parasternal mid-papillary muscle level short-axis view (b) parasternal level long-axis view (c) apical long-axis two-chamber view (d) apical long-axis four-chamber view.

including single plane area-length, biplane area-length, bullet formula, Simpson's rule, modified Simpson's rule, and disc summation. In an attempt to standardize measuring methods in 1989, the American Society of Echocardiography (ASE) [60] recommended a standard set of models and algorithms based on the dimensions and area measurements in the images. The methods can be divided into those using single plane and those using biplane views of echo images in calculations. The ASE recommends the use of the biplane method in which the dimensions and area measurements obtained are from paired apical Long Axis (LA) views (both two and four chamber) that may be considered nearly orthogonal. This technique is known as the 'modified Simpson's rule' or the 'method of discs' in which the calculation of volume involves the summation of the areas of the 20 elliptical discs from their diameters a_i and b_i as shown in Figure 2.4.

These discs are derived by dividing the LV longest length, L, into 20 equal

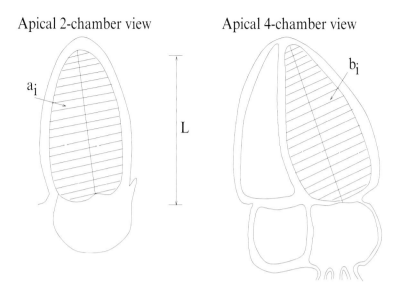

Figure 2.4: Biplane left ventricular volume measuring using the modified Simpson's rule or the method of discs. Reprinted with permission from [110] © 1998 IEE.

sections in both images. The volume is then calculated as:

$$V = \frac{\pi}{4} \sum_{i=1}^{20} a_i b_i \frac{L}{20} \qquad (2.4)$$

For routine use however, the single plane method is preferable. It can be performed either by the 'area-length' method using the LA apical 2-chamber view (Figure 2.5(a)) [60] [65]:

$$V = 0.85 \frac{A^2}{L} \qquad (2.5)$$

or by the 'modified ellipsoid model' using the SA mid-papillary muscle level view (Figure 2.5(b)) [62]:

$$V = \left(\frac{7.0}{2.4 + D} \right) D^3 \qquad (2.6)$$

where D is the average diameter of the LV endocardial boundary.

The LV diameter measurement at the diastole itself, irrespective of whether or not it accurately measures the LV volume, is one of the most valuable single measurements which is useful for judging the overall size of the LV. For the evaluation of LV systolic function, the volume ejection fraction can be computed from Equation (2.3) using ESV and EDV. Therefore, selecting the images at the end diastole and end systole for this measurement demands a uniformity of approach. Although there are more accurate methods for selecting these

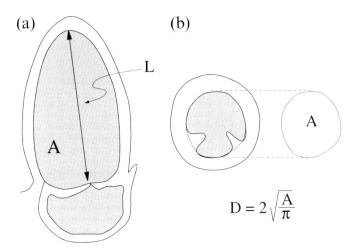

Figure 2.5: Single plane left ventricular volume measuring by (a) area-length method. Reprinted with permission from [110]. © 1998 IEE. (b) Modified ellipsoid model.

frames based on the ECG and phonocardiogram described in [60], the smallest and largest cavity areas are less satisfactory alternatives. The study of the LV regional wall motion and wall thickening from 2-DEs is usually done by dividing the LV cavity into a series of radial segments, ranging from 4 to 360, beginning at the cavity centroid and then analysing the endocardial and epicardial movements at each segment [68] [69] [7]. There is also a clinically acceptable algorithm for LV mass evaluation (known as the area-length method) based on the area measurement from the SA mid-papillary muscle level and the length measurement from LA 2-DE images [60] and using the following equation:

$$LVM = 1.05 \left(\left(\frac{5}{6} A_1 (L + t) \right) - \left(\frac{5}{6} A_2 L \right) \right) \qquad (2.7)$$

in which A_1 and A_2 are the areas enclosed by the epicardium and endocardium respectively, t is the LV wall thickness (assumed constant) and L is the length of the LV cavity (Figure 2.6).

2.3 Review of LV Boundary Extraction Techniques Applied to Echocardiographic Data

Fundamentally, there are two different groups of approaches for LV boundary extraction from echocardiographic images. In one group, boundary extraction takes place before the image formation process using the raw Radio Frequency

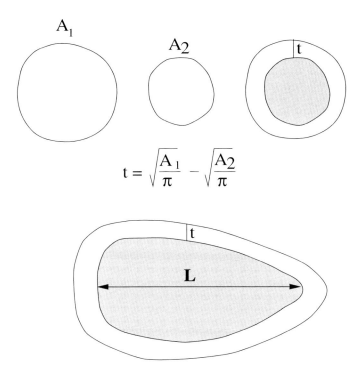

$$t = \sqrt{\frac{A_1}{\pi}} - \sqrt{\frac{A_2}{\pi}}$$

Figure 2.6: Left ventricular mass measurement by area-length method.

(RF) scan lines. This technique in which only the blood-tissue interface is identified is called Acoustic Quantification (AQ). In the second group of approaches, boundary extraction takes place on the two-dimensional echocardiographic image itself using various general signal and image processing techniques. These are usually referred to as Image Processing-Based approaches.

In this chapter, we are interested in the Image Processing-Based LV boundary extraction approaches and will concentrate only on the image processing of 2-DE images. For completeness, however, the principles of the AQ-based methods will be reviewed briefly first, which will also reflect the natural limitations and drawbacks of all AQ-based algorithms.

2.3.1 Acoustic Quantification Techniques

Acoustic Quantification [96] [105] [72] [94] is solely based on the processing of the raw RF signal of each scan line in order to discriminate between blood and surrounding tissue. In fact, this technique attempts to define the endocardial boundary by locating the transition from a tissue with low echo activity (blood) to a tissue with high echo activity (myocardium). Different parameters within the RF signal features can be used for this discrimination including Integrated Backscatter (IB), tissue transfer function and calculating the statistics of the scatters. However, IB measurement and thresholding, which is a measure of the average energy reflected from a particular part of tissue, is the classic and basic method used [72] [96]:

$$IB = \int_{f_l}^{f_h} \left| \frac{R(f)}{T(f)} \right|^2 df \qquad (2.8)$$

in which:
f = frequency
f_l = lowest frequency in the signal
f_h = highest frequency in the signal
$R(f)$ = spectrum of the (received) reflected RF signal
$T(f)$ = spectrum of the transmitted pulse.

As with any threshold method, AQ creates a new surface which has a value one at locations where the reflected energy is above the threshold (tissue) and zero at locations where the reflected energy is below the threshold (blood). Since it does not perform any higher level tasks of selecting desired edges, rejecting undesired edges, and filling gaps to form continuous borders, an observer must outline the region in which quantitation is to be performed. Thus, the method is actually semi-automated. Since AQ is unable to identify the epicardial boundary, the method is neither able to estimate regional wall motion nor perform wall thickening estimates [105]. Another problem with the AQ method is that it is not able to distinguish between the true endocardial boundary edges and those belonging to papillary muscles and valves. This reduces the accuracy of the final quantitative measurements based on the endocardial boundary derived by this technique.

2.3.2   Image-Based Techniques

Most of the research into echocardiographic LV contour extraction has focused on image processing-based techniques. This is due to the promising benefits in quantitative assessment of cardiac structure and function which can be obtained by image processing of 2-DEs which are not achievable by AQ or even by other cardiac imaging modalities [113].

Image processing of 2-DEs is naturally based on the various image processing techniques developed separately for different image processing purposes in many other disciplines. However, due to many difficult problems associated with 2-DE images including image data variability, the granular appearance of images (called speckle noise), dropouts and discontinuities of the LV borders, existence of such intra-cavity structures as chordae tendineae, papillary muscles and valves, as well as a variety of abnormalities, the results obtained using conventional image processing techniques have been repeatedly reported to be unsatisfactory and more sophisticated algorithms and knowledge-based techniques are needed. Various algorithms have been proposed which take advantage of the *a priori* knowledge of either the imaged geometry or the noise

characteristics. Moreover, most of the proposed approaches utilize user interaction as the most reliable source of additional knowledge.

In general, image-based LV contour extraction schemes can be classified,
based on the processing strategies used, into three main groups namely: Edge-
based strategy, Radial search-based strategy (also known as Center-based strategy), and Sequential frame-based strategy [89]. The aim of this section is to
introduce each one of these strategies and to monitor their advantages and
disadvantages.

2.3.2.1 Edge-Based Strategy

The edge-based strategy for LV boundary extraction in 2-DE images is basically
the general method for object boundary identification in the images and scenes.
It usually comprises the four main components illustrated in Figure 2.7.

In this strategy, the edge map of the input image is firstly generated (usually
from the pre-processed image) using a general two-dimensional edge operator.
The main problem at this stage is selecting a proper threshold value to determine the LV boundary edge points [115] [89] [78]. When the appropriate
threshold value is selected and the edge map of the image is produced, there
are the problems of edge classification and edge linking. Edge classification
deals with the very difficult problem of differentiating all the relevant edges
that correspond to the desired LV boundary from those which belong to the
other structures or noise. This step usually needs *a priori* knowledge to be
considered which could be based on geometrical and morphological information about the imaged structure (LV cavity) or even based on user interaction.
In some of the edge-based approaches, edge classification takes place on radial lines emanating from the LV center point. It should be noted that this
is different from edge detection on the radial lines which we refer to as radial
search-based strategy.

The final step is the closed LV boundary definition using the classified edge
groups which usually involves post-processing of the edges and an interpolation
technique to fill the gaps between the edge groups in the missing boundary
regions.

Depending upon the edge operator, the edge classification, and the edge
linking techniques used, various edge-based LV boundary extraction algorithms
have been proposed [77] [75] [115]. In [77], edge detection was performed according to Marr and Hildreth's theory [134] which is based on a Laplacian-
of-Gaussian (LoG) kernel. The edges were grouped into a set of curves by
a linking procedure which was based on edge connectedness. Classification of
the edge groups was then carried out by considering the anatomical and spatial
information of the LV chamber in an Artificial Neural Network (ANN) framework. The classified edge-segments from different views were then used for the
recovery of the LV surface using deformable models in [77].

Chu *et al.* [75] used a (41×41) $\nabla^2 G$ (LoG) operator to produce a low
resolution edge map. Using the edge map, an edge classification was then
carried out for each one of the endocardial and epicardial boundaries inside the

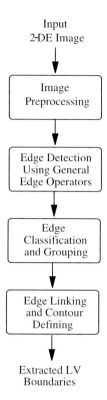

Figure 2.7: General block diagram of the edge-based LV boundary extraction strategy.

search limits by defining the zero crossings on radial lines emanating from the manually defined center point. Further processing to remove false edge points and missing regions was carried out on a distance angle plot. A one-dimensional (1-D) median filter (window size 5) was used to remove spurious edge points and the final closed boundaries were defined using a linear interpolation.

The edge-based strategy, in general, is very sensitive to image quality and variability [88] [115] [71]. The approaches based on this scheme usually suffer from very noisy effects and signal dropouts in 2-DE images. The edge maps produced usually contain many inconsistent noise-related edge segments with no continuous contour for the myocardial boundary. As indicated by Han *et al.* [89] and Chu *et al.* [75], this type of approach is not effective in complex echo images due to the high noise content and signal dropout. The problem of edge detection in 2-DE images will be discussed in more detail in Section 2.3.3.2.

2.3.2.2 Radial Search-Based Strategy

When a sequence of frames of 2-DE images is observed on a video monitor, it is very apparent that the basic motion of the LV borders is radially oriented. In other words, the motion is almost parallel to the radii and the orientation

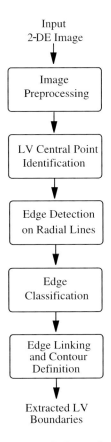

Figure 2.8: General block diagram of the radial search-based LV boundary extraction strategy.

of the borders is almost perpendicular to the radii in any direction and at any instant of the heartbeat. This observation has been the main motivator for many researchers to use the radial search-based or center-based strategy for LV boundary extraction from 2-DE images.

In this technique, the center of the region that corresponds to the LV cavity is used as the origin of a set of radial lines which are usually (but not necessarily) equally spaced in the angle. The LV cavity is then intensity sampled over these radial scan lines and the LV boundary edge points are searched for along each intensity profile. Depending upon the edge detection technique used, there is usually more than one extracted potential edge on each scan line which implies the need for an edge classification procedure for the final LV boundary definition. The final closed LV boundaries are then usually defined using the classified edges and an interpolation technique or using active contour models and energy minimization techniques. A general block diagram of the radial search-based strategy is shown in Figure 2.8.

Depending upon the techniques used for each block, various radial search-based LV boundary extraction algorithms have been developed [90] [86] [85] [81] [82] [98] [80].

In [90], the center of the LV cavity was initially defined using a trained Artificial Neural Network (ANN) and then refined using a model-based procedure. This center estimation approach will be explained in Section 2.4. LV boundary edge points were then searched for on 60 radial scan lines using another set of trained ANNs. Finally, edge classification and closed boundary identification were carried out using knowledge-based snakes and energy minimization by dynamic programming.

Dias *et al.* [81] [82] and Friedland *et al.* [85] used the radial search-based strategy in a probabilistic framework in which the LV boundary edge points on radial lines were assumed as one-dimensional non-causal first-order Markov Random Fields (MRF). In the algorithm developed by Friedland *et al.* [85], simulated annealing was used to optimize the location of edge points along 64 radial lines, each of which was treated as a 1-D MRF. Additionally it incorporated temporal information from previous frames. The LV cavity was manually selected by locating a pointer in it in a preprocessed reduced resolution image. Then the cavity boundary was approximated by calculating a 4 parameter elliptic model using the Star algorithm and a 1-D Hough Transform. A High Probability zone which will contain the edge points was defined by scaling the elliptic model by factors of 1.6 and 0.7. Each radial line within the High Probability zone produced one random variable in the 1-D cyclic MRF.

The simulated annealing process provided a global minimum of the energy function:

$$E = \alpha_1 E_1 + \alpha_2 E_2 + \alpha_3 E_3 + \alpha_4 E_4$$

where α_i = empirically defined constant and:

- E_1: Optimal Edge Detector element – provided optimal edge detection along each radii

- E_2: Radial Smoothness element – provided smoothness between neighboring radii

- E_3: Maximal Volume element – provided maximization of cavity volume

- E_4: Temporal Continuity element – provided temporal continuity with the previous frame

Once the energy function was defined the annealing schedule was determined and then the iterative optimization took place.

Detmer *et al.* [80] designed and used different 1-D matched filters along 60 radial lines from a manually selected center to detect LV endocardial boundary edge points. For each search line an intensity template was created by aligning the boundary points on that line and then averaging the spatially corresponding lines from the 8 images in the training set. To calculate the edge locations each of the radial lines was cross correlated with its template. The positive peaks in the matched filter output were possible endocardial points. The ranks of each peak's amplitude and radius within each radial output were calculated in order to use the probability density functions to calculate the most likely candidate for the edge point. Finally outliers were rejected by calculating the mean and standard deviation of the radii of the detected edge points and rejecting all those more than 1 standard deviation from the mean.

The radial search-based strategy has the advantage of reducing the boundary searching problem from two dimensions to one dimension which is an important factor in reducing the processing time. Moreover, edge detection on radial lines, which are usually perpendicular to the boundary, produces better edge estimates and makes it unnecessary to use directional operators. Previous utilization of the radial search-based strategy has shown, in general, its superiority to the edge-based methods, but most work has failed to solve the following common problems. First, the center of the LV cavity has to be identified before the process begins. In most of the previous articles this is done manually by a human operator using a pointing device [82] [80] [75] [85] [79] [95] [98]. Automatic LV center defining has been addressed by a number of researchers and this will be discussed separately in Section 2.4. Another common problem with the radial search-based strategy is the high noise sensitivity of edge detection on radial lines [89]. This is basically due to limiting the knowledge used for edge detection to only one-dimensional intensity information in a two-dimensional image.

2.3.2.3   Sequential Frame-Based Strategy

The sequential frame-based strategy is basically a semi-automatic approach designed for LV boundary extraction in a sequence of frames of 2-DE images. It is based on the fact that there is only small inter-frame displacement for the LV boundaries in a sequence of frames. In this strategy, the expert observer has to initialize the algorithm in the first frame or the frames coincident with end-systole and end-diastole by indicating the LV epicardial and endocardial boundaries, or at least the narrow regions of interest in which the real boundaries are expected to lie. Boundary detection in the defined regions is usually done using a general 2-D edge operator or on radial scan lines using a 1-D edge operator. The initialized LV boundaries (or the computer generated boundaries in the initialized regions of interest) are then mapped to the next frame in order to define the new regions of interest in that frame and the process is then repeated in a loop for the entire image sequence. Figure 2.9 shows the general block diagram of the sequential frame-based LV boundary extraction strategy.

A typical example of the sequential frame-based algorithm can be found in [76] where initialization was carried out by the user specifying a rough epicardial boundary on the end-diastolic frame. Canny's edge detector [74] was then employed to produce image gradients. Final epicardial boundaries were defined using a multiple active contour model with the internal and external energies[1] E_{int} and $E_{ext} = E_{grad} + E_{time}$ respectively, together with the energy

---

[1] Detailed discussions of these deformable models can be found in Chapters 3, 4 and 8.

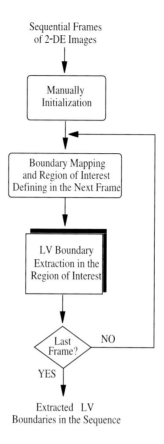

Figure 2.9: General block diagram of the sequential frame-based LV boundary extraction strategy.

minimization which was achieved by solving the Euler–Lagrange equation associated with the total energy. After the epicardial borders had been detected on the entire sequence, they were used to define the Region of Interest and to initialize the endocardial border detection process. Other examples of the sequential frame-based strategy can be found in [71] and [114].

The dependency on user interaction in the sequential frame-based strategy, is the main drawback of the technique. This is not only time consuming, but also introduces another source of variability whose effects on the final result can be difficult to evaluate.

The review of the three general image-based LV boundary extraction strategies in this section and the comparison of their advantages and disadvantages show that the radial search-based technique is the most appropriate strategy for LV boundary extraction from 2-DE images if the important problems of automatic LV center point identification and the noise sensitivity of edge detection on radial scan lines were solved appropriately. Also the idea of using the information in the neighboring frames (time domain) in the sequential frame-based strategy is an important knowledge source which can be considered and adopted in the framework of the radial search-based strategy. This idea will be developed in the following sections of this chapter.

2.3.3   2-DE Image Processing Techniques

Most of the previously published works on image processing-based LV boundary extraction schemes can be classified into one or more of the three previously introduced general strategies. Referring to the block diagrams of these strategies in Figures 2.7 to 2.9, there are some basic image processing procedures common to all of these approaches, the most important ones being pre-processing and edge detection. The aim of this section is to provide a brief review of the application of these general signal and image processing techniques to 2-DE images.

2.3.3.1   Pre-processing of 2-DEs

Image pre-processing is of special importance in 2-DE image analysis where there is a large amount of noise in the raw echo images due to the various artifact sources. The goal of image pre-processing is mainly to enhance the real edges by reducing the image noise in order to improve the accuracy of the subsequent image processing steps. The most common procedures for echocardiographic image enhancement are image smoothing and histogram modification. Another common process which usually takes place in the pre-processing step is data size reduction either by Region of Interest defining or by image decimation. This is also an important task for reducing the process time and getting closer to the long-term goal of real-time (or nearly real-time) automatic cardiac functional assessment using echo images.

Since the imaged object in 2-DEs is large (cardiac LV), the information in the 2-DE images is naturally confined to the lower frequency bands. Therefore, such procedures as decimation and image smoothing in the pre-processing stage do not greatly reduce the quality of the 2-DE data [85].

− Image Smoothing
The main purpose of image smoothing is to reduce the high level of various kinds of image noise in the 2-DE image. It also has the drawback of blurring the real edges and cardiac borders in the image. Image smoothing can be accomplished in the spatial or temporal domains.

Space domain image smoothing is the most common approach for noise reduction in 2-DE images [79] [75] [71] [114] [103] [100] [89]. In this technique, each pixel in a 2-DE image is replaced with the linear or nonlinear combination of the values of the pixels in its immediate surrounding $n \times n$ neighborhood which is referred to as the smoothing window. For instance, the neighborhood might consist of the pixel itself and its eight immediately adjacent neighbors ($n = 3$).

Linear space domain smoothing is performed by replacing each pixel in the image with the average of the window pixel values [75] [114] [103] [100] [89]. The degree of smoothing and also the blurring effect can be controlled either by changing the size of the window or by assigning weights to the pixels in the window according to their distance from the smoothed pixel. Window sizes that have been used in different studies range from (3×3) [100], (5×5) [100], or even up to (41×41) [75]. The larger the window size, the more noise reduction will be achieved with a subsequent increase in blurring effect.

Nonlinear spatial domain operators, in particular median filters, introduce more effective noise reduction with fewer blurring effects [80] [71]. Median filters are, however, computationally expensive. Since the blurring effect degrades the spatial resolution of the image, it may be helpful to make the nature of the smoothing operation dependent upon the resolution characteristics of the original image. For example, as explained in Chapter 1 the axial resolution in 2-DEs is much finer than the lateral resolution. Considering this point, a smoothing approach has been reported in [97] which was referred to as lateral filtering. The approach consists of smoothing over greater distances perpendicular to each B-scan line and shorter distances along the line itself. This is analogous to using a neighborhood of smaller size in the axial direction and larger size in the lateral direction.

In addition to the above methods, images may also be smoothed over time [91] [73] [104] using temporal averaging. With ECG gating, the frames obtained at the same point in the cardiac cycle can be averaged over time to produce a single composite cardiac cycle at each sample time with improved SNR characteristic. This procedure is based on the assumption that the only difference between the several gated sequential images is the amount of the noise in a particular pixel. This method of smoothing also suffers from blurring effect due to the patient and probe motions relative to each other in the period of imaging. In a study to define the optimal number of the averaged frames, Vitale *et al.* [104] noticed that the maximum noise reduction can be obtained by image averaging over 40 cardiac cycles and no more remarkable reduction was obtained by increasing the cycle numbers. They reported, however that using only 10 cycles produces about 90% of that maximum noise reduction value with less blurring effect [104]. A further disadvantage of this approach is that a composite echocardiographic image is formed from images from several cardiac cycles, thus reducing the ability of this approach to depict dynamic events.

– Histogram Modification

The second class of image enhancement technique which is frequently applied to 2-DE images is histogram modification [99] [80] [71] [92] [87] [83]. The image histogram (i.e., the frequency of occurrence of gray values in the image) of a typical 2-DE image will show a large number of low gray value (dim) pixels with a progressive decrease in the number of high gray value (bright) pixels (Figure 2.10(b)).

An image histogram can be manipulated in different ways including background subtraction, linear contrast stretching, and histogram equalization. It should be noticed that all processing techniques that enhance an image will re-

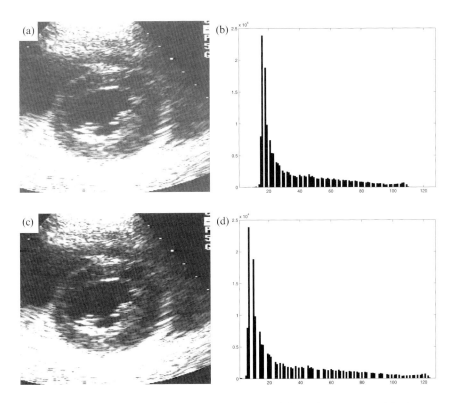

Figure 2.10: (a) An example 2-DE image and (b) its histogram, (c) the same image after background subtraction and linear contrast stretching, (d) the histogram after modification.

sult in a change in the image histogram. By histogram modification, however, we mean the technique that can be defined in terms of its effect upon the image histogram.

The aim of histogram modification is to make some image feature, such as endocardial or epicardial boundaries, more visually apparent. Background subtraction is the most simple method of histogram enhancement in 2-DEs in which a fixed value is subtracted from the gray value of each pixel in the image [99] [80] [71]. For those pixels with negative results the gray value is set to zero. Background subtraction affects the image histogram by shifting it to the left (toward zero) and appears as a change in the image contrast (ratio of maximum to minimum gray values). The background or the fixed value is usually specified as a fraction of the maximum gray value in the image, or as the mean gray value of a Region of Interest. If the Region of Interest is selected within the left ventricular cavity, background subtraction will improve the contrast between the myocardium and cavity and reduce the inter-patient variability, and also compensate for the differences in the setting of the ultrasound imaging system [80] [71].

Linear contrast stretching is another technique for histogram modification in 2-DEs in which the gray value of each pixel is multiplied by a constant [71] [92]. If the new value for a pixel is greater than the maximum acceptable value, it is replaced by the maximum value. This process results in a linear expansion of the gray scale and produces a histogram that has the same overall shape but is wider than the original histogram. Linear contrast stretching, combined with background subtraction, is particularly helpful in extending the image histogram over the entire range of possible gray values [80]. Figures 2.10(a) and 2.10(b) show an example 2-DE image and its histogram. The same 2-DE image is shown in Figure 2.10(c) after histogram modification which includes background subtraction and linear contrast stretching. The modified histogram is also shown in Figure 2.10(d). In this example, the minimum gray value in the image is selected as the background value.

Another histogram modification technique is histogram equalization which is a non-linear approach. This technique which attempts to make all gray levels occur with approximately equal frequency is rarely used for 2-DE image modification [87].

– Region of Interest Defining

The Region of Interest (RoI) is the part of the image in which the desired structure lies. RoI defining is a knowledge-based technique for data size reduction relying on the manually or automatically defined rough estimates of the position of the desired structure. In some semi-automatic approaches for 2-DE image analysis, [114] [75] [71], the Regions of Interest of the features (e.g. epicardial and endocardial borders) are defined manually in the first frame or in the end-diastolic and end-systolic frames of a cardiac cycle. These restricted areas are then "floated" from frame to frame providing only small portions of the echo image to be processed for the moving structural information. RoI defining not only provides the advantage of reduced computation costs, but also, it makes the subsequent detection procedure more reliable. Regions of Interest for epicardial and endocardial boundaries or for left ventricular center point and papillary muscles have also been defined automatically using some frequently occurring features in the areas with clearly visible cardiac structures, [85] [86] [89] [90] [92] [106]–[112].

An example of a Region of Interest which is automatically defined for the left ventricular endocardium in an LA four-chamber view is shown in Figure 2.11.

– Image Sub-Sampling

Image sub-sampling is another method of image size reduction. Contrary to the RoI defining method in which the image resolution is left unaffected, image sub-sampling reduces image size at the expense of losing part of the image resolution. One straightforward method for image sub-sampling is saving every other pixel of the image in both directions and blotting out the rest. This produces a new image with a size of one fourth of the original image. To prevent aliasing, it is necessary that the original image is low pass filtered

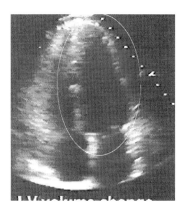

Figure 2.11: An example of the automatically defined Region of Interest for the left ventricular endocardium in an LA view 2-DE image.

before sub-sampling. This process can be repeated for further reduction in the data size, resulting in more decay in the image resolution. In [85] a 7×7 Hamming FIR low pass filter was applied to the image before sub-sampling for a $(4 : 1 \times 4 : 1)$ image reduction.

Another approach to sub-sampling is subdividing the original image into non-overlapping $n \times n$ blocks. A new reduced image can then be formed by mapping these blocks to pixels in the new image in different ways [90] [89]. In [89], the reduced image which was called a "feature picture" was formed by mapping the difference between the maximum and minimum intensity values within the 3×3 blocks of the original image into the corresponding pixels in the reduced image. In [90], the mean gray value of the pixels in each 2×2, 16×16, and 32×32 block were mapped to the corresponding pixels in the reduced images. These reduced size and resolution images were usually used for feature extraction and defining rough Regions of Interest in the original resolution image.

Figure 2.12(b) illustrates a reduced resolution image which is defined from the original image shown in Figure 2.12(a) by mapping the average gray value of non-overlapping 8×8 blocks to the corresponding pixels in the reduced image.

2.3.3.2 Edge Detection in 2-DE Images

Another important image processing task in all the general LV boundary extraction strategies is edge detection. Typical edge operators applied to echo images include the 3×3 Sobel operator [102], a 3×3 approximation of the Laplacian operator [84], 41×41 Laplacian of Gaussian operator [75], 5×5 Canny edge operator [76] and Marr-Hildreth's edge detection algorithm [77]. Basically, these edge operators are based on the first-order or the second-order derivative of the image. The extrema of the first derivative correspond to the zero crossing of the second derivative and the sharp variations in the image intensity. As the size of the operator increases, more globally significant edge

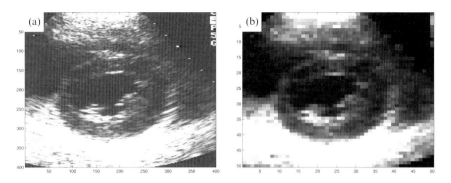

Figure 2.12: (a) An example 2-DE image in the original resolution. (b) The image after resolution reduction by a factor of $(8{:}1 \times 8{:}1)$.

segments are detected, at the price of mis-locating the edge places.

The many noisy effects which are naturally brought up in the two-dimensional echocardiographic images (the most important being the intrinsic granular structure known as speckle noise), signal dropouts and the existence of such intra-cavity structures as papillary muscles and heart valves with the same echo activity as the heart muscle, make conventional edge detection techniques inappropriate for LV boundary edge detection in echo images. This is shown in the study by Linker *et al.* [93]. They applied Roberts, Sobel, Prewitt and compass edge detectors to the short axis views echo images. In conclusion they reported that "... the standard sequence of edge detection used in image processing, consisting of smoothing, edge operator and thresholding, is less suited to ultrasound images than to standard density images."

In another study, Adam *et al.* [71], applied the Sobel edge operator, with an interactively defined optimal thresholding level to a 4-chamber apical 2-DE. In their results they reported that, no continuous contour could be drawn for the myocardial wall in the edge map of the image produced. Similar results illustrating the inadequacy of conventional edge and border detection techniques in echocardiographic data can also be found in [75]. These studies showed that more sophisticated techniques are required for LV boundary identification in 2-DE images.

Noise sensitivity of edge detection is even worse, when one-dimensional edge operators are applied to the radial scan lines emanating from the LV center in the radial search-based strategy. This is basically due to limiting the knowledge used for edge detection to only one-dimensional intensity information instead of using the two-dimensional image information. Different signal processing techniques have been employed to improve the noise sensitivity of edge detection on radial lines by taking advantage of the *a priori* knowledge of either the imaged geometry or the noise characteristics. For example the anatomical and geometrical information is used for snake initialization in [90] and [98] which is then followed by a dynamic programming-based energy minimization technique to select a particular edge point out of the multiple extracted candidate edges over the radii. In [85] simulated annealing and in [81] and [82] 'improved multi-grid dynamic programming' together with the noise characteristics were used for final edge detection.

The accuracy of these and similar algorithms depends on the initialization of the snakes, the experimentally selected snake parameters (energy weights) and the processing time allowed for energy minimization. This data dependency, makes the final extracted LV boundaries dependent on many variables.

In Section 2.5, we will develop a multiscale edge detection technique which introduces a final single edge point considering the spatial image information in the Wavelet Transform domain framework.

2.4 Automatic Fuzzy Reasoning-Based Left Ventricular Center Point Extraction

Key feature points of the left ventricle in various cardiac imaging modalities play important roles in automatic border identification and consequently in automatic quantitative assessment of cardiac function. Examples of these feature points are the end-systolic cardiac apex point in the X-ray ventriculograms which has been used for overall end-systolic LV boundary extraction [101], and the Left Ventricular Center Point (LVCP) in 2-DE images which has been frequently used for initialization of boundary detection algorithms [89] [86] [90] [106] [80] [75] [79] [95] [81] [82] [107]–[112] [129]. LVCP is also an important reference point for quantitative analysis of LV wall motion, [69] [68], and in automatic identification of papillary muscles in SA 2-DE views [92].

A robust, reliable and reproducible automatic LVCP approximation in both SA and LA echocardiographic views is then the first step towards the automatic quantification of the cardiac function and the LV wall motion analysis and would remove subjectivity from the center-based algorithms and would provide completely automatic methods.

One common approach for LVCP estimation is to assume the LVCP as the center of gravity of the ventricular chamber which appears as a dark hole surrounded by bright strips in the image [89] [86]. In [89] the center detection takes place in a reduced resolution image called Feature Picture (FP). Each pixel in the FP is given by the difference between the maximum and minimum pixel values in the 3×3 windows in the original image. The FP is then thresholded using a histogram-based threshold selection algorithm. The LV is detected in the FP by placing overlapping circles on the image. The diameter of these circles is chosen to be larger than the gap in the lateral walls of the LV due to dropout. If the circle entirely covers a dark region, and no more than 2 of 8 equiangular radial lines from the circle center intersect with the image boundary before passing through a bright region, then that circle is defined as an LV candidate point. The LV is defined as the largest labeled region and its center is given by the center of gravity of this region.

Similarly in [86], the authors identify the center of the largest dark hole in the image as LVCP. This is done using an iterative procedure which removes the small bright areas due to noise from the image first, and then LVCP is given by the midpoint of the longest ray which fits into this dark area. The accuracy of the center of gravity method depends on the accuracy of the ventricular chamber segmentation, which itself is one of the ultimate goals of echo image analysis. As discussed in Chapter 2 of [11], pulse-echo imaging is based on the line of sight, and only the specular reflectors which are perpendicular to the incident wave can be imaged properly. This image degradation, which can be clearly seen in parasternal SA views of the left ventricle in the lateral wall and intra-ventricular septum regions, makes LV cavity segmentation from echo images a difficult task and is the main source of error in those center detection approaches which rely on the center of gravity detection of the segmented LV cavity.

In another approach in [90] and [106], a circular approximation for LV is considered and used along with the strong intensity edge points from myocardial boundaries (mostly epicardium) at some regions inside the image. In [90] an initial estimate of the LVCP is obtained using a trained ANN which is then used in a radial search process to determine strong edge points in three regions of the posterior and anterior walls. These are used to set up the circular approximation of the epicardium from which the LVCP is subsequently refined.

In [106], large "circular-arc" matched filters are used to locate the epicardial and endocardial boundaries in the posterior and anterior wall regions during systole. Then the LVCP is calculated as the midpoint of the two epicardial boundary estimates. The estimated endocardial boundary is used to refine the initial LV center location. Although the use of the epicardial boundary for LVCP detection is more accurate than the center of gravity definition for a segmented dark area of the LV, its success depends on the accuracy of the epicardial boundary definition in the anterior wall region which is not always free of error.

In the rest of this section, we present a robust knowledge-based LVCP estimation algorithm which is applicable to both SA and LA echocardiographic images. This algorithm is a modified version of the method presented by Setarehdan and Soraghan in [129]. The most distinctive characteristic of the algorithm is the adaptation of the *fuzzy reasoning* techniques in the LVCP detection module. By applying the descriptive features acquired from a human expert observer through fuzzy reasoning, the pieces of evidence are combined to give a reliable approximation of the LVCP. In essence, the approach mimics a human's ability to locate and integrate small but crucial features. In comparison to the previous methods which rely only on the local edge information in a crisp way, the method described in this section uses both local edge information (the strong specular reflections from the posterior muscle-pericardium interface and also posterior and anterior muscle-blood interfaces) and global intensity and position information in a fuzzy-based framework.

2.4.1 LVCP Extraction System Overview

As a gray tone image, a 2-DE possesses different kinds of ambiguities and is "fuzzy" in nature. The fuzziness in a 2-DE arises from both grayness ambiguity and spatial (geometrical) ambiguity. Grayness ambiguity means "indefiniteness" in deciding a pixel as white or black. For example, in most cases there are regions in the image in which it is extremely difficult to answer the question: "Is a given pixel dark enough to belong to the LV cavity?". The grayness ambiguity results from many different phenomena such as low contrast resolution, speckle noise, shadowing, and anisotropy of the tissue. Spatial ambiguity, on the other hand, refers to indefiniteness in shape and geometry of a region in the image. The spatial (geometrical) ambiguity mainly results from the natural and diseased object variability, low axial, lateral, and elevational resolutions, and mirror images.

When the regions or object boundaries in an image are ill-defined (fuzzy), like the problem under consideration, the use of traditional image processing methods such as segmentation and thresholding which involve hard decisions will produce less satisfactory results. Furthermore, more reliable results are expected by allowing the image features such as pixel gray values, pixel locations, boundary segments and neighborhood information to be fuzzy subsets of the image.

A block diagram of the fuzzy-based automatic LVCP extraction system is illustrated in Figure 2.13. The system comprises three distinctive stages of: image pre-processing, fuzzy-based candidate pixel defining, and final LVCP estimation using template matching and fuzzy decision-making.

The pre-processing stage involves Region of Interest defining, image decimation and image enhancement. In the second stage, some imprecise descriptive features of LVCP such as LVCP is a *dark* pixel inside the LV cavity, LVCP is usually located in the *central* part of the image plane and LVCP is usually *close* to the vertical and horizontal 'LV center lines', are firstly translated to fuzzy subsets of the image using appropriately defined fuzzy membership functions. Fuzzy methods are then applied to the fuzzy subsets to produce a combined fuzzy subset representing the most potential candidate pixels for LVCP. The third stage involves a template matching technique to determine the most likely LVCP among the candidate pixels. This procedure takes into account the neighborhood information of LVCP in the reasoning process. This is achieved by defining appropriate templates which are based on the most seen general patterns of the dark neighborhood of the LVCP inside the LV cavity. Template matching defines a new fuzzy subset of the image which is combined with the previous resulting fuzzy subset to estimate the final LVCP.

2.4.2 Stage 1: Pre-Processing

Image pre-processing is an important and necessary step in any automatic algorithm for echocardiographic image processing. This is mostly due to the very noisy nature of echocardiographic data. Pre-processing in the present system includes both data size reduction and image enhancement. Data size

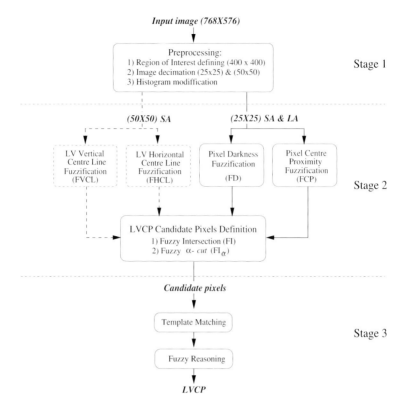

Figure 2.13: Block diagram of the automatic fuzzy reasoning-based LVCP extraction system.

reduction takes place in two distinct steps. First, the active echo cone (the ultrasound image itself) is separated from the rest of the picture (the patient identification and the information regarding the set-up of the system) as a fixed size (400×400) Region of Interest. This portion which covers approximately 40% of the input image is derived by considering all the typical frames of echo images in the data set. This can be redefined according to the different configurations of the different ultrasound devices.

The second data size reduction step which involves image decimation now takes place on the Region of Interest. Experiments were conducted to study the minimum acceptable scale reduction with acceptable LVCP estimation. As a result, a decimated image of size (25×25) is made from the Region of Interest by mapping non-overlapping (16×16) blocks to pixels in the reduced resolution image with values given by the average of the pixels in the blocks. This image decimation effectively reduces the processing time, and yet preserves those descriptive LVCP features (see Section 4.5) which are important in the framework of the fuzzy system. Therefore, the rest of the LVCP extraction procedure will take place on this reduced resolution image. In the case of SA view images, a second reduced resolution image of size (50×50) is also generated

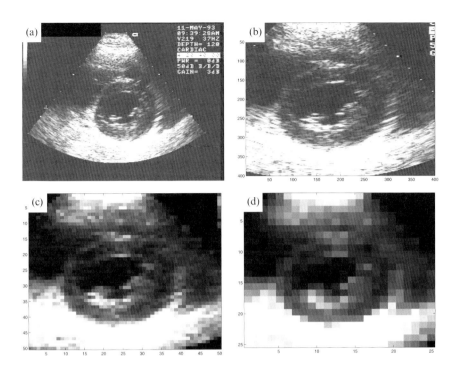

Figure 2.14: ROI extraction process: (a) Input image of size (768×576) pixels, (b) Region of Interest of size (400×400) pixels, (c) (50×50) and (d) (25×25) reduced resolution images after histogram modification.

in a similar way. This will be used only for approximating the location of the epicardial boundary in the regions with strong specular reflections, usually in the posterior and anterior wall regions. This is because the accuracy of the identification of these LVCP features in any further reduced image was visibly found to be unsatisfactory.

Image enhancement involves a histogram modification using background subtraction and linear contrast stretching, which is applied to all reduced images. By choosing the least gray value in the image as the background this process extends the histogram of the input image over the entire range of possible gray values to take full advantage of the gray scale range.

Figure 2.14(b) illustrates the Region of Interest extracted from the input image shown in Figure 2.14(a). The reduced resolution images of size (50×50) and (25×25) after enhancement are also shown in Figures 2.14(c) and 2.14(d) for this image, respectively.

2.4.3 Stage 2: LVCP Features Fuzzification

Expert systems derive their power from knowledge. The heart of any expert system is the knowledge it contains, and it is the effective use of this knowledge that makes its reasoning successful. In this section, we discuss the most prominent features of LVCP in the standard SA and LA views of 2-DE images which can be used as a reliable knowledge source for reasoning. The descriptive LVCP features which we will consider in the reasoning are obtained from an expert human observer. These are based on the intensity, positional and morphological information related to the left ventricle and its central point in 2-DE images.

In the typical 2-DE images considered in this study the left ventricular cavity always appears as a dark hole surrounded by bright pixels. This is due to the low echo activity of blood compared with the myocardial tissue. Therefore, LVCP is always expected as a dark pixel in the image. In regard to the positional appearance of LVCP, when the aim of echocardiography is the study of the LV structure and function, it is necessary for each echo image to cover the entire LV. For this reason the LV cavity is deliberately placed in the central part of the frame in the standard SA and LA views. As a result, the central region of the image frame is the most probable location for the LVCP. Another most prominent feature of the LV cavity in SA views is the very bright part of the image in the myocardium-pericardium interface in the posterior wall region. This bright region provides the sharpest contrast of the image along the curvature of the posterior wall. As will be shown shortly, this is a very helpful source of knowledge in the LVCP detection module. Similarly, but with less importance, there is a sharp contrast region in the image along the epicardial boundary in the anterior wall region. This is usually expected due to the strong specular reflections from myocardium in this region which is perpendicular to the ultrasound wave and very close to the ultrasound imaging probe.

In addition to the above descriptive pixel-wise information, a human observer also uses neighborhood information for LVCP locating. We will also consider this knowledge by defining appropriate templates for the dark neighborhood of the LVCP in Section 2.4.4. Similar to most human reasoning processes which are qualitative in nature and involve imprecise and fuzzy logic, we use the rich assortment of fuzzy logic operators and functions for reasoning based on the fuzzy data. In the following, we describe the procedure of generating appropriate data driven fuzzy membership functions which allow us to convert LVCP and image properties from real numbers to fuzzy subsets of the image.

2.4.3.1 Fuzzy Center Proximity

In order to define an appropriate fuzzy membership function to fuzzify the positional information of the LVCP in 2-DE images, all the real SA and LA images in the data set were considered in a statistical study. This is in essence similar to the method of "generating fuzzy rules by learning from examples" explained in [120]. An expert observer was asked to identify the location of the LVCPs in all the images of the data set which we will call the "reference" LVCPs in the rest of this chapter. As expected, most of the expert-defined reference LVCPs were located in the central part of the image plane in the

(400×400) Region of Interest.

Next, the smallest possible circular region which is in the center of the image plane is defined such as to cover almost all the reference LVCPs. This circle defines the *potential* region for LVCP in the image plane. A second circle with the same origin is then also defined to encircle only 90% of the expert defined reference LVCPs in the data set. This is the *more likely* region for LVCP. In this fuzzification procedure we would like to consider the highest membership value (unity) to the pixels residing in the *more likely* region and no membership value (zero) to the pixels outside the *potential* region. For the pixels residing in the *potential* but not in the *more likely* region a monotonically decreasing membership is considered as the pixel's distance from the center increases.

Based on the above study and discussion, the fuzzy membership function of the center proximity, f_{CP}, which produces the fuzzy subset fuzzy center proximity (FCP) of the and defines to what degree any pixel in the image plane is similar to the LVCP based on only its positional information, is then defined as follows:

$$\mu_{CP}(i,j) = f_{CP}(r_{ij}) = \begin{cases} 1 & r_{ij} \leq r_a; \\ \frac{r_b - r_{ij}}{r_b - r_a} & r_a \leq r_{ij} < r_b; \\ 0 & r_b < r_{ij}; \end{cases} \qquad (2.9)$$

where $\mu_{CP}(i,j)$ is the membership value of the (i,j)th pixel in the fuzzy subset FCP, r_{ij} is the distance of the (i,j)th pixel from the central pixel (x_c, y_c) in the image plane $(r_{ij} = \sqrt{(i - x_c)^2 + (j - y_c)^2})$, and r_a and r_b are the radii for the *more likely* and *potential* circular areas.

When the *more likely* and *potential* regions are mapped to the reduced resolution image of size (25×25) pixels, the following values for the parameters are obtained: $r_a = 4$, $r_b = 11$, $x_c = 13$ and $y_c = 13$. By applying the f_{CP} function to the pixels in the image plane, the fixed fuzzy subset FCP for all the images in the data set is defined as:

$$FCP = \{(i,j), \mu_{CP}(i,j)\}, \qquad i, j = 1, 2, ..., 25 \qquad (2.10)$$

Figures 2.15(a) and 2.15(b) illustrate the fuzzy membership function f_{CP} and the resulting fixed fuzzy subset FCP respectively.

2.4.3.2 Fuzzy Darkness (FD)

In this sub-section we will define a fuzzy membership function to generate a fuzzy subset of the input image describing the degree of *darkness* of each pixel. The definition of such a fuzzy membership function which converts the pixel intensity values from real numbers to corresponding fuzzy grades depends on the purpose of the image analysis. In the present scheme, we would like the fuzzy membership function to describe how a given pixel is similar to the typical pixels coincident with LVCP considering only its intensity. With this aim, in a statistical study, the intensity gray value of the pixels coincident with the expert

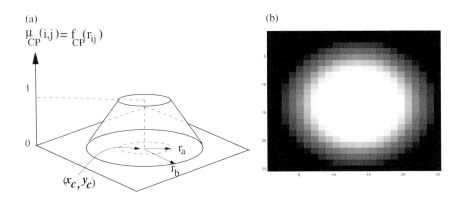

Figure 2.15: (a) Fuzzy membership function f_{CP}, defined for the *center proximity* property of LVCP. Reprinted with permission from [129]. © 1997 Elsevier Science. (b) the fixed fuzzy subset FCP defined for all images in the data set.

defined reference LVCPs were examined on the entire pre-processed database of 2-DE images. It is found that the gray value of the LVCP pixel (after pre-processing) is almost always less than 30 (on a scale of 0 to 127). Thereafter, in approximately 90% of the cases, the gray value of the LVCP pixel was not more than 10. It is important to notice that these values were obtained on the pre-processed data (including decimation and histogram modification).

Based on this study, we defined the fuzzy membership function of the *darkness* property of LVCP, f_D, as shown in Figure 2.16(a). By applying this function to the decimated image, any pixel with a gray value less than 10 will have the maximum grade of unity in the fuzzy subset FD of the image. Also, any pixel with a gray value of more than 30 will have the minimum grade of zero.

For the pixels with a gray value of between 10 and 30, the membership value varies linearly between zero and one inversely. The degree of *Darkness* or the membership value of the (i, j)th pixel, $\mu_D(i, j)$, can then be defined as:

$$\mu_D(i,j) = f_D(g_{ij}) = \begin{cases} 1 & g_{ij} \leq 10; \\ 1.5 - 0.05 g_{ij} & 10 \leq g_{ij} < 30; \\ 0 & 30 < g_{ij}; \end{cases} \tag{2.11}$$

where g_{ij} is the gray value of the (i, j)th pixel. The fuzzy subset FD can then be expressed as:

$$FD = \{(i,j), \mu_D(i,j)\}, \quad i, j = 1, 2, ..., 25 \tag{2.12}$$

Figure 2.16(b) demonstrates an example of a fuzzy subset FD which is obtained by applying the fuzzy membership function f_D to each pixel of the image in Figure 2.14(d).

As an important point in the definition of the fuzzy membership function f_{CP} above, it should be noticed that the definition of the *potential* region, which

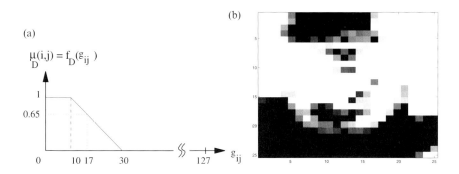

Figure 2.16: (a) Fuzzy membership function f_D, defined for the *darkness* property of LVCP. (b) an example fuzzy subset FD defined for the echo image in Figure 2.14(d). Part (b) is reprinted with permission from [129]. © 1997 Elsevier Science.

covers all the reference LVCPs in the data set, ensures that we have considered all the possible locations for the LVCP in our fuzzy-based system. Also, by considering only 90% of the reference LVCPs in the definition of the *more likely* region, a reduction of 65% is obtained in the radius of this region ($r_a = 4$ pixels) compared to the radius of the *potential* region ($r_b = 11$ pixels) in the (25×25) reduced image. In our study, however, no significant reduction in the radius of the *more likely* region was observed (in the (25×25) reduced image), by considering slightly smaller portions (instead of 90%) of the reference LVCPs to define the size of this region.

2.4.3.3 Fuzzy Vertical Center Line (FVCL)

The very high contrast region along the epicardial boundary in the posterior wall region is a prominently-occurring feature in the SA views. This phenomenon in the myocardium-pericardium interface, which is attributed to the speckle noise [106], is a good indicator of the location of the epicardial boundary along the posterior wall. In a study on the images of the data set, it was observed that the LVCP is always in the vicinity of the vertical line passing through the lowest point of the curve made by this high contrast region in the image. This is not far from expectation. Recall from basic geometry that, due to the approximately circular shape of the LV in SA views and since the above-mentioned vertical line is perpendicular to the tangent to the LV at the lowest point $A(x_c, y_1)$ (see Figure 2.17), it should pass through the center of the circle in the ideal case. This line which we call the Vertical Center Line (VCL) together with the border of the high contrast region and point $A(x_c, y_1)$ are shown schematically in Figure 2.17.

The key steps toward VCL identification in any given SA view which is carried out on the reduced resolution image of size (50×50) are as follows:

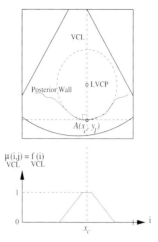

Figure 2.17: Schematic of SA view echo image which illustrates the relationship between the LVCP, the lowest point of the border of the posterior high contrast region $A(x_c, y_1)$ and the Vertical Center Line (VCL).

1. In the lower half of the image ("half-image" for short) in which the posterior wall region is usually expected, the maximum pixel value is firstly identified. A threshold t_1 is then set to the $1/3$ of this maximum value.

2. Any column in the "half-image" which has at least one pixel with gray value higher than t_1, is considered as a column with a possible coincident with the high contrast region. For such a column, the location of the intensity edge is calculated using the robust multiscale edge detection technique of Section 2.5. For the columns with no pixel with a gray value higher than t_1 (usually in the lateral parts of the image), a "neutral" edge point is considered in the first row of the "half-image". An example of the extracted and "neutral" edge points is shown in Figure 2.18(a).

3. The extracted and 'neutral' edge points are then median-filtered (window size $W = 5$) and interpolated to form the boundary of the high contrast region which includes parts of the epicardial boundary in the posterior wall region (Figure 2.18(b)).

4. The lowest point of the extracted contour is then identified. If there is more than one equal lower point, the median one is selected. The vertical line passing through this point is the VCL which is shown in Figure 2.18(c).

Due to the various imprecise assumptions in above process including the circularity of the LV and the uncertainty confined to edge detection in the noisy environment, we define and use a fuzzy version of the VCL in the LVCP extraction module. In this fuzzification we consider the fact in the ideal case that any pixel closer to the VCL is more likely to be the LVCP. Also, the

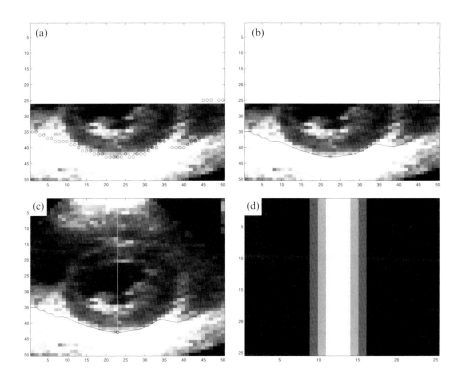

Figure 2.18: An example Fuzzy Vertical Center Line (FVCL) definition process. (a) Posterior high contrast region edge detection, (b) extracted boundary after median filtering, (c) the lowest point of the extracted boundary together with the vertical center line, (d) the fuzzy subset FVCL of the image. Part (d) is reprinted with permission from [129]. © 1997 Elsevier Science.

maximum width of the fuzzy line need not to be wider than 50% of the width of the typical LV cavities. Considering many examples of the reduced resolution image (25×25) from the data set (see Figure 2.14(d)), it was found that, on average, 7 pixels is a reasonable number for the width of the fuzzy VCL. Based on these assumptions, the fuzzy membership function f_{VCL} which defines the degree of *closeness* of any pixel in the image plane to the VCL can be defined as:

$$\mu_{VCL}(i,j) = f_{VCL}(i) = \begin{cases} 1 - \frac{|i-x_c|}{4} & |i - x_c| \leq 3; \\ 0 & 3 < |i - x_c|; \end{cases} \quad j = 1, 2, ..., 25 \quad (2.13)$$

where $\mu_{VCL}(i,j)$ is the degree of *closeness* of pixel (i,j) to the VCL and x_c is the position of the VCL as shown schematically in Figure 2.17. The fuzzy subset $FVCL$ can then be expressed as follows:

$$FVCL = \{(i,j), \mu_{VCL}(i,j)\}, \quad i, j = 1, 2, ..., 25 \quad (2.14)$$

which is shown in Figure 2.18(d) for the example image considered here.

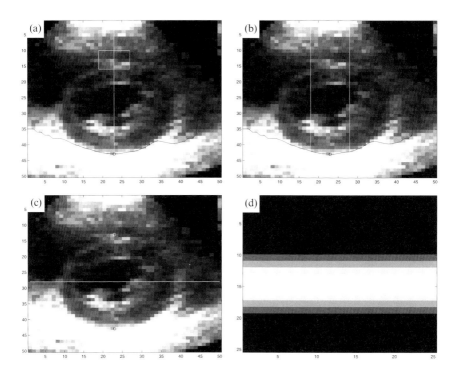

Figure 2.19: An example of the Fuzzy Horizontal Center Line definition process. (a) Position of the anterior high contrast region relative to the VCL, (b) columns coincident with the anterior high contrast region, (c) the extracted edge in the anterior high contrast region together with the Horizontal Center Line, (d) the fuzzy subset fuzzy horizontal center line of the image.

2.4.3.4   Fuzzy Horizontal Center Line

Due to the strong specular reflections from the epicardium in the anterior wall region, which is virtually perpendicular to the ultrasound wave and very close to the ultrasound probe, a comparatively sharp contrast region in this part of image is usually expected in SA views. This is another most prominent feature in the image and a reliable knowledge source which can be efficiently used in the LVCP extraction module. This anterior high contrast region is naturally in the opposite side of the posterior high contrast region, hence very close to the previously defined vertical center line (VCL). This fact, which can be clearly seen in the example image in Figure 2.19(a), is also confirmed by considering many example frames in the data set.

   To define the location of the anterior high contrast region, which belongs to epicardial boundary, the column representing the VCL in the (50×50) reduced resolution image and some of its neighboring columns (the region between the two vertical lines shown in Figure 2.19(b)) is firstly intensity-averaged to reduce the speckle noise and to provide a strong edge signal. The combined signal is

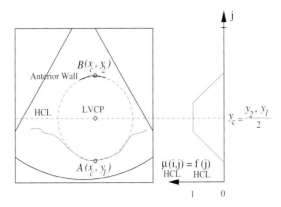

Figure 2.20: Schematic of SA view echo image which illustrates the relationship between the LVCP, points $A(x_c, y_1)$ and $B(x_c, y_2)$ and the Horizontal Center Line.

then processed by means of the robust multiscale edge detection technique of Section 2.5 to extract the epicardial boundary edge point in the anterior wall region which is the sharpest intensity edge in the combined signal. The resulting anterior wall edge for the example image of Figure 2.19(a) is shown in Figure 2.19(c). The two extracted epicardial boundary edge points in the anterior and posterior wall regions define a horizontal line which passes through the vicinity of LVCP as shown in Figure 2.19(c). This line which we call the Horizontal Center Line (HCL) together with the two epicardial boundary edge points in the anterior and posterior wall regions, $B(x_c, y_2)$ and $A(x_c, y_1)$, are shown schematically in Figure 2.20.

For the same reasons as VCL, we define and use a fuzzy version of HCL in the LVCP extraction module. Again we consider the fact in the ideal case that any pixel closer to HCL is more likely to be the LVCP. Based on similar assumptions to those explained in the case of VCL, the fuzzy membership function f_{HCL} which defines the degree of *closeness* of any pixel in the image plane to HCL can be defined as:

$$\mu_{HCL}(i,j) = f_{HCL}(j) = \begin{cases} 1 & |j - y_c| \leq 1; \\ 1.25 - \frac{|j-y_c|}{4} & 1 < |j - y_c| \leq 4; \\ 0 & 4 < |j - y_c|; \end{cases} \qquad (2.15)$$

$$i = 1, 2, ..., 25 \qquad (2.16)$$

where $\mu_{HCL}(i,j)$ is the degree of *closeness* of pixel (i,j) to the HCL and $y_c = (y_2 + y_1)/2$ is the position of the HCL as shown schematically in Figure 2.20. The fuzzy subset $FHCL$ can then be expressed as follows:

$$FHCL = \{(i,j), \mu_{HCL}(i,j)\}, \qquad i, j = 1, 2, ..., 25 \qquad (2.17)$$

which is shown in Figure 2.19(d) for the example image considered here. There is an obvious difference between the definitions of the two fuzzy membership functions f_{HCL} and f_{VCL} comparing Equation (2.15) to Equation (2.13). The difference is a wider covering area for $FHCL$ compared with $FVCL$. The reason for a wider $FHCL$, is the lower degree of accuracy in locating point $B(x_c, y_2)$ due to the poor intensity contrast in the anterior wall region compared with the intensity contrast in the posterior wall region.

2.4.3.5   Combined Fuzzy Subset Definition

The four image fuzzy subsets defined in the last sub-sections are all based on the LVCP properties which were extracted using the knowledge of a human observer based on the image features in typical 2-DE images. Each subset represents the degree of similarity of a pixel to LVCP considering a different property. In this sub-section, the aim is to unify the information contained in these fuzzy sets using fuzzy logic set operators.

The fact is that any pixel which has all the properties together, or equivalently has a higher membership value in all fuzzy sets, is more likely to be the real LVCP. This implies that the intersection of the fuzzy sets, $FI = FCP \cap FD \cap FVCL \cap FHCL$, should be calculated. In the case of LA views, $FI = FCP \cap FD$ since $FVCL$ and $FHCL$ are defined for SA views only.

The set intersection operator in fuzzy logic is defined by the fuzzy min operator which selects the minimum of the membership values for each element from all the input fuzzy sets. Therefore, the membership values of any pixel in the resulting intersection fuzzy set, FI, is calculated as follows:

$$\mu_{FI}(i,j) = min\Big(\mu_{FCP}(i,j), \mu_{FD}(i,j), \mu_{FVCL}(i,j), \mu_{FHCL}(i,j)\Big);$$
$$i,j = 1,...,25 \quad (2.18)$$

The intersection fuzzy set FI, therefore, can be expressed as:

$$FI = \{(i,j), \mu_{FI}(i,j)\}, \quad i,j = 1,2,...,25 \quad (2.19)$$

Figure 2.21 shows an example fuzzy set FI which is the fuzzy intersection of the four fuzzy subsets $FCP, FD, FVCL$ and $FHCL$ shown in Figures 2.15(b), 2.16(b), 2.18(d) and 2.19(d) respectively.

2.4.3.6   Fuzzy α-cut for Candidate LVCPs Definition

As Figure 2.21 shows, most of the pixels in the combined fuzzy set FI have zero or very small membership values (dark pixels). Moreover, there are few pixels with comparatively *high* membership values (bright pixels). The pixels with higher membership values in FI, which are the most likely candidate LVCPs, are separated and considered for further processing. This is done by a "soft thresholding" method known as fuzzy α-cut. A fuzzy α-cut of a fuzzy set can be understood as a new fuzzy set whose elements have membership values greater than "approximately α". The new membership values are generated from the old membership values using a continuous non-decreasing mapping

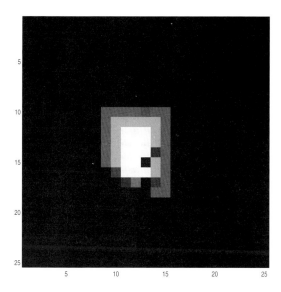

Figure 2.21: An example Fuzzy Intersection subset. It is the fuzzy intersection of the four fuzzy subsets FCP, FD, $FVCL$ and $FHCL$ shown in Figures 2.15(b), 2.16(b), 2.18(d) and 2.19(d) respectively.

function, $f_{\tilde{\alpha}}$, defined from $[0\ 1]$ to $[0\ 1]$. Therefore, the membership values of the fuzzy α-cut of the fuzzy set FI can be expressed as:

$$\mu_{FI_{\tilde{\alpha}}}(i,j) = f_{\tilde{\alpha}}\Big(\mu_{FI}(i,j)\Big); \quad i,j = 1,2,...,25 \tag{2.20}$$

where $FI_{\tilde{\alpha}}$ is the "soft thresholded" fuzzy set.

The study of many example FI fuzzy sets and their corresponding reference LVCPs from the data set showed that the membership value for the pixels coincident with the reference LVCP in FI is never less than 0.5. Moreover in most of the cases these pixels have a membership value greater than 0.9 in FI. According to this study, we defined and used the mapping function $f_{\tilde{\alpha}}$ shown in Figure 4.10(a) for soft thresholding of the fuzzy set FI. According to the definition of Fuzzy α-cut this is a simple realization of $f_{0.\tilde{7}}$ and implies that the membership value of the LVCP candidate pixels is always greater than "approximately 0.7". Application of $f_{0.\tilde{7}}$ to the fuzzy set FI guarantees that all the non-zero membership values in $FI_{\tilde{\alpha}}$ are greater than "approximately 0.7". Figure 2.22(b) demonstrates an example fuzzy set $FI_{0.\tilde{7}}$ which is calculated for the fuzzy set FI of Figure 2.21. The resulting LVCP candidate pixels for this example are shown in Figure 2.23. The soft thresholding technique explained above has the advantage over the simple thresholding method of preserving the relative importance of the pixels. This can be clearly seen in the different pixel gray values in the example fuzzy set $FI_{\tilde{\alpha}}$ in Figure 2.22(b).

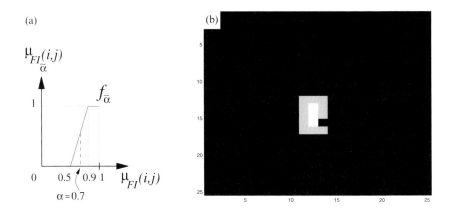

Figure 2.22: (a) A simple realization of the mapping function $f_{0.7}$, (b) An example fuzzy set $FI_{0.7}$ which is the fuzzy α-cut of the fuzzy set FI shown in Figure 2.21.

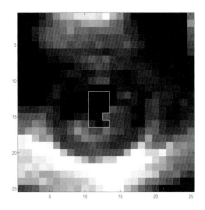

Figure 2.23: LVCP candidate pixels identified and superimposed on the example image.

2.4.4 Template Matching

So far, the knowledge used for describing the pixel coincident with the LVCP was solely based on pixel-wise information. A human operator, on the other hand, also considers regional and neighborhood information for more accurate and robust reasoning. This usually involves considering the dark area inside the LV cavity and virtually defining its center of gravity excluding intra-cavity structures like papillary muscle and valves. The final decision is made considering all the pixel-wise and neighborhood information together in a human fuzzy reasoning method.

In this section we will concentrate on the available LVCP neighborhood information used in the final LVCP extraction process. In particular, we will define and use appropriate templates for the dark LVCP neighborhood in standard 2-DE images. The rationale behind the use of the template matching technique is that there is usually a frequently occurring general pattern of dark LVCP neighborhood in the standard views of echo images. For example, in SA parasternal mid-papillary muscle level echo images the blood pool is roughly a dark circular region with two lateral lower parts missing due to the existence of papillary muscles. In LA echo images, the LV chamber always appears as a dark vertical ellipsoidal shape, both in the two-chamber and four-chamber views.

Template matching is generally used to locate known objects in an image or to search for specific patterns within an image [119]. A template is defined as an ideal representation of the object (or pattern) to be identified. The template matching process usually involves moving the template to every position in the image and evaluating the degree of similarity at each position. This is usually done by computing the *generalized convolution* of the image and the template which is defined as [106]:

$$A \otimes T_{(i,j)} = < A, T_{(i,j)} >; \quad for \ all \ (i,j) \in R_t \tag{2.21}$$

where A is the input image, $T_{(i,j)}$ is the template with its center positioned at pixel (i,j), R_t is the region of the template and $< . >$ represents the *inner product*. According to the image algebra [118] [106] the inner product of the two images A and B is defined as:

$$< A, B >= \sum_{(i,j)} A(i,j) B(i,j); \quad for \ all \ (i,j) \in \{Image \ domain\} \tag{2.22}$$

The main problem with the template matching technique, in general, is its computational complexity. This has less effect in the present system, because we will apply it to only the small number of LVCP candidate pixels in $FI_{\tilde{\alpha}}$.

2.4.4.1   Template Definition

The selection of an appropriate template is an important task at this point. Although the above-mentioned general patterns of dark neighborhood are expected, at least in the normal cases, there are also some states where these general shapes are not observed for different reasons. The most obvious of these are severe diseased states where a regional wall motion abnormality may distort the ventricle from its normal shape. Also there are obvious changes in the shape and size of the LV pattern from patient to patient or in different instants of the heartbeat. Before describing the study we carried out for template definition, it is important to notice that the amount of distortion in the normal left ventricle shape caused by diseased states, and also the changes in its size, reduces greatly when the image resolution reduces from (400×400) to (25×25) in the pre-processing stage. In other words, the distortions which can be seen in the original resolution (and are not so important from the viewpoint of LVCP detection), are not so visible in the reduced resolution image.

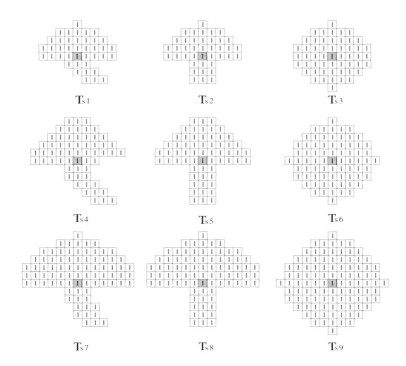

Figure 2.24: Different data driven templates defined for the dark neighborhood of LVCP in the SA echo images. The central pixel is identified for each template.

As a result, the overall shape of the LV cavity in the reduced resolution image approximates the most frequently seen normal patterns. This allows us to define and use a fixed size and shape template in the (25×25) reduced resolution image. The study of template selection includes a statistical assessment of the performance of different data driven nominated templates applied to the images in the data set which will be covered in Section 2.4.4.4. After reconsidering the dark area of the LV cavity in conjunction with the expert defined reference LVCPs in all reduced resolution images, 3 different shapes of templates were proposed in 3 different sizes, giving a total of 9 nominated templates, $T_{S1} - T_{S9}$, for SA echo images as shown in Figure 2.24.

In a similar way, 2 different shape templates were defined in 3 different sizes for LA echo images giving a total of 6 nominated templates, $T_{L1} - T_{L6}$, which are illustrated in Figure 2.25.

As Figures 2.24 and 2.25 show, each template is defined by a different combination of *unity* values in the template region with the center of the template identified by a dark pixel. Therefore, the convolution $A \otimes T_{(i,j)}$ produces the sum of the gray values of all the image pixels covered by the template, with the

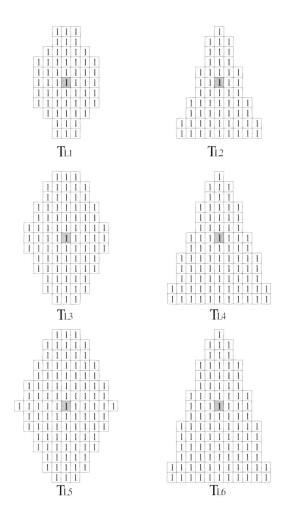

Figure 2.25: Different data driven templates defined for the dark neighborhood of LVCP in LA echo images. The central pixel is identified for each template.

center of the template located at pixel (i, j). This is computed for all candidate LVCPs in $FI_{0.7}^{-}$. Since, the aim is to match the template to the dark LVCP neighborhood, the smaller the convolution value for a candidate pixel, the more likely that it is the real LVCP. Equivalently, the average pixel gray values over the template can be used for this purpose.

2.4.4.2   LVCP Neighborhood Information Fuzzification

Let us assume for the present that T_o is the selected best performance template among the nominated candidate templates for each group of SA and LA 2-DE image views. The statistical performance analysis of the different nominated templates for the appropriate template selection is carried out and will be explained in the next section. The following procedure describes the application of the selected template T_o to the input image in order to identify the neighborhood information for each candidate pixel in the image domain:

Initialize a matrix $N(25, 25)$ to zero;

For i=1,2,...,25 (loop for each column)

> **For** j=1,2,...,25 (loop for each row)
>
>> **If** $(i, j) \in_{Supp} FI_{\tilde{a}}$
>>
>> $$N(i, j) = \frac{A \otimes T_{o(i,j)}}{\sum\limits_{(i,j) \in R_t} (i,j)};$$
>
> **End**
>
> **End**

End

where A is the (25×25) reduced resolution image, $_{Supp}FI_{\tilde{a}}$ is the location of the non-zero elements in $FI_{\tilde{a}}$, R_t is the template region, and $N(i, j)$ is a (25×25) matrix in which the value of each element $\{(i, j) \in {}_{Supp}FI_{\tilde{a}}\}$ is the average gray value of the image pixels covered by the template $T_{o(i,j)}$ and the value of the other elements is zero.

In order to be able to combine this information with the pixel-wise information contained in $FI_{\tilde{a}}$ in a fuzzy reasoning scheme, we first need to fuzzify N. Since, the smaller the $N(i, j)$ value for any $\{(i, j) \in {}_{Supp}FI_{\tilde{a}}\}$, the more likely the corresponding pixel (i, j) in the image A is the LVCP, the following mapping procedure is used for the neighborhood information fuzzification which provides greater membership values for darker pixels:

$$\mu_{FN}(i, j) = \begin{cases} \frac{N(i,j) - max(N)}{min(N) - max(N)} & if \quad (i, j) \in_{Supp} FI_{\tilde{a}}; \\ 0 & otherwise; \end{cases} \qquad (2.23)$$

where $max(N)$ and $min(N)$ are the maximum and the minimum element values of N respectively. The Fuzzy Neighborhood (FN) information can now be expressed as:

$$FN = \{(i, j), \mu_{FN}(i, j)\}, \quad i, j = 1, 2, ..., 25; \qquad (2.24)$$

2.4.4.3   Fuzzy $\max\limits_{x}\{\min\limits_{i}(\mu_i(x))\}$ for Final LVCP Extraction

This sub-section describes the final LVCP extraction procedure by considering the previously defined LVCP neighborhood and LVCP pixel-wise information in a *fuzzy decision* making scheme. The problem can be explained as follows: we are given a fuzzy goal $FI_{\tilde{a}}$ (pixel-wise information) and a fuzzy constraint FN (neighborhood information) as the basis to form the final decision. Since, the constraint and the goal has the same importance the *fuzzy decision* is a fuzzy set F_d on the image domain as [116]:

$$F_d = FN \cap FI_{\tilde{\alpha}} \tag{2.25}$$

that is:

$$\mu_{Fd}(i,j) = \min\left(\mu_{FN}(i,j), \mu_{FI_{\tilde{\alpha}}}(i,j)\right); \quad i,j = 1,2,...,25 \tag{2.26}$$

Since we are interested in a final crisp "optimal" solution to the problem, we define the "maximizing solution" to (2.26) [116] [121] [117] as described in Section 3.7. Therefore the final decision (i_c, j_c) can be expressed as:

$$\max_{(i,j)}\left(\mu_{Fd}(i,j)\right) = \left\{(i_c,j_c), \mu_{Fd}(i_c,j_c) \geq \mu_{Fd}(i,j) \ i,j = 1,2,...,25; \right\}; \tag{2.27}$$

The pixel identified by (i_c, j_c), which has the highest membership value μ_{Fd} over F_d, is the LVCP in the (25×25) reduced resolution image.

To compensate for the image decimation stage, the coordinates of the LVCP in the full size input image are then calculated as:

$$
\begin{aligned}
x_c &= (16 \times i_c) - 8, \\
y_c &= (16 \times j_c) - 8,
\end{aligned} \tag{2.28}
$$

2.4.4.4 Performance Analysis of the Templates

The performance analysis of the different nominated templates and appropriate template selection involves a statistical analysis of the accuracy of the automatic LVCP extraction algorithm when each template is employed by the system one at a time. For this analysis, we compared the computer generated LVCPs with the expert defined reference LVCPs in the whole data set for each nominated template. The standard used for comparison is similar to that used in [106] and [92], except that instead of assuming a fixed number for the diameter of the left ventricular myocardium in different cases and for different instants of the cardiac cycle, it is defined for each frame individually by the expert observer. This increases the accuracy of the measurements and produces a better comparison. In this standard the distance between the reference LVCPs and the estimates made by the automated method are calculated in the real size images. A maximum distance of 10% of the diameter of the left ventricular myocardium is considered "Acceptable" while a difference more than 10% is considered "Poor". A similar standard is defined for the accuracy measurement in LA echo images. In each LA frame, the minor and major radii of the ellipsoidal approximation of the left ventricular myocardium are manually defined. An ellipsoidal region for the acceptable results is then defined such that its minor and major diameters are within 10% of those manually defined with its center equal to the expert defined reference center of the LV. The above-mentioned procedure for templates performance analysis is summarized as follows:

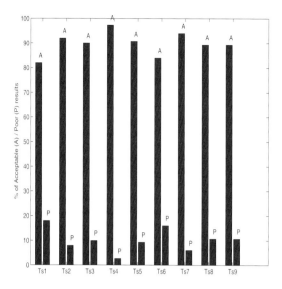

Figure 2.26: Percentage of "Acceptable" and "Poor" results obtained by different templates on SA images of the data set.

For $i=T_{first},...,T_{last}$ (Loop for each nominated template)

Initialize variables Ac_i (acceptable results) and P_i (poor results) to zero;

   For $F=F_{first},...,F_{last}$ (Loop for each echo frame in the data set)
      Compute (x_c, y_c) (Coordinates of the extracted LVCP)
      Compare (x_c, y_c) to (x_r, y_r) (Coordinates of the reference LVCP)
      If (Error$\leq$10%) $Ac_i = Ac_i + 1$
      Else $P_i = P_i + 1$
   End

End

The above procedure has been applied to 150 SA and 30 LA frames of real echo images of the data set obtained from different patients and at various instants of the cardiac cycle, employing the nominated templates T_S1-T_S9 and T_L1-T_L6, one at a time. The result of each run in terms of the percentage of "Acceptable" and "Poor" estimates (according to the criteria described above) are shown in Figure 2.26 for SA and in Figure 2.27 for LA echo images.

   The plots also compare the performance of the templates. Since the templates T_S4 and T_L4 have produced more acceptable results in comparison with the other templates, they are selected as the more appropriate templates in shape and size in the present system.

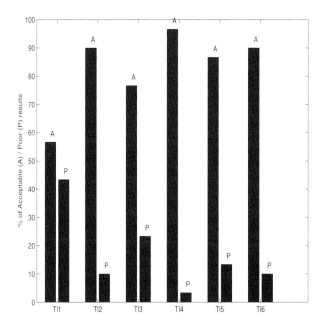

Figure 2.27: Percentage of "Acceptable" and "Poor" results obtained by different templates on LA images of the data set.

2.4.5 Experimental Results

Considering the overall automatic fuzzy-based LVCP extraction system equipped with the higher performance templates T_S4 and T_L4, the results of comparing the automatic system against the expert defined reference LVCPs are shown in the Table 2.1 with more detail. In the case of SA 2-DE images the estimated LVCPs in 146 (97.3%) frames were found acceptable while only 4 frames were in poor agreement with the reference centers. The mean and standard deviation of error for each one of the "Acceptable" and "Poor" groups are shown in the table. The maximum error in the failed cases was not more than 16.71% which means the extracted center was inside the LV cavity and close to the real center. For LA images the estimated centers in 29 (96.7%) frames were found acceptable and for just one frame the estimate was in poor agreement with the expert defined reference center. The maximum error in the failed case was not more than 10.06%. Figure 2.28 shows examples of "Acceptable" computer generated LVCPs in SA and LA echo images. The expert defined estimates are at the center of the circles or ellipses which indicate regions of "Acceptable" approximations. According to the criteria for success explained previously, the radii of the circles are 10% of the epicardial vertical diameter in SA echo images and also the long and short radii of the ellipses are 10% of the long and short diameters of the LV cavity in LA views. The area defined by the circles and the ellipses represents all possible "Acceptable" approximations with an error of less than 10%. Figure 2.29 illustrates examples of "Poor" computer

Image view	Total	Acceptable (error < 10%)	Mean of error	STD of error	Poor (error >10%)	Mean of error	STD of error
SA	150	146	4.98	2.34	4	12.20	1.78
LA	30	29	6.24	2.40	1	10.06	–

Table 2.1: Comparison of the results of the automatic system against the expert defined reference LVCPs. The "mean" and the "standard deviation" of the "Acceptable" and the "Poor" results are given.

generated LVCPs in SA views.

The accuracy of the above method is now compared with the accuracy of the LVCP estimation scheme described in [106]. This method only identifies LVCP in SA systolic echo images. The method in [106] was tested on 207 echo images and produced 28 estimates which were poor (more than 10% error), 55 which were found to be usable (less than 10% but more than 5% error), and 124 which were found to be good (less than 5% error) using a similar criterion described earlier. Thus 179 echoes were "Acceptable" yielding a success of 86.5%. This is to be compared with the new fuzzy-based method presented in this chapter which is applicable to both SA and LA echoes in any instant which has a success of 97.3%.

2.4.6   Conclusion

In this section we have developed the concept of a new fuzzy reasoning-based system for automatic left ventricular center point extraction in both SA and LA 2-DE images. This extraction system used the most descriptive LVCP features acquired from a human expert observer through fuzzy reasoning. The LVCP features used in the system include both local (pixel-wise) information, such as the gray value and positional coordinates of each pixel, and regional (neighborhood) information which was defined based on the most seen patterns of the dark left ventricular cavity in terms of predefined templates.

The statistical analysis of the real 2-DE images in the image database for each case of the pixel-wise LVCP features provided us with an appropriate data driven fuzzy membership function. These were used to convert the underlying feature for each pixel from a real number to a corresponding fuzzy value in terms of fuzzy subsets of the input image. The information in the fuzzy subsets were then unified by means of the fuzzy set operators to introduce a set of the most probable candidate pixels for guiding the subsequent template matching process including the neighborhood information for each candidate pixel. The final result was then defined by integrating the pixel-wise and neighborhood information for each candidate pixel into a fuzzy reasoning framework identifying the pixel which has the combination of the features in a higher value. The method is a simulation of the ability of a human operator to combine different sources of local and neighborhood information to make a final decision.

The system was tested on real SA and LA echo images from the image

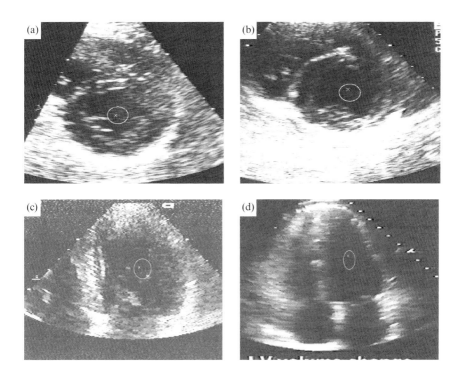

Figure 2.28: Examples of "Acceptable" LVCP estimations in typical SA view echo images (a) and (b), and in typical LA view echo images (c) and (d), with the regions of acceptable estimates superimposed. The computer-generated LVCP estimations are circled. Reprinted with permission from [129]. © 1997 Elsevier Science.

database. The excellent compatibility of the results of our system with the manually defined reference LVCPs (in terms of the very high number of LVCPs residing inside the 10% error region defined by the expert observer over each image) showed the robustness of the system and the effectiveness of the fuzzy reasoning methods in dealing with the very noisy and fuzzy echocardiographic images.

2.5 A New Edge Detection in the Wavelet Transform Domain

The review of the 2-DE based LV boundary extraction strategies in Section 2.3.2 showed that the radial search-based strategy has gained more attention for its advantages over the other image-based LV boundary extraction strategies. However, most of the previous attempts have failed to solve the major problem of the robust edge detection on radial scan lines.

In the review of the edge detection techniques applied to 2-DE images in

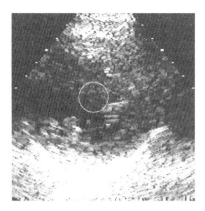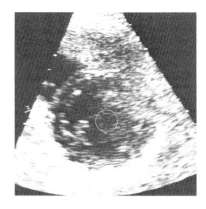

Figure 2.29: Examples of "Poor" LVCP estimations in SA view echo images with regions of acceptable estimates superimposed. The computer-generated LVCP estimations are circled. Reprinted with permission from [129]. © 1997 Elsevier Science.

Section 2.3.3.2 we also noted the inadequacy of the conventional gradient-based edge operators for echocardiographic images, in general, and the inadequacy of 1-D edge operators to radial scan lines in particular [93] [75] [71] [89].

The difficulty of edge detection in 2-DE images is, in general, due to the very noisy nature of the ultrasound data and the existence of various error sources in the 2-DE image formation procedure. In fact, the object regions in the image scene, i.e. cardiac muscle, blood, and the other tissues outside the heart, are made by the Rayleigh distributed granular structure known as speckle noise.

In order to reduce the noise effects, many researchers have applied various sizes of smoothing operators to the images prior or simultaneous to edge detection [75] [71] [85] [91] [80]. In general, the larger the size of the smoothing operator the clearer the edge appears but at the expense of a reduction in the localization precision. Canny [74] showed that there is a natural uncertainty principle between detection and localization performances of the edge operators, in general, in finding noisy step edges in that there is a direct trade-off between the two which can be optimized by fine tuning the size of the operator for any given edge. It should be noticed that, since the signal to noise ratio will be different for the edges at different locations of the image and for different instants of time (different frames), any fine-tuned fixed size optimum operator for a given edge will not be necessarily optimum for the edges in other locations of the image and other frames. This implies that no single size operator is sufficient for every place and time. In fact the use of single scale operators for edge detection in 2-DE images was the main reason for the failure of most of the previous efforts.

In this sub-section we address the concept of the multiresolution edge detection and its application to the edge profiles with poor SNR conditions. The section provides a novel Wavelet Transform based concept in multiscale edge

detection with superior accuracy and robustness compared to the conventional
edge detection techniques.

2.5.1 Multiscale Edge Detection and the Wavelet Transform

Most multiscale edge detectors smooth the input signal at different scales and
detect sharp variation points from their first-order or second-order derivative.
The extrema of the first derivative corresponds to the zero crossing of the second
derivative and to the inflection points of the smoothed signal. In this section
we explain the relation between multiscale edge detection and the Wavelet
Transform and show that by particular assumptions, maxima locating in the
wavelet scales of a signal is equivalent to multiscale edge detection.

The following description of the Wavelet Transform (WT) summarizes that
presented by Mallat and Zhong [126]. The Wavelet Transform can be regarded
as a signal expansion using a set of basis functions, which are obtained from
a single prototype function $\psi(x)$, called the *Mother Wavelet*. By definition, a
function $\psi(x)$ can be considered to be a wavelet if

$$\int_{-\infty}^{+\infty} \psi(x)\,dx = \Psi(0) = 0 \tag{2.29}$$

where $\Psi(\omega)$ is the Fourier transform of the function $\psi(x)$. The family of
wavelets, corresponding to the mother wavelet $\psi(x)$, are functions $\psi_{s,t}(x)$:

$$\psi_{s,t}(x) = \frac{1}{\sqrt{|s|}} \psi\left(\frac{x-t}{s}\right) \tag{2.30}$$

where $s, t \in \mathcal{R}$ $(s \neq 0)$ are the scaling and translation parameters respectively
and the normalization ensures that $\|\psi_{s,t}(x)\| = \|\psi(x)\|$.

The WT of a 1-D real function $f(x) \in L^2(\mathbb{R})$ with respect to the mother
wavelet $\psi(x)$ is defined as:

$$W_\psi f(s,t) = \frac{1}{\sqrt{|s|}} \int_{-\infty}^{+\infty} f(x)\psi\left(\frac{x-t}{s}\right) dx \tag{2.31}$$

which gives a scale-space decomposition of the signal $f(x)$ with s indexing
the scale and t indexing the position in the original signal space. Note that
one must always refer to the wavelet transform of a function with respect to
a *mother wavelet*. Equation (2.31) can also be interpreted by the following
convolution product:

$$W_\psi f(s,t) = f(t) * \psi_s(-t) \tag{2.32}$$

Let us assume that the wavelet $\psi(x)$ is chosen so that $\psi(x) = d\phi(x)/dx$, in
which $\phi(x)$ is a smoothing function. In other words, $\phi(x)$ satisfies the following

condition:

$$\int_{-\infty}^{+\infty} \phi(x)\,dx = 1 \tag{2.33}$$

Also let, $\phi_s(x) = \frac{1}{\sqrt{|s|}}\phi\left(\frac{x}{s}\right)$. Then, Equation (2.32) can be rewritten as:

$$
\begin{aligned}
W_\psi f(s,t) &= f(t) * \left(-s\frac{d\phi_s(-t)}{dt}\right) \\
&= -s\left(f(t) * \frac{d\phi_s(-t)}{dt}\right) \\
&= s\frac{d}{dt}(f(t) * \phi_s(t))
\end{aligned} \tag{2.34}
$$

Equation (2.34) implies that the WT $W_\psi f(s,t)$ is proportional to the first derivative of the input signal $f(x)$ smoothed by $\phi_s(x)$. Therefore, for a fixed scale s, the local extrema of $W_\psi f(s,t)$ along the x variable, corresponds to the inflection points of the smoothed signal $f(x) * \phi_s(x)$. This is the idea exploited in all multiscale edge detectors which smooth the signal at different levels to detect sharp variation points from their first derivative. More details about the similarity between the WT and multiscale edge detection can be found in [126] and [125]. In the particular case where $\phi(x)$ is a Gaussian function, the extrema detection corresponds to a Canny [74] edge detection.

In the multiscale representation of a signal, the details of fine signal variations can be obtained from small scales and the coarse signal information can be obtained from large scales. In order to recover the edge information from the multiscale representation of a signal, some researchers [122] [127] have proposed a coarse scale to fine scale strategy and some others have proposed the opposite direction [74] [134].

In his computational approach to edge detection, Canny [74] proved that the first derivative of a Gaussian function is a very close approximation to the optimum shape for a step edge operator. Having determined the optimal shape for the operator, to achieve the best detection/localization tradeoff in any particular application, Canny's multiscale algorithm marks all edge points produced by the operator at the minimum scale first. Then, it applies a "feature synthesis" approach to edges produced by the operator at the next scale to find edges that are not marked at the previous scales. This procedure is repeated until the largest scale is reached. Canny suggested that the scales of the operators should be determined dynamically by using the local estimation of the noise energy in the region surrounding the candidate edge, and operators of smaller widths should be used whenever they have sufficient signal-to-noise ratio. Canny did not provide sufficient information on determining the range of the scales of operators and the step lengths of different operator sizes. These kinds of methods are not applicable to 2-DE images since the object regions in the 2-DE images are made by (speckle) noise.

Instead, as we will show shortly, the global knowledge in the typical 2-DE image views can be used effectively for appropriate Regions of Interest defined

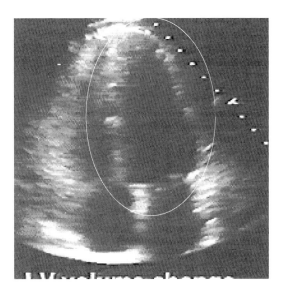

Figure 2.30: An example of the automatically defined Region of Interest for the left ventricular endocardium in a standard LA view 2-DE image.

for LV boundaries in which only one real boundary is expected. An example of such a Region of Interest which is automatically defined for the left ventricular endocardium in a standard LA view 2-DE image is shown in Figure 2.30. The definition of such a Region of Interest ensures that the only useful information in the bounded region is the edges corresponding to the desired boundary. This assumption which is similar to the "recovering only the useful information from scale-space" strategy of [123], allows us to concentrate on the problem of "a single step edge detection in a very noisy environment" in the rest of this section.

2.5.2   Edge Detection Based on the Global Maximum of Wavelet Transform (GMWT)

The technique referred to as the Global Maximum of Wavelet Transform (GMWT) -based edge detection [109] [110] uses the wavelet representation of an edge profile to locate the single step edge included in the signal in poor SNR conditions. It will be shown that this technique automatically defines the appropriate scale (operator size) which provides the best detection/localization trade-off. In this work, we use Mallat's WT algorithm [126] for multiscale representation of the input signal. The non-orthogonal wavelet $\psi(x)$ in Mallat's WT algorithm, which is shown in Figure 2.31(a), is the first derivative of the cubic spline function $\phi(x)$ shown in Figure 2.31(b). Since $\phi(x)$ satisfies Equation (2.33), maxima locating in Mallat's WT is equivalent to a multiscale edge detection. In this part, we first give the definitions of *modulus maxima*, *general maxima*, and *maxima line* in a WT which are taken from [125]:

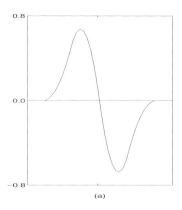
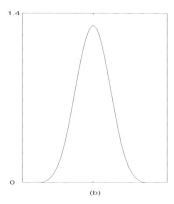

Figure 2.31: (a) Non-orthogonal mother wavelet $\psi(x)$; this wavelet is a quadratic spline and it is the first derivative of the cubic spline function $\phi(x)$ in (b). Reprinted with permission from [110]. © 1998 IEE.

Definition 1: Assuming $W_\psi f(s,t)$ to be the WT of a real function $f(x)$ with respect to a real wavelet $\psi(x)$,

- Any point (s_e, t_e) is called a local extremum if $W_\psi f(s_e, t)$ is locally maximum or minimum at (s_e, t_e) with respect to t.

- A *modulus maximum* is any point (s_e, t_e) such that $|W_\psi f(s_e, t)| < |W_\psi f(s_e, t_e)|$ when t belongs to either the right or left neighborhood of t_e, and $|W_\psi f(s_e, t)| \leq |W_\psi f(s_e, t_e)|$ when t belongs to the other side of the neighborhood of t_e.

- A *general maximum* of $W_\psi f(s,t)$ is any point (s_e, t_e) where $|W_\psi f(s,t)|$ has a strict local maximum within a two-dimensional neighborhood in the scale-space plane (s,t).

- A *maxima line* is any connected curve in the scale-space (s,t) along which all points are modulus maxima.

It has been proven [125] that all singularities of $f(x)$ can be located by following the maxima lines when the scale goes to zero. Moreover, the values of the WT modulus maxima often characterize the Lipschitz exponent of the signal irregularities [125]. Now, we define the *global maximum (minimum)* point of a WT and show how it characterizes the location of the only singularity (step intensity edge) over the signal (each radial intensity profile) which is the case in the present research.

Definition 2: The *global maximum (minimum)* of $W_\psi f(s,t)$ is a point (s_e, t_e) where $W_\psi f(s,t)$ has a strict maximum (minimum) in the whole scale-space plane (s,t).

A global maximum is also a modulus maximum of the WT, as defined by Definition 1, and thus belongs to a modulus maxima line. Let us denote the input signal as $f(x) = u(x - x_e)$ where $u(x)$ is the step function that is,

$$u(x) = \begin{cases} 0 & \text{for} \quad x < 0; \\ 1 & \text{for} \quad x \geq 0 \end{cases}$$

Substituting for $f(x)$ in (2.34) gives

$$W_\psi f(s,t) = s\left(\delta(t - t_e) * \phi_s(t)\right) \tag{2.35}$$

Equation (2.35) shows that for the function $f(x)$ defined above, each scale is made by locating the scaled version of the smoothing operator $\phi_s(t)$ at the edge place. This implies that the maxima curve is a straight vertical line. Since the global maximum also belongs to the modulus maxima line, its location identifies the position of the only singularity of $f(x)$.

Now we give an illustrative interpretation of the relationship between the location of the single positive step edge in the signal, the wavelet scale equivalent to the best selected operator size (therefore, providing a good detection/localization trade-off) and the *global maximum* of the WT. Equation (2.34) can be rewritten as follows:

$$W_\psi f(s,t) = \sqrt{|s|} \int_{-\infty}^{+\infty} \frac{df(x)}{dx} \phi\left(\frac{t-x}{s}\right) dx \tag{2.36}$$

An obvious interpretation of Equation (2.36) is that the magnitude of the WT $W_\psi f(s,t)$ at each point (s,t) is defined by integrating $\frac{df(x)}{dx}\phi\left(\frac{t-x}{s}\right)$ over the range of the support of $\phi\left(\frac{t-x}{s}\right)$.

If $f(x)$ has a local positive step edge (with some oscillations due to noise) at location $x = t_e$, like the signal shown in Figure 2.32(a), then $df(x)/dx$ has more positive parts around t_e than the other places of the signal domain as shown in Figure 2.32(b). According to Equation (2.36), at any given scale s, the WT $W_\psi f(s,t)$ has higher magnitudes whenever the support of $\phi\left(\frac{t-x}{s}\right)$ covers more positive than negative parts. In a particular scale s_e this value reaches its maximum value when the support of $\phi\left(\frac{t_e-x}{s_e}\right)$ covers as much as possible the positive parts of $df(x)/dx$, without paying the cost of covering a domain where $df(x)/dx$ is too negative. This is diagrammatically shown in Figure 2.32(b). Therefore, the *global maximum* of $W_\psi f(s,t)$ appears in the location of the step edge and in a particular scale which is equivalent to the appropriate operator size. The *global maximum* point and the corresponding t_e and s_e for the example signal of Figure 2.32(a) are shown in the 2D and 3D views of the WT in Figures 2.33(a) and 2.33(b) respectively. A similar discussion is valid for a single negative step edge and the *global minimum* point of $W_\psi f(s,t)$.

In practice, the WT scale and translation parameters s and t are discretized and for fast numerical implementations the scale normally varies only along

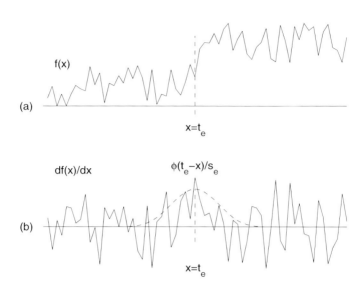

Figure 2.32: The point (s_e, t_e) is the global maximum of $W_\psi f(s,t)$, if $\phi\left(\frac{t_e - x}{s_e}\right)$ covers as much as possible the positive parts of $df(x)/dx$ without paying the cost of covering a domain where $df(x)/dx$ is too negative. (a) The noisy step edge signal. (b) The first derivative of the signal together with the best size of $\phi(x)$ covering mostly the positive parts. Reprinted with permission from [110]. © 1998 IEE.

dyadic sequences $(2^j)_{j\in Z}$. This yields the *discrete dyadic wavelet transform* [128]:

$$W_\psi f(j,k) = 2^{\frac{-j}{2}} \int_{-\infty}^{+\infty} f(x)\psi\left(2^{-j}(x-k)\right) dx \qquad (2.37)$$

where j is the scale index ($j = 1, 2, ...$), and k is the translation (spatial) index ($k = 1, 2, ...$). The main properties of a dyadic wavelet transform are explained in [124]. In numerical applications we are concerned with a finite length discrete input signal $f(k)$ ($k = 1, 2, ..., N$) which is measured at a finite resolution. Therefore it is impossible to compute the wavelet transform at an arbitrary fine scale. By limiting the scale index j to unity, the finest resolution (scale) is normalized to one. The discrete dyadic wavelet transform thus decomposes any signal of N samples over $J = \log_2(N) + 1$ scales.

Experimentally we noticed that, when the signal to noise ratio is too small, at the finest scale 2^1 the signal is dominated by the noise. For this reason, and similar to most multiscale edge detection methods [125], we exclude the finest scale from the calculations of the *global maximum*.

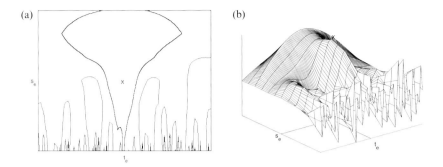

Figure 2.33: Two-dimensional (a) and three-dimensional (b) views of $W_\psi f(s,t)$ for the noisy signal shown in Figure 2.32(a). The global maximum point (s_e, t_e) is marked with a "X". Reprinted with permission from [110]. © 1998 IEE.

2.5.3 GMWT Performance Analysis and Comparison

This sub-section provides a performance analysis and an illustrative and quantitative comparison of the GMWT with the conventional gradient-based Sobel and Laplace edge operators. The Sobel and Laplace edge operators [119] detect an edge using a finite-difference gradient operator but with a degree of smoothing along the direction of the edge component. They are implemented convolving each sample of the signal with the masks given in Equations (2.38) and (2.39) for Sobel and Laplace respectively:

$$[-1 \quad 0 \quad 1] \tag{2.38}$$

$$[-1 \quad 2 \quad -1] \tag{2.39}$$

Figure 2.34 demonstrates the application of the three methods to an example synthetic noisy signal which includes a gradual step edge (five pixels in the slope). The signal before and after contaminating by a Gaussian zero-mean white noise is shown in Figures 2.34(a),(b),(c) and 2.34(d), (e),(f) respectively. The signal to noise ratio for this signal is approximately 2 dB which is defined as:

$$SNR_{dB} = 10 \log_{10} \left(\frac{E\left[(f - \bar{f})^2\right]}{\sigma_N^2} \right) \tag{2.40}$$

where $f(k)$ is the input edge profile with average of $\bar{f}$, $E(.)$ is the expectation function, and σ_N^2 is the variance of the noise.

The results of the convolution of the signal with the Laplace and Sobel operators are shown in Figures 2.34(g) and 2.34(h) respectively. Also the discrete dyadic WT of the signal in all scales are shown in Figures 2.34(i) to 2.34(p) from fine scale (2^1) to coarse scale (2^8) respectively. The threshold values for

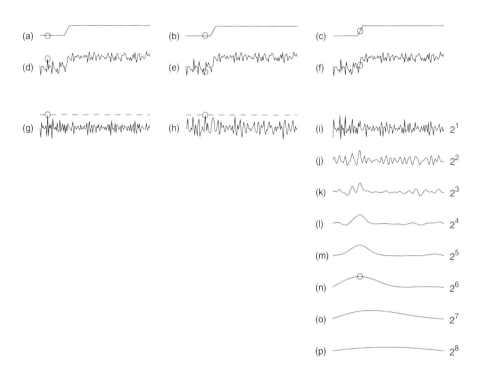

Figure 2.34: A comparative illustration of edge detection by Laplace, Sobel and GMWT in an example noisy signal (SNR ≈ 2dB).

Laplace and Sobel are selected so that they define only one extracted edge point as expected in the signal, similar to GMWT. As shown in Figures 2.34(g) and 2.34(h), the Laplace and Sobel methods have failed to locate the correct edge location. The result obtained using the global maximum of the wavelet transform of the signal which has occurred at the sixth scale (Figure 2.34(n)) is in the correct location.

In order to perform a quantitative relative comparison of the three methods, we applied them to a test data set of different synthetic noisy signals similar to the signal shown in Figure 2.34(d). Each signal in the test data set is a 128 length signal with a single positive step edge of amplitude one at position 32. Gaussian zero-mean white noise with increasing standard deviation from $\sigma_N = 0.1$ to $\sigma_N = 0.4$ in steps of 0.1 is added to the signal. We also let the slope of the step edge vary with parameter $T = 0, 1, 3, 5$, the number of samples in the transient part of the edge. With the above definition of the signal, according to Equation (2.40) the varying standard deviation of the noise results in four different signal to noise ratios, $SNR_{dB} = 12.73, 6.71, 3.19, 0.69$. For each case of the different SNRs and different slopes an ensemble of one hundred different noisy signals was generated to form the test data set. In each test process, the position of the detected edges by Laplace, Sobel and GMWT edge detectors

SNR(dB)	Slope(T)			
	0	1	3	5
12.73	10.07	43.04	48.14	48.99
6.71	39.96	48.22	46.16	48.76
3.19	47.82	50.52	49.18	48.53
0.69	45.99	49.78	44.25	48.55

Table 2.2: RMSE (in terms of number of samples) of the edge detection results on the test data set using the Laplace operator.

SNR(dB)	Slope(T)			
	0	1	3	5
12.73	0.73	0	0.88	6.76
6.71	19.38	9.84	28.45	36.47
3.19	22.26	37.98	38.12	44.94
0.69	40.23	42.08	45.54	44.43

Table 2.3: RMSE (in terms of number of samples) of the edge detection results on the test data set using the Sobel operator.

were compared to the real position of the center of the edge, and the accuracy of the results were measured using the Root Mean Squared Error (RMSE) in terms of the number of samples. The overall comparative results for Laplace, Sobel and GMWT are shown in Tables 2.2, 2.3 and 2.4 respectively.

As seen in the tables, by increasing the slope of the step edge, and also by decreasing the SNR of the signal, the RMSE of the results increases for all three methods. However, GMWT introduces much less error in comparison with Laplace and Sobel as expected. The superior performance of GMWT can be explained by the fact that in this technique edge detection is always carried out by an appropriate window size (scale); however, the operator size in Laplace and Sobel is kept constant for different situations.

According to Table 2.4, the good performance of GMWT is, however, limited to SNR values greater than 3.19 dB. This can be explained partly by the discrete nature of the WT. Since we use a discrete dyadic WT to produce the wavelet scales of the signal, it is obvious that for some cases the most appropriate operator size for the given signal is missed between two dyadic scales, letting the global maximum occur for a noise-related maximum in the wrong scale and wrong place.

SNR(dB)	Slope(T)			
	0	1	3	5
12.73	0.22	0.73	0.71	0.67
6.71	0.56	0.89	0.98	0.93
3.19	0.72	1.08	8.49	1.26
0.69	18.34	23.23	13.29	17.36

Table 2.4: RMSE (in terms of number of samples) of the edge detection results on the test data set using the GMWT technique.

In this section, the study of the results of the application of different sizes of smoothing operators prior or simultaneous to edge detection in 2-DE images in some of the previous works, led us to the development of a new global maximum of the WT-based multiscale edge detection technique of GMWT.

We showed that the GMWT scheme is capable of automatically defining the most appropriate scale (operator size) for approximating the location of a given noisy single step edge. The superior (detection/localization) performance of GMWT in comparison to the conventional Sobel and Laplace edge operators was demonstrated quantitatively by the application of the three methods to a test data set of different synthetic noisy edge profiles.

In the next section, we will combine the fuzzy-based LVCP extraction algorithm with the multiscale edge detection technique of GMWT to develop a fully automatic radial search-based LV boundary extraction (LV cavity segmentation) in 2-DE images.

2.6   LV Segmentation System

In this section, we describe a new automatic Left Ventricular Endocardial (LVE) boundary extraction system from sequences of LA 2-DE images. When such a sequence of frames is observed on a video monitor, it is apparent that the basic motion of the LVE is radially-oriented. In other words, the motion is almost parallel to the radii and the orientation of the borders is almost perpendicular to the radii in any direction and at any instant of the beat. This observation is the main reason that the center-based or radial search-based strategies have been used for LVE extraction from different views of 2-DEs by many researchers in the past. In this approach, the LVE edge points are searched for on radial lines emanating from the left ventricular center point. The center-based strategy also has the advantage of reducing the boundary searching problem from two dimensions to one dimension, and hence reducing the processing time.

The new automatic system comprises four main components: (1) overall LVCP approximation for the frames of a complete cardiac cycle, (2) 3D radial intensity sampling over the entire sequence, (3) LVE edge detection on radial intensity profiles for all frames and (4) spatial/temporal processing of the extracted edge points and Cubic B-Spline LV boundary approximation.

2.6.1   Overall Reference LVCP

An automatic fuzzy-based method for estimating the location of the Left Ventricular Center Point in a single 2-DE frame was presented in Section 2.4. The technique is a modified version of the algorithm developed by Setarehdan *et al.* [129]. In LVE detection in the 2-DE frames of a complete cardiac cycle, we wish to relate all boundary edge point information to one reference center point. This overall reference LVCP is achieved using the mean of all the LVCP in the sequence frame.

2.6.2 3D Non-Uniform Radial Intensity Sampling

The second major block in the system is 3D non-uniform radial intensity sampling. Moving outward in any direction from the automatically defined LVCP, there is an intensity change in the LVE region from dark to bright due to the higher echo activity of the heart muscle in comparison to the blood. The aim of the LVE detection procedure is to find the place of this intensity change in all directions. This requires that the left ventricular area is intensity sampled over the M radial scan lines in all the N input frames of a complete cardiac cycle.

To our knowledge, all of the previous center-based approaches have used equi-angular radial intensity sampling of the LV cavity, even for LA views (for example see [85]). For an SA view in which the LV cavity has a near circular appearance this makes sense. For a normal apical LA view, however, in which the cavity has an elliptical shape in the vertical direction, we propose a non-uniform intensity sampling by considering smaller angles between the radii at the two far ends of the ellipse. The aim of the non-uniform intensity sampling in LA views is to produce an almost equal resolution in all places of the cavity regardless of their distance from the reference LVCP which increases the accuracy of the LV boundary extraction process in the apex and valve regions with an almost twice longer distance from the center point in comparison with the closest lateral regions.

Figure 2.35 illustrates an example of automatically defined non-uniformly distributed radial scan lines superimposed on a 4-chamber LA 2-DE image.

This is carried out over an elliptical Region of Interest (RoI) covering the whole LV cavity and centered at the overall LVCP. To define the angle of the ith scan line, we use the polar form of the ellipse equation:

$$
\begin{aligned}
y &= b\ sin(\theta) \\
x &= a\ cos(\theta)
\end{aligned}
\tag{2.41}
$$

in which y and x are the Cartesian co-ordinates of each point on the ellipse, b and a are the major and minor radii of the ellipse respectively, and θ is the independent polar variable. The angle of the ith radial scan line, θ_i, is then defined by:

$$
\theta_i = tan^{-1}\left(\frac{y}{x}\right) = tan^{-1}\left(\frac{b}{a}tan\left(\frac{2\pi(i-1)}{M}\right)\right), \quad i = 1, 2, ..., M
\tag{2.42}
$$

where M is the total number of the scan lines. Note that Equation (2.42) becomes a uniform intensity sampling if $a = b$. The major radius of the elliptical RoI, b, is defined as the distance between the overall reference LVCP (ellipse center) and the top of the image plane. This overestimated major radius of the LV cavity ensures that the elliptical RoI vertically covers the whole LV cavity. The minor radius of the elliptical LV cavity usually appears to be half of its major radius [130]. For the same reason as explained above with an overestimation we set the minor radius a, to 0.67 of b to ensure that the

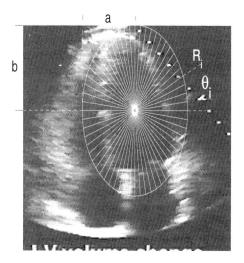

Figure 2.35: Non-uniform radial intensity sampling in an apical LA view 2-DE. (smaller angles between the radii at the two far ends of the elliptical region). Reprinted with permission from [110]. © 1998 IEE.

elliptical RoI covers the whole LV cavity in the horizontal direction as well. For $a = 0.67b$, Equation (2.42) provides a non-uniform distributed radii over the RoI with the maximum and minimum inter-radii angles of approximately $9°$ (in the lateral sides of ellipse) and $4°$ (in the top and bottom sides of ellipse) respectively. These values are independent of the absolute values of a and b.

After defining the fixed radial scan lines, the image sequence is intensity-sampled over them in all frames of the cardiac cycle and the resulting intensity profiles are stored in a three-dimensional (3D) matrix as follows:

$$\mathbf{f} = [f(n)_{i,j}, \ g_{min} \leq f(n)_{i,j} \leq g_{max}] \ \text{ for } \ \begin{matrix} n = 1, ..., R_i & \text{pixel (sample)} \\ & \text{index} \\ i = 1, ..., M & \text{radial index} \\ j = 1, ..., N & \text{frame index} \end{matrix} \qquad (2.43)$$

where R_i is the length of the ith scan line and g_{min} and g_{max} are the minimum and maximum gray values in the image sequence.

2.6.3 LV Boundary Edge Detection on 3D Radial Intensity Matrix

Referring to Figure 2.35, it is very apparent that moving outward from LVCP in any direction, there is only one real positive intensity step edge expected on each scan line which belongs to the LVE. This allows us to concentrate on the problem of a single positive step edge detection in a very noisy signal. We

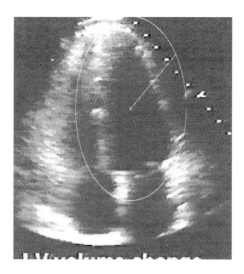

Figure 2.36: A real 4-chamber 2-DE with an example radial scan line superimposed on the image. Reprinted with permission from [110]. © 1998 IEE.

addressed this problem in Section 2.5 and developed a new global maximum of the WT-based multiscale edge detection technique.

We also showed in Section 2.5 that the GMWT scheme is capable of automatically defining the most appropriate scale (operator size) for approximating the location of a given noisy single step edge. The superior (detection/localization) performance of GMWT in comparison with the conventional Sobel and Laplace edge operators was also demonstrated quantitatively by the application of the three methods to a test data set of different synthetic noisy edge profiles.

In this sub-section we first demonstrate the application of GMWT to a real example of an intensity profile, which is achieved by intensity sampling of the LV cavity over a radial line. Figure 2.36 illustrates such an example with the radial scan line superimposed on the real image. Figure 2.37 shows the corresponding intensity profile and its discrete dyadic wavelet transform in all available dyadic scales underneath. The location of the global maximum point of the wavelet transform which occurs on the 3rd scale is indicated by an "O" on the radial scan line in both Figures 2.36 and 2.37. The three-dimensional illustration of the wavelet transform of the signal is also shown in Figure 2.38.

By applying the three edge operators of Laplace, Sobel and GMWT to the 2-DE image of Figure 2.36, we now compare their performance with each other in Figure 2.39. The superior performance of the GMWT for the real 2-DE images is obvious from this example.

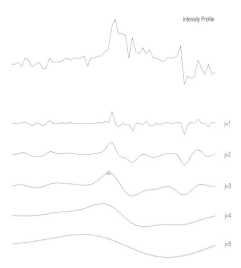

Figure 2.37: The intensity profile over the scan line shown in Figure 2.36 and its wavelet transform scales with the global maximum point found and marked on the 3rd scale. Reprinted with permission from [110]. © 1998 IEE.

2.6.4   Post-Processing of the Edges and Closed LVE Approximation

When the extracted LVE edge points of some example sequences were reviewed, it was found that there always exist some inconsistent rough elements. In reality, however, heart contours are continuous and smooth with continuous motion in time. This implies that further processing needs to be carried out on the extracted candidate edges. Many different techniques have been used for removing the erroneous edge points and smoothing the raw extracted LV boundaries including, spatial/temporal 2D mean filtering [114], Gaussian spatial smoothing [95], and Fourier domain analysis on either the spatial dimension [131] or temporal dimension or both [132]. Since the aim of the present work is LV volume change assessment in time, both spatial and temporal processing of the LVE in a sequence of frames are considered using two-dimensional nonlinear median filters. A 5×5 two-dimensional median filter was experimentally found appropriate for spatially/temporally refining the erroneously extracted boundary edge points.

The final closed boundaries are extracted using the spatially/temporally processed edge points together with a uniform cubic B-spline approximation [133] technique. Given a set of data points, Cubic B-spline approximation defines a smooth closed boundary which passes not through the data points but very close to them. This approximation method is used rather than interpolation because any given echo image and LVE is "fuzzy". In fact, it is meaningless to define a single pixel in the image as an exact location of the boundary edge point and this is the main cause of the inter-observer variability.

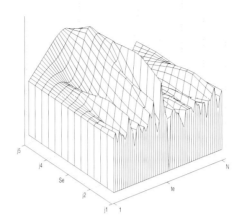

Figure 2.38: The three dimensional illustration of the wavelet transform of the intensity profile over the scan line shown in Figure 2.36. Reprinted with permission from [110]. © 1998 IEE.

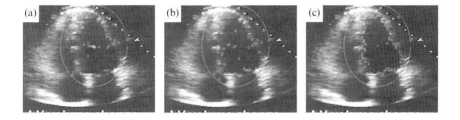

Figure 2.39: LVE edge points extracted on 60 radial scan lines using: (a) Laplace edge operator, (b) Sobel edge operator, and (c) GMWT technique. Reprinted with permission from [110]. © 1998 IEE.

The application of the cubic B-spline approximation method for LVE definition, provides much more visually acceptable boundaries compared to interpolation techniques. Figures 2.40(a) and 2.40(b) demonstrate two examples of the final LVEs computed by the technique developed here in typical LA apical views.

2.6.5 Automatic LV Volume Assessment

The final closed LVEs can now be used together with the ASE recommended biplane or single plane strategies to compute the LV volume at any instant of cardiac cycle. In this work we use the single plane "area-length" method and its approximating formula (see Figure 2.5(a)) to calculate the LV volume in each frame. This method needs the enclosed area A and the longest diameter of the oval shape L to be measured from the extracted borders first. This is

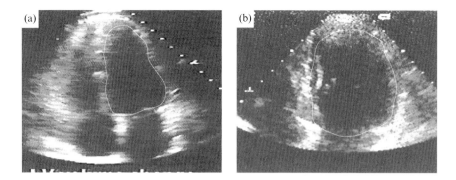

Figure 2.40: Typical examples of the extracted LVE (a) in a 4-chamber (b) in a 2-chamber apical LA 2-DE. Reprinted with permission from [110]. © 1998 IEE.

a simple calculation given the coordinates of every point of the LVE border. By approximating end-diastole and end-systole by the largest and the smallest cavity areas respectively [60], the LV stroke volume, SV, and the ejection-fraction ratio, EF, can also be calculated using the following formulae:

$$SV = EDV - ESV \tag{2.44}$$

$$EF = \frac{SV}{EDV} \tag{2.45}$$

Figure 2.41(a) demonstrates an example of computer-generated LV volume changes in one complete cardiac cycle (29 frames) which is repeated three times to display the cyclic nature of the process. The first derivative of the LV volume changes which includes important diagnostic information is also calculated and shown in Figure 2.41(b). The EDV, ESV, SV, and EF for this example are $124.73 ml$, $114.84 ml$, $9.90 ml$, and 7.93% respectively. Also, the maximum and minimum values of the derivative which show the maximum rates of filling and emptying of the LV chamber in the diastole and systole phases are 3.46 and -7.01, respectively.

2.7 Conclusions

In this chapter we have focused on the concept of quantitative analysis of cardiac function by automatic LV cavity segmentation in standard 2-DE images. The physiology and anatomy of the human heart was initially reviewed. The standard echocardiographic views of the heart and the recommended standard models and methods for quantification of cardiac function using 2-DE images were studied. From this study we found that the recommended methods are commonly based upon the segmentation of the LV cavity and its centroid.

By reviewing the previous efforts for LV cavity segmentation in the 2-DE images it was then concluded that segmentation in 2-DE images is one of the

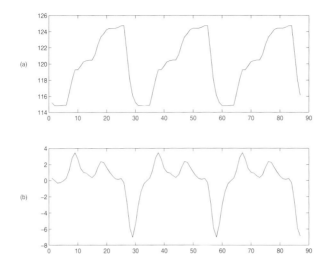

Figure 2.41: (a) LV volume changes measured (in a cardiac cycle and repeated three times) by the "area-length" method and using the LVE boundaries computed by the present algorithm in a cardiac cycle. (b) First derivative of the volume changes which includes important diagnostic information. Reprinted with permission from [110]. © 1998 IEE.

most difficult image processing tasks due to many particular problems in the image formation process of the 2-DEs. This review also showed that the center-based strategy has attracted more interest than the other strategies. This is basically due to the advantage of reducing the boundary searching problem from two-dimensions to one-dimension which is an important factor in reducing the processing time. Moreover, edge detection on radial lines, which are usually perpendicular to the boundary, produces better edge estimates.

Previous utilization of the center-based strategy, however, has usually failed to solve the following common problems. First, the center of the LV cavity has to be identified before the process begins. Second, edge detection on radial lines is more sensitive to noise due to limiting the knowledge used for edge detection to only one-dimensional intensity information in a two-dimensional image.

To solve the first problem, we developed a novel automatic fuzzy reasoning-based Left Ventricular center point estimation algorithm, which is applicable to both standard Short Axis (SA) and Long Axis (LA) 2-DE images, in Section 2.4. As for the second problem, a multiresolution edge detection scheme based on the Global Maximum of Wavelet Transform (GMWT), was developed in Section 2.5. It was shown that GMWT is capable of automatically defining the most appropriate scale (operator size) for approximating the location of a given noisy single step edge in a very noisy signal.

By combining the two robust algorithms of fuzzy-based LVCP extraction and the wavelet transform-based multiresolution edge detection technique, a fully automatic LV cavity segmentation from 2-DE images was developed in Section 2.6.

2.8   Acknowledgments

The authors would like to express their gratitude to Professor H. Dargie (professor of cardiology) and Dr T. McDonagh (medical doctor) from the Cardiology department of the Western Infirmary in Glasgow for supplying the echo images and the manual interpretation of the data. They would also like to thank Elsevier Science and the IEE for permission to use text and images from [110] and [129] in this chapter.

Chapter 3

Segmentation and Quantification Techniques for Fitting Computer Vision Models to Cardiac MR, CT, X-Ray and PET Image Data[1]

Jasjit S. Suri

3.1 Introduction

The field of medical imaging has experienced an explosive growth in recent years (1990–99) due to several imaging modalities, such as X-ray, computer tomography (CT), magnetic resonance imaging (MRI), positron emission tomography (PET) and spectral positron emission computer tomography (SPECT) (see Stytz *et al.* [135] for an extensive survey). The digital revolution and the processing power of computers combined with these modalities have helped humans understand to some extent the complex anatomy of the heart and its behavior. There are still, however, some unresolved problems which are linked to computer vision-pattern recognition (CVPR) and clinical cardiology research. The importance of cardiovascular research has increased, due to the inter-linking of effects arising from non-cardiovascular diseases. In the United States alone, the budget for cardiovascular research was $269 billion in 1997. This points towards the national concern and the degree of importance of cardiovascular research. As reported by the American Heart Association (AHA) [136] and the Herald Newspaper, UK [137], heart disease claims an enormous number of lives.

Imaging has played a major role in understanding the heart's behavior [138], [139]. The full advantage of the diagnostic capability of any imaging system lies in its integrated components, their relationship to each other and a thorough understanding of each component. Though cardiac imaging has been accomplished through several modalities, the most popular being cardiac MRI (see Zerhouni *et al.* [140], Axel *et al.* [141], [142], Creswell *et al.* [143], Barth *et al.* [144]), cardiac CT (see Richey *et al.* [145], Huang *et al.* [146], Seppi *et al.* [147], Ritman *et al.* [148]), cardiac nuclear (see Behren [149], Strauss *et al.* [150], Leitl *et al.* [151]) and cardiac ultrasound (see Heather [152], Herlin

---

[1]This chapter is based on material previously published in *Pattern Analysis and Applications* [139] [550].

et al. [153], [154]), this chapter deals with CVPR techniques applied to any of these cardiac imaging modalities. No matter which cardiac imaging modality one uses, boundary estimation is of the highest clinical importance.

A quantitative evaluation of the left ventricle (LV) wall motion is required both for mathematical modeling of cardiac mechanics and evaluation of cardiac performance. For example, LV modeling is required for finite element analysis of cardiac stress and deformation [155], [156]. Another example where LV modeling is needed is in the area of cardiac electrical activation [157]. Cardiac functional analysis and its performance require accurate boundary estimation. This helps cardiologists in studying different kinds of cardiomyopathy. The cardiac quantification can be done manually, but it is very tedious to trace these boundaries for each time frame of the cardiac cycle and for large, voluminous data sets. As a result, cardiologists are very interested in accurate and automatic boundary estimation. This chapter presents tools and segmentation techniques for LV contouring and LV surface estimation from different imaging modalities.

LV boundary estimation is not new to CVPR and clinical cardiac researchers. Its existence was established when cardiac imaging began (see the following three books published in the space of two years, each on cardiac angiography: Moodie *et al.* [24], Mancini [25], Moore [26]). These boundaries help cardiologists find the volume of the LV chamber, which is helpful in computing the ejection fraction[2] (the ratio of the difference in the heart volumes during end-diastole and end-systole times to the end-diastole time) of the heart [27]. These boundaries, when traced from frame to frame of the cardiac cycle, are very useful in studying the behavior of the heart in relation to coronary heart disease (CHD). The time-course of LV volume is an indicator of cardiac performance. Researchers have also tried modeling the contraction and expansion process of the LV. This modeling can be more accurately accomplished if the LV chamber boundaries are estimated reliably, accurately and quickly in real-time. To actually estimate these boundaries, which is not an easy process, segmentation must first be done. In medical applications, the shape of the LV varies considerably among patient studies and over time.

This chapter is limited to the following three major categories: first, a system for imaging the heart using X-rays, its major components, risks and procedure; second, post-processing of these imaging modalities to automatically estimate the boundaries of the LV using model-based CVPR techniques and to compare them among different researchers; and third, a discussion of LV wall motion estimation techniques in 2-D, LV wall thickness, LV volume measurements in 3-D and LV tracking. There will also be a comparison of the CVPR techniques applied to cardiac CT/MR/Nuclear Medicine and it will be shown how they fit into cardiac X-rays or vice versa. What are similarities between different algorithms when applied to cardiac CT, MR or X-rays? A secondary goal of this chapter is to present and understand a collection of ready-references of CVPR techniques applied to cardiac CT, MR, ultrasound,

---

2 $\frac{ED_{vol} - ES_{vol}}{ED_{vol}}$

Nuclear Medicine and X-rays. Another goal is to understand how pattern recognition-based techniques have been more successful for learning about the heart's behavior. Readers in the field of cardiac imaging will encounter the following new concepts in this chapter: (**1**) how active contour LV modeling is similar to learning LV modeling; (**2**) how some low-level techniques can be usefully incorporated into both active contour modeling and learning LV modeling algorithms to design the overall system robustly and accurately; (**3**) how different cardiac imaging modalities (CT, MR, ultrasound and X-rays) are inter-related when it comes to CVPR; (**4**) key characteristics of model-based LV segmentation; and (**5**) the power of hand-drawn boundaries to model the LV shape in temporal and spatial domains.

As shown by Suri [28], the variability in heart rates, sizes, positions and orientations, gray scale variations in data sets, noise due to the varying modulation transfer function of the X-ray imaging set-up, interference of other thoracic structures within the LV and the large number of cardiac abnormalities have caused different CVPR researchers to pursue different paths for segmentation and contouring of the LV. The goal of any LV diagnostic imaging system is to build a fast, accurate, robust, low-cost and reliable system for estimating the borders of the LV. Due to all of these complexities, it is obvious that one particular model alone is not enough for accurate or robust border estimation; it is necessary to depend on many sources of information, but the question is, which combination of CVPR techniques should be used?

Having discussed the importance of cardiac boundary estimation, the goals of this chapter and what factors contribute to making an efficient cardiac software imaging system, the remaining part of this section focuses on the classification tree for cardiac LV segmentation. With the current state-of-the-art CVPR algorithms, and the models proposed for LV border estimation, the classification tree can be built on the foundation of three main classes: low-level, mid-level and high-level. This can be seen in Figure 3.1.

All the computer vision models and techniques covered under this classification tree will be discussed later in this chapter, the layout of which is as follows: Sub-section 3.2 presents the cardiac anatomy and data acquisitions. Low-level and medium-level algorithms are presented in Sub-section 3.3. A survey on high-level CVPR algorithms is presented in Sub-section 3.4. Sub-section 3.5 presents LV apex modeling. Sub-section 3.6 presents the integration of low-level features in boundary models for LV modeling. The validation techniques for LV boundary estimation are presented in Sub-section 3.7. The LV convex hulling process is discussed in Sub-section 3.8. Eigen analysis in LV modeling is presented in Sub-section 3.9. Neural Network models for LV processing are discussed in Sub-section 3.10. A comparison between active and training-based systems is presented in Sub-section 3.11. Sub-section 3.12 presents details on LV wall motion, LV volume and LV tracking. Finally, conclusions regarding design issues and considerations related to accurate LV modeling, both in terms of hardware and software, are presented in Sub-sections 3.13.1 and 3.13.2, respectively.

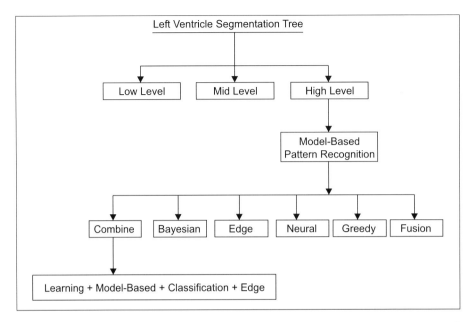

Figure 3.1: Classification tree for LV segmentation techniques: integration of low, medium and high-level computer vision algorithms.

3.2   Cardiac Anatomy and Data Acquisitions for MR, CT, Ultrasound and X-Rays

The section has the following parts: Sub-section 3.2.1 presents cardiac anatomy and the circulation system. Data acquisitions in cardiac MR, CT, Ultrasound and X-rays are presented in Sub-section 3.2.2. Since this chapter is geared more towards cardiac X-rays, cardiac catheterization and its risks will be discussed in Sub-section 3.2.2.2. Sub-section 3.2.2.3 presents the LV data acquisition system using X-rays and finally Sub-section 3.2.2.4 presents the drawbacks of cardiac catheterization.

3.2.1   Cardiac Anatomy

Figure 3.2 shows the 3-D anatomy of the heart. The top figure shows the base of the heart from the posterior view. The bottom figure shows the surface of the heart. Also clearly seen are the left and right ventricles, left and right atria, left and right pulmonary arteries, left and right superior pulmonary veins and the coronary sinus. For details, see Netter [158].

Figure 3.3 shows cut sections of the heart with its muscles. This consists of three layers of tissues: the myocardium (the innermost layer), the endocardium (the middle layer) and the epicardium (the outermost layer). The muscular part of the interventricular septum is clearly seen. Also observed are the left and right papillary muscles (note the shape difference seen in the papillary muscles

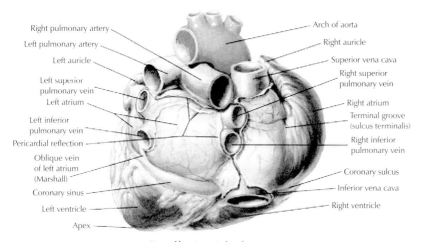

Base of heart: posterior view

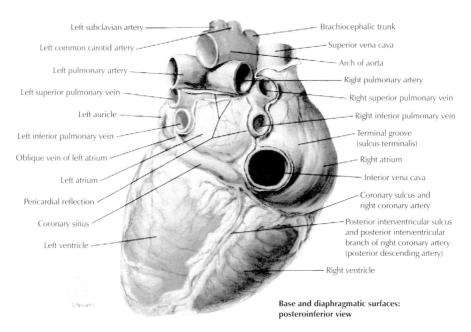

Figure 3.2: 3-D anatomy of the heart. From [158]. © 1995, Havas. Reprinted with permission from Havas MediMedia; illustrated by Drs. John A. Craig and Carlos Machado. All rights reserved.

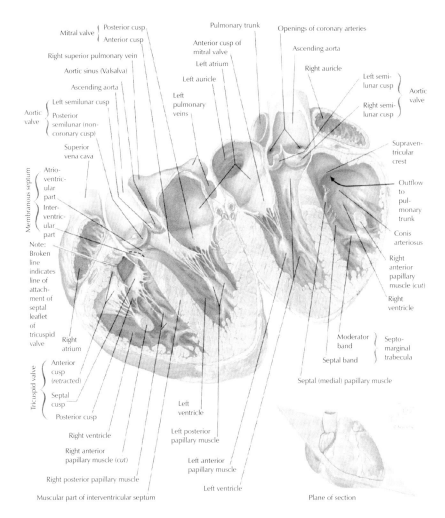

Figure 3.3: 3-D anatomy of the heart with cut sections. From [158]. © 1995, Havas. Reprinted with permission from Havas MediMedia; illustrated by Drs. John A. Craig and Carlos Machado. All rights reserved.

on the left and right sides of the heart). The important aspect to observe is the thickness of the muscles of the LV. This could be one of the reasons which causes a delay and the low contrast seen in the apical zones in cardiac X-ray images.

Figure 3.4 shows the circulatory system of the heart. The main function of the heart is to pump blood. The left atrium receives oxygenated blood from the lungs and pumps it throughout the left ventricle. The left ventricle then pumps it to the entire body through the aorta and its distributing branches. Deoxygenated blood is then received in the right atrium and is sent to the lungs via the right ventricle for oxygenation.

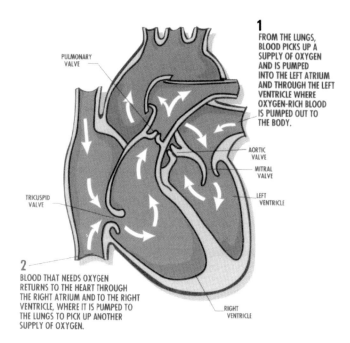

Figure 3.4: Circulatory system of the heart. The blood picks up a supply of oxygen that is pumped into the left atrium, through to the left ventricle where blood rich in oxygen is pumped out to the body (see point 1). Blood that needs oxygen returns through the the right atrium, to the right ventricle, where it is pumped to the lungs to pick up another supply of oxygen (see point 2) (Courtesy of Dr. Malvika Suri).

3.2.2   Cardiac MR, CT, Ultrasound and X-Ray Acquisitions

In this sub-section we will discuss briefly the presentation of LV using different modalities and then focus mainly on the cardiac X-rays. Thus the layout of this section is as follows: different views of LV using different modalities are discussed in Sub-section 3.2.2.1. The risks of cardiac catheterization are presented in Sub-section 3.2.2.2. The LV data acquisition system for X-rays is presented in Sub-section 3.2.2.3. Finally, the drawbacks of the cardiac catheterization technique are discussed in Sub-section 3.2.2.4.

3.2.2.1   Different Views of LV Using MR, CT, Ultrasound and X-Ray

Some sample images of the long axis and short axis views of the LV using Magnetic Resonance will be shown. A comparison between the end-diastole (ED) and the end-systole (ES) frames of the cardiac cycle in MR imaging will also be shown.

Figure 3.5 shows a comparison of different modalities for scanning the left ventricle. The first row shows short- and long-axis views of the LV using Magnetic Resonance. The second row shows a CT image of the LV using non-gated and gated imaging. The third row shows X-ray images of the LV in the end-diastole and end-systole frames. The last row shows short- and long-axis views of the LV in ultrasound. For details on the image generation process for ultrasound, MR and CT images, readers are referred to Chapter 1.

Figures 3.6 to 3.10 show sample MR images of the heart in different views and different techniques. Figure 3.6 shows the horizontal long-axis view in the axial plane of the left ventricular outflow tract in the leftmost panel. The middle panel of Figure 3.6 is the long-axis view in the coronal plane. The rightmost panel of Figure 3.6 shows the vertical long-axis view in the sagittal plane. Figure 3.7 shows the horizontal long-axis view in the axial plane for end-diastole and end-systole in MR images. Figure 3.8 shows the short-axis view of the left ventricle for the end-diastole and end-systole frames. Figure 3.9 shows a single slice multi-phase (16) series of MR images acquired during the cardiac cycle from ED to ES. They are FAST (Field Echo type) cardiac MR images. Figure 3.10 shows a single slice, multi-phase bright blood series of MR images (15 images) of the short-axis of the left ventricle.

3.2.2.2   X-Ray Cardiac Catheterization and its Risks

Cardiac catheterization (CC) involves inserting a pigtail catheter into the LV chamber of the heart through one of the arteries passing through the groin of a human. In 1940, this procedure was introduced to the medical field of cardiovascular research for the purpose of heart treatment and diagnosis (for details, see Hood *et al.* [16] and Zisserman *et al.* [17]). During this procedure, a contrast agent or dye is inserted through the catheter, which causes it to mix with blood in the LV chamber of the heart. During the bolus injection of this contrast agent, the X-ray source is turned on and the dosage is passed through the human chest (from posterior to anterior) covering the LV chamber in a right anterior oblique (RAO) view of 30 degrees to yield projection images called ventriculograms (LVgrams). The RAO projection is recommended and used by most investigators to correct foreshortening of the projected long-axis[3] of the chamber and to visualize the plane of the mitral valve in order to grossly detect the presence of mitral regurgitation[4]. Since the procedure is invasive, there must be an awareness of its risks and complications. Details of these risks can be seen in Conti *et al.* [18], but some of the most common ones are presented briefly here: (**1**) death, (**2**) arrhythmias (irregular heartbeat), (**3**) profound hypotension (low blood pressure), (**4**) complications involving the arterial system, (**5**) accidental perforations of the heart, (**6**) catheter problems, (**7**) embolism (plaque dislodging from one place and blocking another artery/vein), (**8**) bleeding and (**9**) ventricular fibrillation (rapid irregular beating of the ventricle).

---

[3]The segment joining the mid point of the aortic valve plane and the apex.
[4]Backwards motion.

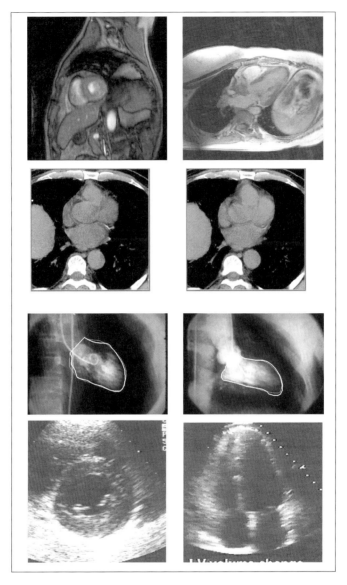

Figure 3.5: Comparison of LV images from different modalities. **Row − 1, Left**: MR cardiac short-axis view of the LV. **Row − 1, Right**: MR cardiac MR long-axis view of the LV. **Row − 2, Left**: Nongated CT image of the LV. **Row − 2, Right**: Gated CT image of the LV. **Row − 3, Left**: X-ray cardiac sample image of LV (ED frame). **Row − 3, Right**: X-ray cardiac sample image of LV (ES frame). **Row − 4, Left**: Ultrasound parasternal mid-papillary muscle level, short-axis view. **Row − 4, Right**: Ultrasound apical long-axis, four-chamber view (MR and CT Data, Courtesy of Marconi Medical Systems, Inc., Cardiac X-ray images from [28], Ultrasound Data, Courtesy of S. K. Setarehdan, University of Strathclyde, Glasgow, UK).

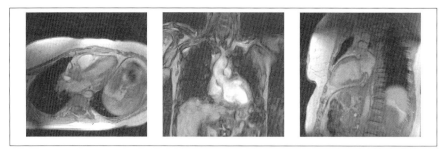

Figure 3.6: **Left**: Horizontal long-axis view in the axial plane of the left ventricular outflow tract. **Middle**: Long-axis view in the coronal plane. **Right**: Vertical long-axis view in the sagittal plane. FAST (Field Echo type) cardiac MR images with the following parameters: T_E=3.8 ms, T_R=915 ms, FoV=30 cm, Matrix Size=256 × 256, NSA=2, Flip Angle=35, Thick=5 mm, Gap=0 mm (MR Data, Courtesy of Marconi Medical Systems, Inc.).

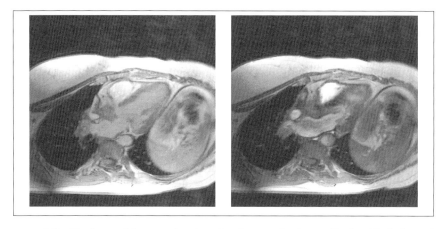

Figure 3.7: Horizontal long-axis view in the axial plane. **Left**: End-diastole. **Right**: End-systole. FAST (Field Echo type) cardiac MR images with the following parameters: T_E=3.8 ms, T_R=915 ms, FoV=30 cm, Matrix Size=256 × 256, NSA=2, Flip Angle=35, Thick=6 mm, Gap=0 mm (MR Data, Courtesy of Marconi Medical Systems, Inc.).

3.2.2.3   LV Data Acquisition System

A cardiac imaging X-ray acquisition system is shown in Figure 1.9. The major components of the system are an X-ray source, an image intensifier, a cine or video camera and an analog-to-digital converter (ADC) (a detailed version can be seen in Shung *et al.* [19]). A high enough voltage is applied to the X-ray source, which produces the X-ray beam. The beam is made to pass through the chest of the patient and is received by the detector. Note that the X-ray beam source and the detector axis are aligned along the same common line, called the axis of the tube. The LV is made to lie in the center of the

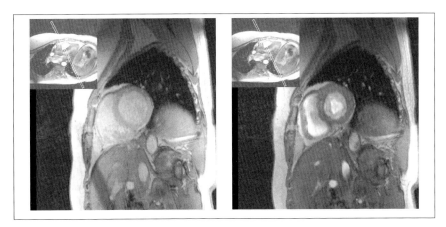

Figure 3.8: Short axis of the left ventricle in MR images. **Left**: End-diastole. **Right**: End-systole. FAST (Field Echo type) cardiac MR images with the following parameters: T_E=3.8 ms, T_R=915 ms, FoV=35 cm, Matrix Size=256 × 256, NSA=2, Flip Angle=35, Thick=6 mm, Gap=0 mm (MR Data, Courtesy of Marconi Medical Systems, Inc.).

X-ray beam. The image intensifier converts the X-ray beam into an optical image. For a clear delineation of the LV to be imaged from its neighboring tissue, a radio opaque contrast agent, such as an iodine compound, is injected into the organ to absorb part of the X-ray beam energy. This brings out a relatively high or brighter region compared with the surrounding background in the image produced by the image intensifier. The function of the silvered mirror is to focus the incoming X-ray beam into the cine camera, which is placed transversely to the direction of the incoming X-ray beam. The remainder of the light comprising the image is partially transmitted through the silvered mirror along the axis of the detector (image intensifier) and into the lens of a video camera. Usually, the video camera produces an analog signal resulting from scanning the image produced by the image intensifier. Alternatively, images produced by the image intensifier can be projected in a video camera. The analog signal is simply a voltage level which corresponds to the pixel value in the image. The analog-to-digital converter (ADC) converts this voltage, which represents the gray scale of a pixel as a digital value. Typical X-ray ventriculograms for end-diastole (ED[5]) and end-systole (ES[6]) frames are shown in Figure 3.5 (third row) and Figure 3.12.

3.2.2.4 Drawbacks of Cardiac Catheterization

Though CC provides definitive anatomical information not obtainable from other imaging modalities and is relatively economical and effective for studying cardiac disorders, it has a weakness, which controls the dynamic of the dye

---

[5]This is the last time frame of the expansion stage or diastole cycle.
[6]This is the last frame of the contraction stage or systole cycle.

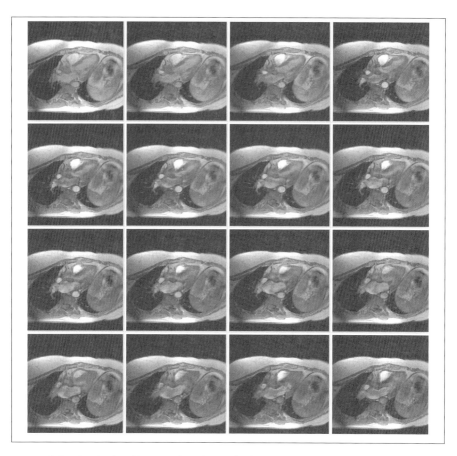

Figure 3.9: A single slice, multi-phase (16) series of images acquired during the cardiac cycle from ED to ES. FAST (Field Echo type) cardiac MR images with the following parameters: T_E=3.8 ms, T_R=915 ms, FoV=35 cm, Matrix Size=256 × 256, NSA=2, Flip Angle=35, Thick=6 mm, Gap=0 mm (MR Data, Courtesy of Marconi Medical Systems, Inc.).

flow into the LV chamber. This dynamic has put an extra burden on the post-processing of the LV gray scale data. As a result, this has led CVPR researchers to model the LV modeling process in a special way. The most critical drawback in CC is its low quality[7], especially in the apical[8], anterior wall and inferior wall zones (see Figure 3.11, right) for the labeling of the LV in projection ventriculograms. There are several reasons for poor quality in the LV apex: first, the contrast agent is unable to reach the apex zone of the LV due to curling of the catheter, as shown in Figure 3.11, left (for details on catheter design, the reader is referred to the excellent US patent by Rickerd [20] and Stephen *et al.* [21]), which is necessary to avoid irritation to the patient;

---

[7]Particularly in the apical zone of the left ventricle.
[8]Bottom one third of the LV.

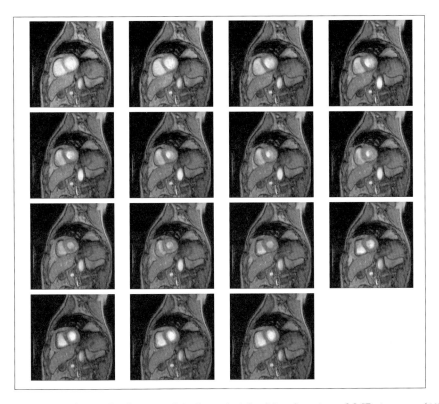

Figure 3.10: A single slice, multi-phase bright blood series of MR images (15 images) of the short-axis of the left ventricle (MR Data, Courtesy of Marconi Medical Systems, Inc.).

second, the contrast agent is unable to reach the apex if the LV is extremely large in size; third, the abnormality of the LV shape causes an irregularity that contributes to the poor propagation of the contrast agent towards the apex (see MacCallum [22] and Mall [23]); fourth, the dynamics of blood mixing with the contrast agent are not homogeneous in the LV chamber because of the muscle resistivity. Some boundary muscle tissues are thick and resist the penetration of the contrast agent towards the LV apex. The LV anterior and LV interior wall zones do not receive enough of the dye either. The inferior wall of the LV chamber is particularly poor in quality because of the superposition of the diaphragm over the LV. (Later, it will be shown by Suri *et al.* [246] how to separate the diaphragm from the LV in LVgrams.) In addition, the projection of the ribs over the LV in the LVgrams is another cause of poor contrast. Motion artifacts and noise due to the scattering of X-ray radiation by tissue volumes not related to the LV also contribute to the low quality of LVgrams. All of these factors pose a great challenge in LV segmentation and modeling. Having discussed the classification tree for LV segmentation, cardiac anatomy and different views of the LV along with the acquisition details, we now present

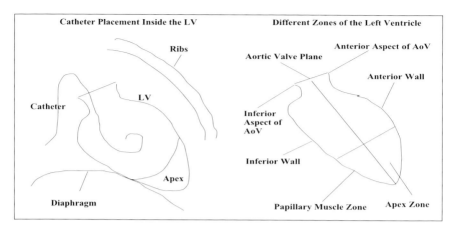

Figure 3.11: **Left**: Position of the catheter in the LV chamber. Also seen are the diaphragm and ribs. **Right**: Labeling of the LV parts: anterior wall, apex zone, inferior wall, aortic valve plane and the longitudinal axis. AoV stands for aortic valve plane [28].

the software tools and techniques for LV segmentation.

3.3   Low- and Medium-Level LV Segmentation Techniques

This sub-section is divided into four subparts: (**1**) LV segmentation based on histogramming and thresholding. Here dynamic histogramming, histogram selection using discriminant analysis, interactive thresholding and histogram peak clustering will be discussed; (**2**) LV edge detection. The major techniques include region growing, facet modeling, wavelet transform and spatial and temporal edge detection; (**3**) maximum likelihood based on matched filter using heuristics taken from the field of artificial intelligence; (**4**) mathematical morphological approaches for LV segmentation and their shortcomings. We conclude by summarizing the drawbacks of these techniques and how model-based imaging brings changes in LV segmentation and its analysis.

3.3.1   Smoothing Image Data

Smoothing was the first step performed before any post-processing could be done on the LVgrams. The edge information could be lost by smoothing and hence would require the use of edge-preserving filters. Higgins *et al.* [160] addressed this using a region-sharpening technique for their cardiac data set. This technique consisted of two template reconstructions followed by the application of a template on the image. Wilson and Bertram [161] developed a technique to pre-flatten contrast and mask images that reduced artifacts. Their cardiac cycle could be displaced with a narrower gray scale compared with the original gray

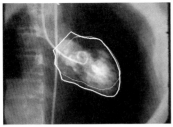
(a1) ED Frame: GT & computer est.

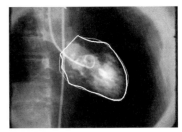
(a2) ED Frame: GT & computer est.

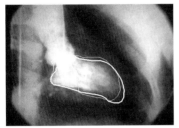
(b1) ES Frame: GT & computer est.

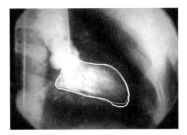
(b2) ES Frame: GT & computer est.

Figure 3.12: X-ray ventriculograms. **Top**: ED frames, **Bottom**: ES frames; GT stands for ground truth boundary, shown with a thick boundary. The thin boundary is a computer estimated technique [28].

scale images. Nagao *et al.* [162] proposed a smoothing algorithm which looked for the most homogeneous neighboring area around each point in a picture and then gave each point the average gray level of the selected neighboring area. The algorithm removed noise in a flat region without blurring sharp edges or destroying details of the boundary of the region. Subtraction schemes for noise reduction were first proposed by Vonesh *et al.* [163]. The segmentation algorithm consisted of a first-order gray scale histogram computation on the image data. Gray scale standard deviation and gray scale standard deviation normalized to a mean gray scale were used as primary measures of artificial noise. Vonesh reported that different image data had low noise content compared with the original gray scale ultrasound data set. Morphology-based smoothing was first implemented by Lamberti *et al.* [164] followed by Lee [201] and Suri [28]. Gray scale morphological [187] smoothing consisted of gray scale opening followed by gray scale closing.

3.3.2 Manual and Semi-Automatic LV Thresholding

The smoothing algorithm covered in the previous sub-section affects the thresholding process. Once the smoothing process was complete, a threshold was selected so that all pixels having gray scale intensities greater than the threshold were cardiac structures and other pixels were the background pixels (low intensities). These methods considered the dye-injected region to be the foreground (brighter region), but since the catheter and ribs had high gray scale values, they seemed to be taken into the foreground after the threshold. Several threshold-based methods have been developed to separate the LV by finding the minimum between two modes in a histogram of using gray scale LVgrams (see Weszka *et al.* [165], Tananka [166], De Jong *et al.* [167], Reiber [168], Han *et al.* [169], Nakajima *et al.* [171], Hideya *et al.* [170], Muhammed [172], Jang [173], Capozzi *et al.* [174]). All these methods were either semi-automatic or not accurate and robust enough to produce reliable boundaries. Wollschlaeger *et al.* [175] developed a frame-by-frame LV contour detection algorithm based on low pass filtering and interactive thresholding. Wollschlaeger *et al.* 's algorithm consisted of the following steps: (**1**) image processing generated raw contours. This step involved smoothing and low pass filtering with a filter size of 10×10. These filtered ED and ES LV images were thresholded interactively based on regions outside and inside the LV. The output of this process was an LV binary image. The raw LV contour around this binary LV region was then drawn using a graphics pad. This raw contour was further smoothed using a median filter of size 5×5. (**2**) The raw contours were then used to define the refined contour (Wollschlaeger *et al.* called it a "real contour"), using contrast values at the border of the LV. In that step, Wollschlaeger *et al.* drew 100 scan lines at each LV vertex from inside (high contrast value) to outside (low contrast value) with the left ventriculogram (LVG) in the background. The arctangent function was then fitted to the gray level variation along each scan line corresponding to each vertex of the LVG. Wollschlaeger *et al.* called the process densogram analysis and defined the real contour as being at the 25% level of the total amplitude of the function above the lower plateau. This threshold was based on empirical results. (**3**) Finally, the real contours were smoothed again. Wollschlaeger *et al.* 's method involved user interaction at two major stages. The raw contour generation used interactive thresholding and then a graphics pad to trace the binary output. Wollschlaeger *et al.* 's method did not discuss the relationship between the 25% threshold point and the heart size. In other words, the question was how to validate that a large LV would also have the same 25% threshold point on the fitted arctangent curve from the lower plateau of all parts of the LV contour (LVC). In the fuzzy region where the diaphragm overlapped the LV, the gray scale distribution would yield many false alarms and the 25% value of the fitted curve might not be correct for those parts of the LVC. In addition, Wollschlaeger *et al.* computed LV borders of the systole phase of the heart cycle (contraction phase) by direct interpolation of ED and ES boundaries, which might not be the right estimate for varying heartbeats of the same patient. Wollschlaeger *et al.* 's technique did not discuss the geometric method as to how the 100 chords (scan lines) were drawn along the LVC. Since this was a crucial stage of border detection, automation of this stage could reduce variability and bring an improvement in speed. Some other interactive thresholding schemes applied to echocardiograms can be seen in Revanakar *et al.* [176], [177], [178].

Adam *et al.* [71] also used a semi-automated technique for boundary estimation in echocardiograms which used a combination of several low-level computer vision techniques. This system consisted of two stages: stage one consisted of four steps called filtration, LV center of gravity computation, mean gray level computation around the LV and amplification of the gray level intensities by a Gaussian function along the long axis of the LV. Stage two consisted of the actual border detection. This stage (also called the low-level stage) has the following steps: sectoring the LV into 8 parts radially from the center of the LV outwards; placement of the $N \times N$ square-sized boxes on these radial vectors and computing the mean and standard deviation of the gray level distribution in these squares; computing the likelihood of the pixel being a border point for the inner three squares and given as: $P_i = K_1 \mu_i + K_2 \sigma_i + K_3 \delta \mu_i$. The point of maximum P_i was the border point (also called the pointer) and serves as the pointer for the next step of iteration. Finally, the second step was repeated until the square size was reduced to a 1×1 pixel size. Adam *et al.* fitted the cubic spline in the end to smooth the borders and used the root mean square error as the method of computation of the boundary error which Adam *et al.* called the success index.

3.3.3 LV Dynamic Thresholding

Of the earlier works in thresholding, Chow *et al.* [179] developed a LV boundary detection algorithm in cardio-angiograms using dynamic thresholding. The fundamental assumption of Chow *et al.* was based on the probability distribution of the intensity for any small region of a picture which consisted solely of the object or the background. The distribution was Gaussian in nature (as established by Lee [201]). Chow *et al.* 's algorithm consisted of the following steps: (**1**) dividing the image into smaller overlapping regions and then computing its histograms; (**2**) choosing the histograms which had large variances, showing that the variance of the region was a function of the variance of the contrast agent, mean value of the contrast agent and fractions of the area of the region by the object; (**3**) for selected histograms, finding the distribution parameters, namely the mean, the variance and the fraction of the area of the object and background in that region and these parameters, then underwent the bimodality histogram test; and (**4**) the threshold was estimated using the maximum likelihood function by solving a quadratic equation of the form: $Ax^2 + Bx + C = 0$. Chow *et al.* 's algorithm was definitely a statistical procedure to estimate the threshold, but it was not robust enough to handle the gray scale distribution of X-ray cardiac data sets. The histogram of the left ventriculograms did not have a Gaussian distribution. Furthermore, Chow *et al.* 's experiments only took the background and the object, which was not the case when the diaphragm interfered with the left ventricle in LVgrams.

3.3.3.1 Dynamic Thresholding Based on Discriminant Analysis

Otsu [180] developed a better thresholding method for finding a threshold for gray scale images, which was based on discriminant analysis and the statistical distribution of gray scale intensities. The positive features of Otsu's method were: (**1**) selection of an optimum threshold by discriminant criteria to maximize the separability of the resultant classes in gray levels, (**2**) requirement of the zeroth and first order moments along with class variances and (**3**) straight-forward extension of the method to multi-threshold problems. A technique based on peak clustering for refining the histogram was given by McAdams [181].

3.3.4   Edge-Based Techniques

In 1981, Fu and Mui [182] published a survey paper summarizing a set of segmentation techniques, in which they pointed out that segmentation techniques thus far were strongly application dependent. For example, in medical imaging, edge detection techniques were favored by most researchers in chest X-rays, whereas thresholding and clustering techniques were widely used by researchers in cell image segmentation. Semantic and *a priori* information about the type of images was critical to the solution of the segmentation problem. Fu and Mui pointed out that one of the best and most useful methods of segmentation was the combination of spatial and semantic information with edge detection and thresholding or clustering techniques for image segmentation. After a short time, Haralick and Shapiro [183] also published a survey paper summarizing a set of segmentation techniques. Haralick and Shapiro classified the segmentation techniques as measurement space-guided spatial clustering, single-linkage region growing schemes, hybrid-linkage region growing schemes, centered-linkage region growing schemes, spatial clustering schemes, and split-and-merge techniques. In this sub-section edge-based techniques based on facet least squares, wavelets and gradient-based techniques will be discussed.

3.3.4.1   Facet-Based LV Edge Detection

Haralick's work continued in low level edge detection and was applied in cardiac image processing. For example, Haralick's [184], [185] zero crossing work was very useful in diaphragm detection. In this work, an edge occurred on a pixel if, and only if, there was some point in the pixel's area with a negatively sloped zero crossing of the second directional derivative taken in the direction of a non-zero gradient at the pixel's center. Haralick used a functional form consisting of a linear combination of the tensor products of discrete orthogonal polynomials of up to the third degree. Haralick assumed that in each neighborhood of the image, the underlying gray tone intensity function f took the parametric form of a polynomial in row and column coordinates. Haralick also assumed sampling of the digital picture function as a regular equal-interval grid sampling of the square plane which was the domain of f. Thus, in each neighborhood, f took the facet model form:

$$f(r,c) = K_1 + K_2\,r + K_3\,c + K_4\,r^2 + K_5\,rc + K_6\,c^2 + K_7 r^3 + K_8\,r^2 c + K_9\,rc^2 + K_{10}\,c^3\,,$$
$$(3.1)$$

where the coefficients K_1 to K_{10} changed from one neighborhood to another and were estimated using a Least Square error surface fit. A pixel was marked as an edge if, in the pixel's immediate area, there was a zero crossing of the second directional derivative taken in the direction of the gradient and the slope of the zero crossing was negative. The advantage of the cubic fitting model was that the residual error was small since the polynomial was of a high degree. Also, this edge detector was less sensitive to noise compared with traditional edge detectors, like those of Sobel and Prewitt. The edge-based technique was also presented by Davis [186]. Another choice of edge detection based on morphology was by Lee and Haralick [187].

3.3.4.2 Wavelet-Based LV Edge Detection

Setarehdan and Soraghan [107], [189], [190] addressed the issue of LV boundary extraction in echocardiogram images using a combination of fuzzy logic (see Zadeh [191]) and multi-resolution edge detection. Setarehdan and Soraghan's algorithm consisted of two major steps. First, the point inside the LV cavity was estimated using knowledge of standard echo views and heart morphology. This point was important since the radial lines were made to originate from this point outward. It was along these radial lines that an edge was searched using the wavelet transform. The acceptable error for center point detection was 10%. In the second step, Setarehdan and Soraghan searched for a global maximum of the wavelet transform $W(f(s,t))$ in the scale-space domain which corresponded to a positive edge. Equation (3.2) shows the wavelet transform of the function $f(s,t)$, where s is the scale and t is the support index. Setarehdan and Soraghan computed the first derivative of a function and took its wavelet transform. If the wavelet transform yielded a maximum, then that position was an edge. This, however, depended upon the factor s, called the index of the scale. The maximum s value depended on the length of the signal and on the scales together in the scale-space plane.

$$W(f(s,t)) \quad = \quad \sqrt{(|s|)} \int \frac{df(x)}{dx} \phi(\frac{(t-x)}{x}) dx \qquad (3.2)$$

The radial search-based strategy has the advantage of reducing the boundary searching problem from two-dimensions to one-dimension, which is an important factor in reducing the processing time. Moreover, edge detection on radial lines, which is usually perpendicular to the boundary, produces better edge estimates and makes it unnecessary to use directional operators. A common problem with the radial search-based strategy is the high noise sensitivity of edge detection over radial lines. This is basically due to limiting the knowledge used for edge detection to only one-dimensional intensity information in a two-dimensional image (see the results in Figure 3.13).

3.3.4.3 Gradient-Based Techniques

Tu and Goldgof [192] proposed an edge detection technique to extract boundaries in deformable objects. Their data set consisted of 3-D cardiac images in the time domain. Tu and Goldgof pointed out that it was very difficult to compare and evaluate the plethora of edge operators because some operators

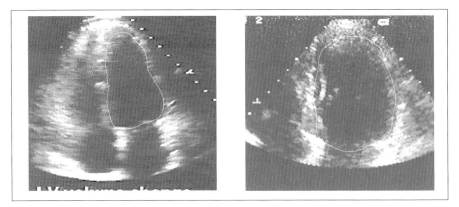

Figure 3.13: Typical examples of extracted LVE. **Left**: in a 4-chamber view. **Right**: in a 2-chamber apical LA 2DE view. (Courtesy of S. K. Setarehdan, University of Strathclyde, Glasgow, UK).

found more edges but responded strongly to noise, while others could be noise-insensitive but missed some crucial edges. Tu and Goldgof proposed the idea of spatio-temporal edge detection to extract boundaries of deformable objects where the time domain was another dimension similar to the space dimension. The capability of estimating the discontinuity in the time domain enabled the spatio-temporal edge operator to have a higher gradient magnitude. For this reason, Tu and Goldgof claimed that these operators had a higher gradient magnitude and were given as follows: for the 3-D edge detector, Tu and Goldgof simply extended the 2-D gradient operator to the third and fourth dimensions. If f was the original gray level signal and i, j and k are the unit vectors in the positive x, y and z directions, then Tu and Goldgof gave the 3-D extension as $\nabla f(x, y, x) = \frac{\partial f}{\partial x}i + \frac{\partial f}{\partial y}j + \frac{\partial f}{\partial z}k$ where $|\nabla f(x,y,x)| = \sqrt{(\frac{\partial f}{\partial x})^2 + (\frac{\partial f}{\partial y})^2 + (\frac{\partial f}{\partial z})^2}$. Tu and Goldgof simply added the fourth dimension to the time t for the 4-D edge detection, i.e., $\nabla f(x, y, x) = \frac{\partial f}{\partial x}i + \frac{\partial f}{\partial y}j + \frac{\partial f}{\partial z}k + \frac{\partial f}{\partial t}v$, where $|\nabla f(x,y,x)| = \sqrt{(\frac{\partial f}{\partial x})^2 + (\frac{\partial f}{\partial y})^2 + (\frac{\partial f}{\partial z})^2 + (\frac{\partial f}{\partial t})^2}$. Note $\frac{\partial f}{\partial x}$, $\frac{\partial f}{\partial y}$ and $\frac{\partial f}{\partial z}$ are the partial differentiation of function f in the x, y and z directions. In discrete terms, the values are the difference in gray scale intensities of the pixels taken into consideration. Tu and Goldgof presented the edge detector formula for 3-D and 4-D data sets, but there was no performance validation of these detectors. Tu and Goldgof did not compare the edges with the standard boundaries drawn by the cardiologist and, hence, the performance of the edge detectors could not be predicted.

3.3.4.4   Statistical-Based Matched Filtering

Detmer *et al.* [80] presented a matched filter-based approach to endocardial border estimation in echocardiograms. A maximum likelihood method was used to choose the endocardial border points from the matched filter output peaks obtained from radial intensity profiles centered within the ventricle. The theory of matched filtering has been comprehensively reviewed by Turin [193]. The mathematical operation was simply a cross-correlation of a reference signal (called the template in spatial applications) with the input signal to be processed. The template is a model of the signal to be detected, which in Detmer *et al.*'s case was the amplitude profile of the ultrasonic echo across the endocardial border. The essential feature of a matched filter was that the resulting output signal was maximized when the input signal best matched the template. The vector form of the computations yielded a rapid execution by an array processor. Detmer *et al.*'s algorithm consisted of seven steps: (**1**) median filtering using 9×9 pixels was done to smooth the image. (**2**) Background subtraction, i.e., the smoothed image subtracted from the original image, took place. (**3**) Extraction of intensity profiles along radial lines originating from the center of the image was computed. (**4**) Matched filtering on each intensity profile by cross-correlation with the border template was done. Detmer *et al.* observed that the positive peak in the matched filter output appeared as bright regions along the radial lines. The location of the peak, the radial distance and the amplitude of the peak were stored. (**5**) Since the distribution was independent, the joint probability of a peak being a border point was the product of amplitude rank and radius probabilities. The border point was the point with the maximum joint probability. (**6**) Selection of the maximum peak along the borders took place. (**7**) Removal of outlying border points by choosing a new centroid of the current border and repeating the process was performed. The mean boundary distance between the estimated boundaries and the hand-drawn outlines computed by Detmer *et al.* for endocardial borders was 3.32 mm. Detmer *et al.*'s study, however, used fairly high-quality transesophageal images. Also, Detmer *et al.*'s algorithm generated endocardial boundaries which excluded the papillary muscles.

3.3.4.5 LV Detection Based on Artificial Intelligence

Grattoni *et al.* [194] presented a sequence of steps to outline the LV cavity from the ED angiographic images in RAO projection in the human heart. Grattoni called the LV processing "sui-generis", which meant they were subject to great variations from case to case. Grattoni's algorithm consisted of four major steps: (**1**) low pass filtering or averaging to smooth the LV images; (**2**) non-linear filtering by a Sobel operator to compute the gradient directions; (**3**) thresholding the gradient image by keeping certain parts of the edges by computing the maximum of the gradient magnitude in the directions of its maximum rate of change of the gradient; and (**4**) using a heuristic boundary follower to connect the edge-based information. Grattoni used the A* algorithm from artificial intelligence. The problem was solved by looking at the LV contour as a set of segments of designated length (stroke) obtained on the gradient image. Thus, the search for the true contour was reduced to finding the optimized path in a weighted graph, whose stated space had been implicitly defined as the set of all strokes (nodes of the graph) that was used by the successor operator. The successor operator consisted of a procedure that searched all strokes inside a 32×32 window (search region). Here, search regions were opened over the gradient image as a function of position and direction of the parent node. Successors were obtained by an algorithm which linked contour points, filling gaps of $l \leq 2$ pixels to form smooth curves. Each stroke was accepted only if $l \leq 4$ pixels. Note that the search procedure for the optimal path on the graph was provided by the heuristic information about the behavior of the LV contour. Grattoni did mention the issue of large variability in shapes from case to case, but the algorithm presented did not handle this. The A* algorithm is acceptable for a heuristic search, but the inherent problem with this method is that if the number of strokes is large, then one needs to have a pre-filtering step to reduce the processing steps. This would pose a great challenge. Grattoni did not discuss it.

3.3.5   Mathematical Morphology-Based Techniques

3.3.5.1   Marker-Based

Beucher [196] developed a watershed segmentation algorithm for segmenting pictures using the tools provided by mathematical morphology. This methodology was based on the marking of the objects to be segmented. The marking provided a marker set which was used to modify the gradient of the image. Then, using a geodesic transformation [199], a new gradient image was produced. The main characteristic of this modified gradient image was that its minima fitted the various connected components of the marker set exactly. The second step consisted of the watershed morphological transform over the gradient image. This watershed transformation produced a partition of the image into homogeneous regions called a catchment basin. Every catchment basin contained only one marker and its boundary corresponded to the pixels of the image where the contrast was locally maxima. As a result, the transformed image exhibited the contours of the marked objects. Beucher showed segmentation techniques on traffic lane images (page 80 of [196]) which worked very well on those images because there was already information about the lanes. The markers were able to pick up the lanes well. The problem was too simple. What happened when one lane started to interfere with another lane in the traffic images? What happened when the fuzzy zone started to appear by overlapping one of the side traffic lanes? In such cases, the distinguishing markers were very difficult to generate and no technique was presented. Some *a priori* knowledge could have helped to solve part of the problem. Another problem was what happened when traffic lanes started to vanish with distance? In other words, the contrast values started to decrease in the image from one end to the other. Under such conditions, the markers would be of the right size and the watershed algorithm would pick up false edges. This can also be seen happening in LVGs. Overlapping of the diaphragm near the inferior zone of the LV causes contrast values to start to decrease with distance down the longitudinal axis of the LV.

3.3.5.2 Neighborhood Graph-Based

Vincent and Soille [198] and Beucher [197] developed a watershed segmentation algorithm for segmenting objects from noisy images. Vincent and Soille proposed a robust and accurate method for segmenting gray scale images of corneal endothelial tissues. The algorithm consisted of the following steps. Step one consisted of the extraction of the markers of the corneal cells using a dome extractor based on morphological gray scale reconstruction. Step two consisted of watershed segmentation yielding binary images of the corneal cell network. The condition of the corneal cells was decided on the histogram of the cell sizes and the number of neighbors. Vincent and Soille then constructed the neighborhood graph of the corneal cells that presented information about the granulometric analysis of the distribution of the cells with a large number of neighbors in the tissue. Lastly, Vincent and Soille presented the model that could identify dead corneal endothelial tissues. The first step consisted of a morphological filter to remove the impulse noise while preserving the valley (dark lines between the two cells). This step was a great location to start for cell images because the valley lines separated the two cells well.

How good is watershed segmentation in LVG processing? In LVGs, the concept of division hardly exists because the dye barely propagates down the LV or near the anterior and inferior walls, thus making the division line barely visible. Step two of Vincent and Soille's approach was marker reconstruction. This would go well with endothelial cell images and with LVGs, but the size of the marker could be a problem in the case of LVGs. Marker size was an important factor in searching for edges in the next step. If the marker was too small, then there was a very high likelihood of obtaining a false edge in the left ventriculogram. A narrower marker meant a large Region of Interest for the edge search. In LVG, a marker was likely to be small in size because the dye area was small inside the LV. As for the cells, they were very tiny, so even a small marker was enough in that case. Step three, the most crucial step, was the watershed segmentation. In this technique, the lines which divide the two regions were computed. The two regions are considered to be catchment basins or valleys. One can imagine water starting to fill these catchment basins and when it reaches the peak, those points become the dividing points between the two basins or regions. This technique is popular and simple, but the issue is in which region one wants to apply the watershed algorithm. In the case of cell images, valley lines (which, as pointed out in step one, are visible) were picked up rapidly by the watershed algorithm. In the LVG case, the valley lines were barely there, so the watershed segmentation did not give the correct edge. Watershed lines were very likely to have the position of an edge at the wrong location. The approach taken by Suri [28] was analogous to the watershed where he finds the shoulder edges in the elliptical band of the LV in the left ventriculograms. This elliptical band already incorporated global shape information because it was generated from the classifier boundaries [201]. In addition, Suri [28] used the knowledge of the changing gradient angles along the curvature of the walls. These gradient angles were not a simple gradient operation, but were based on a facet model and cubic fitting approach. Lastly, Vincent and Soille used only normal patient studies for their population, while Suri used both normal and abnormal patient studies.

3.3.6   Drawbacks of Low-Level LV Segmentation Techniques

The majority of low-level techniques were based either on plain thresholding, histogramming or radial edge estimation. These techniques totally depended upon the local characteristics of the spatial distribution of intensities. They lacked modeling of spatial neighborhood interdependence and temporal coherence. Not much prior distribution was used. A few examples, like Haralick's facet model and Setahedran's wavelet transform, are effective model-based edge techniques. These models can be used in integration with high-level techniques. Wavelet transform has dominated the mammography field. Interested readers can see Mallat [124] and Wang *et al.* [200]. Low-level techniques were seen to emerge as a sequence of steps and the idea of involving hand-drawing was not used extensively. As a result, the concept of fitting mathematical equations to justify the approach did not exist. All of the above drawbacks were compensated by model-based pattern recognition cardiac imaging, which is discussed in the next sub-section.

3.4   Model-Based Pattern Recognition Methods for LV Modeling

Model-based cardiac computer vision and pattern recognition methods are methods where mathematical models are built on the basis of anatomical knowledge such as shapes, position, size and orientation. The main idea behind model-based techniques is choosing a mathematical model which resembles the LV shape and then tailoring the mathematical model to fit the data. In this fitting process, the fitting parameters are estimated using part of the LV data, preferably off-line. These off-line parameters are then used in modeling the new LV data. The greatest asset of the model-based CVPR techniques is the ability to dynamically update during the fitting process. Another feature of model-based techniques is that no matter what the data size was, there was no load on the user. The model was made to automatically adjust the data size by changing the dimensions of the mathematical equations. These CVPR models have the ability to learn the shape, study shape correspondences and use neighboring information to develop time analysis. The ability to incorporate low-level features in these mathematical models is one of the extraordinary features of the model-based CVPR techniques. In brief, model-based techniques have helped in the integration of imaging modality, anatomical knowledge, integration of experience and learning ability of the LV: their shapes, sizes, position, orientation and movements. The interesting point about model-based CVPR techniques is that in the last two decades (1979–99), there has been an explosive growth in model-based LV segmentation and its modeling. In this sub-section it will be shown that these model-based approaches are faster, more accurate, reliable, robust and noise insensitive.

Model-based CVPR techniques will be covered as follows: Sub-section 3.4.1 presents active contour-based models utilizing energy. Sub-section 3.4.2 presents the training models. Sub-section 3.4.3 presents the polyline method for the performance evaluation of model-based techniques. Sub-section 3.4.4 presents a discussion on data analysis using the greedy approach method.

3.4.1 LV Active Contour Models in the Spatial and Temporal Domains

3.4.1.1 Energy Minimization Concept

In 1988 Wikins and Terzopoulos [209] published a paper titled "Snakes: Active Contour Models", which presented an energy-minimizing spline guided by external and image forces that pulled the spline towards features such as lines and edges in the image. The energy-minimizing spline was named a "snake" because the spline moved softly and quietly while minimizing the energy. Snakes were an example of the more general technique of matching a deformable model to an image by means of energy minimization. A starting contour was first placed by the user and then the snake deformed itself into conformity with the nearest salient contour. Snakes did not solve the entire problem of finding the salient image contour but relied on another mechanism to place itself somewhere near the desired contour. The active contour model differed from the traditional approaches to edge detection and edge linking in that the active contour model was based on a variational approach which was dynamic because of the iterative nature of the differential equation. The total energy of the snake was given as:

$$E_{snake} = \int E_{int} + \int E_{ext} , \qquad (3.3)$$

where $\int E_{int}$ and $\int E_{ext}$ were the internal and external energies of the contour, respectively. The internal energy of the contour could be taken as the energy of the spline and this energy was composed of two terms: the first term was the first order derivative of the parametric curve given as $v_s(s)$. This term acted like a membrane. The second term was the second derivative of the parametric curve given as $v_{ss}(s)$. This term represented a thin plate. These terms were controlled by the constants $\alpha(s)$ and $\beta(s)$. On the basis of this reasoning, the internal energy term was given mathematically[9] as:

$$E_{int} = \frac{\alpha(s) \, |v_s(s)|^2 + \beta(s)|v_{ss}(s)|^2}{2} . \qquad (3.4)$$

Note that since it was an energy term, the first and second order terms were squared, added and divided by a factor of 2. Snakes had flexibility since they

---

[9]The variational-based principle was used for solving the energy minimization equation. For details, see Wikins *et al.* [209].

could be dynamically controlled, but there were inherent drawbacks when they were applied to low contrast images, those which had a lot of noise, or those which had objects with sharp bends and corners. The snake's accuracy to minimize energy depended upon the external energy, which in turn depended upon image forces or image energy. This was the function of the image gradient. In LVgrams, the image gradient was very poor and not in its correct place, thus this energy contributed little to pushing the snake curve towards the ideal contour drawn by the cardiologist.

3.4.1.2   Application of Snakes to MR Cardiac Data Set

Singh *et al.* [210] discussed an algorithm for LV segmentation in cardiac MR slices based on information propagation in space and time. Here, the information being propagated was the initial hand-drawn contour in one of the reference slices selected. The propagation criterion in space was based on the minimization of energy (in the spirit of the active contour model). The final estimated 2-D LV contour at $(z + 1)^{th}$ slice used information at z^{th} slice in depth, similarly, the 2-D LV contour at $(t + 1)^{th}$ time used information at t^{th} time. Singh decomposed the internal energy term into two components, E_{int1} and E_{int2}. The first and second terms of internal energy were the first and second order partial differential of the entire parametric curve, i.e., $\int_s |v_s(s)|^2 ds$ and $\int_s |v_{ss}(s)|^2 ds$. Thus, the final expression of internal energy in the discrete case as the summation of its two components $E_{int} = \alpha_1 E_{int1} + \alpha_2 E_{int2}$ was:

$$E_{int} = \alpha_1 \sum_s |v(s) - v(s-1)|^2 + \alpha_2 \sum_s |v(s+1) - 2v(s) + v(s-1)|^2 . \quad (3.5)$$

Similarly, the external energy terms were broken into two terms, E_{ext1} and E_{ext2}. The term E_{ext1} was derived from the fact that the intensity of all points on the LV boundary is almost constant for a given slice. If the intensity at the point $(x(s), y(s))$ was given as $I((x(s), y(s))$ and the constant intensity as I_c, then the external energy term was given as $\sum_s \{|I(x(s), y(s)) - I_c| - K\}$, where K was a constant positive value. The second term of the external energy was derived from the intensity gradient and was given as $\int_s \nabla I(x(s), y(s))^2$, where ∇ denoted the gradient operation in x and y directions represented by S_x and S_y. Combining the first and second terms of external energy in the discrete case, $E_{ext} = \beta_1 E_{ext1} + \beta_2 E_{ext2}$ was:

$$\begin{aligned} E_{ext} &= \beta_1 \sum_s \{|I(x(s), y(s)) - I_c| - K\} \\ &+ \beta_2 \sum_s \{-[S_x * I(x(s), y(s)]^2 + [S_y * I(x(s), y(s)]^2\} . \end{aligned} \quad (3.6)$$

Note that $v(s) = (x(s), y(s))$ represented the parametric representation of the contour, I_c was the density of the pixel. β_1 and β_2 were the constants.

Since Singh's algorithm was in the spirit of Kass's algorithm of active contouring, a very key difference will be presented. In Singh's implementation, energy minimization was done on *a fraction* (five pixels) of the entire LV contour, rather than on the *entire contour*. This process was similar to Shah's algorithm [226]. The fractional curve could be unstable when the central pixel was at a sharp curvature due to noise; however, Singh imposed a configuration and this condition was nullified. Singh remarked that the performance of the algorithm was very good. If the gap between slices (inter-slice distance) was large, it was possible that the wrong segmentation of LV could occur, which could be due to noise or other structures. The system was semi-automatic. Energy minimization was not optimal and the weighting parameters α_1, α_2, β_1, β_2 were entered manually. In such a process, parameter selection could be improved by taking a large database and picking the global shape information of the LV in MR using the cardiologist's assistance.

Another form of snakes, called coupled snakes, was first given by Richens *et al.* [211]. The new aspect about Richens' work was the following: given a contour, one can find the energy of the contour. Using the same formula, one can couple two contours (strong contours) to estimate the third contour (called the weak contour). The reason for doing this was that images taken from the diastolic stage of ventricular filling can often provide a weaker signal from the inside of the ventricle due to the lower blood flow and as a result, the endocardial border is less prominent. Richens' method guided the contour of the weak image using the contours of the two strong images, before and after the weak image.

3.4.1.3 Cardiac Active Contouring in Time

In ultrasound imaging, Chalana *et al.* [76] applied the snake model as developed by Kass. The two energy components for the total energy of the contour as given by Kass were $E_{snake} = \int E_{int} + \int E_{ext}$, where $\int E_{int}$ and $\int E_{ext}$ were the internal and external energies of the contour, respectively. Internal energy was accounted as:

$$E_{int} \quad = \quad w_1(s)|V_s(s)|^2 + w_2(s)|V_{ss}(s)|^2. \tag{3.7}$$

Chalana *et al.* modified the above equation as follows: Here, the first and second terms of the internal energy were given as the first and second partial differential terms of degrees one and two. These two terms were given as $V_s(s,r)$ and $V_{ss}(s,r)$. Note these terms are exactly the same as presented by Kass previously. The first and second order surfaces with respect to r were given as $V_r(s,r)$ and $V_{rr}(s,r)$. The in-plane constraints were given as $V_{sr}(s,r)$. Since all these terms reflected energy, thus they were normed, squared and integrated with respect to parameters s and r and were given as:

$$E_{in} \quad = \quad \int\int w_1 \, ||V_s(s,r)||^2 + w_2 \, ||V_{ss}(s,r)||^2 + w_3 \, ||V_r(s,r)||^2 ds dr \tag{3.8}$$

$$+ \int\int w_4 \, ||V_{rr}(s,r)||^2 + w_5 \, ||V_{sr}(s,r)||^2 ds \, dr \ .$$

Note the elastic (stretching) and bending terms in the third dimension, V_{sr} were the energy of interaction between in-planes and between planes; s was the normalized contour length and had a value between 0 and 1 and r was the in-plane index and also took a value in between 0 and 1. Chalana *et al.* modified Kass' external energy term as:

$$E_{ext} = E_{grad} + E_{time}, \qquad (3.9)$$

where $E_{ext} = -w \int \int G_\sigma * || \bigtriangledown I(x(s,r), y(s,r), r)|| \, ds \, dr$ and E_{time} was given as:

$$
\begin{aligned}
E_{time} = & -w_t \int \int (v(s,r) - v(s, r - \epsilon)) \, ds \, dr \\
& + w_t \int \int (v(s, r - \epsilon) - v(s,r)) \, ds \, dr \,.
\end{aligned} \qquad (3.10)
$$

Note that the first term was for the systole (r to $r - \epsilon$) cycle, while the second term was for the diastole ($r - \epsilon$ to ϵ) cycle, ϵ represented incremental change. The above equations could be solved using the Euler-Lagrange method as solved by Kass.

Limitations of Chalana's Method: (**1**) the active contour model assumed that the image sequences were registered with respect to each other, but actually, the transducer and patient did move during the scanning process. Chalana *et al.*'s model did not use temporal gradient information, so it was acceptable to use the active contour model independently for each time frame. However, if one used the time information model, then the active contour model required a pre-registration step. (**2**) Chalana's first version of the active contour model relied only on gradient information derived by Canny's operator. Certainly Canny's operator was a good choice, but too simple and non-robust for highly noisy ultrasound images, which require a reliable LV contouring system. (**3**) Lastly, the user interface problem existed, i.e., it required user interaction at the first stage. One solution would be to use Setarehdan and Soraghan's [107] approach of estimating a center point in the LV using fuzzy logic and then computing the raw edges using the wavelet transform. This raw edge boundary can now undergo the regularization term as used by Chalana *et al.* in the boundary estimation process of a fetal head in ultrasound images. So far, an attempt has not been made in ultrasound images, where a combination of several algorithms can be used, just like a Bayesian approach for edge detection can be utilized in conjunction with fitting and regularization to approach this problem.

3.4.1.4 Fourier Snakes

In the elasticity domain, Szekely *et al.* [213] developed a Fourier parameterized model to create Fourier snakes in 2-D and elastically-deformable Fourier surface models in 3-D. By using the Fourier parameterizations followed by a statistical analysis of a training set, Szekely defined the mean organ models and their eigen deformations. An elastic fit of the mean model in the sub-space of eigen-modes restricted possible deformations and found an optimal match between

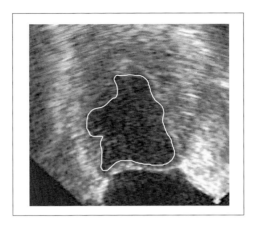

Figure 3.14: Application of level sets to an ultrasound LV image. Courtesy of Chenyang Xu, Johns Hopkins University, Baltimore, MD. For further details on level set methods, see Chapter 4.

the model surface and boundary candidates. This work was very similar to Cootes *et al.* [227]. Its comparison will be postponed until training models in the point domain have been dealt with. Similar work can be seen in Clarysse *et al.* [214].

3.4.1.5   Level Set Approach to LV Boundary Estimation

With the evolution of differential geometry and partial differential equations, fast marching methods have started to be used in applications for LV boundary estimation (see the application of WM/GM boundary estimation by Suri in Chapter 4). The idea is to capture the LV topology in time using fuzzy clustering and force the user-defined contour towards the final position. An example of such a modeling is shown in Figure 3.14.

3.4.1.6   Superquadratic Fitting

Superquadratic fitting-research at INRIA[10]: Superquadratic fitting is popular in cardiac imaging. Bardinet *et al.* [215], [216], Ayache [217] and Staib *et al.* [218] fitted a deformable superquadratic to segment 3-D cardiac CT and SPECT images. These models were then refined using the volumetric deformation technique known as free form deformations (FFD). The complete algorithm can be summarized as follows: (**1**) extraction of the 3-D data points in the time sequence of slices, (**2**) superellipsoid fitting to find the set of parameters so that the superellipsoid best fits the above 3-D data points. The fitting satisfied the equation $F = 1$ and F was given as:

$$\left\{\left[\left(\frac{x}{a_1}\right)^{\frac{2}{\epsilon_2}} + \left(\frac{y}{a_2}\right)^{\frac{2}{\epsilon_2}}\right]^{\frac{\epsilon_2}{\epsilon_1}} + \left(\frac{z}{a_3}\right)^{\frac{2}{\epsilon_1}}\right\}^{\frac{\epsilon_1}{2}} , \qquad (3.11)$$

---

[10]Institut National de Recherche en Informatique et Automatique; Research Reports of INRIA can be ftp'ed from: ftp.inria.fr/INRIA/publication/pub-ps-gz/RR

where a_1, a_2 and a_3 were constants. ϵ's are the parameters of shape change. Note the left hand side is the equation of the superellipsoid surface. If one looks carefully, $\frac{x}{a_1}$, when squared and added to the squared of the term $\frac{y}{a_2}$, was the equation of the ellipse in a 2-D plane. In the above equation, the power was changed from 2 to $\frac{2}{\epsilon_2}$. Adding the third dimension, one gets $\frac{z}{a_3}$ with the power $\frac{2}{\epsilon_1}$. The whole expression was raised to the power of $\frac{\epsilon_1}{2}$. Therefore, the whole idea was to change an ellipse to an ellipsoid, controlling the shape by ϵ's. (**3**) The refinement stage, the so-called FFD, where the Least Squares fitting was performed between the object and the box, was done. A good physical analogy for FFD is to consider a parallelepiped of clear, flexible plastic in which is embedded an object, or several objects, which is to be deformed. The object is imagined to be flexible, so that it deforms along with the plastic that surrounded it. Mathematically, the FFD was defined in terms of a tensor product trivariate Bernstein polynomial. If one imposes a local coordinate system on a parallelepiped region in three orthogonal directions, any point $\mathbf{X}$ has (s, t, u) coordinates in this system so that $\mathbf{X} = \mathbf{X}_0 + s\mathbf{S} + t\mathbf{T} + u\mathbf{U}$, where s, t, u can all be computed using linear algebra. On imposing a grid of control points $\mathbf{P}_{ilk}$ on the parallelepiped and letting it form $l+1$, $m+1$ and $n+1$ planes in $\mathbf{S}, \mathbf{T}, \mathbf{U}$ directions, then these points lie on the lattice and their locations are defined as: $\mathbf{P}_{ijk} = X_0 + \frac{i}{l}\mathbf{S} + \frac{j}{m}\mathbf{T} + \frac{k}{m}\mathbf{U}$. The deformation was specified by moving $\mathbf{P}_{ijk}$ from their undisplaced lattice positions. The deformation function was defined by a trivariate tensor product polynomial. The deformed position $\mathbf{X}_{ffd}$ was thus given as:

$$\mathbf{X}_{ffd} = \sum_i \sum_j \sum_k C_l^i \left(1 - s\right)^{l-i} s^i \; C_m^j \left(1 - t\right)^{m-j} t^j \; C_n^k \left(1 - u\right)^{n-k} u^k \; \mathbf{P}_{ijk} \; ,$$

(3.12)

where $\mathbf{P}_{ijk}$ denoted the volumetric grid of the control points, (s, t, u) denoted by the local coordinates of the object points in a frame defined by the box of control points and (l, m, n) denoted the degrees of the Bernstein polynomials. C_l^i, C_m^j and C_n^k were the coefficients. The results of Bardinet's algorithm are shown in Figures 3.15 and 3.16.

INRIA vs. University of Washington (UW), Seattle: UW Seattle has implemented algorithms in the area of LV image analysis and modeling. In step one, INRIA performed superellipsoidal fitting to the LV data set, while UW performed Bayesian model fitting using training data collected from hand-traced boundaries. In step two, INRIA performed the Least Squares free-form deformation to smooth the boundaries, while UW did the Least Squares calibration, which is also a smoothing step. The ultimate goal of FFD and calibration is the same. However, the number of parameters estimated in the UW case were 10,000 to 40,000, while INRIA solved for no more than 300 parameters. Although INRIA did present the 3-D views of the surfaces of the epicardium and endocardium, no validation was presented in 2-D which could validate the 3-D reconstruction.

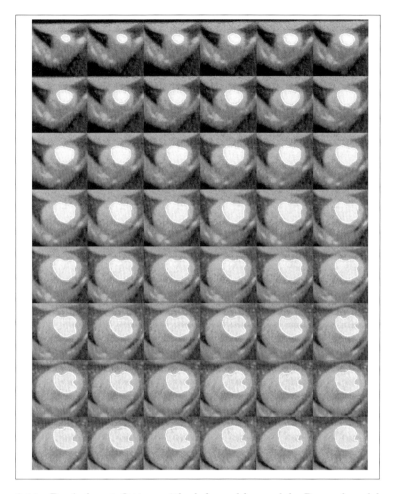

Figure 3.15: Dog's heart fitting with deformable model. Reproduced by permission of Oxford University Press from [216].

3.4.1.7 LV Fourier Decomposition

In active modeling, Staib *et al.* [220] presented a parametrically deformable contour model to represent a closed contour using an elliptic Fourier decomposition method, given by:

$$
\begin{bmatrix} x(t) \\ y(t) \end{bmatrix} = \begin{bmatrix} a_0 \\ b_0 \end{bmatrix} + \sum_{k=1}^{\infty} \begin{bmatrix} a_k \ b_k \\ c_k \ d_k \end{bmatrix} \begin{bmatrix} cos\,kt \\ sin\,kt \end{bmatrix} , \tag{3.13}
$$

where $x(t), y(t)$ were the points on the contour, a_k, b_k, c_k, d_k were the raw coefficients of the Fourier expansion. Upon examining these more carefully, one sees: $x(t) = a_0 + a_1\,cos(t) + b_1\,sin(t) + a_2\,cos(2t) + b_2\,sin(2t)...$, where a_0, a_1, b_1, a_2, b_2 are Fourier constants. Similarly, one has $y(t)$ as: $y(t) = b_0 +$

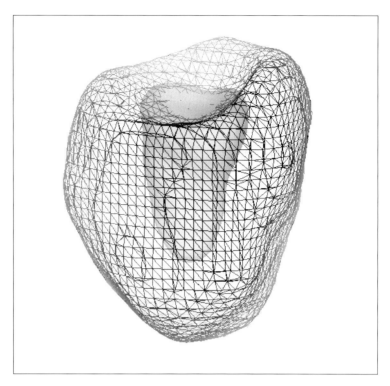

Figure 3.16: 3D display of the epicardium and the endocardium of the LV Reproduced by permission of Oxford University Press from [216].

$c_1\,cos(t) + d_1\,sin(t) + c_2\,cos(2t) + d_2\,sin(2t)...$, where b_0, c_1, d_1, c_2, d_2 are Fourier constants. Thus, the elliptical properties were expressed using the Fourier expansion. If the elliptical parameters were given by a vector $\mathbf{p}$, then the parameters $\mathbf{p}$ were computed from the hand-drawn boundaries of the object from the given population. In step two, Staib did the matching using correlation, where the ellipse was the template and a search procedure was done on the gradient of the image, $\bigtriangledown I$. Staib then found $\mathbf{p}$, which maximized the probability $P(\bigtriangledown I|\mathbf{p})$. This method can be considered a combination of training and fitting: training because the $\mathbf{p}$ was computed from the training population and fitting because the algorithm tried to maximize $P(\bigtriangledown I|\mathbf{p})$, to obtain the final contour. Staib called this a parametric deformable model because the final contour was estimated after the deformation of the initial contour using the probabilistic approach to maximize the posterior estimate (similar to Lee [201]) of the parameter vector $\mathbf{p}$. It has been seen that success in cardiac imaging was being dominated by use of a combination of training, fitting and estimating good priors.

3.4.1.8 LV Ballooning

Miller *et al.* [221] presented another technique called ballooning, which was in the spirit of a deformable model. In this technique, a polygon was approximated to a sphere and geometrically deformed a balloon model until the balloon surface conformed to the object surface in 3-D CT data. The segmentation process was formulated as the minimization of a cost function, where the desired behavior of the balloon model was determined by a local cost function associated with each model vertex. The cost function was a weighted sum of these three terms: a deformable potential that expanded the model vertices towards the object boundary, an image term that identified features such as edges and opposed balloon expansion, and a term that maintained the topology of the model by constraining each vertex to remain close to the centroid of the neighbors. Careful observation of this technique showed that the balloon model was like a weighted error reduction based on pixel gradient intensities, while the push-pull forces acted like constraints on the boundary and became deformed as per the desired shape.

3.4.1.9 Hierarchical LV Modeling

Chen and Huang [222] proposed a hierarchical motion model that was able to combine various cardiac motion and deformation models into one. They fitted a superquadratic model to LV data. By fitting the superquadratic model to the ground truth data, the deformation parameters are estimated by fitting the Least Squares model to the initial estimated LV contours. Spherical harmonic surfaces were closed surfaces that were functions on the sphere and could be decomposed into a set of orthogonal functions. The parameterization of the spherical harmonics can be done by two numbers, "m" and "n" and are continuous, orthogonal, single valued and complete on the sphere. In the spherical coordinate system, the basis functions are $U_{nm}(\phi, \theta)$ and $U_{nm}(\phi, \theta)$. Mathematically, these basis functions are defined as a Legendre polynomial given as: $U_{nm}(\phi, \theta) = cos(m\phi) \times P_{nm}(Cos(\theta))$ and $V_{nm}(\phi, \theta) = sin(m\phi) \times P_{nm}(Cos(\theta))$, where $P_{nm}(x) = (1 - x^2)^{\frac{m}{2}} \frac{d^m}{dx^m} . P_n(x)$. Chen and Huang took the standard approach to reconstruct the shape of the LV where the major component was a radius $r(\phi, \theta)$ which was given as a function of the product of the basis function and its coefficients. Thus, if A_{nm} and B_{nm} were the coefficients of the basis function, then the radial factor was mathematically given as:

$$r(\phi, \theta) = \sum_{n=1}^{N} \sum_{m=0}^{M} A_{nm} U_{nm}(\phi, \theta) + B_{nm} V_{nm}(\phi, \theta). \qquad (3.14)$$

The idea behind the model was to develop a closed surface with its functional properties. Chen's hierarchical decomposition was an excellent example of the conversion of the seemingly complex estimation procedure of the coupled parameterization into coarse-to-fine estimation sub-procedures. Chen and Huang used displacement field computation in their hierarchical model, which was complex to estimate from time-varying data in order to establish the frame-to-frame correspondence. Chen and Huang did propose a good definition of the longitudinal axis that passed through the centroid of the LV surface with orientation in such a direction that the sum of the squared distances between the axis and the individual points was at a minimum. This definition seemed justified for LV shapes which were elliptical in nature. There were two major drawbacks to this method. (**1**) The whole idea of the long axis was to determine the position of the apex. In abnormal patient studies with cardiomyopathy, aneurysms in the apical zone or in anterior or inferior walls, the long axis will not determine the apex of the LV. (**2**) The criterion[11] of estimating the LV centroid to let the long axis pass through the centroid would lead to the wrong direction. It is important not to ignore the idea that the long axis must fall in the bottom third of the LV cup whose curvature is maximum with respect to the aortic valve plane.

3.4.1.10   LV Polar Active Contouring

Revankar and Sher [223] presented the boundary estimation algorithm in ultrasound images based on the constraints of context, distance from the approximate contour and image gradient, all in polar coordinates. Revankar's algorithm found the optimal contour locations in all radial directions (other authors who used radial approaches were Detmer *et al.* [80] and Setarehdan [190]) according to all of the above constraints. When the algorithm's greedy nature is discussed later, the similarities and differences between Revankar's, Shah's and Suri's algorithms will be discussed. Another method of graph theory and a combination of mathematical morphology for estimating the boundary of the LV in ultrasound images can be seen in Wei [224]. Finally, in deformable models, O'Donel *et al.* [225] presented a deformable periodic generalized cylinder for simultaneously modeling and tracking closed contours which exhibited a repeating motion.

3.4.1.11   Energy Minimization Using the Greedy Approach

Williams and Shah [226] developed an algorithm based on the greedy nature for contour estimation of objects in images based on energy minimization and curvature. They assumed that the initial curve of the object was given. The greedy algorithm moved all the vertices of the initial contour towards the final or destination contour vertex by vertex in such a way that the total energy of the contour was at a minimum. At each vertex of the initial contour, a window, which could be the candidate for the new location where the energy was at a minimum, was searched for. The greedy cycle was repeated in such a way that each vertex was tested for a fixed number of movements set as the threshold by the user. After each greedy cycle, each vertex was given the chance to move to a new location so that the total energy was at minimum. The energy coefficients were based on the curvature, which was based on the

---

[11]Singular.

central difference. Williams and Shah used six different ways to estimate the curvature used in the greedy algorithm, one of which was energy minimization to constrain the contour to its right position. These approaches lacked full usage of the oscillation behavior of LV. There was not much usage of temporal information and correspondence. The technique was spatially constrained in each slice of the CT or MR or projection, echo or ultrasound images. In the next sub-section, another concept will be discussed which involves the physics of the LV motion.

3.4.1.12   Finite Element Models

In finite element LV modeling, the mathematical equations taken resemble the laws of physics, such as the pendulum equations of motion. Because the LV nature has an expansion and contraction process, researchers have tried modeling the LV as a second order motion equation. McInerney *et al.* [228], [229], presented a deformable model for medical image analysis. This was interesting research since there were distinctive similarities between active contour models and training-based modeling. Here we will discuss the algorithm used for LV modeling. McInerney's algorithm was summarized in a three step process. Step one consisted of user interaction to gather global shape information, like the center of the LV and size collection in each successive slice (just like Singh's algorithm [210]). In step two, image model construction, which consisted of fitting physics-based deformable models and solving the potential energy terms and dynamic equations, was done. The last step consisted of the refinement stage or smoothing process. McInerney *et al.*'s fitting process used deformable surface models to fit the data. They made the model dynamic as the data was time-varying. This dynamic formulation had the following two advantages: First, the data fitting process was shown as a smoothly animated display, and second, the user was made to interact with the model by applying a constraint force to pull it out of the local minima toward the correct shape. McInerney's deformation model, defined in the spatial and temporal domain at the point location, was represented by $\mathbf{x}(u, v, t)$. The model was simulated with a mass and damping densities. The deformation energy yielded internal elastic forces, and the potential energy term was minimized when these forces equilibrated against externally applied forces. The model stabilized when the first and second order differentials were set at zero. The fitting process was governed by a second order partial differential equation. This equation followed the law of physics of the pendulum where the first term was a second order term given as $\frac{\partial^2 \mathbf{x}}{\partial t^2}$ premultiplied by the mass of the LV. The second term was a single order term given as $\frac{\partial \mathbf{x}}{\partial t}$ pre-multiplied by the damping force γ. The last term represented the elastic forces which resist deformation. All these terms were added and equalized to external forces f_{ext} derived from the image data. Thus the final equation was given as:

$$\mu \frac{\partial^2 \mathbf{x}}{\partial t^2} + \gamma \frac{\partial \mathbf{x}}{\partial t} + \delta \epsilon_p = f_{ext} , \qquad (3.15)$$

where ϵ_p was the potential energy term and this energy was the deformation energy of a thin plate under tension. This term consisted of a partial differential equation premultiplied by constants. The first and the second terms were the first order differential equation in the u-v plane and were given as $|\frac{\partial \mathbf{x}}{\partial u}|$ and $|\frac{\partial \mathbf{x}}{\partial v}|$. The second and third terms were the partial differential equation of the second order given as $|\frac{\partial^2 \mathbf{x}}{\partial^2 u}|$ and $|\frac{\partial^2 \mathbf{x}}{\partial^2 v}|$. The last term was given as the cross energy term $|\frac{\partial^2 \mathbf{x}}{\partial u \partial v}|$. Now by changing these terms to energy by squaring the amplitude and adding them together, the final expression of potential energy becomes:

$$\epsilon_p(\mathbf{x}) = \int \int \alpha_a |\frac{\partial \mathbf{x}}{\partial u}| + \alpha_b |\frac{\partial \mathbf{x}}{\partial v}| + \beta_b |\frac{\partial^2 \mathbf{x}}{\partial^2 u}| + \beta_c |\frac{\partial^2 \mathbf{x}}{\partial u \partial v}| + \beta_d |\frac{\partial^2 \mathbf{x}}{\partial^2 v}|\} \, du \, dv. \quad (3.16)$$

Note that the constants were the terms which caused the stretching, twisting and bending. These terms were very critical in LV modeling, which were used manually by Singh. For details on these parameters, see Samadani [233]. Another attempt to model the LV using finite element analysis was done by Nielsen [230], [231]. For a good understanding of finite element analysis, the reader is recommended to see Zienkiewicz *et al.* [232].

3.4.1.13   Moment of Inertia Models

Grattoni *et al.* [194], [195] addressed the minimum-radial-inertia method for LV contour motion analysis in cineangiographic image sequences. Grattoni's work could be categorized as model-based work like the snakes. Here, every vertex of the contour was assumed to be radially connected and was described in an analytical form by means of periodic cubic splines. A detailed critique of Grattoni *et al.* can be found in the first chapter of Suri [28].

3.4.2   Model-Based Pattern Recognition Learning Methods

3.4.2.1   LV Segmentation Using Bayesian Classification

Lee [201], [202] used a pixel-based Bayesian approach to LV boundary estimation in LVgrams, where the gray scale values of the location throughout the cardiac cycle were taken as a vector (see Figure 3.17). Lee assumed that the distribution was bi-variate normal. For each observed vector, one class was assigned according to the ground truth, which was available by filling the LV region surrounded by the hand-drawn LV boundary. Mathematically, the problem was posed as: given gray scale images in systole N_s (or diastolic cycle N_d), classify a pixel at a location (x, y) having gray scale values $g_1, ...g_{N_s}$ (feature vector) to class c belonging to classes $1, 2, ...N_s, N_{s+1}$, where the class number c maximizes:

$$P(c|\mathbf{X}) = \frac{P(\mathbf{X}|c)P(c)}{P(\mathbf{X})}, \quad (3.17)$$

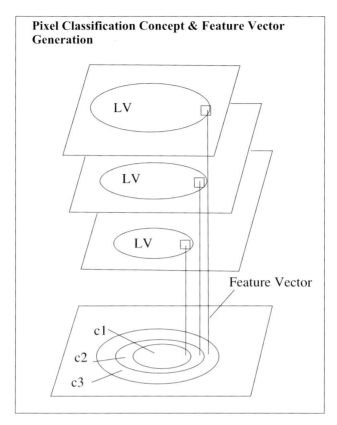

Figure 3.17: Pixel classification approach. Formation of the feature vectors **X** during the cardiac cycle. The projected LV's make different classes during the systole (or diastole). Note, c1, c2 and c3 represent three classes.

where $P(\mathbf{X}|c)$ is the class conditional probability that followed a multi-variate normal distribution and $P(c)$ was the prior class probability. The ground truth of a pixel through F frames of the cardiac cycle generated 2^F possible classes, but far fewer than 2^F classes were actually required in order to represent all existent classes. Due to the different heart rates (i.e., the variable number of frames in the cardiac cycle for different studies), Lee allowed different dimensions of the observation vector. Lee simultaneously segmented all the frames from ED through ES to the next ED, instead of separately segmenting each frame. Lee assumed that each pixel was statistically independent in the same frame but later modified that assumption by considering the nearest neighbor. The training system developed by Lee is partially shown in Figure 3.18.

   The left half consisted of the Bayes' classifier training system, which accepted gray scale LVgrams and LV hand-drawn boundaries. The output was classification parameters which were then applied on-line to the raw LVgram to estimate the initial pixel-based classification region. Using connected component analysis followed by boundary tracing, the system yielded the initial

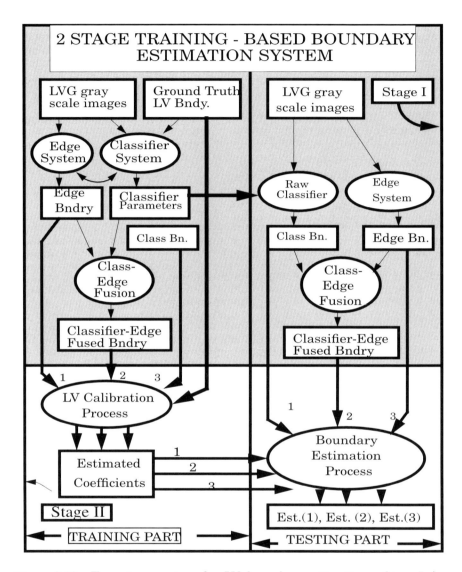

Figure 3.18: Two stage system for LV boundary estimation. Stage I (upper half, shown with darker background) consists of three approaches: pixel-classification approach, edge detection approach, and classification-edge fusion approach. Stage II (lower half, shown with lighter background) consists of the calibration stage, which smooths the raw boundaries produced in stage I. Left Half: Off-line training system. Right Half: On-line boundary estimation.

classification boundaries. The rest of the features of the overall system will be seen when we discuss CVPR techniques in more detail. For performance and error computation of the detected LV boundary, Lee compared the classifier boundary with the manually traced boundary using the Hausdorf distance measure, given as: $e(A, B) = maxmax\ i\{d(a_i, B)\}, max\ j\{d(b_j, A)\}\}$, where $d(a_i, B) = min\ j||b_j - a_i||$. Here, A and B are the 2-D shapes of the LV region. Note, $d(a_i, B)$ is the minimum distance from point a_i to all the points in shape B. Similarly, $d(b_j, A)$ is the minimum distance from point b_j to all the points in shape A. The Hausdorf distance is very popular in mathematical morphology for shape quantification (for further details, see Haralick *et al.* [244]). Because of the low gray scale contrast in the apical zone of the LV, Bayes' classifier boundaries were not close to the ground truth boundaries in that region. Furthermore, the boundaries produced by the classifier did not reflect the true LV shape and sometimes the ED and the ES boundaries could hardly be distinguished. The automatic contour tracing system (ACTS) model presented by Lee [202] modeled the heart motion by specifying an inner bound and outer bound of the motion between any two frames in terms of morphological operations. With these motion constraints, ACTS bounded the LV region in one frame of the cardiac cycle based on the classifier detected LV boundary in another frame (see Chapter 4 of Lee [201]). This can be called time-dependent or inter-frame dependent modeling. In the training-based point modeling of Sub-section 3.4.2.3, it will be seen that these classification boundaries can be further improved using calibration systems. Note that in Lee's technique, the posterior probability needs to be maximized given the image information. This is the formulation in a Bayesian sense. Similar to this, Wilson [205] studied the prior terms exhaustively in boundary estimation problems.

3.4.2.2 Probability-Based Surfaces

In probability-based approaches, van Bree [206] attempted to find the LV borders using a combination of probability surfaces and dynamic programming. Van Bree's algorithm can be summarized as follows. First, there was the building of the probability surfaces from a database of hand-drawn boundaries after the LV boundaries were corrected for translation and rotation. The second step consisted of generating the extraction lines (also called search lines) for the design of the search matrix. These search lines originated from the interior of the LV and extended radially towards the outer region (background). The third step consisted of smoothing the search matrix, followed by dynamic programming, to search for the optimal path of the LV border. Van Bree's method was an attempt towards a more sophisticated algorithm for boundary estimation. However, in step three of van Bree's approach, searching for the optimal path depended upon the search lines originating from the LV center, which in turn depended upon the ribbon band generated from the entire database. If the thickness of the ribbon band was large, then the position of the right edge point corresponding to the wall led to a *false alarm*. On the contrary, if the ribbon band was small, the search was accurate and fast. In other words, if the database had very large variabilities, the estimation would not be robust. This was exactly the case in Lee's Bayesian classifier [201], [202]. One way to make it robust was by combining several algorithms, in addition to using pixel-classification techniques. These are regularization algorithms, such as low contrast edge-detection algorithms, which will be discussed in Sub-section 3.6. Pope *et al.* [207], [208] also used dynamic programming to locate the optimal path through a search matrix for LV border estimation. A different approach than Bayesian was energy minimization, as will be presented in the next sub-section.

3.4.2.3   Training-Based LV Point Modeling

Lee's Bayesian classifier [201] was explored for LV border estimation in Sub-section 3.4.2.1. Those image processing boundaries could not handle the low contrast of the apex, the anterior wall, the inferior wall or the poor quality of LV images. Thus, the automatic contour tracing system (ACTS) system did not yield an accurate LV boundary [201]. Suri *et al.* [236] modeled the LV using two training-based systems in which the training coefficients were produced by taking hand-drawn and classifier boundaries and reducing the error among them. In the *identical coefficient* method, each vertex was associated with a set of coefficients. The calibrated x-coordinate for that vertex was computed as the linear combination of raw x-coordinates of the LV boundary using the coefficients associated with that vertex. The calibrated y-coordinate of that vertex was similarly computed as the same linear combination of raw y-coordinates of the LV boundary.

Two Coefficient Methods: IdCM and InCM   This sub-section presents the mathematical statements of the two calibration methods for bias correction of the classifier boundaries produced by the Bayesian classifier [201]. This classification scheme will not be discussed here, but interested readers can look at the dissertation by Lee [201].

Definitions of Identical and Independent Coefficient Methods: in the *Identical Coefficient* method, each vertex is associated with a set of coefficients. The calibrated x-coordinate for that vertex is computed as the linear combination of raw x-coordinates of the left ventricle boundary using the training coefficients associated with that vertex. The calibrated y-coordinate of that vertex is similarly computed as the *same* linear combination of raw y-coordinates of the left ventricle boundary. In the *Independent Coefficient* method, the calibrated x-coordinate is computed as the linear combination of raw x- *and* raw y-coordinates of the left ventricle boundary, using the training coefficients associated with that vertex. The calibrated y-coordinate of that vertex is computed with a *different* linear combination of raw x- *and* y-coordinates. The problem of calibration then becomes a problem of determining the coefficients of the linear combination which can be accomplished by solving a regression problem. The initial (x, y) coordinates of the left ventricle are converted from pixels to millimeters using a magnification correction factor. This factor is computed by keeping a grid of lead wires of known millimeter size or a kugel of known diameter (in mm) over the ventriculograms. The kugel is approximately the same size as the left ventricle (approximately 70 millimeters). These input raw and ground truth boundaries are initially in an irregularly spaced vertex polygon format with 100 vertices and unit dimensions in millimeters. Thus there is a need to change the polygons to equally spaced vertices, as will be discussed next.

Data Correspondence: Interpolation and Resampling Due to the variation in left ventricle sizes, resampling and interpolation for each of these polygons into polygons with equally spaced vertices was performed. Note here, since there is no prior information about the motion such as uniform expansion or contraction, the simplest case was taken by using equal-sampling-normalization, similar to the approach taken by Duncan *et al.* [302]. The interpolation was done with respect to the arc length. The arc length for a vertex is defined as the distance traveled along the left ventricle contour to that vertex, starting from the anterior aspect of the aortic valve (i.e, clockwise direction). Thus the arc length for the last vertex is the perimeter of the left ventricle contour. Since the original contour having P_1 vertices is sampled into P_2 vertices, the interval length between the vertices of the sampled contour is given as: $\frac{\mathcal{P}}{(P_2-1)}$, where $\mathcal{P}$ is the perimeter of the left ventricular contour, given as: $\mathcal{P}=\sum_{i=2}^{P_1}\sqrt{(x_i-x_{i-1})^2+(y_i-y_{i-1})^2}$. As a result of this resampling[12] and interpolation process, every vertex number of a ground truth boundary corresponds to the same vertex of the classifier boundary. This resampling and linear interpolation is done in an automatic way, where the user only needs to specify the total number of boundary vertices to be sampled and a list of frames of the cardiac cycle which need to be sampled. In this case, two frames were chosen for sampling, the end diastole (first frame) and the end systole (last frame), and the number of sampled boundaries vertices are P_2. Note that the AoV plane is known. This means the (x, y)-coordinates for the anterior aspect of the aortic valve and the inferior aspect of the aortic valve are known, which is called two-feature correspondence.

Justification of Two- and Three-Feature Correspondence Note that the above data correspondence scheme takes the prior information of the aortic valve (AoV) plane (similar to the way taken by van Bree *et al.* [206]) between the classifier and the ground truth boundary, while the remaining vertices are equally arc sampled and interpolated. This correspondence uses two features: the first and last point of the left ventricle contour. There are other features on the left ventricle contour which can also be used for data correspondence, e.g., the apex point (the farthest point from the mid AoV plane to the bottom one-third of the left ventricle). There are two ways to incorporate the apex

---

[12]Note carefully that there are three symbols used here: P_1, P_2 and $\mathcal{P}$ representing total points on the unsampled contour, total points on the sampled contour and the perimeter of the contour.

information in the data correspondence: either one must find the apex from the gray scale images, or use the ground truth apex as delineated by the cardiologist. Estimating the apex from the gray scale images is a very difficult process, since the apex zone is the most uncertain zone in the LVgrams (as it is known that there is no gray scale information present). The ES gray scale apex is even harder to estimate than the ED gray scale apex. This is because during the ES frame, the dye is emptying from the left ventricle chamber and the contrast level further decreases in the apex zone. Rather than estimating the apex using the pattern recognition technique, Suri *et al.* [101] developed schemes to estimate the ES apex using the dependence approach (not covered in this chapter). Using the prior information of the ground truth, the ES apex as delineated by the cardiologist, and the observed ED apex, Suri estimated the ES apex using a training-based system. This estimated ES apex can now be used for the data correspondence for ES frame boundaries. Suri *et al.* [240] also developed a robust apex estimation scheme where they estimated the apex using a weighted iterative least squares algorithm. This apex can be used as the third feature in data correspondence. Suri *et al.* [249] also recently developed a forced calibration algorithm where the left ventricle contour was forced to pass through the apex point. This can be thought of as putting a penalty on the apex point and letting the left ventricle contour pass through the apex. Thus this method is very similar to using three feature points (or three point correspondence): two points from the AoV plane and the third as the apex. Using this concept, the two wall curves can be independently equally arc sampled on both sides of the apex point. Currently being developed is a robust three feature data correspondence. The three point correspondence is another alternative method and can be considered as an option if the apex information is available. In this chapter, the data correspondence will be obtained by taking only the two feature points, which is a reasonable assumption, given that there is no prior information about the apex position or the source of classifier boundaries. Thus one can consider the above correspondence to be a simple case of a non-rigid correspondence. Using this relaxed assumption, one will see that hardly any information is lost around the left ventricle contour except a little near the apex. Using the two feature correspondence, the learning of the global left ventricle shapes based on the first layer of the neural network was performed, yielding results up to the expectation of the cardiologists. This involves the IdCM and InCM calibrations, which are stated mathematically in the next sub-section.

Identical Coefficient Method (IdCM) for Any Frame:
Let $g'_n = [x_1, x_2, ..., x_P]_n$ and $h'_n = [y_1, y_2, ..., y_P]_n$ be the row vectors of x-coordinates and y-coordinates, respectively, for the ground truth boundaries for patient n. Let $r'_n = [x_1, x_2, ..., x_P]_n$ and $s'_n = [y_1, y_2, ..., y_P]_n$ be the row vectors of x-coordinates and y-coordinates, respectively, for the classifier boundary for any patient n, where $n = 1, ..., N$. For the calibrated boundary estimation in left ventriculograms using the *Identical Coefficient* method, it is:

- **Given**: Corresponding pairs of ground truth boundaries $\mathbf{R}$ $[2N \times P]$, and the classifier boundaries $\mathbf{Q}$ $[2N \times (P+3)]$, respectively:

$$
\mathbf{R} = \begin{pmatrix} g_1^{'} \\ h_1^{'} \\ \dots \\ g_N^{'} \\ h_N^{'} \end{pmatrix} \qquad
\mathbf{Q} = \begin{pmatrix} r_1^{'} \; 1 \; \underbrace{u_{11} \; u_{21}} \\ s_1^{'} \; 1 \; \underbrace{v_{11} \; v_{21}} \\ \dots \\ r_N^{'} \; 1 \; \underbrace{u_{1N} \; u_{2N}} \\ s_N^{'} \; 1 \; \underbrace{v_{1N} \; v_{2N}} \end{pmatrix}
$$

where (u_{11}, v_{11}), (u_{1N}, v_{1N}) and (u_{21}, v_{21}), (u_{2N}, v_{2N}) are the coordinates for the anterior aspect and inferior aspect of the AoV plane of the left ventricle from the ground truth boundary, the known information of the starting and ending points of the contour. The last three columns constitute the translation offset effect (unity padding) and the pair u_{1n}, u_{2n} are the x-coordinates for the starting and ending vertex. Similarly, the pair v_{1n}, v_{2n} are the y-coordinates for the starting and ending vertex.

- Let $\mathbf{A}$ $[(P+3) \times P]$ be the unknown regression coefficient matrix.

- The problem is to estimate the coefficient matrix $\mathbf{A}$, to minimize $\| \mathbf{R} - \mathbf{Q}\mathbf{A} \|^2$. Then for any classifier boundary matrix $\mathbf{Q}$, the calibrated vertices of the boundary are given by $\mathbf{Q}\hat{\mathbf{A}}$, where $\hat{\mathbf{A}}$ is the estimated coefficient matrix.

Note the coefficients that multiply $g_n^{'}$ also multiply $h_n^{'}$, hence the name *Identical Coefficient* method. Also note that the new x-coordinates for the nth boundary depend only on the old x-coordinates from the nth boundary and the new y-coordinates from the nth boundary depend only on the old y-coordinates from the nth boundary.

Independent Coefficient Method (InCM) for Any Frame:
As before, let $g_n^{'}$ and $h_n^{'}$ be the row vectors of x- and y-coordinates for any patient n. Let $r_n^{'}$ and $s_n^{'}$ be the row vectors of x- and y-coordinates of the classifier boundary. For the calibrated boundary estimation in ventriculograms using the *Independent Coefficient* method, it is:

- **Given**: Corresponding ground truth boundaries $\mathbf{R}$ $[N \times 2P]$, classifier boundaries $\mathbf{Q}$ $[N \times (2P+5)]$, respectively:

$$
\mathbf{R} = \begin{pmatrix} g_1^{'} \; h_1^{'} \\ \dots \\ g_N^{'} \; h_N^{'} \end{pmatrix} \qquad
\mathbf{Q} = \begin{pmatrix} r_1^{'} \; s_1^{'} \; 1 \; \underbrace{u_{11} \; v_{11} \; u_{21} \; v_{21}} \\ \dots \\ r_N^{'} \; s_N^{'} \; 1 \; \underbrace{u_{1N} \; v_{1N} \; u_{2N} \; v_{2N}} \end{pmatrix}
$$

where (u_{11}, v_{11}), (u_{1N}, v_{1N}) and (u_{21}, v_{21}), (u_{2N}, v_{2N}) are the coordinates of the anterior aspect and inferior aspect of the AoV plane of the left ventricle from the ground truth boundary. The padding explanation is the same as in the previous sub-section, except that the pair (x, y) for the starting and ending points are on the same row. This this makes the total number of padding columns to be five.

- Let $\mathbf{A}$ $[(2P + 5) \times 2P]$ be the unknown regression coefficient matrix.

- The problem is to estimate the coefficient matrix $\mathbf{A}$, to minimize $\| \mathbf{R} - \mathbf{Q A} \|^2$. Then for any classifier boundary matrix $\mathbf{Q}$, the calibrated vertices of the boundary are given by $\mathbf{Q\hat{A}}$, where $\hat{\mathbf{A}}$ is the estimated coefficient matrix.

Note that the new (x, y)-coordinates of the vertices of each boundary are a *different* linear combination of the old (x, y)-coordinates for the polygon, hence the name *Independent Coefficient* method. The above two methods are different in the way the calibration model is set up. The classifier boundary matrix $\mathbf{Q}$ in IdCM is of size $\underbrace{2N \times (P + 3)}$, while in InCM, it is of size $\underbrace{N \times (2P + 5)}$.

For IdCM, the number of coefficients estimated in the $\hat{\mathbf{A}}$ matrix is $\underbrace{(P + 3) \times P}$.

For InCM, the number of coefficients estimated is $\underbrace{(2P + 5) \times 2\,P}$. Thus the

Independent Coefficient method requires around four times the number of coefficients of the *Identical Coefficient* method to be estimated. This difference could represent a significant factor for the data size in the ability of the technique to generalize rather than memorize. For this reason, one first optimizes both calibration techniques before they undergo greedy fusion.

Identical and Independent Optimization Calibrations: Training and Estimation. Once the data has been interpolated and equally arc sampled, one applies the regression model [236] to find the off-line training coefficient matrix $\mathbf{A}(\mathrm{t})$ to minimize the error function ϵ^2_{ifr}:

$$ \epsilon^2_{ifr} \quad = \quad \| \mathbf{R}(t) - \mathbf{Q}(t)\, \hat{\mathbf{A}}(t) \|^2 \ . \tag{3.18} $$

Generalizing for any frame t of the systolic cycle, minimizing $\hat{\mathbf{A}}$ is given by the normal equation: $\qquad \hat{\mathbf{A}}_{tr} = \underbrace{(\, \mathbf{Q}^T \mathbf{Q}\,)^{-1}\, \mathbf{Q}^T \mathbf{R}}\ . \tag{3.19}$

The above equation is solved using the singular value decomposition (SVD) (see Press *et al.* [256] and Haralick *et al.* [244]). Given the test set $(\mathbf{Q}_{te})$ or training set $(\mathbf{Q}_{tr})$, one can estimate the calibrated boundary as:

$$ \underbrace{\hat{\mathbf{R}}_{te} = \mathbf{Q}_{te}\, \hat{\mathbf{A}}_{tr}}, \ \& \ \underbrace{\hat{\mathbf{R}}_{tr} = \mathbf{Q}_{tr}\, \hat{\mathbf{A}}_{tr}}\ . \tag{3.20} $$

Thus the estimated matrices for the IdCM and InCM test sets are:

$$ \underbrace{\hat{\mathbf{R}}_{id} = \mathbf{Q}_{te}\, \hat{\mathbf{A}}_{id}}, \ \& \ \underbrace{\hat{\mathbf{R}}_{in} = \mathbf{Q}_{te}\, \hat{\mathbf{A}}_{in}}\ . \tag{3.21} $$

Note, if P_2 is the sampled vertices, then $\hat{\mathbf{R}}_{id}$ is of dimension $2N \times P_2$ and $\hat{\mathbf{R}}_{in}$ is of dimension $N \times 2P_2$.

Cross-Validation Technique: the input to the calibrator is the left ventricle boundary data which is represented by polygons of N studies, F frames and $P_1 = 100$ vertices. This used a *cross-validation* procedure for estimating the error of the calibration system. The procedure took a database of N patient studies and partitioned this database into K equal sized subsets. For all the K *choose L* combinations, the system was trained using L subsets and applied the estimated transformation on the remaining $(K - L)$ subsets. The mean error of the transformed boundary was then computed from these $(K - L)$ subsets coming from all K *choose L* combinations. These experiments consisted of varying the calibration parameters: N, K, L, P. Six different sets of K values (corresponding to each protocol) were chosen for training the system. Because of the small number of available patient studies in the database (N=291) and the large number of parameters (about 200 times N) in the transformation, there was a danger of memorization rather than generalization in the estimation of the transformation parameters. Therefore, it was essential that the number of vertices (P in the left ventricle polygon) were carefully chosen. As P decreased, the generalization improved but the representation of the true left ventricle shape became worse, thereby causing higher error with respect to the ground truth. As P increased, generalization was lost but representation of the true left ventricle shape improved. With the other parameters K, L and N fixed, there was an optimal number of boundary vertices P^* balancing the representation error with the memorization error. This protocol finds the *optimal number*. The estimated boundary using the two calibration algorithms undergo performance measure using the polyline metric method, as discussed in Sub-section 3.4.3.

The Greedy Algorithm: LV Calibration by Vertex. The idea is to obtain a fused boundary which has an error lower than the the two fusing boundaries. The nature of the fusion process has a greedy approach to obtain one fused boundary. This fused boundary in each iteration needs to be compared to the ideal boundary and the process repeated until no further reduction of the error can be done. First of all, the need for the greedy approach will be discussed and then it will be illustrated by the ball-basket method of implementation. A comparison will also be made between Cootes's [227] and the author's approaches.

Need for the Greedy Algorithm: as discussed before, there is not enough information in the apical zone and left ventricle walls of the gray scale ventriculograms. The above two calibrations help to stretch the initial classifier boundaries closer to the ground truth boundaries [236], thereby removing the bias errors in shape, position and orientation. These two calibration algorithms are sensitive to the number of data vectors (N) and dimensions of the data vectors (P). As a result, one calibration technique performs better than the other for the same frame of the cardiac cycle. This is seen particularly in the apical zone and the papillary muscle zone, where the dye is unable to propagate and mix well with the blood. Since the left ventricle ground truth boundaries were used for training the system, the same database of left ventricle contours can be used in the greedy technique. The two boundary calibration estimates (vertex-by-vertex) from the above calibration algorithms can be fused to produce a boundary closer to the boundary traced by the cardiologist. A fixed subset of estimated vertex positions from IdCM and InCM techniques was selected, which, when fused together, minimized the resulting error between the final estimated polygon boundary and the physician-traced left ventricle boundary. This idea will now be illustrated using a ball-basket method.

Ball-Basket Method: consider two baskets (say, b_1 and b_2), each containing the same number of balls P_2. Let the color of the balls in the b_1 basket be white and those in the b_2 basket be black. These balls can be imagined to represent the vertices of the left ventricle boundary. The goal is to fuse these two baskets in such a way that the fused basket (representing the fused boundary) has the greatest resemblance to the ideal basket (ideal boundary). In the first cycle, the algorithm consists of searching for that white ball from basket b_1 which when combined with the remaining $P_2 - 1$ black balls in basket b_2 will yield a lower error than when no ball was transferred. One such greedy cycle is shown in Figure 3.19, on the left. Finally, one such ball is transferred from basket b_1 to basket b_2 (see Figure 3.19, left). Now, the greedy cycle is repeated until no more balls are found, which improves the performance of the system (see Figure 3.19, right, row # 3 (cycle 2), row # 4 (cycle 3)).

The Greedy Algorithm Implementation. The greedy algorithm consists of three basic steps. First, fusion of the IdCM and InCM boundary data, second, polyline performance (see Sub-section 3.4.3) to compute the errors and third, the vertex selection. The input to the fusion process is two sets of boundaries $\hat{\mathbf{R}}_{id}$ and $\hat{\mathbf{R}}_{in}$ which need to be fused. The fusion is done by selection of that vertex (or column) of InCM boundary which contributes to a reduction in error. The Polyperformance() function takes two sets of boundaries: the fused boundary $\hat{\mathbf{R}}_{com}$ and the original ground truth $\mathbf{R}_{gt}$ consisting of $P_1 = 100$ vertices and computes the mean error (as discussed in Sub-section 3.4.3). The third function is the argmin() function or vertex selection function that takes the error associated with P_2 vertices and finds that vertex number from InCM LV boundary that yielded the least error in each greedy cycle.

Greedy Algorithm. Let S, S_{id} and S_{in} be three sets consisting of all vertices, IdCM pool vertices and InCM pool vertices, respectively. Let $\hat{\mathbf{R}}_{id}$ ($2N \times P_2$) and $\hat{\mathbf{R}}_{in}$ ($N \times 2P_2$) be the estimated boundary matrices from the IdCM and InCM techniques with P_2 samples vertices. Let $\mathbf{R}_{gt}$ ($N \times 2P_1$) and $\mathbf{R}$ ($N \times 2P_2$) be the matrices consisting of (x, y)-coordinates from the original ground truth with $P_1 = 100$ and sampled P_2 vertices, respectively. Initially all the vertices are considered in the IdCM pool and the error is computed. Its error is denoted by ϵ_{id}. Now select that vertex from the IdCM pool which when fused with the InCM pool vertices yields an estimated boundary error lower than ϵ_{id}. This procedure is repeated until there is no further improvement. If ϵ is the error at any time in the greedy *do-while loop* and $\mathcal{F}$ is the set consisting of all the frames, then the greedy *do-while loop* for any frame t in the set $\mathcal{F}$, consists of the following steps.

The Greedy Boundary Calibration()

For each $t \in \mathcal{F}$

    $S_{id}=S$; $S_{in}=\phi$, $\epsilon=0$ greedyCounter$=0$

    While ($\epsilon \leq \epsilon_{id}$) **do**

        greedyCounter++

          For each $i \in S_{id}$,   /* total vertices are P_{id} */

            $S_{id} = S_{id} - \{i\}$; $S_{in} = S_{in} \bigcup \{i\}$

            Combine IdCM ($\hat{\mathbf{R}}_{id}$) and InCM ($\hat{\mathbf{R}}_{in}$)

               Using S_{id} **and** S_{in}

            $\hat{\mathbf{R}}_{com} = $ Combine($\mathbf{R}_{id}, \mathbf{R}_{in}, N, P_2, S_{id}, S_{in}$, greedyCounter)

            Performance Evaluation using Original GT:

            Error for index i

            $\epsilon_i = $ Performance($\hat{\mathbf{R}}_{com}, \mathbf{R}_{gt}, N, P_1, P_2$)

          End /* end of the for loop */

          ArgMin Computation: Min. error and best vertex j selection

          $(\epsilon_{min}, j) = $ ArgMin($\epsilon[i]$, $P_{id} - greedyCounter$)

          if ($\epsilon_{min} < \epsilon$)   **then** $S_{id} = S_{id} - \{j\}$; $S_{in} = S_{in} \bigcup \{j\}$ **else** break;

End

    End /* end of the while loop */

End /* end of all the frames of systolic heart cycle */

The advantage of the above algorithm is that the initial error is decided from either of the above coefficient methods. Note, this is implemented independently for each frame of the cardiac cycle.

Comparison Between Cootes's [227] and Suri's [550] Techniques. As stage one and stage two of Suri's system have been discussed, his methodology will now be compared with Cootes's technique: (**1**) Cootes used knowledge of the expected shape combined with information from the areas of the image where good wall evidence could be found to infer the missing parts of the left ventricle. In Suri's approach, he also used the Least Squares (independent of each frame) to infer the position of the parts of the boundary where there is less contrast or left ventricle information (the apex zone of the left ventricle or bottom $(\frac{1}{3})^{rd}$ region of the left ventricle) by using the knowledge of the top $(\frac{2}{3})^{rd}$ region of the left ventricle where there is good evidence of the left ventricle data points. (**2**) For the final shape estimation, Cootes used a weighted iterative algorithm where weights were proportional to the standard deviation of the shape parameter over the training set. This is more like Weighted Least Squares where the initial guess was the first stage: Least Squares. The termination process of the iteration depended upon the Mahalanobis distance D_m when compared to the constant, say, D_{max}. The idea behind the iterative algorithm was to improve the accuracy of the border detection. In Suri's method, the

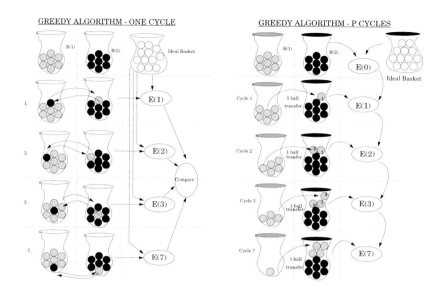

Figure 3.19: **Left**: One greedy cycle where the best vertex (ball) is selected out of basket b_1. E's denote the errors when compared with the ideal basket. **Right**: Basket b_2 filling up after each greedy cycle.

second stage is the greedy algorithm which fused the two sets of boundaries to yield boundaries closer to the ideal boundary (as traced by the cardiologist). First, one optimized for that P number of vertices which yields the best left ventricle shapes from the *Identical* and *Independent Coefficient* methods. These methods are based on Least Squares models. Thereafter, the greedy algorithm can be considered as an iterative process where one selects that vertex of the left ventricle boundary from one estimation technique which, when fused with another boundary (other estimation technique), will yield an error lower than the error of either of the two methods. The greedy algorithm does not give up unless it has checked all the vertices on the boundary. (**3**) In Suri's approach, the initial error is not a guess but the error which is the better of the two existing errors, unlike in Coote's method, where the initial guess is taken as the mean shape with the addition of the weighted principal axis of the ellipsoid. Cootes first finds the mean shape, then the eigen vectors of the covariance matrix of the deviation. Thus, any shape is approximated as:

$$\mathbf{x} = \bar{\mathbf{x}} + \mathbf{P}\,\mathbf{b}\,, \tag{3.22}$$

where $\bar{\mathbf{x}}$ is the mean shape, $\mathbf{P}$ is the matrix of the eigen vectors and $\mathbf{b}$ is the vector of the weight matrix. In the greedy method, if the fusing boundary vertices have a large error compared with the the ideal boundary (traced by the cardiologist), then the greedy algorithm rapidly picks the vertices. The important aspect about the greedy algorithm is: one does not have to repeat the *Identical Coefficient* method and the *Independent Coefficient* method calibrations. Once these runs are over, one then just chooses vertices (switching columns between two boundary data matrices) in such a way that in each greedy cycle, one is heading closer to the ground truth boundaries until all the vertices are checked. (**4**) Another similarity between Cootes's and Suri's methods is that both methods use a point model, which means that the starting analysis of the boundaries are the vertices or points. The only difference is in the dimension of the matrices. Finally, Cootes uses the Mahalanobis distance for performance, while Suri uses the polyline distance metric as discussed in the next sub-section.

3.4.3 Polyline Distance Measure and Performance Terms

Several methods have been developed for measuring the left ventricle wall motion (see details in [280]). Sheehan *et al.* [292] developed a centerline method for quantitative assessment of the ventricular boundary. Sheehan measured the motion along 100 chords constructed perpendicular to a centerline drawn midway between the end-diastole and the end-systole left ventricle contours. The centerline method was developed to find the extent of the local left ventricle wall motion. The algorithm consists of the following principle: if the two left ventricle polygons are end-diastole and end-systole boundaries, the end-diastole having a larger number of points on it, then one first linearly interpolates the larger contour to get 200 points and then for each tuple of three points on this contour, a perpendicular is drawn to the tangent of the circle passing through these three points. The centers of these perpendicular chords constitute the centerline. This distance is a function of the area swiped between two left ventricle boundaries. The performance of the training algorithm is measured by the error of closeness between the estimated boundary and the ideal boundary as traced by the cardiologist. The error of closeness is measured using a stable method based on vector calculus called the polyline metric as derived below.

3.4.3.1 Derivation of Polyline Metric

The polyline metric actually is based on the ratio of the average area between two polygons *to* the average perimeter of the two polygons. Suri's assumption prior to the polyline distance error computation was that the polygons have equal perimeters and the vertices are equally spaced along the perimeter; i.e., the two arc intervals on the two contours are the same. Using this assumption, Suri mathematically showed that the ratio of the average area between the polygons to their perimeters actually is the average polyline distance error between the two polygons.

Let the two polygons be B_1 and B_2 consisting of the total points[13] P_1 and P_2 having interval lengths of l_1 and l_2, respectively. This is shown in Figure 3.20. Let the perpendicular distances from each of the vertices (of polygon B_1) to the

---

[13]Note that the reader should not get confused with the symbols of P_1 and P_2 used before. There is no relationship between the symbols used in this section and those used in the section on Data Correspondence (3.4.2.3). The idea here is to explain how to compute the polyline error given two polygons B_1 and B_2 consisting of P_1 and P_2 number of vertices.

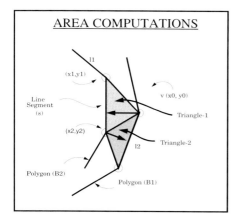

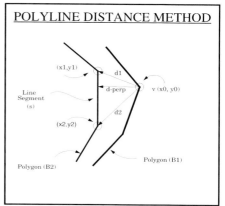

Figure 3.20: **Left**: Figure showing the area of the triangles between the two polygons. **Right**: Geometry of the polyline distance computation.

opposite interval sides of the polygon B_2 be d_n, where, $1 \leq n \leq P_1$. Similarly, let d'_m be the perpendicular distances from each of the vertices (of polygon B_2) to the opposite interval sides of the polygon B_1, where, $1 \leq m \leq P_2$. Thus the areas of the triangle with a height d_n and base l_2 are $\frac{1}{2}l_2 d_n$. Similarly, the area of the triangle with height d'_m and base l_1 is $\frac{1}{2}l_1 d'_m$. The total area $\bar{A}$ between two polygons is computed by computing the sum of the area of all the triangles whose bases lie on the polygon B_1 and the sum of the area of all the triangles whose bases lie on the polygon B_2 and is given as:

$$\bar{A} \;=\; \sum_{n=1}^{P_1} \frac{1}{2}\, l_2\, d_n + \sum_{m=1}^{P_2} \frac{1}{2}\, l_1\, d'_m \;. \tag{3.23}$$

Similarly, one can compute the average perimeter of the two polygons as:

$$\bar{P} \;=\; \frac{l_2 P_1 + l_1 P_2}{2} \;. \tag{3.24}$$

Taking the ratio of Equation (3.23) to Equation (3.24) one gets:

$$\frac{\bar{A}}{\bar{P}} \;=\; \frac{\sum_{n=1}^{P_1} \frac{1}{2} l_2\, d_n + \sum_{m=1}^{P_2} \frac{1}{2} l_1\, d'_m}{\frac{l_2 P_1 + l_1 P_2}{2}} \;. \tag{3.25}$$

Using the above assumption, $l_1 \approx l_2$, Equation (3.25) reduces to:

$$\frac{\bar{A}}{\bar{P}} \;=\; \frac{\sum_{n=1}^{P_1} d_n + \sum_{m=1}^{P_2} d'_m}{P_1 + P_2} \;. \tag{3.26}$$

It will be shown that this is what the polyline distance method computes and will be represented from now on as $D_s(B_1{:}B_2)$. The polyline distance $D_s(B_1 : B_2)$ between two polygons representing boundary B_1 and B_2 is symmetrically defined as the average distance between a vertex of one polygon and the boundary of the other polygon. To define this measure precisely, one first needs to define a distance $d(v, s)$ between a point v and a line segment s. The distance $d(v, s)$ between a point v having coordinates (x_o, y_o) and a line segment having end points (x_1, y_1) and (x_2, y_2) is:

$$d(v, s) \;=\; \begin{cases} \min\{d_1, d_2\}; & if \;\; \lambda < 0, \lambda > 1 \\ |d^\perp|; & if \;\; 0 \le \lambda \le 1, \end{cases} \qquad (3.27)$$

where

$$\begin{aligned} d_1 &= \sqrt{(x_0 - x_1)^2 + (y_0 - y_1)^2} \\ d_2 &= \sqrt{(x_0 - x_2)^2 + (y_0 - y_2)^2} \\ \lambda &= \tfrac{(y_2 - y_1)(y_0 - y_1) + (x_2 - x_1)(x_0 - x_1)}{(x_2 - x_1)^2 + (y_2 - y_1)^2} \\ d^\perp &= \tfrac{(y_2 - y_1)(x_1 - x_0) + (x_2 - x_1)(y_0 - y_1)}{\sqrt{(x_2 - x_1)^2 + (y_2 - y_1)^2}}. \end{aligned} \qquad (3.28)$$

Note, d_1 and d_2 are the distances from the vertex v to the end points of the segment s. λ is the distance along the vector of the segment s, while $d^\perp$ is the perpendicular distance along the vector orthogonal to the segment s. The polyline distance $d_b(v, B_2)$ from the vertex v to the boundary B_2 is defined by:

$$d_b(v, B_2) \;=\; \min_{s \,\in\, sides\ B_2} d(v, s). \qquad (3.29)$$

This step is a confirmation that is being chosen as the closest segment on B_2 from the vertex v. The distance $d_{vb}(B_1, B_2)$ between the vertices of polygon B_1 and the sides of polygon B_2 is defined as the sum of the distances from the vertices of the polygon B_1 to the closest side of B_2.

$$d_{vb}(B_1, B_2) \;=\; \sum_{v \,\in\, vertices\ B_1} (v, B_2) \qquad (3.30)$$

Reversing the computation from B_2 to B_1, one can similarly compute $d_{vb}(B_2, B_1)$. Using Equation (3.30), the polyline distance between polygons, $D_s(B_1 : B_2)$ is defined by:

$$D_s(B_1 : B_2) \;=\; \frac{d_{vb}(B_1, B_2) + d_{vb}(B_2, B_1)}{(\#vertices \in B_1 + \#vertices \in B_2)}. \qquad (3.31)$$

This equation is basically the same as Equation (3.26), where the numerator is the sum of all the perpendicular distances for both the polygons, while the denominator is the sum of the total number of vertices on the two polygons. This mathematical expression $D_s(B_1 : B_2)$ signifies how far one left ventricle wall is away from the other and is very helpful in wall motion estimation, for example, the wall motion measurement between the end-diastole and end-systole left ventricle boundaries. This expression is used in computing how far the estimated left ventricle boundaries are away from the ideal boundaries and it represents an average error measure.

3.4.3.2   Justification of Using Polyline

The IdCM and InCM optimization algorithms are based on the vertex-to-vertex distance error, while the performance measure of the estimated boundaries is based on the slightly closer measure called the polyline distance measure. The polyline distance measure basically finds the average distance from the vertex to a polygon. Computationally, they are slightly different measures, but from the cardiologist's point of view, the polyline measurement tool does not foresee the algorithm or technique from which the estimated boundaries are coming from, e.g., the estimated boundaries could come from either the pixel classifier scheme, regression scheme or neural network scheme or any segmentation technique. Since the earlier method developed by Sheehan [292] computed the minimum distance as the perpendicular distance between the two contours (left ventricle polygon), Suri uses similar grounds to estimate the shortest distance from a vertex to the opposite polygon. It was seen that the polyline distances were superior to current methods. These advantages are as follows: (**1**) the method is very stable and computes the error based on the geometry of the triangles and vector calculus, which is the ratio of the average area to the average perimeter as shown in the mathematical derivation. (**2**) The polyline distance error has an added advantage. If there are cups or cusps in the polyline, then the algorithm can easily spot them. Since the algorithm looks for those perpendiculars whose λ lies between 0 and 1 to satisfy the condition of closeness, there is no possibility of any error. (**3**) Since prior to the polyline error computation, the curves (left ventricle polygons) undergo equal arc sampling and interpolation, thus there exists a one-to-one correspondence between the estimated and ground truth vertices of the curves. (**4**) This is a non-iterative computation and thus saves time, unlike Bolson and Sheehan's method [291], [292], where one has to do the computations again to smooth the curves to improve the accuracy. (**5**) In Bolson and Sheehan's [292] method, one has to compute the tangents by fitting the circle through three points. The circle fitting algorithm is very sensitive to the number of points taken on either side of the vertex (see Haralick *et al.* [244]). In the polyline method, there is no fitting involved. Also, Suri showed in [101] that the polyline method is more accurate than the centerline method to the third decimal place. (**6**) Another advantage of the polyline algorithm is that it can easily find out whether the distance computed for every vertex is positive or negative, positive when going from one vertex to the opposite polygon and vice versa. This is very useful in finding out if the part of the curve is on the inside or outside. (**7**) The polyline algorithm is in conjunction with the swapping mechanism which makes the process symmetric[14]. So, the average statistics give a better estimate of the mean error when computed from one polygon to another and vice-versa. (**8**) Another advantage is that the correct bias errors at every vertex are computable. Since not only the closest perpendicular is computed, but also the coordinate position and its bias relative to the vertex on the opposite polygon, thus one can use this

---

[14]One could compute the polyline error when going from one boundary to the opposite boundary and vice-versa.

distance to correct the bias errors in calibration algorithms by making the optimization algorithm the weighted Least Squares algorithm, where the weights are inversely proportional to the polyline bias errors. This is building a technique by which one can use these errors and build a constrained optimization problem. (**9**) One of the major advantages of the polyline distance measure is the coherence with the ejection fraction computation. For example, if the ES left ventricle shape is totally convex and inside the ED left ventricle shape, then the ejection fraction number truly reflects the polyline distance error. As 95% of the ES left ventricle lies inside the ED left ventricle, the polyline distance error will reflect very close approximations for sweeping the area between left ventricle shapes for volume computations. Thus, the primary advantage of the contour extraction and quantification can be studied better and the cardiologist can establish a better clinical relevance. Even though the polyline distance measure and optimization algorithms are computing a measure which is computationally slightly different, this difference in terms of error can be accepted by cardiologists, considering the fact that the polyline distance method not only computes a similar mean error measure to the centerline [101] technique to the third decimal but has advantages, superiority and stability compared with other methods.

3.4.3.3 Mean Error (e_{NFP}^{poly}) or Measure of Agreement

The performance of the calibration algorithms is evaluated by computing the boundary error on the test data set ($\mathbf{Q}_{te}$). Using the definition of the polyline distance between the two polygons, one can now compute the mean error of the overall calibration system. It is denoted by e_{NFP}^{poly} and defined by:

$$e_{NFP}^{poly} = \frac{\sum_{t=1}^{F} \sum_{n=1}^{N} D_s(G_{nt}, C_{nt})}{F \times N}, \qquad (3.32)$$

where $D_s(G_{nt}, C_{nt})$ is the polyline distance between the ground truth G_{nt} and calibrated polygons C_{nt} for patient study n and frame number t. Note, F and N are the total number of frames and points, respectively. This term is very significant, as it represents how far the estimated boundary and the ideal boundary are from each other on an average over the entire population of patient studies, frames and vertices. This term will be used to analyze the estimated data and the training performance of the cross-validation procedure. Equation (3.32) is very relevant in the optimization technique. For each set of $P = P_2$ number of points, e_{NFP}^{poly} is computed and the operating point is estimated which corresponds to the best fitted shape. Using the definition of the polyline distance between two polygons, the standard deviation can be computed as:

$$\sigma_{NFP}^{poly} =$$

$$\sqrt{\frac{\sum\limits_{t=1}^{F}\sum\limits_{n=1}^{N}\sum\limits_{v\in\ vertices\ G_{nt}}\left(d_b(v,C_{nt})-e_{NFP}^{poly}\right)^2 + \sum\limits_{v\in\ vertices\ C_{nt}}\left(d_b(v,G_{nt})-e_{NFP}^{poly}\right)^2}{N\times F\times(\#vertices\in B_1+\#vertices\in B_2)}}$$

$$(3.33)$$

3.4.3.4   Error Per Vertex and Error Per Arc Length

Using the polyline distance formulaes, one can compute the error per vertex (EPV) from one polygon (ground truth) to another polygon (calibrated). This is defined as the mean error for a vertex v over all the patients and all the frames. The *error per vertex* for a fixed vertex v, when computed between the ground truth G and the calibrated boundary C, is defined by:

$$e_v^{GC} = \frac{\sum_{t=1}^{F}\sum_{n=1}^{N} d_b(v,G_{nt})}{F\times N} .$$

$$(3.34)$$

Similarly, one can compute the *error per vertex* between the calibrated and the ground truth using Equation (3.29). *Error Per Arc Length* (EPAL) is computed in the following way: For the values e_v^{GC} where $v=1,2,3,\ldots P_1$, one constructs a curve f^{GC} defined on the interval $[0,1]$ which takes the value e_v^{GC} at point x, which is the *normalized arc length* to vertex v and whose in-between values are defined by linear interpolation. One computes the curve f^{CG}, between the calibrated boundary and the ground truth boundary in a similar way. One then adds algebraically these two curves to yield the final *error per arc length*, given as: $f = \frac{f^{GC}+f^{CG}}{2}$. Note that the EPV is a very useful term, as it tells the error between the estimated vertex and the ideal vertex over the entire population. This is particularly useful in the apical zone of the left ventricle. EPAL is a better representation of EPV since it is normalized over the entire contour. The EPAL is equally significant in the apical zone of the left ventricle, as it shows how much improvement the training algorithms performed to remove the bias errors of the classifier boundaries around the entire contour.

3.4.4   Data Analysis Using IdCM, InCM and the Greedy Method

The database population consisted of 291 patient studies, out of which 135 studies had acute myocardial infarction with the top 50% in quality used on a scale of 0 to 10, where 0 is rejected and 10 is considered excellent. The number of studies during acute infarction, that then underwent follow-up studies over the course of one year was 35. The number of studies from Japan which were normal and had a diagnostic cardiac catheterization was 27. The Japanese patients' left ventricle images represented the top 50% in quality; the remainder of the 94 studies were from the Catheterization Laboratory, at the University of Washington Medical Center, Seattle, Washington. These studies represented

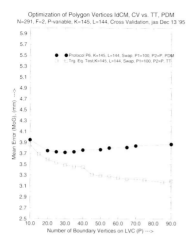
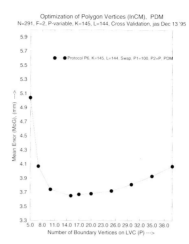

Figure 3.21: Vertex optimization using the polyline distance metric. **Left**: IdCM (identical coefficient method), cross-validation vs. training equals testing (TT), **Right**: InCM (Independent Coefficient method). Note, the IdCM operating point is 30 vertices and the InCM operating point is 15 vertices.

the top 30% in quality. Suri used this knowledge to build his training system. The performance of the system can be judged by evaluating the error measures on the test data $\mathbf{Q}_{te}$ set. This sub-section discusses the performance of IdCM, InCM and the greedy methods. All of the performance evaluation is with respect to the original ground truth boundaries having $P_1 = 100$ vertices.

3.4.4.1 Data Analysis 1: Vertex Optimization for Cross-Validation

One finds the mean error as a function of the number of polygon boundary vertices on the left ventricle contour. The optimization curve and operating point are shown in Figure 3.21. This database consists of $N=291$ patient studies and the selected number of partitions of $K=145$. One now varies the number of vertices P_2 on the left ventricle polygon by varying it from 10 vertices to 90 vertices with 5 vertex increments. If $L=144$ is the training sets, then for each combination there are $K-L$ test set boundaries on which the error is computed. Suri chose the number of vertices P_2 to minimize the error on the test set. Since there are $^K C_L = 145$ trials, each trial has $(K-L)$ subsets, each subset consists of $\frac{N}{K}$ patients (in a protocol, if $\frac{N}{K}$ is not a perfect division, then for the last trial in $^K C_L$ combinations, one has $(K-L+r_p)$ patients as a testing set, where r_p is a remainder number of $\frac{N}{K}$) and each patient consists of P_2 vertices and $F=2$ frames. Thus one gets the total number of points as: $F \times {}^K C_L \times (K-L) \times \frac{N}{K} \times P_2$, resulting in: $N \times F \times P_2 \times \frac{(K-1)!}{(K-L-1)!\,L!}$ points for each (N, K, L, P_2) tuple. Since one is computing the polyline distances, the number of operations is $N \times F \times P_1^2 \times P_2 \times \frac{(K-1)!}{(K-L-1)!\,L!}$. It can be seen Figure 3.21 that the *optimal* number of vertices in InCM is about *half* the optimal number of vertices in IdCM, the reason being that the number of coefficients that have to be estimated in InCM is about *four* times the number of coefficients that have to be estimated in IdCM.

3.4.4.2   Data Analysis 2, 3: Cumulative Distribution of $(\frac{ED+ES}{2})$ Errors and Error Per Arc Length Along the Left Ventricle Contour

Here the cumulative distribution of end frame errors $(\frac{ED+ES}{2})$ from both the calibration methods using IdCM and InCM is shown (see Figure 3.22). This figure demonstrates the mean *error per arc length* along the LVC. The x-axis shows the length of the arc starting from AAV. The ordinate shows the error at each vertex in mm. As seen in the plot, the mean *error per vertex* is largest near the middle of the normalized arc length which is close to the apex of the left ventricle. Thus the error is at a maximum in the apex region. One sees that the greedy algorithm does *best* in the apex zone compared with the IdCM and InCM methods. The *error per vertex* shows that in the ED frame, the apex zone error is reduced by **8.5** mm (from **12.5** mm to about **4** mm), while in the ES frame, the apex zone error is reduced by **3 mm** (from **9** mm to **6 mm**). The corresponding mean error over the ED and ES frames of the pixel-based boundaries was **6.4** mm, which is reduced to **3.8** mm in IdCM and **3.5** mm in the greedy algorithm. As per Suri's assumption, the error is least at the end points of the LVC since the AoV plane is known, thus the *error per vertex* curve drops at both ends. Suri's results show that 81% of the patient boundaries had a mean $(\frac{ED+ES}{2})$ less than 4.0 millimeters using the greedy calibration technique.

3.4.4.3   Data Analysis 4: ED and ES Errors vs. InCM Pool Vertices

Here the effect of the greedy calibration scheme is shown. Figure 3.23 shows the drop in the ED and ES frame errors when the IdCM pool vertices are transferred to the InCM pool. This is implemented using the greedy *do-while loop*, where some columns (or vertices) of the IdCM matrix $\hat{\mathbf{R}}_{id}$ are replaced by the corresponding columns (or vertices) of the InCM matrix, $\hat{\mathbf{R}}_{in}$. Figure 3.23 (right) shows that the greedy algorithm reduced the error by **0.3** mm over IdCM. It is also observed that the best number of vertices for IdCM is 30, while for InCM it is 15. The best performance over all three techniques is by the greedy algorithm with the number of vertices being 30. In the greedy calibration technique, the error does not rise very sharply after 30 vertices but rises gradually by $(\frac{1}{100})^{th}$ of a millimeter from 30 vertices to 40 vertices.

3.4.4.4   Discussion of Training-Based LV Point Modeling

The greedy algorithm for error correction fuses two sets of estimated boundaries: those produced by the *Identical Coefficient* method and those produced by the *Independent Coefficient* method. If these two estimated boundaries have large errors with respect to the ground truth (ideal or hand-drawn boundary),

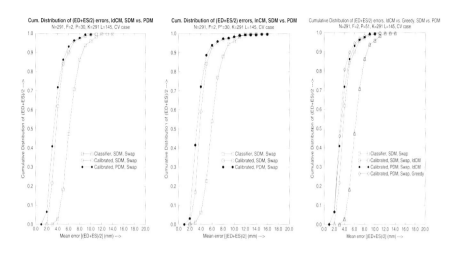

Figure 3.22: Cumulative distribution vs. mean error of $\left(\frac{ED+ES}{2}\right)$ errors. **Left**: Identical coefficient method. **Middle**: Independent Coefficient method. **Right**: Greedy vs. IdCM. The curves show that 80% of the patient estimated boundaries have an error $\leq$ 4 mm in IdCM, while 72% of the patients have an error $\leq$ 4 mm in InCM, and 81% of the patients have error $\leq$ 4 mm in the greedy algorithm. Partition Protocol Parameters: N=291, F=2, K=145, L=144, P_1=100, P_2=30.

then the greedy algorithm rapidly identifies those vertices which are too far from the ideal vertices, significantly reducing the boundary error. Nevertheless, the true shape of the left ventricle depends upon the number of optimized boundary vertices selected on the left ventricle contour. If the number of vertices is less than the optimum number, the true left ventricle shape may not be represented. On the other hand, if the number of vertices is larger than the optimized boundary vertices, the shape becomes more accurate, but generalization is lost. Therefore, one must first optimize the IdCM and InCM techniques and then fuse the best results together. Consequently, the error will always improve, but the drop in the error will depend upon the following factors: (**1**) the number of vertices on the LVC; (**2**) the initial errors of the IdCM and InCM boundary data before the fusion starts, which in turn depends upon the number of data vectors N for training the calibration model; (**3**) the starting error value (ϵ) before the greedy loop starts (in this case, the starting value is the best error for the IdCM boundary data).

These preliminary results indicate that the three sets of calibration algorithms significantly reduced the boundary error over the image processing algorithms. In other words, given any method for finding a digitized contour (computer-based estimates) in the plane for a certain class of images and the corresponding set of expert (or ground truth) contours, these three calibration

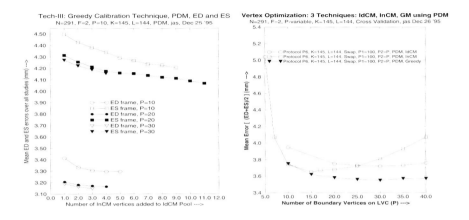

Figure 3.23: Greedy performance: **Left**: Plot showing the reduction in the error for ED and ES frames when some vertices are calibrated using IdCM and others using InCM. With the increase InCM pool, the error drops. **Right**: In a comparison of the three calibration techniques, greedy does the best. Partition protocol parameters: $N=291$, $F=2$, $K=145$, $L=144$, $P_1=100$, $P_2=30$. The mean error used for IdCM=**3.8** mm, InCM=**3.9** mm and Greedy=**3.5** mm. So, the greedy algorithm improves by **0.3** mm over the IdCM method. Note, SDM means shortest distance method, PDM means polyline distance method and swap means repeating the process of distance computation from one boundary to another and vice-versa.

algorithms will polish the computer-based estimates so that they are in better agreement with the expert (here, the cardiologist). However, the left ventricle boundary calibration system can be made more robust by padding information or features like the apex information to the **Q** matrix (classifier data) to improve the accuracy [101]. This algorithm requires no operator assistance; furthermore, the algorithm is relatively simple and can be implemented on any commercial imaging system.

3.4.4.5   Conclusions on the Greedy Calibration Algorithm

Three sets of calibration algorithms have been presented, the *Identical Coefficient* method, the *Independent Coefficient* method and the greedy calibration method. The *greedy calibration algorithm* for calibrating the initial pixel-based classifier boundaries takes the best of the other two calibration methods. The mean error over the ED and ES frames using a *cross-validation* protocol and polyline distance metric is **3.5** millimeters over the database of **291** patient studies. The greedy algorithm is a considerable improvement over the *Identical Coefficient* method by **0.3** millimeters, which is significant for the accuracy of the overall calibration system. The greedy algorithm performs best in the apex zone of the left ventricle where the dye is unable to propagate, reducing the error by approximately **8.5** mm. Thus it can be seen that the calibration constitutes a significant last step for boundary estimation. One could say that the training algorithm alone used in this research is not a sophisticated method such as neural networks, but a plain Least Squares trained for bias correction. If one looks at the entire system of boundary estimation, it fits very well: a Bayesian classifier as a raw boundary estimator followed by a calibrator for bias correction. Also proposed was a constrained Least Squares method based on eigenvalues for bias correction which propagates good boundary information from the end-diastole frame to the end-systole frame. These constrained methods are very powerful along with the training methodology as discussed in this chapter, which is very promising for medical contour extraction in several medical imaging modalities, not just in X-rays. The apex extraction feature will be pursued more accurately, which will make the entire design more robust when used with the two stage boundary estimation system.

LV boundary fusion algorithms. The boundary calibration system employed two different techniques: the *Identical Coefficient* method (IdCM) and the *Independent Coefficient* method (InCM), named after the manner in which each technique estimates the parameters. The above two coefficient algorithms did improve apical and wall errors over the initial boundaries, but were not robust enough to handle the LV boundary estimation process to yield a boundary error closer to the desired accuracy of 2.5 mm. These calibration algorithms were sensitive to the number of data vectors (N) and the dimensionality of the data vectors (P) (see Takeshita *et al.* [237] for the effect of sample size on bias errors). As a result, one calibration technique performed better than the other for the same frame of the cardiac cycle. This was especially clear in the apical zone and in the papillary muscle zone (see Figures 3.3 and 3.12), where the dye was unable to propagate and mix well with the blood. Using the LV ground truth boundaries in the database of LV contours, Suri *et al.* [238] took advantage of the global shape by *fusing* the two boundary calibration estimates (vertex-by-vertex) from the above calibration algorithms to produce a fused boundary closer to the boundary traced by the cardiologist. Suri selected a *fixed* subset of estimated vertex positions from the IdCM and InCM techniques which, when fused together, minimized the resulting error between the final estimated polygon boundary and the physician-traced LV boundary. Suri used the ball-basket model where they transferred the vertices (balls) from one basket (the IdCM boundary) to another basket (the InCM boundary) until the error reduction scheme was no longer permitted. This was an iterative process.

Suri vs. Cootes's point training model. There are many similarities between Cootes's [227] method and Suri's [238] technique. (1) Cootes used the knowledge of the expected shape combined with information from the areas of the image where good wall evidence could be found to infer the missing parts of the LV. Suri also used Least Squares (independent of each frame) to infer the position of the parts of the boundary where there was less contrast or LV information (apex zone of the LV or the bottom $(\frac{1}{3})^{rd}$ region of the LV) by using the knowledge of the top $(\frac{2}{3})^{rd}$ region of the LV where there was good evidence of the LV data points. (2) For the final shape estimation, Cootes used a weighted iterative algorithm where weights were proportional to the standard deviation of the shape parameter over the training set. This was more like Weighted Least Squares (WLS), where the initial guess was the first stage, the Least Squares. The termination process of the iteration depended on the Mahalanobis distance D_m when compared to the constant D_{max}. The idea behind the iterative algorithm was to improve the accuracy of the border detection. In Suri's method, the second stage was the greedy algorithm that fused the two sets of boundaries to yield boundaries closer to the ideal boundary (as traced by the cardiologist). First, Suri optimized for the P number of vertices which yielded the best LV shapes from the *Identical* and *Independent Coefficient* methods. Thereafter, the greedy algorithm could be considered a process where a vertex was selected from one estimation technique which, when fused with another boundary (another estimation technique), yielded an error lower than the error of either of the two methods. The greedy algorithm did not give up unless it had checked all the vertices on the boundary. (3) In Suri's approach, the initial error was not a guess but the best of the two existing errors, whereas in Cootes's method, the initial guess was taken as the mean shape with the addition of the weighted principal axis of the ellipsoid. Cootes first found the mean shape, then the eigenvectors of the covariance matrix of the deviation. Thus, any shape was approximated as:

$$\mathbf{x} = \bar{\mathbf{x}} + \mathbf{P}\,\mathbf{b} \, , \qquad\qquad (3.35)$$

where $\bar{\mathbf{x}}$ was the mean shape, $\mathbf{P}$ was the matrix of the eigen vectors and $\mathbf{b}$ was the vector of weight matrix. In the greedy method, if the fusing boundary vertices had large errors compared with the ideal boundary (traced by the cardiologist), then the greedy algorithm rapidly picked the vertices. The important aspect about the greedy algorithm was that one did not have to repeat the IdCM and InCM calibrations. Once these runs were over, there was a need to choose vertices (switching columns between two boundary data matrices) in such a way that in each greedy cycle, the algorithm was heading closer and closer to the ground truth boundaries until all the vertices were checked. (4) Another similarity between Cootes's and Suri's methods was that both methods used a point model, which meant that the starting analysis of the boundaries were the vertices or points. The only difference was in the dimensionality of the matrices. Finally, Cootes used the Mahalanobis distance for performance, while Suri used the polyline distance metric. The greedy algorithm did a very effective job in the walls for the ED and ES frames and it even did well for the apical area of the ED frames, but it did not achieve a very accurate apex position in the ES frames. It did not pick up the rotational effect of the LV, which meant that the ES apex must be near the ED apex and around 45 degrees to the ED long axis. In the next section work on LV apex modeling will therefore be discussed.

3.5 Left Ventricle Apex Modeling: A Model-Based Approach

Modeling the LV apex is as important as modeling the LV boundaries. Due to the problems highlighted above, apex modeling is particularly cumbersome. Suri *et al.* [101] developed a relationship between the ED apex and ES apex using the same greedy approach. Suri first estimated the ED boundaries using the IdCM and the InCM models without apex information. Later, the regression model was used to estimate the transformation parameters required in the ES apex estimation. Regression in time utilized the training ground truth ES apex coordinates and the training ED apex coordinates, along with the coordinates of the selected ED boundary vertices. Suri used the same greedy algorithm for the ED boundary vertex selection, subject to the minimization of the error between the estimated ES apex position and the ground truth ES apex position. Note that the training ED apex and ES apex positions were determined from the estimated ED and ES frame boundaries. The apex position was given as that vertex on the bottom $(\frac{1}{3})^{rd}$ LV boundary, which was farthest from the midpoint of the AoV plane. This estimated ES apex was then padded to the classifier ES raw boundary and the boundary calibration was repeated using the training-based system. This system reduced the error further, as compared to the plain IdCM and InCM algorithms [236]. The basic reason was that an accurately determined ES apex was used to bring the LV to its correct position. Apex determination using the ground truth boundaries based on curvature change can be seen in Brower [239]. Having discussed the need for LV apex modeling, we will now discuss how this is being done. The layout of this section is as follows: Sub-section 3.5.1 presents the motivation behind implementing the ruled surface for LV apex modeling. The statement problem on the ruled surface is discussed in Sub-section 3.5.2. The coefficient estimation of the ruled surface is given in Sub-section 3.5.3. The Iterative Weighted Least Squares based on the Huber weight function is discussed in Sub-section 3.5.4. Experimental design for the ruled surface method is presented in Sub-section 3.5.5. The results of the ruled surface experiments are presented in Sub-section 3.5.7. Finally, some conclusions on LV apex modeling are given in Sub-section 3.5.8.

3.5.1 Longitudinal Axis and Apex Modeling

The left ventricle changes its shape under varying pathological conditions. Quantitative assessment of the 3-D geometry of the left ventricle (LV) may help to discriminate between different pathological conditions. The LV motion during the heart cycle involves (i) translation, (ii) rotation, (iii) wringing and (iv) movement of the endocardial circumference towards the center of the ventricular chamber. These motions are not uniform throughout the cardiac cycle. Moreover, the complexity increases because of large variations in the heart size, heart rate, position of the patient during the catheterization procedure, noise artifacts, and gray scale variation in the ventriculograms (cardioangiograms) [267], [201], [291]. For example, during systole, the mitral valve plane in an adult with normal cardiac function descends one to two centimeters towards the apex, but the apex barely moves up towards the center of the heart.

The apex point is the farthest point along the longitudinal axis (LA) from the aortic valve (AoV) plane. To keep track of the changing shape at the apex, one must keep track of the apex points of the LA. During the systole and diastole periods of the cardiac cycle, the heart's motion causes the LA to change its length and inclination (position). When these *automatically mea-sured longitudinal axes* are observed frame by frame, they fall into two classes. Most are small perturbations from the axis that a physician would delineate. A few have very large perturbations and are called *outliers*. Because outliers have an unusually great influence on *least square estimators* [244], it would be inappropriate to use a Least Squares estimation in such a situation. Therefore, the next sub-section determines the apex points of the LA in each frame of the cardiac cycle by robustly estimating the ruled surface coefficients using an iterative reweighted least squares (IRLS) fit.

3.5.2   Ruled Surface Model

Given the noisy *perturbed automatically measured* LA data of the LV, one must robustly estimate the ruled surface and its coefficients using an itera-tive reweighted least squares method. From the fitted surface, one can then produce fitted estimates of the *measured longitudinal axis*. First the noise model for the measured apex data for any frame f is given and then the same model is expressed in matrix form, for the complete cardiac cycle. Let $[x(f), y(f)], f = 1, \ldots, F$ denote the coordinates of the automatically measured LA apex (denoted by vertex v_a in Figure 3.24) for the cardiac cycle having F frames. The measured $[x(f), y(f)]$ coordinates for frame f are assumed to follow a Gaussian noise model, given by:

$$\left[\underbrace{x(f)\ y(f)}_{1\times 2} \right] = \sum_{j=0}^{2} B_j(f) \left[\underbrace{a_j\ b_j}_{1\times 2} \right] + \left[\underbrace{\eta_x(f)\ \eta_y(f)}_{1\times 2} \right], \qquad (3.36)$$

where $\{B_0(f) = 1, B_1(f) = f, B_2(f) = f^2\}$ is the basis set. $\eta_x(f) \sim \mathcal{N}(0, \sigma_x^2(f)), \eta_y(f) \sim \mathcal{N}(0, \sigma_y^2(f))$. $\sigma_x^2(f)$ is the variance of the noise for x-coordinate for frame f. $\sigma_y^2(f)$ is the variance of noise for y-coordinate for frame f. The Gaussian noise perturbing two different frames is assumed to be independent. It is also assumed that the x-coordinate and y-coordinate noise are indepen-dent. Let $\boldsymbol{\alpha}=(a_0, a_1, a_2)^T$ and $\boldsymbol{\beta}=(b_0, b_1, b_2)^T$ be the coefficients associated with the x and y coordinates of the apex, respectively. If all the frames of the cardiac cycle are taken into account and represented in a matrix form, this is: $\mathbf{V}=[\mathbf{X}\ \mathbf{Y}]^{F\times 2}$, where $\mathbf{X} = [x(1), \ldots, x(F)]^T$ and $\mathbf{Y} = [y(1), \ldots, y(F)]^T$. Note here that $\mathbf{V}$ is simple a matrix consisting of two vectors $\mathbf{X}$ and $\mathbf{Y}$ side by side of length F. Let F_{in} and F_{out} be the set of inlier and outlier frames, $\#F_{in} + \#F_{out} = F$, where F is the total number of frames in the cardiac cycle. $F_{com} = \{F_{in} \cup F_{out}\}$ is called the Combined Data. It is also assumed that $\#F_{out} \le \frac{1}{4}\#F_{in}$. The above model can be represented in matrix form as:

$$[\ \mathbf{V} \ ] = [\ \mathbf{XY} \ ]^{F \times 2} = [\mathbf{B}\psi]^{F \times 2} + [\ \boldsymbol{\eta}_x \ \boldsymbol{\eta}_y \ ]^{F \times 2} , \qquad (3.37)$$

where $\psi = [\ \boldsymbol{\alpha} \ \boldsymbol{\beta} \ ]^{3 \times 2}$ are the coefficients associated with the x- and y-coordinates. $\mathbf{B}\psi$ is the matrix holding the true unperturbed coordinates of the cardiac cycle. $\mathbf{V}$ is the matrix holding the longitudinal axis data, since it consists of the observed apex or aortic coordinates for the complete cardiac cycle. $\mathbf{B}$ is the basis matrix for the given cardiac cycle:

$$\mathbf{B} = \begin{pmatrix} 1 \ 1 \ 1^2 \\ . \\ 1 \ f \ f^2 \\ . \\ 1 \ F \ F^2 \end{pmatrix}^{F \times 3} .$$

The distribution of the noise vector $\boldsymbol{\eta}_x$ $(F \times 1)$ for the cardiac cycle has a mean 0 and covariance Σ_x, given as: $\boldsymbol{\eta}_x \sim \mathcal{N}(0, \Sigma_x)$. Similarly, the distribution of the noise vector $\boldsymbol{\eta}_y$ $(F \times 1)$ for the cardiac cycle has a mean 0 and a covariance Σ_y, given as: $\boldsymbol{\eta}_y \sim \mathcal{N}(0, \Sigma_y)$. The covariance matrix Σ_x for the $\boldsymbol{\eta}_x$ is given as:

$$\Sigma_x^{F \times F} = \begin{pmatrix} \sigma_x^2(1) & 0 & . & . & . & . \\ 0 & . & 0 & . & . & . \\ . & 0 & . & . & . & . \\ . & . & . & \sigma_x^2(f) & . & 0 \\ . & . & . & . & . & . \\ . & . & . & . & 0 & \sigma_x^2(F) \end{pmatrix} , \qquad (3.38)$$

where the variance for frame f is given as:

$$\sigma_x^2(f) = \begin{cases} \sigma_{in}^2 \ \text{for} \ f \in F_{in} \\ \sigma_{out}^2 \ \text{for} \ f \in F_{out} \end{cases} \qquad (3.39)$$

where $\sigma_{out}^2 \gg \sigma_{in}^2$, i.e., the noise in the outlier frames (F_{out}) is much larger than the noise in the inlier frames (F_{in}). The covariance for the y-coordinate (Σ_y) is defined in the same way as Σ_x. Note, the Gaussian noise perturbing two different frames is assumed to be independent.

The problem is to estimate $[\hat{x}(f), \hat{y}(f)]$, $f = 1, \ldots, F$, the coordinates of LA apex or aortic points using an iterative least square robust procedure (IRLS). In matrix notation it is estimated: $\hat{\mathbf{V}} = [\hat{\mathbf{X}} \ \hat{\mathbf{Y}}] = [\mathbf{B}\hat{\psi}]^{F \times 2}$ where, $\hat{\mathbf{X}} = [\hat{x}(1), \ldots, \hat{x}(F)]^T$ and $\hat{\mathbf{Y}} = [\hat{y}(1), \ldots, \hat{y}(F)]^T$. $\hat{\psi}(3 \times 2)$ is the estimated coefficient matrix. The problem thus reduces to estimating $\hat{\psi}$ using an iterative least square robust procedure.

LONGITUDINAL AXIS AND RULED SURFACE
Example of Systole Cycle (Contraction phase)

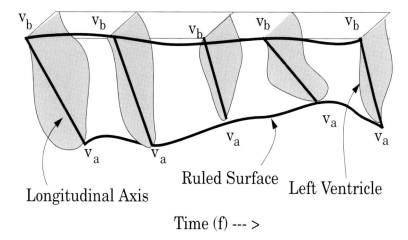

Figure 3.24: Generation of the ruled surface from the motion of the longitudinal axis in time. Longitudinal axis (or long axis) is the segment joining the starting vertex v_a and ending vertex v_b.

3.5.3   Ruled Surface s_r and its Coefficients

Consider the ruled surface (see Figure 3.24) generated by the LA during the cardiac cycle. This ruled surface is modeled in the quadratic parametric form given in Equation (3.36). Let the apex and aortic end vertices of the LA for a frame f in the cardiac cycle be $[x_a(f),\, y_a(f)]$ and $[x_b(f),\, y_b(f)]$, respectively. The ruled surface is given mathematically as:

$$s_r(f, \lambda) = (1 - \lambda)\begin{bmatrix} x_a(f) \\ y_a(f) \\ f \end{bmatrix} + (\lambda)\begin{bmatrix} x_b(f) \\ y_b(f) \\ f \end{bmatrix}, \qquad (3.40)$$

where λ, $0 \leq \lambda \leq 1$, is the variable designating a position along the LA and $f = 1, \ldots, F$ is the frame number. Thus, the ruled surface equation is a function of the end coordinates of the LA, which in turn is a function of $\psi = \begin{bmatrix} \alpha & \beta \end{bmatrix}$, the apex coefficient matrix and $\zeta = \begin{bmatrix} \gamma & \delta \end{bmatrix}$, the similarly defined aortic[15] coefficient matrix. Since the estimation for the apex coefficients and aortic coefficients is similar, a generic (x, y) is used in the remainder of this chapter, not distinguishing between (x_a, y_a) and (x_b, y_b).

---

[15] A similar procedure is adapted for the aortic coordinates of the longitudinal axis of the left ventricle. The coefficients pair used is $\zeta = \begin{bmatrix} \gamma & \delta \end{bmatrix}$.

3.5.4 Estimation of Robust Coefficients and Coordinates of the Ruled Surface

The coefficient matrix of the ruled surface is robustly estimated using the iterative re-weighted least squares procedure, in which low weights are assigned to the outliers which have high residual error and high weights are assigned to the inliers which have low residual error. This weighting has the effect of reducing the influence of the outliers on the estimated coefficients. At each iteration, a weighted least squares problem is solved. The weight matrix for the first iteration is taken to be the identity matrix. The weights for each successive iteration are a function of the residual errors of the previous iteration. Convergence is achieved in fewer than 10 iterations. Sub-section 3.5.4.1 describes the weighted least square (WLS) estimation. Sub-section 3.5.4.2 describes the complete iterative reweighted least squares algorithm.

3.5.4.1 Weighted Least Square (WLS) Estimate, $\hat{\psi}_w$

The weights for the current iteration are a function of the normalized residuals of the estimated x- and estimated y-apex coordinates from the previous iteration. Here, an assumption is made that the weights are given. The next sub-section discusses the determination of the weights at each iteration. Thus given the matrices for the Combined Data $\mathbf{V}$, the basis matrix $\mathbf{B}$, the diagonal weight matrix $\mathbf{W}$, the weighted least squares problem is to determine $\hat{\psi}_w$ to minimize the weighted residual squared error function ϵ_w^2, defined by:

$$\epsilon_w^2 = \| \mathbf{W} (\mathbf{V} - \mathbf{B}\,\hat{\psi}_w) \|^2 . \tag{3.41}$$

The estimated apex coordinate matrix $\hat{\mathbf{V}}$ is given by the product of $\mathbf{B}$ and the estimated coefficients $\hat{\psi}_w$ given as:

$$\hat{\mathbf{V}} = \mathbf{B}\,\hat{\psi}_w . \tag{3.42}$$

To determine the $\hat{\psi}_w$ that minimizes ϵ_w^2, the partial derivative of ϵ_w^2 is taken with respect to $\hat{\psi}_w$ and equate the result to 0. Solving for the coefficient matrix, $\hat{\psi}_w$, results in:

$$\underbrace{\hat{\psi}_w}_{3\times 2} = \underbrace{(\mathbf{B}^T\,\mathbf{W}^T\,\mathbf{W}\,\mathbf{B})^{-1}}_{3\times 3}\underbrace{(\mathbf{B}^T\,\mathbf{W}^T\,\mathbf{W}\,\mathbf{V})}_{3\times 2} . \tag{3.43}$$

3.5.4.2 Iterative Reweighted Least Squares Algorithm

The following are the iterative steps to estimate the robust coefficients.

1. *Normalized residual error computation:*
   The expression is derived for the raw residual error with respect to the x-coordinate and the same procedure is adapted for the y-coordinate. If $\mathbf{r}_x$ and $\mathbf{r}_y$ are the raw residual error vectors for the x-coordinate and the

y-coordinate, respectively, then the joint raw residual error matrix for the cardiac cycle is given as $\mathbf{r}=[\mathbf{r}_x\ \mathbf{r}_y]$, where, $\mathbf{r}_x = [r_x(1),\dots,r_x(F)]^T$ and $\mathbf{r}_y = [r_y(1),\dots,r_y(F)]^T$. The expression for $\mathbf{r}$ is given as:

$$\mathbf{r} = [\mathbf{V} - \mathbf{B}\,\hat{\psi}_w]^{F\times 2} \tag{3.44}$$

$$= [\mathbf{V} - \mathbf{B}\,\underbrace{(\mathbf{B}^T\,\mathbf{W}^T\,\mathbf{W}\,\mathbf{B})^{-1}(\mathbf{B}^T\,\mathbf{W}^T\,\mathbf{W}\,\mathbf{V})}_{3\times 2}].$$

Thus, $\mathbf{r}_x$ and $\mathbf{r}_y$ can be given as:

$$\begin{cases} \mathbf{r}_x = [\mathbf{X} - \mathbf{B}\,\underbrace{(\mathbf{B}^T\,\mathbf{W}^T\,\mathbf{W}\,\mathbf{B})^{-1}(\mathbf{B}^T\,\mathbf{W}^T\,\mathbf{W}\,\mathbf{X})}] \\ \mathbf{r}_y = [\mathbf{Y} - \mathbf{B}\,\underbrace{(\mathbf{B}^T\,\mathbf{W}^T\,\mathbf{W}\,\mathbf{B})^{-1}(\mathbf{B}^T\,\mathbf{W}^T\,\mathbf{W}\,\mathbf{Y})}]. \end{cases} \tag{3.45}$$

Each component is normalized of the raw residual error $\mathbf{r}_x$ by an estimate of its root mean square error. The root mean square error for $\mathbf{r}_x$ can be computed from the covariance of the raw residual error. By definition, $\mathrm{COV}(\mathbf{r}_x)=E[(\mathbf{r}_x - E[\mathbf{r}_x])(\mathbf{r}_x - E[\mathbf{r}_x])^T]$. Here, E stands for the expectation. Let the projection operator be defined as:

$$\mathbf{P} = \mathbf{B}\,\underbrace{(\mathbf{B}^T\,\mathbf{W}^T\,\mathbf{W}\,\mathbf{B})^{-1}\mathbf{B}^T\,\mathbf{W}^T\,\mathbf{W}}. \tag{3.46}$$

Thus the raw residual vector $\mathbf{r}_x$ ($F \times 1$) reduces to:

$$\mathbf{r}_x = [\mathbf{X} - \mathbf{P}\,\mathbf{X}] = [(\mathbf{I} - \mathbf{P})\,\mathbf{X}]. \tag{3.47}$$

Note, $[(\mathbf{I} - \mathbf{P})]$ is of dimension $F \times F$. If α_{true} (3×1) are the true coefficients, then substituting $\mathbf{X} = \mathbf{B}\alpha_{true} + \eta_x$ and using the fact that $\mathbf{P}\,\mathbf{B}=\mathbf{B}$, the covariance of $\mathbf{r}_x$ can be expressed as:

$$COV(\mathbf{r}_x) = (\mathbf{I} - \mathbf{P})\,E[\eta_x\,\eta_x^T](\mathbf{I} - \mathbf{P})^T. \tag{3.48}$$

Since by assumption $E[\eta_x\,\eta_x^T]= \sigma_x^2\mathbf{I}$, this is: $COV(\mathbf{r}_x)= (\mathbf{I}-\mathbf{P})\,\sigma_x^2\mathbf{I}\,(\mathbf{I}-\mathbf{P})^T$. The interest is in the diagonal elements of the product of the matrices: $(\mathbf{I}-\mathbf{P})(\mathbf{I}-\mathbf{P})^T$. Let $\mathbf{Q}=(\mathbf{I}-\mathbf{P})(\mathbf{I}-\mathbf{P})^T$. Expanding the right hand side and taking the diagonal elements, results in:

$$diag[\mathbf{Q}] = diag[\mathbf{I} - \mathbf{P} - \mathbf{P}^T + \mathbf{P}\mathbf{P}^T]. \tag{3.49}$$

Since the diagonal elements of $\mathbf{P}$ and $\mathbf{P}^T$ are the same, thus the above equation reduces to: $diag[\mathbf{Q}]=diag[\mathbf{I} - 2\mathbf{P} + \mathbf{P}\mathbf{P}^T]$. Let:

$$diag[\mathbf{Q}^{F\times F}] = [q_{11}\dots q_{ff}\dots q_{FF}], \tag{3.50}$$

then the element q_{ff} of $\mathbf{Q}$ can be expressed as:

$$q_{ff} = 1 - 2p_{ff} + \sum_{k=1}^{F} p_{fk}^2 \tag{3.51}$$

$$= (1 - p_{ff})^2 + \sum_{k=1,k\neq f}^{F} p_{fk}^2,$$

where p_{ff} is the diagonal element of $\mathbf{P}$ and p_{fk} is the off-diagonal element of $\mathbf{P}$. Now the $\text{COV}(\mathbf{r}_x)=\sigma_x^2\,\mathbf{Q}$. Thus, the variance of the raw residual error for frame f is: $\text{var}[r_x(f)]=\sigma_x^2\,q_{ff}$ and its standard deviation is: $\sigma[r_x(f)]=\sigma_x\sqrt{q_{ff}}$.

The estimate of the noise σ is based on the raw residual vector $\mathbf{r}_x$. Consider $E[\mathbf{r}_x^T\,\mathbf{r}_x] = E[\text{trace}(\mathbf{r}_x^T\,\mathbf{r}_x)]$. As "$E$" and trace commute, $E[\mathbf{r}_x^T\,\mathbf{r}_x] = \text{trace}\{\sigma_x^2\,(\mathbf{I} - \mathbf{P})\}$, so that:

$$E[\mathbf{r}_x^T\,\mathbf{r}_x] = \sigma_x^2\,\text{trace}(\mathbf{I} - \mathbf{P}) = \sigma_x^2\,(F - 3). \tag{3.52}$$

Since the trace of a projection operator is the dimension of the space to which it projects and $\mathbf{P}$ projects to a three dimensional subspace, one can estimate $\hat{\sigma}_x^2$ from the raw residual error as: $(\frac{\mathbf{r}_x^T\,\mathbf{r}_x}{F-3})$. Thus: $\hat{\sigma}_x=\sqrt{\frac{\mathbf{r}_x^T\,\mathbf{r}_x}{F-3}}$. Similarly, $\hat{\sigma}_y=\sqrt{\frac{\mathbf{r}_y^T\,\mathbf{r}_y}{F-3}}$. Thus one can express $\hat{\sigma}_x[r_x(f)]$ and $\hat{\sigma}_y[r_y(f)]$ as:

$$\hat{\sigma}_x[r_x(f)] = \sqrt{\frac{\mathbf{r}_x^T\,\mathbf{r}_x}{F-3}(q_{ff})} \tag{3.53}$$

$$\hat{\sigma}_y[r_y(f)] = \sqrt{\frac{\mathbf{r}_y^T\,\mathbf{r}_y}{F-3}(q_{ff})} \tag{3.54}$$

Thus the normalized residuals $\mathbf{r}_n$ are:

$$\mathbf{r}_n = \begin{pmatrix} r_{nx}(1) & r_{ny}(1) \\ \cdot & \cdot \\ \cdot & \cdot \\ r_{nx}(F) & r_{ny}(F) \end{pmatrix}^{F\times 2} \tag{3.55}$$

$$= \begin{pmatrix} \frac{r_x(1)}{\sigma[r_x(1)]} & \frac{r_y(1)}{\sigma[r_y(1)]} \\ \cdot & \cdot \\ \cdot & \cdot \\ \frac{r_x(F)}{\sigma[r_x(F)]} & \frac{r_y(F)}{\sigma[r_y(F)]} \end{pmatrix}^{F\times 2}. \tag{3.56}$$

In matrix notation, the normalized residuals $\mathbf{r}_n$ can be expressed by first defining the diagonal matrix $\mathbf{S}$ as:

$$\mathbf{S}^{F\times F} = \begin{pmatrix} \frac{1}{\sqrt{q_{11}}} & 0 & 0 & 0 & 0 \\ 0 & \frac{1}{\sqrt{q_{22}}} & 0 & 0 & 0 \\ 0 & 0 & \cdot & 0 & 0 \\ 0 & 0 & 0 & \cdot & 0 \\ 0 & 0 & 0 & 0 & \frac{1}{\sqrt{q_{FF}}} \end{pmatrix}^{F\times F}. \tag{3.57}$$

Then, the normalized residual matrix $\mathbf{r}_n$ ($F \times 2$) for the cardiac cycle is given as:

$$\underbrace{\mathbf{r}_n}_{F\times 2} = [\mathbf{r}_{nx}\ \mathbf{r}_{ny}]^{F\times 2} = \underbrace{\mathbf{S}}_{F\times F}[\frac{\mathbf{r}_x}{\hat{\sigma}_x}\ \frac{\mathbf{r}_y}{\hat{\sigma}_y}]^{F\times 2}. \tag{3.58}$$

2. *Huber's weight assignment (**W**):*
   The weights for each frame f are based on the normalized residual error and Huber's weight formula, given as:

$$w(f) = min \left(\frac{H_x + H_y}{\mid r_{nx}(f) + \mid r_{ny}(f) \mid} , 1 \right) \qquad (3.59)$$

where H_x and H_y are a Huber's function [241] for x- and y-coordinates and is given as a product of the tuning constant (T_c) and the median of the normalized absolute residuals is given as:

$$H_x = T_c \, med(\mid r_{nx}(f) \mid), 1 \le f \le F \qquad (3.60)$$
$$H_y = T_c \, med(\mid r_{ny}(f) \mid), 1 \le f \le F.$$

Note, "med" is the median computation over F frames of the cardiac cycle. The range of the tuning constant (T_c) is shown in Table 3.1. The weights depend upon the absolute value of the normalized residual error. If the residual error is high, then low weights are assigned and vice versa. The weight matrix **W** is given as:

$$\mathbf{W}^{F \times F} = Diag(w(1), w(2), w(3), ..., w(F)). \qquad (3.61)$$

3. *Robust Coefficient Estimation $\hat{\psi}_{robust}$:*
   Since IRLS is an iterative process, at the cth iteration, the weight matrix is denoted by $\mathbf{W}_c$. The robust coefficient vector $(\hat{\psi}_{robust})_c$ is computed using Equation (3.43):

$$\underbrace{(\hat{\psi}_{robust})_{c+1}}_{3 \times 2} = \underbrace{(\mathbf{B}^T \, \mathbf{W}_c^T \, \mathbf{W}_c \, \mathbf{B})^{-1}}_{3 \times F} \times \\ \underbrace{(\mathbf{B}^T \, \mathbf{W}_c^T \, \mathbf{W}_c \, \mathbf{V})}_{F \times 2}. \qquad (3.62)$$

This equation can be solved using a singular value decomposition [256]. Steps (1), (2) and (3) are iterated and convergence is achieved in fewer than 10 iterations. Thus, the robust coefficients are: $\hat{\psi}_{robust} = (\hat{\psi}_{robust})_{10}$.

3.5.4.3   Estimation of Robust Coordinates, $(\hat{\mathbf{X}} \, \hat{\mathbf{Y}})$

The apex coordinates of the LA can be derived from the robust coefficients given in Equation (3.62). The estimated $(\hat{x}, \hat{y})$ coordinates of the apex of the longitudinal axis data are:

$$\underbrace{\hat{\mathbf{V}}}_{F \times 2} = \underbrace{[\hat{\mathbf{X}} \, \hat{\mathbf{Y}}]}_{F \times 2} = \underbrace{[\mathbf{B} \, \hat{\psi}_{robust}]}_{F \times 2}. \qquad (3.63)$$

Parameters	Values
Small inlier noise (σ_{in}^2)	0.0, 1.0, 2.0, 3.0, 4.0, 5.0, 6.0,...,10.0 (mm^2)
Large outlier noise (σ_{out}^2)	50.0, 70.0, 80.0,..,100.0 (mm^2)
Total number of outliers (n_o) per case	0%–20% (0 to 12 axis frames/any cycle)
Weights in IRLS fit	0–1
Tuning Constant (T_c)	$2.0 \leq T_c \leq 3.5$
Total number of trials (T_o)	100
Total number of studies (N)	40 (Clinical Data)

Table 3.1: Parameters used in longitudinal axis generation and fitting.

3.5.5 Experiment Design

To test the technique, a controlled set of experiments were performed with synthetic data and a set of experiments on clinical data. Sub-section 3.5.5.1 describes the synthetic data generation process, Sub-section 3.5.5.2 the error measure of the ruled surface for Inlier Data and Sub-section 3.5.5.3 the robust procedure *efficiency*. Finally, the relationships are discussed of the ruled surface error measure with input random perturbation and on the robust procedure. Also shown is the effect on the robust efficiency of increasing the number of outliers. The clinical data consists of hand delineated boundaries drawn by the cardiologist or the trained technologist and the hand delineated apex coordinates and its serial number starting from the anterior aspect of the aortic valve (AAV). Each data file for a patient study consists of F frames and each frame consists of a polygonal boundary with 100 vertices starting from the AAV.

3.5.5.1 Synthetic Data Generation Process

There are two kinds of data sets generated, Inlier Data sets, consisting of $(F - n_o)$ frames and Combined Data sets, consisting of F frames, of which $(F - n_o)$ is the number of inlier frames and n_o is the number of outlier frames. n_o is an experimental parameter and is fixed between 0% to 20% of F. The set of n_o outlier frames $F_{out}=\{f_1, f_2, f_3, ..., f_{n_o}\}$ is selected at random by sampling the set $\{1, ..., F\}$ without replacement. Once the sets of inlier and outlier frames are generated, the synthetic Inlier Data and Combined Data were then generated using Equations (3.36) and (3.37). The variation of Inlier (σ_{in}^2) and Outlier noise (σ_{out}^2) is shown in Table 3.1. An ordinary least squares fitting was applied to the Inlier Data. A robust iterative reweighted least squares was applied to the Combined Data. The ratio of their errors measures the efficiency of the robust procedure.

3.5.5.2 Error Measure of a Ruled Surface ($\hat{Q}_\psi^{in}$) & ($\hat{Q}_\psi^{com}$)

The performance of the *robust ruled surface procedure* can be evaluated in terms of the error measure of the ruled surface. The error measure of the estimated ruled surface from the Inlier Data for patient study n is defined as the expected value of the squared difference between the *true* apex coordinates of the LA and the *estimated* apex coordinates of the LA using LS fit. The error measure for the Combined Data for study n is defined as the expected value of the squared difference between the *true* apex coordinates of the LA and the robustly estimated apex coordinates of the longitudinal axis. The expression is first given for the error measure of the ruled surface for Inlier Data with respect to coefficient α (x-coordinate). The following notational conventions are used: let $Q^{in}_{\alpha n}$ be the error measure for the Inlier Data of a patient study n with respect to α and let $Q^{com}_{\alpha n}$ be the error measure for the Combined Data for study n, with respect to α. First, the expression is derived of the error measure of study n for Inlier Data in terms of frame number f, the true x-coordinate of the apex, $x^{true}_n(f)$, and the estimated x-coordinate of the apex, $\hat{x}^{in}_n(f)$ and the total trials, T_o and then the expression for the mean error measure over all the studies N is given. The expressions for the y-coordinate are similar and hence the total error measure can be computed by adding the x- and the y-coordinate errors. Note as before, F_{in} and F_{out} are the sets of inlier and outlier frames. The squared difference between the true x-coordinate and the estimated x-coordinate of the apex from Inlier Data for any inlier frame f for study n is:

$$(x^{true}_n(f) - \hat{x}^{in}_n(f))^2 .$$

Here, "in" represents Inlier Data. By definition, the error measure of Inlier Data over the frames $f \in F_{in}$ for study n ($Q^{in}_{\alpha n}$) is:

$$Q^{in}_{\alpha n} = E[(x^{true}_n(f) - \hat{x}^{in}_n(f))^2] . \tag{3.64}$$

"E" represents expectation. Thus, the *estimated error measure* for study n over all the frames f with respect to α for T_o trials is:

$$\hat{Q}^{in}_{\alpha n} = \frac{1}{T_o} \sum_{t=1}^{T_o} \left[\frac{1}{F - n_o - 3} \sum_{f \in F_{in}(t)} (x^{true}_n(f) - (\hat{x}^{in}_n(f))_t)^2 \right] , \tag{3.65}$$

where $F_{in}(t)$ is the set of inlier frames for the trial number t. Note that t only subscripts the term $\hat{x}^{in}_n(f)$. Taking into consideration all studies N, the *mean estimated error* is:

$$\hat{Q}^{in}_{\alpha} = \frac{1}{N} \sum_{n=1}^{N} \left[\frac{1}{T_o} \sum_{t=1}^{T_o} \left[\frac{1}{F - n_o - 3} \sum_{f \in F_{in}(t)} (x^{true}_n(f) - (\hat{x}^{in}_n(f))_t)^2 \right] \right] .$$

Repeating the above steps (Equations (3.64), (3.65), (3.66)), for the y-coordinate, this gives the mean error measure with respect to β (the y-coordinate) as:

$$\hat{Q}^{in}_{\beta} = \frac{1}{N} \sum_{n=1}^{N} \left[\frac{1}{T_o} \sum_{t=1}^{T_o} \left[\frac{1}{F - n_o - 3} \sum_{f \in F_{in}(t)} (y^{true}_n(f) - (\hat{y}^{in}_n(f))_t)^2 \right] \right] .$$

Thus the mean estimated error measure of a ruled surface from Inlier Data taking both the x-and y-coordinates of the apex is:

$$\hat{Q}_\psi^{in} = \hat{Q}_\alpha^{in} + \hat{Q}_\beta^{in} .\qquad(3.66)$$

Now the expressions are derived for the joint mean error measure of the robust ruled surface from the Combined Data with respect to ψ. In this study, the squared difference between the true x-coordinate and the estimated x-coordinate of the apex for the Combined Data for a given study n is:

$$(x_n^{true}(f) - \hat{x}_n^{com}(f))^2 ,$$

where "com" stands for the Combined Data. By definition, the error measure of Combined Data, over the frames $f \in F_{com}$ for study n ($Q_{\alpha n}^{com}$) is:

$$
\begin{aligned}
Q_{\alpha n}^{com} &= E\,[\,(x_n^{true}(f) - \hat{x}_n^{com}(f))^2\,] && (3.67)\\
&= \frac{1}{F-3} \sum_{f \in F_{com}(t)} (x_n^{true}(f) - \hat{x}_n^{com}(f))^2 .
\end{aligned}
$$

Thus, the *estimated error measure* for study n over all the frames f with respect to α for T_o trials is:

$$\hat{Q}_{\alpha n}^{com} = \frac{1}{T_o} \sum_{t=1}^{T_o} \left[\frac{1}{F-3} \sum_{f \in F_{com}(t)} (x_n^{true}(f) - (\hat{x}_n^{com}(f))_t)^2 \right] ,\qquad(3.68)$$

where $F_{com}(t)$ is the set of frames in the Combined Data. Taking all the studies N into consideration, the *mean estimated error* ($\hat{Q}_\alpha^{com}$) is:

$$\hat{Q}_\alpha^{com} = \frac{1}{N} \sum_{n=1}^{N} \left[\frac{1}{T_o} \sum_{t=1}^{T_o} \left[\frac{1}{F-3} \sum_{f \in F_{com}(t)} (x_n^{true}(f) - (\hat{x}_n^{com}(f))_t)^2 \right] \right].\qquad(3.69)$$

Repeating the above steps (Equations (3.67), (3.68), (3.69)) for the y-coordinate results in:

$$\hat{Q}_\beta^{com} = \frac{1}{N} \sum_{n=1}^{N} \left[\frac{1}{T_o} \sum_{t=1}^{T_o} \left[\frac{1}{F-3} \sum_{f \in F_{com}(t)} (y_n^{true}(f) - (\hat{y}_n^{com}(f))_t)^2 \right] \right].\qquad(3.70)$$

Thus the mean estimated error measure of a ruled surface from *Combined Data* taking both the x-and y-coordinates of the apex is:

$$\hat{Q}_\psi^{com} = \hat{Q}_\alpha^{com} + \hat{Q}_\beta^{com} .\qquad(3.71)$$

3.5.5.3 Efficiency of a Robust Procedure (η^ψ)

The statistical efficiency of a robust procedure measures how well the robustly computed x- and y-coordinates of the end vertices for data *with outliers* compared with the non-robustly computed x- and y-coordinates of the apex vertices for data *without outliers*. This can be defined as the ratio of the *mean error* of inlier data having $(F - n_o)$ frames, to the *mean error* of the *Combined Data* having F frames. Thus the estimated statistical efficiency $\hat{\eta}^\psi$ is basically the ratio of $\hat{Q}_\psi^{in}$ to $\hat{Q}_\psi^{com}$: $\hat{\eta}^\psi = \frac{\hat{Q}_\psi^{in}}{\hat{Q}_\psi^{com}}$. Having derived the expression of quality measure for the inlier data set, combined data sets and efficiency, the next section derives the expression for the analytical error measure.

3.5.6　Analytical Error Measure, AQ^{in} for Inlier Data

In this sub-section, the equations are derived for the analytical error measure of the ruled surface in terms of variance of inlier noise (σ_{in}^2) and the projection operator $(\mathbf{P})$. For simplicity, the expression will be derived for the x-coordinate of the apex, with respect to $\boldsymbol{\alpha}$. The same procedure is adapted for the y-coordinate of the apex, i.e., with respect to $\boldsymbol{\beta}$. The analytical error measure of the ruled surface is computed by finding the expected value of the experimentally estimated error.

$$AQ_{\boldsymbol{\alpha}}^{in} = E\,[\hat{Q}_{\boldsymbol{\alpha}}^{in}] \tag{3.72}$$

Using the notation and the definition of the error measure for the Inlier Data discussed in Sub-section 3.5.5.2, results in $(Q_{\boldsymbol{\alpha}n}^{in})$ over all the frames $f \in F_{in}$ resulting in:

$$Q_{\boldsymbol{\alpha}}^{in} = E\,[(x^{true}(f) - \hat{x}^{in}(f))^2], \tag{3.73}$$

where these symbols have the same meaning as before. The *estimated error measure* over all the frames $f \in F_{in}$ with respect to $\boldsymbol{\alpha}$ is:

$$\hat{Q}_{\boldsymbol{\alpha}}^{in} = \left[\frac{1}{F - n_o - 3} \sum_{f \in F_{in}} (x^{true}(f) - \hat{x}^{in}(f))^2 \,. \right] \tag{3.74}$$

Changing the above expression into the matrix form results in:

$$\hat{Q}_{\boldsymbol{\alpha}}^{in} = \left[\frac{1}{F - n_o - 3} \parallel \mathbf{X}_{in}^{true} - \hat{\mathbf{X}}^{in} \parallel^2 \right] \,. \tag{3.75}$$

$\mathbf{X}_{in}^{true}$ and $\hat{\mathbf{X}}^{in}$ are both $(F - n_o) \times 1$ vector. Substituting Equation (3.75) in Equation (3.72), the analytical error measure with respect to $\boldsymbol{\alpha}$ is:

$$AQ_{\boldsymbol{\alpha}}^{in} = E\,[\frac{1}{F - n_o - 3} \parallel \mathbf{X}_{in}^{true} - \hat{\mathbf{X}}^{in} \parallel^2]. \tag{3.76}$$

Now, the value of $\hat{\mathbf{X}}^{in}$ in terms of known quantities, $\mathbf{X}_{in}^{true}$, σ_{in}^2, and a projection operator $\mathbf{P}$ can be derived as: the estimated x from the Inlier data $(F - n_o$ frames) using the plain least square (LS) procedure is given as:

$$\hat{\mathbf{X}}^{in} = \mathbf{B}\,\hat{\boldsymbol{\alpha}}^{in} \tag{3.77}$$
$$= \mathbf{B}(\mathbf{B}^T\mathbf{B})^{-1}\mathbf{B}^T\mathbf{X}^{in}, \tag{3.78}$$

where $\hat{\boldsymbol{\alpha}}^{in}$ is the coefficient associated with the x-coordinates. Now since this is a LS procedure, the weight matrix $\mathbf{W}$ equals identity, $\mathbf{I}$, thus the projection operator is: $\mathbf{P} = \mathbf{B}\,\underbrace{(\mathbf{B}^T\mathbf{W}^T\mathbf{W}\mathbf{B})^{-1}\mathbf{B}^T\mathbf{W}^T\mathbf{W}}$ reduces to: $\mathbf{P} = \mathbf{B}\,(\mathbf{B}^T\mathbf{B})^{-1}\mathbf{B}^T$.

Thus, $\hat{\mathbf{X}}^{in} = \mathbf{P}(\mathbf{X}^{in}) = \mathbf{P}(\mathbf{X}_{in}^{true} + \boldsymbol{\eta}_x)$. This results in: $[\mathbf{X}_{in}^{true} - \hat{\mathbf{X}}^{in}] = [\,(\mathbf{I} -$

$\mathbf{P}) \, \mathbf{X}_{in}^{true} - \mathbf{P} \boldsymbol{\eta}_x \,$]. Taking the transpose of $[\mathbf{X}_{in}^{true} - \hat{\mathbf{X}}^{in}]$ and multiplying by itself yields:

$$
\begin{aligned}
[\mathbf{X}_{in}^{true} - \hat{\mathbf{X}}^{in}]^T \, [\mathbf{X}_{in}^{true} - \hat{\mathbf{X}}^{in}] \;=\; & \mathbf{X}_{in}^{true\,T} \, (\mathbf{I} - \mathbf{P})^T \, (\mathbf{I} - \mathbf{P}) \, \mathbf{X}_{in}^{true} - (3.79) \\
& \mathbf{X}_{in}^{true\,T} \, (\mathbf{I} - \mathbf{P})^T \, \mathbf{P} \boldsymbol{\eta}_x + \\
& \boldsymbol{\eta}_x \mathbf{P}^T (\mathbf{I} - \mathbf{P})^T \, \mathbf{X}_{in}^{true\,T} + \\
& \boldsymbol{\eta}_x^T \mathbf{P}^T \, \mathbf{P} \boldsymbol{\eta}_x \,.
\end{aligned}
$$

On taking the expectation of the above four terms and using $\mathrm{E}\,[\boldsymbol{\eta}_x] = 0$, $\mathrm{E}\,[\boldsymbol{\eta}_x^T] = 0$, the analytical quality measure reduces to:

$$
\begin{aligned}
AQ_\alpha^{in} \;=\; & \frac{1}{F - n_o - 3} \, E\,[\mathbf{X}_{in}^{true\,T} \, (\mathbf{I} - \mathbf{P})^T \, (\mathbf{I} - \mathbf{P}) \, \mathbf{X}_{in}^{true}] \\
& + \frac{1}{F - n_o - 3} \, E\,[\boldsymbol{\eta}_x^T \, \mathbf{P}^T \, \mathbf{P} \, \boldsymbol{\eta}_x] \,. \qquad (3.80)
\end{aligned}
$$

where $\mathbf{X}_{in}^{true}$ are the ideal coefficients. The term $E[\boldsymbol{\eta}_x^T \, \mathbf{P}^T \, \mathbf{P} \, \boldsymbol{\eta}_x]$ can be determined using the property that $\mathbf{P} = \mathbf{P}^T$, $\mathbf{P}^2 = \mathbf{P}$ and using the fact that E and *trace* commute to:

$$
\begin{aligned}
E\,[\boldsymbol{\eta}_x^T \, \mathbf{P}^T \, \mathbf{P} \, \boldsymbol{\eta}_x] \;=\; & E\,[\boldsymbol{\eta}_x^T \, \mathbf{P}^2 \, \boldsymbol{\eta}_x] \\
=\; & E\,[\,trace\,(\boldsymbol{\eta}_x^T \, \underbrace{\mathbf{P} \boldsymbol{\eta}_x})\,] \\
=\; & E\,[\,trace\,(\underbrace{\mathbf{P} \boldsymbol{\eta}_x} \, \boldsymbol{\eta}_x^T)\,] \\
=\; & trace\,(E\,[\mathbf{P} \, \boldsymbol{\eta}_x \, \boldsymbol{\eta}_x^T]\,) \\
=\; & trace\,(\mathbf{P} \, E\,[\boldsymbol{\eta}_x \boldsymbol{\eta}_x^T]) \\
=\; & trace\,(\mathbf{P} \, \sigma_{in}^2 \mathbf{I}) \\
=\; & \sigma_{in}^2 \, trace\,(\mathbf{P} \, \mathbf{I}) \\
=\; & \sigma_{in}^2 \, trace\,(\mathbf{P}) \\
=\; & \sigma_{in}^2 \, \sum_{f \in F_{in}} p_{ff} \,. \qquad (3.81)
\end{aligned}
$$

Substituting this last term in the analytical error measure and using the property that the expectation of a constant is a constant, this finally results in:

$$
\begin{aligned}
AQ_\alpha^{in} \;=\; & \frac{1}{F - n_o - 3} \, [\mathbf{X}_{in}^{true\,T} \, (\mathbf{I} - \mathbf{P})^T \, (\mathbf{I} - \mathbf{P}) \, \mathbf{X}_{in}^{true} + \\
& \sigma_{in}^2 \, \sum_{f \in F_{in}} p_{ff}] \,, \qquad (3.82)
\end{aligned}
$$

where C, the degrees of freedom, takes the value 3 and the unit of AQ_α^{in} is mm^2 and p_{ff} is the diagonal element of the projection operator $\mathbf{P}$ for frame f.

Note here that the analytical error measure is independent of the x-coordinate position. Similar to the above procedure, the analytical error measure can be computed with respect to $\boldsymbol{\beta}$ which turns out to be the same as Equation (3.82). Therefore, the analytical error measure for the apex vertex is the sum of the analytical error measure with respect to the coefficients $\boldsymbol{\alpha}$ and $\boldsymbol{\beta}$ and is given as:

$$
\begin{aligned}
AQ_\psi^{in} \;=\; &\frac{1}{F-n_o-3} \, [\mathbf{X}_{in}^{true\,T} \, (\mathbf{I}-\mathbf{P})^T \, (\mathbf{I}-\mathbf{P}) \, \mathbf{X}_{in}^{true} \,+ \\
&\mathbf{Y}_{in}^{true\,T} \, (\mathbf{I}-\mathbf{P})^T \, (\mathbf{I}-\mathbf{P}) \, \mathbf{Y}_{in}^{true} \,+ \\
&2\,\sigma_{in}^2 \sum_{f \in F_{in}} p_{ff}] .
\end{aligned}
\tag{3.83}
$$

In the above equation, AQ_ψ^{in} is proportional to the variance of the inlier noise (σ_{in}^2) and therefore can be plotted. The experimental and analytical results obtained from Equations (3.71) and (3.83) can be compared by plotting these quantities with respect to random variation, the variance of inlier noise (σ_{in}^2).

3.5.7 Experiments, Results and Discussions

3.5.7.1 Results and Discussions on Synthetic Data

The following relationships are derived between the *error measure* of the *ruled surface* and the input random perturbation. The first four relationships are between the error measure of the ruled surface and the variance of the inlier noise and the last relationship is between robust efficiency and the number of outliers.

1. *Experiment 1*: The variation of the joint mean error measure of the estimated non-robust ruled surface $(\hat{Q}_\psi^{in})$ from the Inlier Data $(F-n_o$ frames) *with* the variance of the inlier noise (σ_{in}^2), keeping the number of trials (T_o) and the total studies N fixed (see curve 1 in Figure 1 in [240]).

2. *Experiment 2*: The variation of the joint mean analytical error measure of the non-robust ruled surface (AQ_ψ^{in}) from Inlier Data $(F - n_o$ frames) with the variance of inlier noise (σ_{in}^2), keeping the number of trials (T_o) and the total studies N fixed (see curve 2 in Figure 1 in [240]).

3. *Experiment 3*: The variation of the joint mean error measure of the estimated robust ruled surface $(\hat{Q}_\psi^{com})$ from the *Combined Data with* variance of the inlier noise (σ_{in}^2), keeping the number of trials (T_o), outlier noise (σ_{out}^2), the total number of outliers (n_o) and the total studies N fixed (see curve 3 in Figure 1 in [240]).

4. *Experiment 4*: The variation of the joint mean error measure of the estimated robust ruled surface $(\hat{Q}_{\psi(nr)}^{com})$ with the variance of inlier noise (σ_{in}^2) after it has gone through the *non-robust procedure*, keeping the outlier noise (σ_{out}^2), the total trials (T_o) and the total studies N fixed (see curve 4 in Figure 1 in [240]).

5. *Experiment 5*: The variation of the mean *estimated statistical efficiency* $\hat{\eta}_s^{\psi}$ *of the robust procedure* with the total number of outliers (n_o) changing from 0% to 20% of F, keeping the variance of inlier noise (σ_{in}^2), the variance of outlier noise (σ_{out}^2), the total trials (T_o) and the total studies N fixed. (For details, see [240].)

From the curves (shown in the figure in [240]), it can be seen that as the inlier perturbation is increased, the error measure of the non-robust ruled surface also increases. This is because the inlier vertices are a function of the input random perturbations. It is also observed that with increasing inlier perturbation, the analytical error measure also increases and has a difference of 0.09 millimeters compared to the experimental value when the standard deviation of the inlier noise is 1 mm^2. Curve 3 in Figure 1 in [240] shows that as the inlier perturbation is increased, the square root of the joint error measure for the combined inlier and outlier data using the non-robust ruled surface is approximately 10.5 mm. This is because the outlier perturbation is 50-100 times larger than the inlier perturbation and the plain least squares estimate is used. As this combined data undergoes the IRLS algorithm, the error measure drops drastically (0.5 mm to 2.2 mm) for the inlier noise with standard deviations between 0.5 mm-1 mm. This demonstrates that the effect of the outliers has been totally removed by assigning low weights to large outliers using the IRLS fit procedure. In experiment 5 (see the curve in [240]), as the numbers of outliers (n_o) increase from 0, the efficiency ($\hat{\eta}^{\psi}$) drops slowly. In this experiment, the inlier noise (σ_{in}^2) is fixed to 1 mm^2, the outlier noise (σ_{out}^2) is fixed to 100 mm^2, the total trials (T_o) are fixed to 100 and the tuning constant (T_c) is fixed to 3.0, for this parametric apex model. As one decreases (or increases) the value of the tuning constant below (or above) 3.0, respectively, $\hat{\eta}^{\psi}$, it drops steeply at a higher number of outliers. For the stability of the efficiency curve, T_c was selected as 3.0. It was also observed that as the outlier noise increased, keeping everything else the same, a good tuning constant for this parameteric apex model lies in the range of 2.0 to 3.0. Thus it is seen that an iterative algorithm is an invaluable tool for the estimation of the robust apex coordinates for fitting the longitudinal axes of the left ventricle. These apex coordinates can then be integrated into the boundary calibration system [101] to improve its accuracy.

3.5.7.2 Results and Discussions on Clinical Data

In this sub-section are briefly discussed the results and performance evaluation of the robust apex coordinates when the IRLS algorithm is run on clinical data sets. The robustly estimated apex location was evaluated by comparing it against the ground truth apex location as delineated by the cardiologist. In cardiological imaging, it is a standard practice to divide the ventricle border into 100 equal length segments and compare the estimated position of the apex on the left ventricle contour (LVC) as the vertex number (also referred to as the serial number), which begins from the anterior aspect of aortic valve (i.e., in a clock-wise direction). Two types of experiments were performed: first, was computed the absolute position error of the estimated serial number to the true serial number as given by the cardiologist. In the second experiment, the mean apex position error was computed over all the patient studies N. If $(\hat{x}_n(f), \hat{y}_n(f))$ is the robust apex coordinates produced by the IRLS algorithm for frame number f and patient study n, and if $(x_n^{true}(f), y_n^{true}(f))$ is the apex coordinates as given by the cardiologist for frame f study n, then the estimated distance between these coordinates $\hat{d}_n(f)$ was given as: $\hat{d}_n(f) = \sqrt{[\hat{x}_n(f) - x_n^{true}(f)]^2 + [\hat{y}_n(f) - y_n^{true}(f)]^2}$. Since $\hat{s}_n(f)$ is the serial number of the robust apex starting from the anterior aspect of the aortic valve, this can be computed as the serial number *on true LVC* whose distance from the robust coordinates is at a minimum. The expression for the robust serial number $(\hat{s}_n(f))$ on true LVC is given as: $\hat{s}_n(f) = \{i \mid \min \hat{d}_n(f), 1 \leq i \leq P\}$, where P is the total number of vertices on the LVC. The mean absolute position error was estimated over all the frames F and studies N by:

$$\bar{e} = \frac{1}{N} \sum_{n=1}^{N} \left[\frac{1}{F} \sum_{f=1}^{F} \mid s_n^{true}(f) - \hat{s}_n(f) \mid \right]. \tag{3.84}$$

The probability of the absolute position error is computed as follows. Let $n(e)$ be the number of times the absolute position error $e_n(f)$ occurs with an error e (say, $e \leq 5$), then the probability $(\mathcal{P}(e))$ that the robust serial number and true serial number differ by e is given as: $\mathcal{P}(e) = \frac{\#n(e)}{NF}$. The results can be seen in the figure in [240]. As the error (e) increases, the number of frames with an error less than e drops. It is seen that about 60% of the frames have an error of 0 (the same as the cardiologist's location) and about 90% of the frames have an error of 1 which is considered to be very close and an excellent result. The bias study plot can be seen in the figure in [240].

3.5.8   Conclusions on LV Apex Modeling

A robust algorithm has been developed for fitting the left ventricle longitudinal axis and estimating its apex coordinates. This method shows that if the cardiac cycle has 15% outliers, the robust procedure has an efficiency of 90%. The algorithms were validated and showed a difference of 0.09 millimeters between the experimental and the analytical errors when the inlier noise is 1 mm^2. This robust algorithm was also demonstrated on clinical data sets and showed that in 90% of the frames, the automatically determined apex location was less than 1% of the total border length distance from the ground truth apex location as delineated by the cardiologist. One concludes that the robust procedure surely aids in removing outliers and smoothing the apex coordinates. These apex coordinates can then be used for improving the accuracy of the boundary estimation system [101].

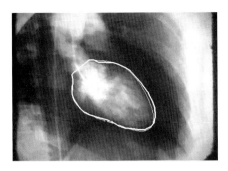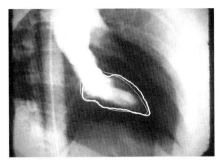

Figure 3.25: Sample results of ED and ES frames of the LV. **Left**: ED frame, **Right**: ES frame.

3.6 Integration of Low-Level Features in LV Model-Based Cardiac Imaging: Fusion of Two Computer Vision Systems

In an attempt to estimate accurately the anterior and inferior walls, Suri *et al.* [246] presented a low-contrast edge detection algorithm for LV boundary estimation. A combination of Least Square cubic fitting [243], [244] edge detection (based on a facet model [184]), morphology [245] and dynamic linking were used to detect the final LV edges. This algorithm is shown in Figure 3.26. To improve the accuracy of the boundary estimation system, Suri then fused the edges from the above system and the edges from the pixel classification algorithm [201]. A fusion algorithm was used vertex by vertex with the classifier boundaries. Finally, the fused classifier-edge boundary underwent calibration [236], [238] to estimate the final LV boundary. This database consisted of 364 patient studies having ED and ES frames. The mean boundary error for the classifier system alone was 5.72 mm and the mean boundary error for the edge system alone was 5.69 mm, while the mean boundary error of the classifier-edge fusion system was 4.8 mm and the mean boundary error after the calibration procedure using the polyline method was 3.7 mm. This was a remarkable improvement in separating the diaphragm from the LV boundary.

3.7 General Purpose LV Validation Technique

Training-based point modeling would be more meaningful if there was a scheme to find out if the estimated boundary was at the correct position. Suri *et al.* [247] developed a general and automatic validation technique that could detect the LV boundaries whose mean end frame boundary errors were above a

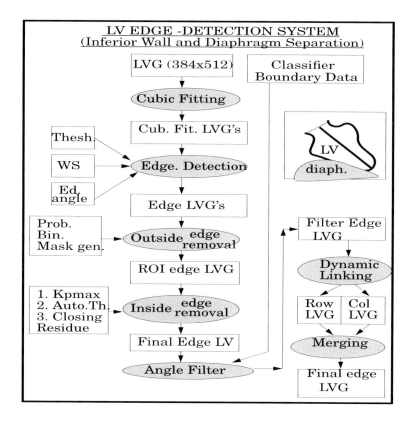

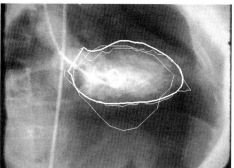

Figure 3.26: **Top**: Algorithm showing the sequence of steps for LV segmentation using the edge detection algorithm. The segmentation separates the LV from the diaphragm. The sequence of steps is: cubic fitting, edge detection and angle determination for the maximum gradient strength position for each pixel location, region growing of angle images, masking of angle images with the region of interest and dynamic linking of broken edges. **Bottom**: results of the above algorithm. Superimposition of these three curves: (i) ground truth (bold curve), (ii) classifier output (perturbed) and (iii) edge-detection algorithm fused with classifier (thin curve).

Comparison of 3 Algorithms w/o, w/, f/ apex					
N=377, K=188, L=187, Test Set=K-L=1, CV case					
Protocol: $^{188}C_{187}$					
$^{K}C_{L}$: Number of Combinations=188					
Training studies = 375, Test studies = 2					
e^{poly}_{NFP}: ($\frac{ED+ES}{2}$) (mm), σ^{poly}_{NFP}: Std. Dev. (mm)					
P	$e^{poly}_{NFP}(\mathbf{w/o})$	σ_{NFP}	$e^{poly}_{NFP}(\mathbf{w/})$	σ_{NFP}	$e^{poly}_{NFP}(\mathbf{f/})$	σ_{NFP}
IdCM	4.09	3.98	3.68	3.42	3.14^*	2.73
InCM	3.92	3.84	3.59	3.36	3.04^*	2.89
Greedy	3.70	3.2	3.4	3.23	2.97^*	2.74

Table 3.2: Chart comparing the three techniques of boundary calibration under three different conditions of the apex. **Left**: when the apex is not known; **Middle**: when the apex is padded in calibration; **Right**: when the apex is forced before calibration. $*$ shows the best performance.

given threshold, R_{th}. For this test, Suri took three inputs: the LV boundary coordinates (x, y), the gray scale left ventriculograms and the binary indicator for the LV region (1 for inside the LV region and 0 for outside the LV region). This boundary rejection scheme was based on the gray scale information near the boundary of the LV. Using a mutually exclusive window of a fixed size centered on the LV boundary vertex and along the LV contour, Suri computed the mean gray level value for part of the window inside the LV region and part of the window outside the LV region. This difference in the mean gray scale intensities (also called contrast values) was associated with the corresponding vertex of the LV observed boundary. The difference in the contrast value at the boundary vertex showed the edge characteristics. If the contrast difference at a vertex was high, this meant that there was a greater likelihood that the vertex had good contrast and was closer to the ideal LV boundary. Polyline errors for such vertices were small. Having a large contrast difference could also mean that the estimated vertex was too far inside the LV (underestimated) and the dye could have ended prematurely, i.e., the inside window had a high gray scale value and the outside window had a low contrast value, accounting for a large contrast difference. Correspondingly, the polyline errors for such vertices were high. On the other hand, if the contrast difference was too low, this meant that the vertex of the boundary was too far inside the LV. This was because the contrast values were high inside the LV, causing the contrast difference to be small. If contrast was too low, this meant that the vertex could be too far outside or far from the ideal LV boundary. This was because both the inside and outside windows had darker regions and thus the contrast difference was small. Both cases of low contrast difference were due to being too far inside the LV (underestimated) or too far outside the LV (overestimated). Cases which were under- or overestimated were the incorrect boundary cases and thus needed to be picked out. The corresponding polyline errors for such boundary cases were high. Therefore, the contrast difference and the polyline errors were very strong information pairs for developing a training-based model which could spot the large-errored vertices of the boundary and the LV boundary as a whole. To implement this training model, Suri regressed the observed contrast values against the polyline distance errors. Since the observed boundary errors were known for the patient study n estimated from any technique, the contrast values were then regressed against the observed errors to compute the rejection training coefficients. These training coefficients were then used to find the predicted errors on the test contrast boundary data (CBD). The predicted errors, which were above the threshold, corresponded to the boundary delineations which were to be rejected. This rejection system was a reliability test because it helped determine the procedure for how reliable the estimated boundaries were.

Advantages of the LV Validation System: (**1**) this determined those LV boundaries from the database (which could be coming from any source) whose error was above a given threshold error. (**2**) The scheme provided feedback to the boundary calibration system so that the system knew which LV boundaries could be rejected. (**3**) It estimated the overall performance of the boundary calibration system without taking the rejected boundaries into consideration. (**4**) It provided a check for the consistency and reliability of the output estimation algorithms (for example: classification algorithm, IdCM algorithm, InCM algorithm or greedy algorithm). Validation in the area of edge detection applied to an echocardiogram can be seen in Zwehl *et al.*[115].

3.8   LV Convex Hulling: Quadratic Training-Based Point Modeling

Recently, Suri *et al.*[249] presented work on convex hulling of the three points (AoV plane and the apex) in a calibration algorithm. The idea was to put a penalty on the apex and let the calibrated LV curve pass through it. This scheme reduced polyline errors in the apex zone, thereby yielding a system error to 2.97 mm over the database of 377 patient studies for the ED and ES frames (see Table 3.2). The convex hull information was linear in nature, so the residual was not too low. To further lower the residuals, Suri *et al.*[250] developed the quadratic nature of the convex hull points and then performed the calibration with an improved method of two calibration schemes by taking the quadratic nature of the convex information. These were the *quadratic identical coefficient* and the *quadratic independent coefficient* methods. The limited database consisted of N=377 patient studies, each having F=2 frames, ED and ES and each having a ground truth and raw polygonal boundary of TS=100 vertices. The mean and standard deviation of the resulting set of $N \times F \times P \times \frac{(K-1)!}{(K-L-1)!\,L!}$ numbers were used to estimate the overall performance. Note here that N, F, P are the patient parameters data size, total number of frames in the cardiac cycle and total vertices on the LV contour, respectively. The calibration parameters were K and L and are the number of partitions in the database and $K - L$ are the test data sets. Using linear calibration, the independent coefficient method without the apex yielded an error of 3.47 mm, while the quadratic calibration with the convex information had a mean error of 2.49 mm. The results can be seen in Figure 3.25. The goal set by the cardiologists was 2.5 mm. All the above training algorithms were fitting based on regression in time. One technique which could also be applied was: the median Least Squares approach developed by Kim [251]. Another technique was Hampel and Holland's [252], [253], [254] iterative reweighted Least Square (IRLS) for robust estimation.

3.8.1 Quadratic Vs. Linear Optimization for Convex Hulling

Suri *et al.* showed the linear calibration with convex information [236], [238], [101], [247], [246] for different data sets (N) ranging from 245 to 377. Using the *cross-validation* protocol discussed in Sub-section 3.4.2.3, the polyline mean error in linear calibrator for InCM was 3.47 mm when $N=291$. Corresponding estimated boundaries are shown in Figure 1 in Suri *et al.* [250]. Here the results are shown for the quadratic calibration under InCM conditions. The optimization curve for cross-validation is shown in Figure 2 (see Suri *et al.* [250]) with a dip when $P = 20$. The corresponding mean error $e_{NFP}^{poly} = 2.49$ mm. The calibration parameters were: $N = 377$, $F = 2$, $K = 188$, $P_1 = 100$, $P_2 = 100$. The mean error when the patient boundary lies both in the training and the testing data (TT case) condition is below 2 mm. The mean error for the InCM technique under four conditions was: without apex: 4.09 mm; with apex alone: 3.59 mm; with apex and AoV (linear): 2.97 mm; with apex and AoV (quadratic): 2.49 mm.

3.9 LV Eigen Shape Modeling

3.9.1 Procrustes Superposition

Sampson *et al.* [255] presented left ventricular shape analysis using eigenvalues when the ED and ES frames of the cardiac cycle were jointly taken into consideration. Sampson *et al.* developed an iterative closest point algorithm for the orientation of the LV hand-drawn contours. Principal modes of variation in the shape were given by the eigen-shapes, the left vectors of the singular value decomposition (SVD) [256]. Sampson's approach to analyzing the hand-drawn contour was powerful. The method began with a mean outline defined by a point-wise average of outlines after they had been oriented in a Procrustes superposition by means of the closest point algorithm. Individual LV outlines were represented by vectors of deviations normal to the mean outlines and variation in the shape was analyzed in terms of SVD. Principal models of variation in shape were given by the so-called eigen shapes. Sampson *et al.* took the SVD for the joint representation of the outline LV shapes of ED and ES and used the scores on a subset of the principal eigen shapes to demonstrate a discriminant analysis distinguishing a sample of "normals" from groups of clinical cases with cardiomyopathy or infarcts associated with coronary heart disease (CHD).

3.9.2 Dimensionality Reduction Using Constraints for Joint ED-ES

Suri *et al.* [258] proposed that the ED and ES shapes could be tied together in the form of constraints. A 3-D high dimensional cluster space could be reduced to a lower dimensionality by propagating information from one time frame to another using SVD. The singular values or eigenvalues which were small did not have much energy. Those components could help in data reduction when the ED and ES shapes were coupled. How the constraints could be used to couple the ED and ES boundaries will be discussed later. In the coupled constrained calibration, the hand-drawn and classifier matrices look like this:

$$
\mathbf{R} = \begin{pmatrix} \underbrace{u_1'}_{ed} & \underbrace{v_1'}_{es} \\ & \cdots \\ & \cdots \\ \underbrace{u_N'}_{ed} & \underbrace{v_N'}_{es} \end{pmatrix}
$$

$$
\mathbf{Q} = \begin{pmatrix} \underbrace{l_1'}_{ed} & \underbrace{m_1'}_{es} & 1\, \underbrace{a_{11}^{ed} b_{11}^{ed} a_{21}^{ed} b_{21}^{ed}}_{} & \underbrace{a_{11}^{es} a_{11}^{es} a_{21}^{es} b_{21}^{es}}_{} \\ & & \cdots \\ & & \cdots \\ \underbrace{l_N'}_{ed} & \underbrace{m_N'}_{es} & 1\, \underbrace{a_{11}^{ed} b_{11}^{ed} a_{21}^{ed} b_{21}^{ed}}_{} & \underbrace{a_{11}^{es} a_{11}^{es} a_{21}^{es} b_{21}^{es}}_{} \end{pmatrix}^{N \times (4P+9)} ,
$$

where the vector for the ground truth is:
$$[u_n'\, v_n'] = [\underbrace{x_1, ...x_P, y_1, ...y_P}_{ed}, \underbrace{x_1, ...x_P, y_1, ...y_P}_{es}];$$
and the vector for the raw boundary is
$$[l_n'\, m_n'] = [\underbrace{x_1, ...x_P, y_1, ...y_P}_{ed}, \underbrace{x_1, ...x_P, y_1, ...y_P}_{es}].$$
Note that $a_{11}^{ed} b_{11}^{ed} a_{21}^{ed} b_{21}^{ed}$ and $a_{11}^{es} a_{11}^{es} a_{21}^{es} b_{21}^{es}$ are the padding[16] for the aortic valve information. Taking all the patients N, the constrained model in matrix notation is:

$$\epsilon_{ccr}^2 = \parallel \mathbf{R}^{gt} - \mathbf{QA} \parallel^2 + \lambda \parallel \mathbf{QAC} \parallel^2, \tag{3.85}$$

where $\mathbf{R}^{gt}$ has the dimension $N \times 4P$, $\mathbf{Q}$ has the dimension $N \times 4P$ and $\hat{\mathbf{A}}$ has the dimension $4P \times 4P$, $\mathbf{C}$ is the constraint matrix $\mathbf{C}$ derived from

---

[16]Process of appending the x- and y-coordinates in the vector.

the given ground truth boundaries and is of the dimension $N \times K_c$ and λ is the weighing factor constant. Equation (3.85) can be rewritten by taking the weighting factor λ inside the matrix and premultiplying with the constrained matrix $\mathbf{C}$. Then using the norm rules, one could rewrite Equation (3.85) as:

$$\epsilon_{ccr}^2 = \| \, [\mathbf{R}^{gt} : \mathbf{0}] - \mathbf{Q}_{tr} \, \mathbf{A} \, [\mathbf{I} : \lambda \mathbf{C}] \, \|^2 , \qquad (3.86)$$

where $\mathbf{I}$ is the identity matrix of the dimension $4\,P \times 4\,P$ and $\mathbf{0}$ is the matrix of all zeros of dimension $N \times K_c$. Note, $[\mathbf{I} : \lambda \mathbf{C}]$ simply means putting together the matrix $\mathbf{I}$ and $\mathbf{0}$. $\mathbf{Q}_{tr}$ represents the matrix of all the classifier boundaries or perturbed boundaries. Appending the ground truth matrix and the constrained matrix, one could rewrite the above Equation (3.86) as:

$$\epsilon_{ccr}^2 = \| \, \mathbf{R}_{*}{}^{gt} - \mathbf{Q}_{tr} \mathbf{A} \, \mathbf{D} \, \|^2 . \qquad (3.87)$$

where $\mathbf{R}_{*}{}^{gt\,17}$ is of the dimension $N \times 4\,(P + K_c)$ and $\mathbf{D}$ is of the dimension $P \times (P + K_c)$. The constrained coefficients using the constraints could be derived using singular value decomposition. Let the SVD[18] of $\mathbf{Q}_{tr}$ and $\mathbf{D}$ be given as $\mathbf{U_1}\,\mathbf{W_1}\,\mathbf{V_1}^T$ and $\mathbf{U_2}\,\mathbf{W_2}\,\mathbf{V_2}^T$, respectively. Substituting these values in Equation (3.87) results in:

$$\epsilon_{ccr}^2 = \| \, \mathbf{R}_{*}{}^{gt} - (\,\mathbf{U_1}\,\mathbf{W_1}\,\mathbf{V_1}^T\,)\mathbf{A}\,(\,\mathbf{U_2}\,\mathbf{W_2}\,\mathbf{V_2}^{\mathbf{T}}\,) \, \|^2 . \qquad (3.88)$$

To minimize Equation (3.88), $\mathbf{U_1}^T$ and $\mathbf{V_2}$ was pre-multiplied and post-multiplied on the left and right hand sides, respectively. Using the orthonormal properties of the SVD matrices, this becomes:

$$\| \, \mathbf{U_1}^T \, \mathbf{R}_{*}{}^{gt} \, \mathbf{V_2} - \mathbf{W_1}\,\mathbf{V_1}^T \mathbf{A}\,\mathbf{U_2}\,\mathbf{W_2} \, \|^2 . \qquad (3.89)$$

Then, to derive the constrained coefficients, the above equation was broken and each component analyzed. Let us define matrices $\mathbf{E}$ and $\mathbf{F}$ as:

$$\mathbf{E} = \mathbf{V_1}^T \mathbf{A}\,\mathbf{U_2} \qquad (3.90)$$

$$\mathbf{F} = \mathbf{U_1}^T \, \mathbf{R}_{*}{}^{gt} \, \mathbf{V_2} . \qquad (3.91)$$

Substituting Equation (3.90) in Equation (3.89) becomes:

$$\epsilon_{ccr}^2 = \| \, \mathbf{F} - \mathbf{W_1}\,\mathbf{E}\,\mathbf{W_2} \, \|^2 . \qquad (3.92)$$

The above Equation for each element could be written as:

$$\epsilon_{ccr}^2 = \sum_{i=1} \sum_{j=1} (f_{ij} - \mathbf{w}_i^1 \, e_{ij} \, \mathbf{w}_j^2)^2 . \qquad (3.93)$$

---

[17]Note that $\mathbf{R}_{*}{}^{gt}$ is obtained by padding the matrix $\mathbf{0}$ to $\mathbf{R}^{gt}$.
[18]Singular Value Decomposition, for details on SVD, see Press *et al.* [256]

There are two possibilities for solving Equation (3.93)[19]. These conditions depend upon the diagonal values $\mathbf{w}_i^1$ and $\mathbf{w}_j^2$. If the diagonal values are both not equal to 0, that is $\mathbf{w}_i^1 \neq 0$ and $\mathbf{w}_j^2 \neq 0$, e_{ij} could be given as:

$$e_{ij} = \frac{f_{ij}}{w_i^1 \, w_j^2} \, . \tag{3.94}$$

The other case arises when any of the diagonal values are equal to zero, i.e., $\mathbf{w}_i^1 = 0$ or $\mathbf{w}_j^2 = 0$. In this case, e_{ij} is forced to be 0 for certain diagonal values and f_{ij}^2 for other diagonal values. Thus, from the above explanation, one could say:

$$\mathbf{E} = \mathbf{W}_1^- \, \mathbf{F} \, \mathbf{W}_2^- \, . \tag{3.95}$$

where $\mathbf{W}_1^-$ and $\mathbf{W}_2^-$ are the inverse matrices of $\mathbf{W}_1$ and $\mathbf{W}_2$, respectively. Finally, the coefficients could be obtained by substituting Equations (3.95) and (3.91) in Equation (3.90).

$$\begin{aligned}
\hat{\mathbf{A}} &= \mathbf{V}_1 \, \mathbf{E} \, \mathbf{U}_2{}^T \\
&= \mathbf{V}_1 \, \mathbf{W}_1^- \, \mathbf{F} \, \mathbf{W}_2^- \, \mathbf{U}_2^T \\
&= \mathbf{V}_1 \, \mathbf{W}_1^- \, \mathbf{U}_1{}^T \, \mathbf{R}_*{}^{gt} \, \mathbf{V}_2 \, \mathbf{W}_2^- \, \mathbf{U}_2^T \tag{3.96}
\end{aligned}$$

Here, $\hat{\mathbf{A}}$ is of the dimension $4\,P \times 4\,P$. Thus finally, the constrained coefficients were given as:

$$\hat{\mathbf{A}} = \mathbf{V}_1 \, \mathbf{W}_1^- \, \mathbf{U}_1{}^T \, \mathbf{R}_*{}^{gt} \, \mathbf{V}_2 \, \mathbf{W}_2^- \, \mathbf{U}_2^T \, . \tag{3.97}$$

Here, $\hat{\mathbf{A}}$ was of the dimension $4\,P \times 4\,P$.

3.10   LV Neural Network Models

Recently, Chiou and Hwang [260] addressed the issue of contour-finding using a combination of neural nets, active contour and Gibbs' sampler, which is called an NNS-SNAKE, named after the neural net stochastic-snake. They used a neural network classifier for building the interior contour, inside which the initial snake was placed. The active contour model was used to alter this snake towards the target contour. Gibbs' sampler basically helped avoid the trapping of the intermediate contours during the slithering operation of the snake. Chiou's algorithm for boundary estimation consisted of three major steps, the first being the interior contour generation using the neural network classifier. In this step, Chiou and Hwang first trained the neural net using contour pixels and non-contour pixels. The neural net was fed by the test data set which output the energy profile image. This image was first binarized and then ANDed with the edge map of the original image. The ANDed image

---

[19]Note that here f represents the element of the matrix $\mathbf{F}$ (not the frame number), similarly, $\mathbf{w}_i^1$, e_{ij} and $\mathbf{w}_j^2$ represent the elements of the matrices $\mathbf{W}_1$ $\mathbf{E}$ $\mathbf{W}_2$.

was then smoothed using the Gaussian kernel and subsequently inverted, which yielded the interior contour. The second step was the generation of the starting contour, which was inside the interior contour, and the running of the active contour model to inflate towards the target contour. In step three, Gibbs' sampling was used to avoid the trapping of the intermediate contour, which could happen with the local minimum of the energy function. This technique was done using the Bayes approach, by taking the prior probability of the shape and the likelihood function of the output of the neural network. Chiou and Hwang used MRI brain images for the training and testing of the neural network to obtain the final contours of the brain inside the brain cavity, slice by slice.

Tseng *et al.* [261],[262] addressed the Least Squares problem that could be solved by using a continuous distance transform neural network (CDTNN). Tseng *et al.* posed an error reduction problem between the observed point in 3-D and the nearest zero point of vector $\mathbf{x}^T$ of the function f, which was given as:

$$||\mathbf{x} - \mathbf{x}^T||^2 = \frac{f(\mathbf{x})^2}{||\bigtriangledown \mathbf{x} \;\; \mathbf{f}(\mathbf{x})||^2} \, ,$$

where $f(x)=0$ for all x belonging to B and where B was the collection of the database points. Tseng *et al.* presented a two layer CDTNN network, where each neuron had a sigmoid non-linearity function and was given as: $\frac{1}{1+e^{-u}}$. The output layer neuron had a sigmoid non-linearity of: $\frac{2}{1+e^{-u}-1}$. Finally, Tseng *et al.* computed the heart motion in echocardiogram images using affine transformation. Since heart motion was deformable, the new surface points could be deformed back to the same shape as the exemplar object. The affine equation was given as:

$$x = \mathbf{Q}(\theta) \; \mathbf{R} \; y + t \; , \tag{3.98}$$

where $\mathbf{R}$'s upper triangle was the scaling and the lower triangle was the shearing of the heart and $\mathbf{Q}(\theta)$ was the rotational matrix.

3.11 Comparative Study and Summary of the Characteristics of Model-Based Techniques

From Sub-section 3.4.2.1 to Sub-section 3.10, the model-based algorithms were discussed for fitting either gray scale or hand-drawn LV data. It was seen that when the gray scale LV data was fitted to the mathematical equation, the assistance of the ground truth boundaries was needed. These hand-drawn boundaries helped to train the mathematical model to yield the fitting parameters applied on the test LV data. The majority of research groups take an ellipsoid or sphere model as the starting point and then tailor these shapes to the LV shapes. In other words, given an ideal shape, one wants to change its shape to the LV shape using the image data. This is primarily shape modeling.

Broadly speaking, model-based techniques can be classified as training-based fitting (or learning-based) and energy minimization (or active contour-based). Suri [264] has attempted to compare these two broadly classified model-based fitting techniques. The differences and similarities between them will now be discussed. (a) Active model segmentation was a two step process. Step one consisted of initial model fitting or reconstruction, where the tuning parameters controlled the twisting, binding and stretching. Step two consisted of the refinement stage, which would bring a smooth appearance to the 3-D surface of the LV. In training-based LV modeling, step one consisted of pixel classification based on the Bayesian approach for each time frame of the cardiac cycle. The output of this stage was the raw or initial boundaries. Step two, called the calibration step, was the smoothing process to remove the bias errors. (b) The second key similarity between active modeling and training-based systems was the global shape extraction. Active modeling had the user extract the initial contours, which were traced by the mouse pointer, whereas in training-based systems, the global shape information was extracted to train the system by using hand-drawn boundaries of the LV. The two major differences between active modeling and training-based modeling are: (a) the fitting procedure was based on dynamic equations using physics-based models of differential equations, while the training system used the learning by maximizing the posterior probability of the Bayesian classifier; and (b) the refinement stage consisted of sub-dividing the finite elements into more smaller triangular meshes to give a smooth appearance, whereas the refinement state in the training-based system consisted of smoothing the output boundaries using the calibration algorithms.

3.11.1   Characteristics of Model-Based LV Imaging

Model-based techniques have the following characteristics:

1. They originate from a mathematical equation resembling an LV shape.

2. These models can easily be framed in the Bayesian domain, where the priors can be estimated from the hand-drawn database.

3. These LV models can be optimized using energy minimization techniques such as: Snakes, Fourier-fitting, Least Squares, Weighted Least Squares or Iterative Weighted Least Squares.

4. These model-based techniques incorporate low-level features to add robustness to the estimation system.

5. The models are less noise sensitive and are easily adaptable to the global shape of the LV.

6. The models can easily be brought into the matrix domain and thus the model's computing power is tremendous. It can handle a huge database of patient studies.

7. These LV-shaped models are easily governed by the eigen shape analysis and yield directional information.

8. These model-based techniques are good buffers between the gray scale data and the hand-drawn data sets.

9. These models have great learning capability and can easily be adapted for Neural Networks.

10. Finally, model-based techniques are robust, accurate, tailorable and easy to integrate into other systems. These models are not only applied in LV segmentation but can be used in LV quantification, as will be discussed in the next sub-section.

3.12 LV Quantification: Wall Motion and Tracking

The CVPR research presented in the previous sub-sections is more valuable if the quantitative tools are robust and accurate. Tool modeling was as necessary as LV segmentation modeling. Researchers have tried to evaluate the 2-D contours segmented from cardiac images (e.g., the motion involved from ED to ES), to estimate the LV wall thickness and the four dimensional LV tracking. Even though quantification techniques have been in existence for quite some time (see Bardeen [268], Dodge *et al.* [269], [270], Marcus *et al.* [271], Chapman *et al.* [272], Jouan [273], Lewis *et al.* [274] and Kim *et al.* [275]), the benefits have not yet reached cardiologists. For example, it has not been possible to establish how LV twisting is related to cardiomyopathy, such as HOCM (hypertrophic obstructive cardiomyopathy), also called asymmetric wall thickening of the LV. Similarly, it has not been established how the torsional component of the LV is related to heart disorder, e.g. RCM (restrictive cardiomyopathy). In regional wall motion, several researchers (see Wynne *et al.* [276], Lehmkul *et al.* [277], Papapietro *et al.* [278], Rickards *et al.* [279], Klausner *et al.* [280], Gibson *et al.* [281]) have attempted to quantify the wall motion. Suri [282] tried to discuss the LV measurement tools necessary for shape and functional analysis of the LV, but here the critical measurement techniques for LV functional analysis will be discussed in detail.

This section has been divided into the following parts. Sub-section 3.12.1 presents LV wall motion and wall thickness measurements. It will also discuss all motion measurement using a directional-based approach (the centerline method), LV curvature measurement using angle change, curvature estimation based on bending energy, LV wall motion estimation using matching and the polyline method for wall-to-wall measurements. Sub-section 3.12.2 discusses the LV volume measurements briefly. Sub-section 3.12.3 presents LV wall motion tracking, where the tracking of the LV walls from frame to frame will be discussed based on endness measure and optic flow.

3.12.1 LV Wall Motion Measurements

3.12.1.1 LV Wall Motion Measurement Using the Directional Component (Centerline)

The directional component of the LV wall was first introduced by Gould *et al.* [290]. Continuing on the same lines, Bolson *et al.* [291] developed a centerline method for quantitative assessment of the LV boundary for wall motion measurement in X-ray ventriculograms. The algorithm measured the perpendicular motion along 100 chords constructed to a centerline drawn midway between the ED and ES LV contours. The centerline method was developed to find the extent of the local LV wall motion. The algorithm utilized the following principle: if the two LV polygons were the ED and the ES boundaries, the ED having a larger number of points on it, the larger contour was first linearly interpolated to get 200 points and then for each tuple of three points on this contour, a perpendicular was drawn to the tangent of the circle passing through these three points. The centers of these perpendiculars constituted the centerline. Further modifications to the centerline method were introduced by Sheehan *et al.* [292]. The application of the centerline was demonstrated in contrast X-ray ventriculography by Sheehan *et al.* [293] in comparing wall motion, variabilities in wall motion, ejection fraction (EF), hypokinesis (slow movement of the myocardial walls) and hyperkinesis (large movement of the muscle walls) in the LV and right ventricle of the human heart. Recently, wall thickening research was presented by Yang *et al.* [294], in which the ED thickness was replaced by the average of the n chords taken on both sides of the current chord, in consideration with the thickness of the chord at $2n + 1$. The above process was called smoothing or interpolation of chords.

3.12.1.2 LV Curvature Measurement

Mancini *et al.* [295] first developed the concept of curvature analysis in shape assessment of the LV. Past traditional methods of wall motion quantification required assumptions about coordinate, reference and indexing systems. Mancini used curvature estimation on hand-traced boundary contours, given as:

$$C \;=\; \frac{1}{r} = \frac{1}{\frac{\delta P}{\delta \theta}}\,, \tag{3.99}$$

where C was the curvature at a given vertex, r was the radius of curvature, δP was the change in the arc length along the LVC and $\delta \theta$ was the change in the angle along the LVC. Mancini pointed out two problems with this curvature analysis. First, if the LVC was noisy (that is, the hand-drawn boundaries were noisy), the differentiation process amplified the noise. This statistical noise could be reduced using seven-point weighted smoothing. The second problem was the quantization error obtained by approximating a continuous curve to a digital (x, y) curve. This was significant when 90° bends were present along the LVC. This was also pointed out by Duncan *et al.* [302] while working with the centerline method, which was also based on curvature. Mancini did propose an interpolation solution to this problem and later computed curvature at every 4th point to avoid the $90°$ bends. Last, Mancini *et al.* proposed three vertex smoothing, where the final value assigned to each point was an average of the value at that point and the values on either side of it. Mancini *et al.* highlighted the curvature analysis comparison of normal and abnormal ventricles at specific phases of the cardiac cycle, not with respect to the overall shape's change from ED to ES.

3.12.1.3 LV Curvature Measurement Using Bending Energy

Duncan *et al.* [300] and Amini *et al.* [301] suggested a bending energy model for comparing the shape change along the LV contour on the boundary data as traced by an expert and obtained from contrast ventriculography. Duncan analyzed 27 normal studies and 16 abnormal studies with acute myocardial infarction and apical aneurysms. The bending energy model was used for finding the curvature along the LV contour, but it did not compute the extent of the wall motion during the cardiac cycle. Duncan also applied the centerline method to find the extent of wall motion from the ED to the ES frame during the systolic heart cycle. Duncan concluded that the bending energy and centerline results were computing two different features of the LV function. The bending energy was computing the curvature along the LV contour, while the centerline method was computing the extent of the wall motion along the LV contour. The bending energy was based on the following principle: given an undeformed state (say, a straight rod), it is necessary to find out how much energy is required to bend the rod to a deformed state. This energy was expressed using the radius of the curvature of the rod or LV contour. Duncan *et al.* used an analogy, that the undeformed state can be taken to be the mean position of the LV contours over the normal N studies and the deformed state can be taken as the current state of a patient study. Thus, the bending energy for each patient study n along the LV contour was given mathematically as:

$$BE(n) = \sum_{k=k_1}^{k_2} [\nu_n(k) - \bar{\nu}(k)]^2,$$

where k was the index for the angular number along the LV contour, and $\nu(k)$ was the curvature for the angular number k. $\bar{\nu}(k)$ was the mean curvature for all the normal patient studies (N) for the angular number k, given as:

$$\bar{\nu}(k) = \frac{1}{N} \sum_{n=1}^{N} \nu_n(k). \tag{3.100}$$

The curvature for the angular k was computed by filtering the curve with a filter $d_c(k)$ and was given as: $\nu(k) = d_c(k)\psi(k)$. The filter $d_c(k)$, which was presented mathematically by Duncan, was first developed by Hamming.

$$d_c = \frac{C \times (m - \alpha)}{m} \left[\frac{c\cos(\alpha\pi c)}{\alpha} + \frac{c\sin(\alpha\pi c)}{\pi\alpha^2} \right], \tag{3.101}$$

m was the number of coefficients of the filter, equal to 9 and c was the tuner of the filter, taken as 0.2. α took the values: $-m \leq \alpha \leq m$. $C = \frac{\pi}{\sum_{-m}^{m} \alpha \, d(\alpha)}$. $d(\alpha) = \psi(\alpha + 1) - \psi(\alpha)$. $\psi(k)$ was given as:

$$\psi(k) = tan^{-1} \frac{y(s_{j+1}) - y(s_j)}{x(s_{j+1}) - x(s_j)}], \quad (3.102)$$

where s_j was the smoothed LV contour in the image plane (x, y) obtained after equal distance sampling and normalization and j was the index with values $1 \leq j \leq 100$.

3.12.1.4   LV Wall Motion Measurement Using the Matching-Based Approach

Duncan *et al.* [302] and Owen *et al.* [303] presented a bending energy-based matching of the contour segments from one frame to the neighboring one. The objective of this matching was to trace the points on the LVC from the ED frame to the ES frame and to ultimately be able to quantify the wall motion from the ED to the ES frame, of the systolic phase. The matching algorithm consisted of two steps. Step one consisted of finding the LV boundary from the gray scale contrast ventriculograms in the time domain. The second step consisted of local segment matching, which took a pair of contours at a time. The matching procedure was based on the following principle: search for a segment on the LVC in a second frame which has undergone the least deformation compared to the segment on the previous LVC. Searching for the segments was done in a circular window. The deformation or bendness was based on the amount of curvature in the segments while moving from the first frame to the second frame. If $\nu_{f1}(s)$ was the curvature of the segment in frame one, and if $\nu_{f2}(s + \delta)$ was the curvature of the segment in frame two at a distance δ along the LVC, then the bendness or bending energy between these states was given as:

$$BE(\delta) = \frac{EI}{2} \int_s [\nu_{f2}(s + \delta) - \nu_{f1}(s)]^2 , \quad (3.103)$$

where EI was taken as a constant. Since the search was within a small window or locally, the process was called local segment matching. Once the match was found, the vector flow field, $\mathbf{d}(s)$ was computed. This flow field was smoothed using the unconstrained method and the displacement vector F was computed using the iterative solution, given as:

$$F = \int \{C_1(s)[u(s) - \mathbf{d}(s)]^2 + \frac{\partial u(s)}{\partial s}\} ds . \quad (3.104)$$

Duncan *et al.* finally compared their shape-based method for quantifying the wall motion with Bolson's centerline [291] method. They claimed that there were problems in the centerline method at sharp curvatures and that it was mathematically unpredictable and unstable. Duncan *et al.* took only one normal study to illustrate their method of quantification of the wall motion. In this study, five contours were traced manually between the ED and the ES frames for a RAO projection in a contrast ventriculogram. Duncan *et al.* did give the algorithm for estimating the LV contours in contrast ventriculogram, which was claimed to be fully automatic, but during the final stage for quantification, manually traced borders were considered for analysis. The Duncan technique refers to Staib's method for automatic boundary determination, which was based on a parametric elliptical deformable model. This method generates the parameters for the ellipse **p** which are finally used for the deformation. The **p** was based on the population of the training data set. The database used by Suri (see Sub-section 3.4.4) had patient studies with acute myocardium infarction, where the bulging of the LV had taken place sideways, that is, in the anterior and inferior or posterior wall zones. Cases were seen to have a bulge in the apical zone also. In such cases, the **p** vector may not have had the right parameters and thus, complete deformation may not have been possible for boundary estimation.

3.12.1.5 LV Wall-to-Wall Distance Measurement Based on the Polyline Metric

Suri, Haralick and Sheehan [238] developed the polyline metric for computing the average error between two polygons. The polyline distance $D_s(B_1 : B_2)$ between two polygons representing boundary B_1 and B_2 was symmetrically defined as the average distance between a vertex of one polygon and the boundary of the other polygon. To define this measure precisely, Suri *et al.* defined the distance $d(v, s)$ between a point v and a line segment s on the opposite segment. The distance $d(v, s)$ between a point v having coordinates (x_o, y_o) and a line segment having end points (x_1, y_1) and (x_2, y_2) was:

$$d(v, s) = \begin{cases} \min\{d_1, d_2\}; & if \ \lambda < 0, \lambda > 1 \\ |d^{\perp}|; & if \ 0 \leq \lambda \leq 1, \end{cases} \tag{3.105}$$

where the parameters were computed using vector calculus. The following are the advantages of the polyline method: (**1**) it is stable and computes the error based on the geometry of the triangles and vector calculus. (**2**) The bias errors at every vertex are computable. Not only the closest perpendicular, but also the coordinate position and its bias relative to the vertex on the opposite polygon are computed. This distance can be used to correct the bias errors in calibration algorithms. (**3**) If there are cups or cusps in the polyline, then the algorithm can easily find them. Since the algorithm looks for those perpendiculars whose λ lies between 0 and 1 and which satisfy the condition of closeness, there is no possibility of error. (**4**) Since prior to the polyline error computation the curves undergo equal arc sampling and interpolation, there exists a one-to-one correspondence between the vertices of the curves. As a result, there is no need for matching of the shapes among the polygons, unlike Duncan's approach [302]. (**5**) It is a non-iterative computation and thus saves time, unlike Bolson and Sheehan's method [291], [292] where one has to do the computations again to smooth the curves to improve the accuracy. (**6**) In Bolson and Sheehan's

[292] method, one has to compute the tangents by fitting the circle through three points. The circle fitting algorithm is very sensitive to the number of points taken on either side of the vertex in consideration (see [244]). In the polyline method, there is no fitting involved. Also, it has been shown [101] that the polyline method is more accurate than the centerline method to the third decimal place. (**7**) It can easily expose whether the distance computed for every vertex is positive or negative, positive when going from one vertex to the opposite polygon and vice versa. (**8**) The polyline algorithm, in conjunction with the swapping mechanism, makes the process symmetric. This is very helpful when computing errors along the LV walls.

3.12.1.6   LV Wall Thickness Measurements Based on the Center Surface

Recently, there was an attempt by Sheehan *et al.* [304] to estimate the wall thickness from ultrasound data sets. The ultrasound image data was acquired by inserting the transesophageal ultrasound probe into the esophagus of the patient. Using the experience of the technologist or the cardiologist in tracing the ED and ES boundaries, the 3-D data points were gathered. Using the hand-drawn data set, the endocardial[20] and epicardial[21] surface of the LV was reconstructed at the ED and ES times. The center surface was then estimated and triangles were assigned to the center surface of the heart. The center surface in 3-D is analogous to the centerline method of 2-D. For quantitative analysis such as wall thickness estimation, the thickness during the ES wall was subtracted from the thickness during the ED wall. The ED (or ES) wall thickness is estimated by taking the ratio of the volume of the prism to the total area of the top and bottom triangles of the prism for ED (or ES). This prism has its base triangle on the endocardial[22] surface and its face triangle on the epicardial[23] surface. The accuracy of this method was highly dependent upon the convergence of the best *center surface* estimation. Also, it would be interesting to see the effect of the size of the triangle meshes and the number of normal computations one has to compute to get accurate center surfaces. Lastly, where there were sharp LV curvature changes, the weighting scheme could be better for normal computations than simply taking the average of the normals of the faces.

3.12.2   LV Volume Measurements

Sandler [283] presented an exhaustive review of 116 references, beginning in 1914, on non-pattern recognition volume estimation techniques and some common problems in LVgrams. Sandler pointed out many factors which influenced the volume estimation from ventriculograms, such as the frame rate, bolus of

---

[20] Inner surface of the LV.
[21] Outer surface of the LV.
[22] Outer surface.
[23] Inner surface.

contrast material, catheter placement, viscosity of the contrast agent and irregularity of the LV.

In the late 1980s, Hoffman *et al.* [284], [285],[286], [287], studied the shape
and dimension of the cardiac chambers using cardiac CT sections. Hoffman
et al. pointed out that the total heart volume remained essentially constant
throughout the cardiac cycle. This constant heart volume relationship appeared to be attributable to a large degree to the reciprocal emptying and
filling of the atria and ventricles and the fixed positioning of the epicardial
(outer surface of the myocardium) apex. 3-D display of congenital heart diseases had been of interest to validate the protocol of constant heart volume
(see Sinak *et al.* [288]).

In cardiac MR, Apicella *et al.* [289] presented a technique to estimate the
LV volume. This was computed by counting the total number of voxels in
the MR slices in the cardiac boundary region. Apicella's technique used three
steps: extraction of the LV region; tissue-blood classification and boundary
estimation; and volume estimation using voxel counting.

Dumesnil *et al.* [296], [297] tried to model the 3-D LV using several synthetic
models: ellipsoidal, spheroid and cylindrical. They then showed that the LV
contraction is inversely related to the ratio of the mid-wall thickness to the
thickness of the wall. Similar research was done by Beier *et al.* [298] that discussed seven different methods for volume estimation. Santos *et al.* [299] also
presented two quantitative ways to measure the LV analysis.

3.12.3   LV Wall Motion Tracking

LV tracking is equally as important as LV wall motion and LV volume measurement. In this sub-section, three major techniques used to track the LV
are discussed. They are based on endness measure computation, contour correspondence and optic flow.

Tracking-based on endness measure: Clary *et al.* [305] and Fritsch *et al.* [306]
used the Deformable Shape Loci (DSL) algorithm to track the LV wall motion
in cardiac nuclear image sequences. Clary placed the DSL manually near the
LV in the first frame of each sequence and allowed it to evolve, which means it
was allowed to position itself optimally with respect to the image information.
The optimal model position in the first frame is used as the initial position
in the second frame. To track the motion over the entire sequence, the final
model configuration in one frame was used as the initial configuration in the
next $t + 1$ time frame. Clary *et al.* defined the term *endness measure*, which
measures the degree of circular osculation (curvature) behavior for a circle of
a particular radius R_o with a boundary at a distance R_o and was given as:

$$K(r, \theta) = \frac{-(r - R_o)}{\sigma_r^3} \; exp[\frac{(r - R_o)^2}{\sigma_r{}^2}] \; exp[\frac{(\theta - \theta_o)^2}{2\theta_\theta{}^2}] \; ,$$

where θ_o was the direction tangent to the medial track, σ_r was proportional to
R_o and θ_θ was a constant and was the derivative of the Gaussian in polar form,

normalized by σ_r to provide zoom invariance and weighted by a decreasing function of the angle swept by an arc along the circle.

3.12.3.1 Sinusoidal Function Tracking

McEachen II *et al.* [307], [308] presented an LV tracking algorithm for analyzing the motion of deforming contours of the endocardial LV wall. McEachen II *et al.* assumed that the motion was periodic, which was not always true. McEachen II *et al.* modeled the LV motion for a particular point i as follows: If m_i was the correspondence between the contour C_i and C_{i+1}, then such a correspondence could be modeled as a sine function and was given as:

$$m_i \; = \; \sum_{r=1}^{R} C_r \; \sin(r w_o t + \phi_r) \; , \tag{3.106}$$

where C_r and ϕ_r are the amplitude and phase of the rth harmonic component of m_i respectively. Note that this was the temporal information of the LV motion. Using this harmonic analysis, McEachen II *et al.* developed a method of filtering the data derived from a shape-based mapping function to obtain a more desirable, smoothly varying mapping function. If the vector $\mathbf{m}_i$ represented the correspondence of point i over F frames during the cardiac cycle $\mathbf{C}$, the diagonal matrix where each element of the matrix represented the confidence of the correspondence for a search region, and $\mathbf{D}$ was the first order differential operator, then the optimal estimate of the correspondence vector $\mathbf{m}_i^*$ was given as:

$$\mathbf{m}_i^* \; = \; (\mathbf{H})^{-1} \mathbf{C} \mathbf{m}_\mathbf{I}^\mathbf{s} \; . \tag{3.107}$$

Therefore, the correspondence could be estimated using the temporal harmonic model, the shape-based correspondence and the spatial smoothness of the differentiation. The whole process was called comb filtering since it was a combination of the above features and the process was considered a filtering process.

3.12.3.2 LV Tracking-Based on Optic Flow

There has been extensive literature published in the area of optic flow. Prominent published work is by Horn *et al.* [309], Spiesberger *et al.* [310], Nagel [311], Mailloux *et al.* [312] and Song *et al.* [313], who applied Horn's technique to 2-D echocardiograms. Lamberti *et al.* [164] then showed analysis of the heart motion using velocity fields. Srikantan *et al.* [314] showed how to recover the myocardial motion from 2-D echocardiograms. Gutierrez *et al.* [315] showed the 3-D LV motion based on optical flow. The whole idea of using the optic flow is to track the LV walls during the heartbeat. Tracking the LV apex is one of the most difficult tasks in pattern recognition, because the gray scale contrast is very poor in the apical zone. One solution is to get the most probable location of the LV apex for every time frame of the cardiac cycle and then estimate the apex motion from frame to frame. Using this concept, Suri *et al.* developed an algorithm for getting the most probable location of the apex based on the convergence of the gradient information representing the dye flow in the ventriculograms. Using the integrated directional derivative approach of Haralick *et al.* [243], Suri *et al.* developed the visual representation of the gradient flow [316] and then computed the average in the window over a database of 300 patient studies for each time frame of the cardiac cycle. This information showed where the apex was most likely to be found. Using that information, one can track the LV apex from frame to frame and can study the apex motion over the cardiac cycle. More research is, however, needed to validate the motion of the LV based on optic flow.

3.13 Conclusions

3.13.1 Cardiac Hardware

The cardiac catheterization procedure needs a more careful design so as to obtain good quality LVgrams. There are significant difficulties: (1) dislodging of the atherosclerotic plaque by the wire can lead to embolism and even myocardial infarction. (2) The procedure time should be minimal to avoid trauma. (3) The movements of the patient are sometimes pertinent. (4) The imaging terms of the image quality need to be considered. (5) The dosage of radiation from fluoroscopy must be controlled. (6) Multiple insertions of the guide wire and catheters must be minimized to avoid thrombosis (blood coagulation). If coagulation commences along the guide wire, coagulated blood can be forced into the heart, which can lead to heart attacks.

Though the goal of boundary estimation can be achieved at the cost of heavy data processing, it may be worthwhile to discuss whether computer processing of large data is the only approach to handling poor-quality data sets (LVgrams). On careful examination, if the LV chamber receives enough contrast agent (dye), the computer processing would be less complex (LV classification, edge detection, calibration). How can the apparatus set-up to inject dye into apical zone be improved? One way would be to change the curvature of the catheter for handling the variability of the LVs. If the LV was more longitudinal, the curvature of the catheter could be changed to let dye flow in towards the apex. On the contrary, if the heart is very wide or huge, would a dual catheter facing opposite walls be a good choice? One catheter could be used for filling the anterior side while the other catheter could be used to fill the inferior side. Another possibility would be to look over the lateral movement of the catheter during the motion of the LV. If the crests and troughs of the LV wall muscles could be detected, the apical zone could then be filled by using computer control. Careful design is feasible by controlling the fluid dynamics inside the LV chamber.

3.13.2   Cardiac Software

In previous sub-sections, the mathematical and algorithmic approaches for LV boundary estimation and LV modeling were discussed. It is still believed that the modeling process needs continued development in active deformable and training-based modeling. The key issues which lead to diversified research directions will be summarized here: (a) active modeling requires significant user interaction. A methodology of a combination of pixel-classification and surface fitting would be a good choice for obtaining the initial contour, which is basically the raw contour the user specifies. (b) Constrained deformable models are useful in LV motion tracking in echocardiograms. As pointed out by McInerney [229], learning techniques are a future direction, which have been established and validated by Lee [201], Suri [28], and Haralick and Sheehan [202], [235]. (c) More validation techniques are needed for the reliability of the algorithms and model developments. Singh *et al.* [210], Wikins *et al.* [209] and McInerney *et al.* [228] showed the implementation of fitting snakes to cardiac data but lacked a validation scheme. Suri *et al.* [247] presented a validation scheme to find whether the estimated curve was at its correct position. (d) Robustness can only be confirmed once the algorithm is able to handle a large volume of data sets with normal and abnormal studies. (e) On-line processes of the training system were very fast (less than 1 sec. on a PC) and active modeling took around 15 minutes, as established and timed by Singh *et al.* [210], although on different data sets.

3.13.3   Summary

An attempt has been made in this chapter to present past and current research work in computer vision, pattern recognition and image processing as applied to LV modeling and analysis. Also, an attempt has been made to cover almost all the cardiac imaging modalities, such as X-ray, CT, MR, PET, SPECT and Ultrasound. Emphasis was placed on state-of-the-art LV imaging algorithms based on model-based techniques which have dominated for the last 15 years. This chapter also showed how high-level models have been replacing low-level techniques and using hand-drawn boundaries to model the LV. Major research successes have been in the learning/training-based and the active contour-based models in segmentation of the LV. The conclusion is that learning techniques such as neural nets and training are the future of global shape extraction for accurate boundary estimation. Incorporating low-level techniques to extract certain features and then fusing them with global shape models are necessary to build a robust LV analysis system. However, there is a lack of validation techniques of LV modeling and a need to have a completely automatic mechanism for all the imaging modalities, as was previously developed in X-ray ventriculograms. Finally, the future challenge of cardiac imaging will be to build a fast, computationally inexpensive, robust cardiac analysis system in two, three and four dimensions.

3.13.4 Acknowledgments

The author would like to thank Springer-Verlag for permission to use material previously published in *Pattern Analysis and Applications.* Thanks to Professor Sameer Singh for valuable suggestions on this chapter. Thanks are also due to Dr. Bardinet of the University of Grenada, for allowing the author to use the dog's heart data sets and to Marconi Medical Systems, Inc., for the MR cardiac data sets.

Chapter 4

Advances in Computer Vision, Graphics, Image Processing and Pattern Recognition Techniques for MR Brain Cortical Segmentation and Reconstruction: A Review Toward functional MRI (fMRI)[1]

Jasjit S. Suri, Sameer Singh, Xiaolan Zeng, Laura Reden

4.1 Introduction

The importance of 2-D and 3-D brain segmentation has increased tremendously due to the recent growth in functional MRI (fMRI), perfusion-weighted imaging, diffusion-weighted imaging, volume graphics, 3-D segmentation, neurosurgical planning, navigation and MR brain scanning techniques. Besides that, recent growth in supervised and non-supervised brain segmentation techniques in 2-D (see Suri [322], Zavaljevski *et al.* [323], Barra *et al.* [324]) and 3-D (see Salle *et al.* [325], Kiebel *et al.* [326], Zeng *et al.* [327], Xu *et al.* [606], Fischl *et al.* [328], Linden *et al.* [329], Stokking [330], Smith [331], Hurdal [332] and ter Haar *et al.* [333]) have brought the engineering community, in areas such as computer vision, graphics, image processing (CVGIP) and pattern recognition, closer to the medical community, such as neuro-surgeons, psychiatrists, psychologists, physiologists, oncologists, radiologists and internists. This chapter is an attempt to review state-of-the-art cortical segmentation techniques in 2-D and 3-D using magnetic resonance imaging (MRI), and their applications. New challenges in this area are also discussed.

MRI, as we already know, has become one of the most common diagnostic tools, especially in the area of neuro imaging. The three main reasons that the field of neurological imaging using MRI has been very valuable both clinically and diagnostically are: first, its ability to yield spatial resolution to a fine level which helps in the detection and delineation of detailed structures (see Hashemi *et al.* [334] and Haacke *et al.* [335]); second, the range of response from

---

[1]This chapter is based on material accepted for publication in *Pattern Analysis and Applications* [826]

the tissues to the MR stimuli[2] allows for the visual differentiation of various classes of internal tissues; and third, the fast acquisitions of the MRI data sets (see Cohen *et al.*[336]).

Cortical segmentation using MRI is one of the most pressing needs for neuro-anatomical analysis because it helps in: (**1**) the quantification of cortical thickness and cortical fold curvatures (see Zeng *et al.*[327]) and (**2**) in determining the spatial inter-relationships of the neuro-anatomical structures (see Crespo-Facorro *et al.*[423], DeCarli *et al.*[396] and Kikinis *et al.*[424]). The quantification of specific regions is required for long-term monitoring of a disease progression or remission (see Rusinek *et al.*[425], Arnold *et al.*[337], Johnston *et al.*[426], Vaidyanathan *et al.*[338] and Clarke *et al.*[339]). Since manual cortical segmentation methods are subject to errors both in accuracy and reproducibility (operator bias) and are time-consuming, we need fast, accurate and robust semi-automatic or completely automatic techniques (see Höhne *et al.*[340], Galloway *et al.*[341], Gerig *et al.*[343] and Kikinis *et al.*[342]).

This chapter focuses on discussing state-of-the-art 2-D and 3-D cortex segmentation techniques, their applications and new challenges. It will also focus on graphical techniques in 3-D to reconstruct the brain. Next, the human brain anatomy and the system which yields the MRI data will be discussed briefly.

4.1.1 Human Brain Anatomy and the MRI System

This sub-section is divided into two. Part one briefly discusses the geometric properties of the cortex and its anatomy and the second part presents the MR brain scanning system.

4.1.1.1 Brain Anatomy, Cortical Geometry, Shapes and Sizes

Figures 4.1, 4.2 and 4.3 show the brain anatomy. As seen in Figure 4.1, the surface of the brain hemisphere in humans is thrown into irregular folds. These ridges are called gyri (singular, gyrus) and the intervening crevices are called sulci (singular, sulcus). A deep sulcus is called a fissure. The arrangement is such that it allows a greater surface area to be accommodated within the same space, which is inside the cranial cavity. For complete details on the anatomy of the brain, see the well written books by Jones *et al.*[427] and by Hendelman [428]. Plate 3 shows four specimen sections of the human brain depicting the white matter and the gray matter areas. Computer generated models of the human cortex are shown in Plate 2 (the algorithms for generating the computer models will be discussed in this chapter). Figure 4.4 and Plate 2 show the anatomy of the human brain in 2-D and 3-D, respectively. On the left in Plate 2, the brain is seen from the superior aspect towards the posterior end showing the frontal, parietal, temporal, occipital and central lobes of the cortex. On the right in Plate 2, the cortex is seen from the posterior end showing the gyrus angularis and gyri occipital. In Figure 4.4 the same areas are seen, now labeled on the MR transverse slices of the brain.

---

[2]Stimulus is singular and stimuli is plural.

Geometry, Shapes and Sizes. Some facts and figures about the human cortex include (for details, see the excellent published work by Griffin [344]): (**1**) the cerebral cortex is a five-layered surface consisting of five lobes: frontal, parietal, temporal, occipital and central; (**2**) the cortical thickness varies between 2 to 3 mm; (**3**) the surface area of the cortex is between 2000 to 2500 cm^2; (**4**) the cortical area during the evolution process increases almost linearly with volume; (**5**) large brains are fissured (gyrencephalic) and small brains are smooth (lissencephalic). For the brain atlas, the reader is referred to the books by England *et al.* [345] and Fischbach [346]. The reader is also referred to the extensive work by Hofman [347], [348], Todd [349] and Prothero *et al.* [350] for detailed information in the area of the shape of the human cortex.

4.1.1.2 Brain Scanning System and the Head Coil

An MRI system and the head coil used for scanning the brain are shown in Figure 4.5, on the left. On the right in Figure 4.5 is an enlarged frontal view of the head coil. This head coil is a receive-only design single channel coil, designed to provide optimum signal-to-noise (SNR) and uniform coverage of the head and brain regions. The head coil design is a 16 rung birdcage configuration, encased in a fiberglass housing around the coil electronics. The anterior aspect of the coil has several openings among the rungs over the region of the eyes, allowing the patient to see out of the head coil. This helps to lessen any claustrophobic feelings the patient may experience. This coil's dimensions are as follows: the inner diameter is 29.5 cm, the outer diameter is 34 cm, the total length of the coil is 44 cm and the electrical area of coverage is 35 cm. Pads are included to position the head and support the neck area. Straps are included to be placed over the head, to remind the patient to lie still during the exam.

The MRI system's most prominent component is the large magnet, and along with it are two sets of the coils, the so-called gradient coils and radio frequency (RF) coils. An MRI image is a map of RF intensities emitted by tissues. This can be briefly explained as follows: the gradient coil is used to inject an out-of-phase pulse to perturb the aligned atoms away from the main magnetic field. As the atoms realign with the main field, they transmit energy back, which is detected by the RF coils which in turn generates an MRI image. For details on the physics of MRI image generation, readers are referred to Chapter 1. For further detailed discussions on the physics in MRI, readers are referred to the following books: Horowitz [351], Hashemi *et al.* [334] and Haacke *et al.* [335]. Details on head coil design can be seen in the US patent by Vaughn [352]. Srinivasan [353] recently presented the design of two types of head coil. One has a symmetrical overlap between the volume head and the surface head coil. The volume coil was of a bird-cage type design. The other type of coil has an asymmetrical overlap between the volume head coil and surface head coil. Studies related to the sensitivity of the RF coils in MR can be seen in Narayana *et al.* [354]. Scanning protocols for collecting brain data will be briefly discussed in Sub-section 4.2 but first, the application and the importance of brain segmentation in the therapy world will be discussed.

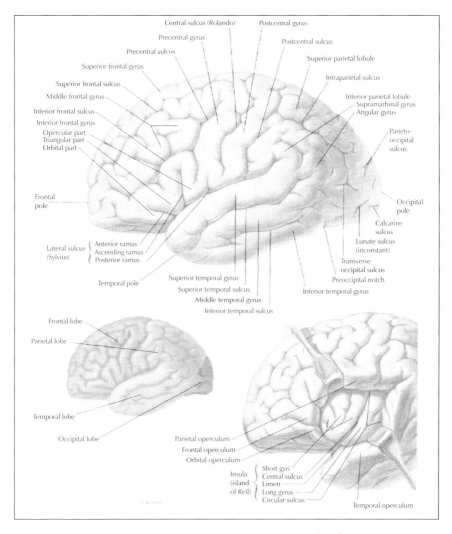

Figure 4.1: 3-D Anatomy of the Human Brain. From [158]. © 1995, Havas. Reprinted with permission from Havas MediMedia, illustrated by Drs. John A. Craig and Carlos Machado. All rights reserved.

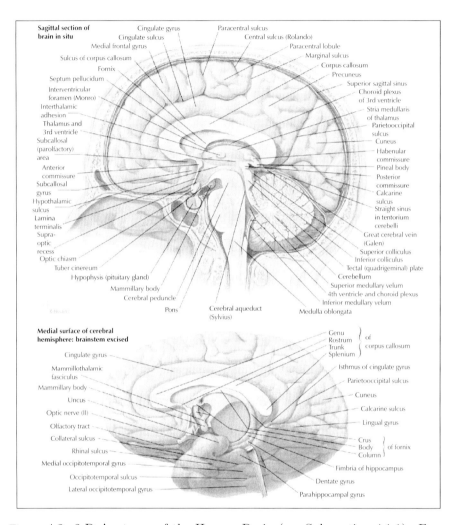

Figure 4.2: 3-D Anatomy of the Human Brain (see Sub-section 4.1.1). From [158]. © 1995, Havas. Reprinted with permission from Havas MediMedia, illustrated by Drs. John A. Craig and Carlos Machado. All rights reserved.

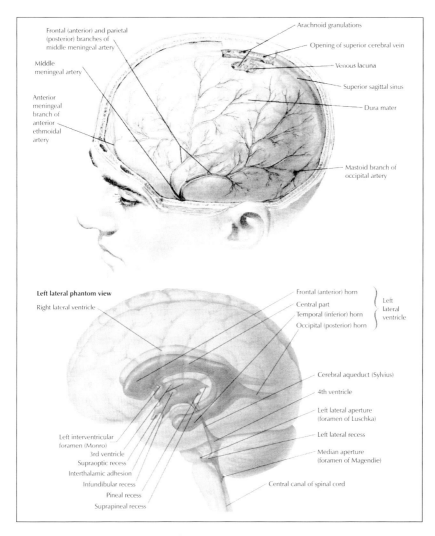

Figure 4.3: **Top**: Vasculature of the human brain. **Bottom**: Cortex and the ventricles in 3-D. From [158]. © 1995, Havas. Reprinted with permission from Havas MediMedia, illustrated by Drs. John A. Craig and Carlos Machado. All rights reserved.

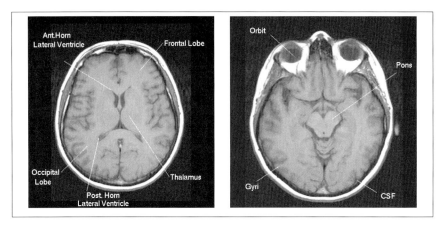

Figure 4.4: MR 2-D transverse brain slices showing the anatomy of the brain and various regions. **Left**: Labeled areas towards the superior aspect of the head: Anterior Horn of the Lateral Ventricle, Frontal Lobe, Occipital Lobe, Thalamus and Posterior Horn of the Lateral Ventricle. **Right**: Labeled anatomical areas lower in the head: Orbit, Pons, Gyri and CSF (Courtesy of Marconi Medical Systems, Inc., Cleveland, OH.)

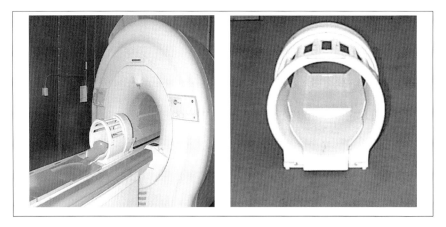

Figure 4.5: **Left**: MRI system with the placement of the head coil on the couch for scanning the human brain. **Right**: Close-up of the frontal view of the head coil (Courtesy of Marconi Medical Systems, Inc., Cleveland, OH.)

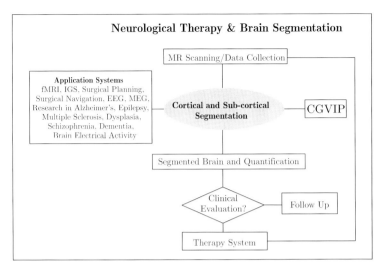

Figure 4.6: The role of MR brain segmentation in neurological therapy and brain imaging applications. MR brain data is collected using a scanning protocol for a particularly desired application. Depending upon the selected data set and the application, a brain segmentation technique is applied using one of the CVGIP and pattern recognition techniques. The output is the segmented brain. On the basis of the clinical evaluation, the patient undergoes therapy. Follow-up may also be necessary, as indicated. Finally, depending upon the therapy, the subject might need another brain scan (feedback loop). As can be seen, the role of brain segmentation, or segmentation of the sub-cortical structures, is the main thrust of the therapy system (fMRI – functional MRI, EEG – Electro-Encephalo-Graphy, MEG – Magneto-Encephalo-Graphy).

4.1.2 Applications of Brain Segmentation

Figure 4.6 discusses the role and importance of brain segmentation in the therapy world, depending upon the neurological conditions. As shown in Figure 4.6, the critical component in the neuro-therapy world is cortical and sub-cortical segmentation. The MR data is collected by scanning the patient's brain. The protocol used depends upon the application's therapy. Brain segmentation and sub-cortical segmentation are performed as per the application, which is then clinically evaluated and the results help to decide the type of therapy needed. Feedback is provided if the patient needs to be scanned again. A follow-up may also be necessary, depending upon the results of the clinical evaluation. We refer readers to the following web sites from McGill University, Montreal [653] and Massachusetts General Hospital, Boston [654] for more detailed discussions on neurological applications. Here, we will discuss in brief the brain segmentation applications. As new technology advances to bridge the gap between radiology, surgery and engineering, we will see the provided diversification of these applications. First we will summarize cortical segmentation applications:

1. *Surgical Planning*: (see Kelly *et al.*[358], Schad *et al.*[359], Peters *et al.*[360], Ayache *et al.*[361], Kikinis *et al.*[363] and Jolesz *et al.*[364]). Here, the main objective is to help the neuro-surgeon to plan the neuro-surgery in an OR[3]; to identify the location of the tumors in 3-D coordinates and the critical trajectories through which the tumors are accessed and removed.

2. *Surgical Navigation*: (see Maciunas *et al.*[365], Grimson *et al.*[383], Kosugi *et al.*[366]). Here, the objective is to navigate using tools (such as the Y-probe) to move towards the target (e.g., a tumor in the brain), while avoiding critical brain structures and their functions during surgery.

3. *3-D Visualization and Interactive Segmentation*: here, the goal is to visualize the anatomy and pathology of the reconstructed brain. This could also be in relation to the reconstructed blood vessels which are used for treatment planning and tumor surgery (see Jaaski *et al.*[368], Höhne *et al.*[340], Suri *et al.*[369], [370], Schiemann *et al.*[371], Saiviroonporm *et al.*[372], Zeng *et al.*[373] and Xu *et al.*[606]).

4. *Multi-Modality Fusion*: here, one can obtain a complete structural segmentation on a patient by combining segmented tissues from different modalities into a single segmented tissue map. For example, one can segment the soft tissue brain along with the vasculature of an MR angiogram, or bone segmented from CT data with a soft tissue brain MR or PET/SPECT functional data with the segmented brain (see the fusion of multi-modalities by Pelizzari *et al.*[375], Henri *et al.*[374] and recently by Stokking *et al.*[376]).

5. *Multi-Modality*[4] *Registration*: there are many ways to perform the registration of medical data sets: manual, atlas-based (see Cuisenaire *et al.*[377]), mutual information-based, etc. For any registration algorithm, one needs the landmark features (see manual segmentation followed by registration in Alpert *et al.*[378]). Here, the landmark features can be identified using segmentation techniques and then used for registration. Neelin *et al.*[379] segmented MR images to create simulated PET images to validate their MRI/PET registration method. Collins *et al.*[380] developed a multi-resolution method to automatically identify and register individual brain regions to a standardized Talairach space. Other researchers who used brain segmentation for registration were Lemieux *et al.*[381] and Hajnal *et al.*[382]. Here, the pipeline consists of converting the acquired MR volume into an isotropic volume, segmenting the brain, interpolating these (using one of these methods - linear, non-linear, sinc, spline, shape, surface-based, volume-based), followed by registration.

---

[3]Operating Room.

[4]By multi-modality, we mean the registration of data sets from different modalities, say, MR with CT, MR with PET, or spatial-MR with functional-MR.

6. *Image-Guided Surgery*: the reconstructed patient's brain anatomy helps neuro-surgeons to interactively guide the surgery (see Höhne *et al.* [384], Tiede *et al.* [385] and the recently published work by Grimson *et al.* [383]).

7. *Research in Pathology Prediction and its Interface with Other Fields, such as Alzheimer's Disease, Epilepsy, Band Heterotopia, Dysplasia, Schizophrenia, Dementia*: some previously developed segmentation methods work well with the brain, in cases where pathologies have predictable appearances, such as with multiple sclerosis (MS) lesions (see Johnston *et al.* [386]), or with other pathologies such as tumors, or structures which are very different from the trained cases. There is a need for semiautomated tools which will incorporate the anatomical expertise (see Clarke *et al.* [339]). Other fields of brain imaging, such as MEG (Magneto-Encephalo-Graphy), EEG (Electro-Encephlo-Graphy), CEP (Cortical Evoked Potentials) and IRS (Infra-Red Spectroscopy) have provided neuro-surgeons and neurologists with a great deal of information in the understanding of brain activity. All of these brain imaging techniques provide valuable tools in studying the functions of the brain (see Wagner *et al.* [387]). These techniques primarily detect or localize regions in the brain which cause a particular activity or actions. The localization of regions in spatial brain data, and the quantification of the regions or areas inside the brain slices, assists the neurosurgeon in understanding a variety of pathological conditions of the brain in a certain set of patients, such as those with Alzheimer's, epilepsy, band heterotopia, dysplasia, dementia, brain aging, brain trauma and schizophrenia (see Brant-Zawadski [389], Drayer [390], Tanabe *et al.* [391], Woermann *et al.* [392], Zubenko *et al.* [393] and the excellent article by Lawrie *et al.* [394] on schizophrenia).

8. *Quantitative Assessment and Treatment Procedures*: for patients who undergo surgery and receive radiation and/or chemotherapy treatment, it is important to make a quantitative evaluation of the treatment strategies, thus the segmentation issue is very critical and helps in further benefitting research into the treatment of such areas as brain tumors. Researchers are always interested in quantifying the depth of sulci, the thickness of the gray matter, the mean and the standard deviation of the cerebral cortex over a large number of patient studies (see Velthuizen *et al.* [395], DeCarli *et al.* [396] and Wright *et al.* [397]). Thus region identification, localization, classification and quantification are needed in the future of fMRI, MEG, EEG and brain imaging in general.

9. *Brain Functional Mapping*: brain segmentation in relation to fMRI measurements (called fMRI) is emerging as a new technological tool for understanding the functions of the human brain (see Carswell [398]). Kim *et al.* [686] recently reviewed the current technical and methodological status of fMRI. In this review, Kim *et al.* discussed a post-processing method for fMRI data. They also presented the potential problems and solutions related to vessels and motion. Golay *et al.* [399] showed the role of brain

segmentation in fMRI. Similarly, Teo *et al.* [514] showed the overlay of fMRI data and the flattened segmented cortex. The fMRI data was collected using the rotating wedge method and expanding ring stimulus (see Figure 10, page 861 of Teo *et al.*). We will discuss the Teo *et al.* method later.

Lotze *et al.* [400] also discussed the segmentation applications in fMRI. They mapped the neural activity (functional data) over the spatial visual cortex surface (topographic data) and compared this with histological data (see Tootell *et al.* [409], [410] and the recent paper by Goldszal *et al.* [401]). We will discuss the fMRI application in some detail at the end of this chapter.

10. *The Brain's Sub-Cortical Segmentation in Relation to the Main Cortex:* another application is in the segmentation of sub-cortical structures in relation to the main cortex. Several authors have attempted this (see Szekely *et al.* [213], Davatzikos *et al.* [565], [566], Fritsch *et al.* [306], Dhawan *et al.* [493], Goualher *et al.* [411], Hill *et al.* [422]). Due to several types of diseases like Alzheimer's Disease and Normal Pressure Hydrocephalus (NPH), the shape of sub-cortical structures such as the ventricles (see Martin *et al.* [416]) and the corpus callosum (see Weis *et al.* [418]) change and therefore, it is important to know the variation of these sub-cortical structures in relation to the main cortex. This helps in determining transcortical pathways in neurosurgery. Segmentation of the hippocampus in MRI brain images was performed by Ghanei *et al.* [419]. Cowell *et al.* (see [420]) showed a stable mathematical model for the corpus callosum and its segmentation. Recently, Worth *et al.* [421] showed semi-automatic ways to segment the lateral ventricles and caudate nucleus in T_1-weighted coronal MR image data sets.

So, we see that there is now a large number of applications for brain segmentation in the different fields of engineering in medicine. Even though cortical segmentation has been one of the top items on the agenda for engineering in medical research, it has not been easy to develop robust and high speed techniques. Some of the main difficulties are: (**1**) *partial volume averaging (PVA)*: this is caused by the finite spatial extent of an imaging system's point spread function (PSF). If there is more than one tissue within the extent of a partial density function or one voxel, then PVA is prominent; (**2**) *tissue inhomogeneity and non-uniformity* (see Meyer *et al.* [403] and Sled *et al.* [405]): this is an intrinsic property that adds to the boundary fuzziness regardless of the imaging system's quality. In other words, it can be said that it is due to the spatial inhomogeneities in the radio-frequency (RF) gain in the RF coil, so the intensities associated with these two tissues overlap, defeating intensity-based classification. Shimming[5] is needed for obtaining good image quality; (**3**) *shading arti-*

---

[5]Shimming is a process of correcting for inhomogeneity in the main magnetic field. The presence of external ferromagnetic objects may also cause inhomogeneity in the main magnetic field. Shimming can be active or passive for correction of inhomogeneity in the magnetic field.

facts (see Nyul *et al.* [407]). There are three sources of artifacts: (i) hardware, (ii) those due to MR physics and (iii) patient-related. The hardware-related artifacts include: zipper[6] artifact, corduroy[7] artifact, dot[8] artifact, data clipping[9] artifact, spurious echo[10] artifact, coherent ghosting[11] artifact and calibration[12] artifact. The MR physics related artifacts include: magnetic susceptibility[13] artifact, chemical shift[14] artifact, truncation[15] artifact, and criss-cross[16] artifact. The patient-related artifacts are motion artifacts due to voluntary or involuntary patient movements; (**4**) *noise randomness:* random noise associated with the MR imaging system; (**5**) *convolutedness and variability of the brain structure:* (see Griffin [344] and Netter *et al.* [158], as shown in Figure 4.1. This is the complex topology causing bends and twists. Besides that, this morphological shape differs from subject to subject; (**6**) *variability in tissue types:* the number of tissue types and connectivity (classes) present in the tissue volume such as optic nerve and blood vessels (see Rademacher *et al.* [429]); (**7**) *size and types of brain tumors:* current techniques are limited to medium to large-sized enhancing intra-cranial tumors (see Velthuizen *et al.* [395]); (**8**) *operator variability:* this is due to variability in tracing (intra-and inter-observer variability) of the cortical boundary/regions for image segmentation algorithms; (**9**) *error susceptibility:* another difficulty is the susceptibility to failures of fully supervised methods; (**10**) *imaging variabilities:* variability in imaging parameters such as the inter-scan interval, voxel dimension, signal-to-noise ratio, position and orientation of the subject in the scanner, also cause complications in the segmentation process; (**11**) *limited availability of shape models*: the absence of explicit shape models that capture the deformations in the human brain anatomy and topology.

Due to the large number of complications in segmenting the human cortex and its extensive volumetric data analysis, the large number of cortical segmentation applications and the large set of neurological disorders, research in cortical 2-D and 3-D segmentation took a different route over the past few years. Another aspect observed from the previous papers was that a particular segmentation technique could be successful in 2-D but was not attempted in 3-D, or was directly handled in 3-D but was never tried in 2-D. Some cortical segmentation techniques were totally geared towards the application they were handling. For example, if speed was a concern (say, in neuro-surgical planning), then direct 3-D segmentation was not used due to its computational expense. We see that most of the techniques were application driven. Hence, one must take the following factors into consideration: (**1**) the application used, (**2**) the

---

[6] This is due to the leaking of RF pulses.

[7] This is the noise burst at any point in the data collection process.

[8] This is a coherent noise source locked to the system frequency.

[9] This is due to the excess of signal reception at the receiver.

[10] This is due to the unwanted NMR signal.

[11] This is due to the instability of the NMR signal.

[12] This is due to the improper alignment of the echoes in k-space.

[13] This is due to the presence of metal or iron content nearby.

[14] This is due to spatial mismapping of frequency-encoded signals.

[15] This is due to an asymmetric sampling aliasing artifact due to the warping of the image.

[16] This is due to the RF excitation pulse of one slice which interfers with the adjacent slice.

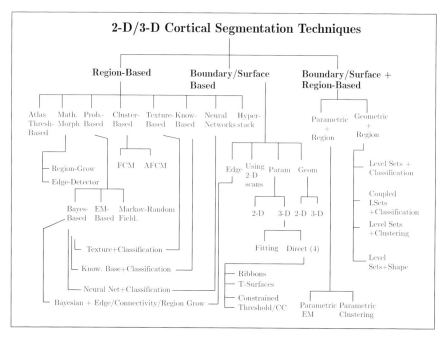

Figure 4.7: Taxonomy of cortical segmentation techniques. The cortical classification tree for 2-D and 3-D cortical segmentation techniques consists primarily of <u>three</u> major techniques: (i) Region-based, (ii) boundary-based and (iii) a fusion of region with boundary/surface based techniques.

kind of supervision needed/not needed, (**3**) the accuracy, (**4**) the robustness desired, (**5**) speed issues and (**6**) the rapid growth of mathematical techniques in engineering in medicine. Cortical segmentation techniques can then be classified into three core classes (see Figure 4.7). These are the techniques which use: (**1**) the regional-based approach, (**2**) the boundary/surface-based approach and (**3**) the fusion of the boundary/surface with the region-based approach.

Since there have been more than 400 publications and several good survey papers written in the area of cortical/sub-cortical segmentation, it is recommended that readers look at the extensive survey papers by Menhardt *et al.* [430], Stytz *et al.* [135], Clarke *et al.* [431], Bezdek *et al.* [466], Golay *et al.* [399], Fu *et al.* [182], Haralick *et al.* [183], Davis [186], Binford [432], Pal *et al.* [433], Suri [139], Kong *et al.* [434], Saeed [435] and Barillot *et al.* [436], [437]. Since it is difficult to discuss all of them, we will briefly talk about the core techniques and the foundations of each type. We will also discuss some salient features of these algorithms, the advantages and disadvantages of these techniques and highlight some references for interested readers but first, we will define the three core classes and discuss the taxonomy.

The first core class consists of region-based 2-D and 3-D segmentation techniques which use region-based information for pixel or voxel classification. Region-based techniques have been in existence for quite some time. In 1976,

Zucker [438] first presented work in region-growing. Since then, several other techniques (see Adams *et al.* [439]) have come into existence. Recently, Justice *et al.* [440] presented a method of using 3-D seeded region growing to solve the segmentation problem. The region-growing process required a threshold on whose basis it was decided whether to merge or to split. This threshold could be computed dynamically and automatically (see Liu *et al.* [441]). In the region-labelling process, a pixel/voxel could be labelled as inside or outside the region. Such a labelling process comes under pixel/voxel classification. One can adapt a probability-based (say, Bayesian) or a cluster-based approach. Note, these techniques could be supervised or non-supervised. This means one can compute the regional statistics in the region defined or for the whole image automatically. We will see later the role of region-based techniques as a stand-alone method or as a regularizer in building robust cortical segmentation techniques.

Region-based techniques are further classifed into the following categories: (**1**) atlas and threshold-based; (**2**) mathematical morphology-based; (**3**) probability-based; (**4**) clustering-based; (**5**) texture-based; (**6**) prior knowledge-based; (**7**) neural network-based; (**8**) region-linking using hyperstack; and (**9**) a fusion of the above techniques. We will now present very brief definitions of these distinctive classes before we go to the next core class of cortical segmentation. Atlas-based techniques are those in which the brain atlases are used as an *a-prior* knowledge for the segmentation and grouping of anatomical structures. Threshold-based techniques are those in which a threshold is selected so that all pixels/voxels having gray scale intensities greater than the threshold are in the foreground region and all the pixels/voxels lower than the threshold are in the background region. Mathematical morphology-based techniques are those that use structuring elements (SE) or masks or kernels as templates to convolve with the image/volumes, followed by binarization using a given function to segment given shapes. The SE and the process of binarization depend upon the morphological operator and the nature of the image. Probability-based methods are those that assign a pixel to a class and are based on the principle of maximization of a posterior (MAP) probability. Clustering-based techniques are those that use the fuzzy membership methods for segmenting the WM/GM[17]. Texture-based techniques use statistical methods to compute textural features to distinguish brain tissues for the segmentation of the cortex. Prior knowledge-based techniques use prior knowledge of different cortical structures of the human brain to segment the human cortex. Neural-network based techniques use altogether a different class of methodology, where one has to train the given MRI volumetric data set to estimate the training parameters which when applied to the test MR data sets, yield segmented shapes in test images/volumes.

The second core class is boundary/surface-based 2-D and 3-D techniques which estimate the boundaries/surfaces of the WM and GM. These techniques can also be supervised and non-supervised, but most are supervised due to the

---

[17]WM/GM: From now on, when we say, WM/GM, this means the interface boundary between the WM and GM.

success of this approach. If it is supervised, then a raw contour or curve/surface is used as a starting point to estimate the interface boundaries/surfaces of the WM/GM. Boundary/surface-based methods are further classified into four classes: (**1**) edge-based approaches; (**2**) 2-D scan-based approaches; (**3**) parametric deformable models (also called classical snakes/surfaces); and (**4**) geometric deformable models (also called level set snakes/surfaces). Edge-based approaches use a continuous approximation of the original image function, so that boundary points can be characterized by a differential property such as image gradient and curvature. The two-dimensional scan-based technique estimates the boundaries of the WM/GM in orthogonal slices using 2-D segmentation methods. These boundaries are then linked and the 3-D cortex is reconstructed. Parametric deformable curves (active contours) are local methods based on the energy-minimizing spline guided by external and image forces which pull the spline towards features such as lines and edges in the image. The classical active contour models can solve the objective function to obtain the goal boundary, if the approximate or initial location of the contour is available. On the other hand, level set methods are active contour energy minimization techniques which solve the computation of geodesics or minimal distance curves. The level set methods are governed by the curvature dependent speeds of moving curves or fronts. Due to the recent growth in parametric deformable models, this sub-class has undergone a lot of exploration and we have thus further divided this class into the following sub-classes: (**1**) constrained parametric 3-D deformable models; (**2**) ribbon-based models; (**3**) Affine Cell Decomposition (ACD)-based (T-surface) models; and (**4**) geometric surface-based models.

The third core class of cortical 2-D and 3-D segmentation is the fusion of regions with boundary/surface-based techniques. This class of cortical segmentation has been the most successful as this technique uses information from two different sources: boundary/surface-based and region-based. Due to its large success, it has recently been given much attention. This fusion of boundary/surface with region-based techniques is further classified into two categories: (i) parametric curve fused with regions; (ii) geometric curve fused with regions. Parametric-based techniques are classified into two types: (**1**) parametric-based techniques with clustering, (**2**) parametric-based techniques with expectation-maximization-based (EM). Geometric-based techniques are classified into four types: (**1**) level sets with Bayesian-classification, (**2**) coupled level sets with classification, (**3**) level sets with clustering and (**4**) level sets with shape modeling. Parametric and geometric contour/surface methods embedded with probability and expectation-maximization-based methods are those that use regional analysis with parametric/geometric snakes/surfaces.

Having discussed the taxonomy of cortical segmentation techniques, we will now focus on the following four major goals/contributions in this chapter. They are: (**1**) to learn about the fast expanding classification taxonomy of cortical segmentation techniques and the links between these core classes. Further, to establish the relationships between low-level computer vision and fast differential geometric techniques for a variety of cortical applications. (**2**) To survey the state-of-the art literature on: (i) region-based 2-D and 3-D cortical segmentation; (ii) boundary/surface-based 2-D and 3-D cortical segmentation; and (iii) the fusion of boundary/surface-based with region-based cortical segmentation techniques for 2-D and 3-D. This also involves discussing the pros and cons of the cortical segmentation techniques (especially from INRIA[18], IRISA[19], UU[20], IMDM[21], MIT[22], JHU[23], UT[24], LBL[25], MNI[26], Yale[27], MMS[28]) and the salient features. Special emphasis is given to how the fusion of regional forces has been successfully incorporated into the topology driven snakes/surfaces in the level set framework using partial differential equations; (**3**) To discuss the validation of cortical segmentation techniques, challenges in cortical segmentation and the future of cortical segmentation. (**4**) Lastly, to provide a comprehensive ready-reference for readers pursuing advanced neuro-imaging research covering the latest state-of-the art literature and techniques, which solve the complex problem of 2-D and 3-D cortical segmentation.

The remainder of this chapter is structured as follows: Sub-section 4.2 presents the state-of-the-art methods used for scanning the human brain. In Sub-section 4.3, we discuss region-based 2-D and 3-D cortical segmentation techniques. Sub-section 4.4 focuses on boundary/surface-based 2-D and 3-D cortical segmentation techniques. The fusion of boundary/surface with region-based 2-D and 3-D cortical segmentation techniques discussed in Sub-section is 4.5. Sub-section 4.7 presents briefly the application of brain segmentation in fMRI. Detailed discussions, validation and new challenges are presented in Sub-section 4.8. Finally, we present conclusions and future aspects of cortical segmentation in Sub-section 4.9.

4.2 Brain Scanning and its Clinical Significance

The computer vision, image processing and pattern recognition algorithms applied to human MR brain images will depend upon the scanning method and the type of application. One segmentation algorithm may not be suitable for every type of brain scan image. For example, WM/GM and CSF may have significant variations in intensity levels when you compare the T_1-, T_2-, and PD-weighted scans as a result of the segmentation algorithm pipeline and the

---

[18]Institut National de Recherche en Informatique et Automatique, Sophia-Antipolis, France

[19]Institut de recherche en informatique et systemes aleatoires, Rennes Cedex, France

[20]Image Science Institute, Utrecht University, Utrecht, The Netherlands

[21]Institute of Mathematics and Computer Science in Medicine, University Hospital Eppendorf, Hamburg, Germany

[22]Massachusetts Institute of Technology, Cambridge, MA, USA

[23]Johns Hopkins University, Baltimore, MD, USA

[24]University of Toronto, Toronto, Canada

[25]Lawrence Berkeley Labs, Berkeley, CA, USA

[26]Montreal Neurological Institute, McGill University, Montreal, Canada

[27]Image Processing and Analysis Group, Yale University, New Haven, CT, USA

[28]Marconi Medical Systems, Inc., Cleveland, OH, USA

techniques that change depending upon the type of application (see Teo *et al.* [514]). Another reason for change in the gray scale contrast in these scans could be due to the quality of the head coils. For example, Wells *et al.* [458] used a correction method prior to segmentation because the brain scans were derived from a low quality head coil. On the contrary, Teo *et al.* [514] do not apply any corrections prior to their segmentation. This sub-section discusses the various types of scanning methods (pulse sequences) that can be used in human brain imaging. For a detailed analysis of optimal pulse sequence design, see Iwaoka *et al.* [414].

Broadly, the brain scanning methods we will discuss are of three types: T_1-weighted, T_2-weighted, and PD-weighted and for each scanning method, we can acquire images of the brain in any of the three orthogonal directions (x, y and z) as well as at oblique angles. The differences between the three scanning methods (see Figure 4.8) depend on the way the T_R (repetition time) and T_E (echo time) are controlled. Usually T_R and T_E are short for a T_1-weighted image, while T_R and T_E are long for a T_2-weighted image. A T_1-weighted scan is useful for studying brain anatomy, such as the shape and structures (morphology) of the human brain, while a T_2-weighted scan is useful for studying human pathology, e.g., to see if the brain has tumors. In a PD-weighted scan, the T_R and T_E are long and short, respectively and it is beyond T_1-weighted and T_2-weighted contributions. Each of these three classes used is based on the brain imaging methods desired. In addition, we will also discuss what kinds of applications they can be used for. T_1-weighted imaging can be acquired using any of the following techniques: (1) FSE (Fast Spin Echo), (2) SE (Spin Echo), (3) RF-FAST (Fourier Acquired Steady State Technique) and (4) FE (Field Echo). T_2-weighted scanning can be done using any of the following techniques:

1. *Fourier-Acquired Steady-State Technique (FAST)*. This is a rapid way of scanning the brain and it uses short T_E and T_R (see Figure 4.9).

2. *Fast Spin Echo (FSE)*. This is a rapid imaging technique that produces T_1-, T_2- and PD-weighted MR images, depending on the T_E and T_R values chosen. Images can be acquired with good resolution using acquisition times that are shorter than conventional Spin Echo techniques. It allows for shorter scan times, although the fat is not suppressed as much as in the Spin Echo technique. Figure 4.10 shows two example images of the brain using T_2-weighted FSE from slice locations 5 and 10 in the head.

3. *Fluid Attenuated Inversion Recovery (FLAIR)*. This kind of pulse sequence is used to suppress the signal from CSF on a T_2-weighted scan (see Figure 4.11[29], on the right). This technique is useful for evaluating patients suspected of having Multiple Sclerosis (see Filippi *et al.* [415]).

4. *Extended Phase Conjugate Symmetry Rapid Spin Echo Sequences (EXPRESS)*. This is a single-shot data acquisition technique, allowing one

---

[29]For details of the definitions on the MR imaging parameters, readers are advised to see Chapter 1.

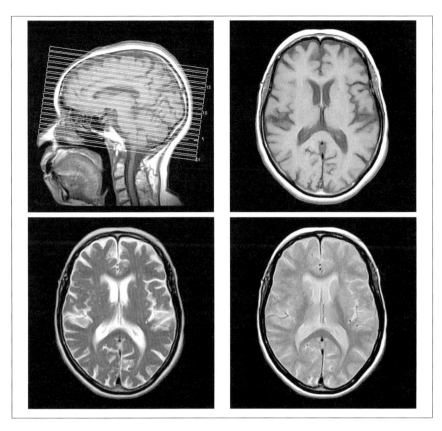

Figure 4.8: Brain images showing the comparison between: **Top Left**: pilot showing the grid lines for scanning the brain. **Top Right**: T_1-weighted image, **Bottom Left**: T_2-weighted image, **Bottom Right**: PD-weighted image (Courtesy of Marconi Medical Systems, Inc., Cleveland, OH.)

to obtain T_2-weighted images within a very short time, such as in breath hold times (see Figure 4.12). EXPRESS sequences collect all the data within one T_R period, resulting in a very short scan time. It is faster to acquire than FSE and useful for scanning the brain and abdominal regions.

5. *Spin Echo (SE)*. This is a type of T_2-weighted scan and is useful for studying brain anatomy and pathology.

6. *Diffusion-Weighted Imaging (DWI)*. This type of scanning can be used for evaluating patients suspected of having a stroke. It is based on the Spin Echo Single-Shot Echo Planar Imaging (EPI) technique. A diffusion gradient is applied in each orthogonal plane. Maps can be created on T_2-weighted diffusion-weighted information. They can also be created from just the diffusion-weighted information, which is the apparent diffusion

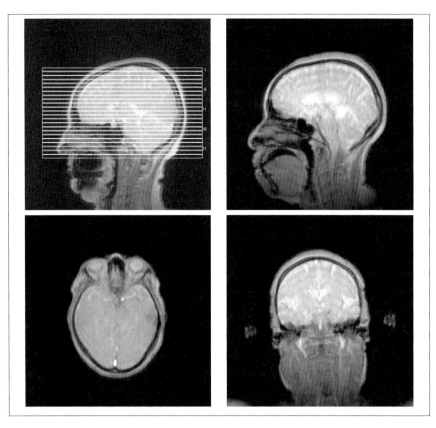

Figure 4.9: FAST-sequence brain images acquired with the following imaging parameters: T_E=3.7 ms, T_R=16 ms, FoV=30 cm, Matrix Size=256 × 256, NSA=1, Flip Angle=20, Thick=10 mm, Gap=0 mm (Courtesy of Marconi Medical Systems, Inc., Cleveland, OH.)

coefficient (ADC) map. In this technique, we acquire data in four different ways: no diffusion-weighted gradient applied, diffusion-weighted gradient applied in the slice, read and phase encode directions. This imaging technique is sensitive to air-tissue interfaces which can create artifacts. It is very useful for detecting ischemic areas. A Single-Shot Spin Echo EPI technique with diffusion-weighting can show damaged tissue as bright areas in the first few hours after a stroke occurs. An example of trace diffusion-weighted brain images is shown in Figure 4.13.

7. *Perfusion-weighted Imaging (PWI)*. Shown here is a T_2^*-weighted technique based on a Field Echo Single-Shot (SS) EPI pulse sequence, allowing many temporal frames to be acquired in a short period of time over multiple spatial locations. A contrast agent (Gadolinium) is injected at the beginning of the scan to study blood flow and how the contrast is distributed throughout the vasculature and tissues in the brain. Samples

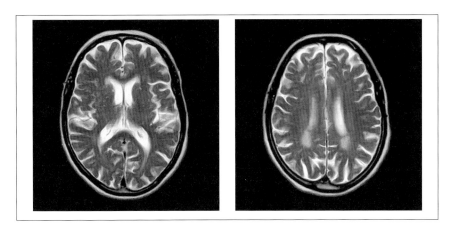

Figure 4.10: FSE T_2-weighted brain images acquired with the following imaging parameters: T_E=105 ms, T_R=3600 ms, FoV=22 cm, Matrix Size=224 × 224, NSA=2, Flip Angle=90, Thick=5 mm, Gap=2 mm. (Courtesy of Marconi Medical Systems, Inc., Cleveland, OH.)

of the brain perfusion images can be seen in Figure 4.14.

8. *fMRI or BOLD (Blood Oxygenation Level Dependent)*. This uses a T_2^*-weighted technique based on a Field Echo Single-Shot EPI pulse sequence, allowing many frames to be acquired in a short period of time over multiple spatial locations (see Figure 4.15). We will discuss fMRI later in Sub-section 4.7.

So, we observe that different scanning techniques can produce the different kinds of gray scale images necessary for 2-D and 3-D brain segmentation techniques, which will be discussed later.

4.3   Region-Based 2-D and 3-D Cortical Segmentation Techniques

Region-based techniques are those which can segment the image/volume into different regions/sub-volumes. Since the human brain consists of multiple classes of tissues, the region-based approach could be either a simple or a complex problem, depending upon what one is trying to segment. For a three class problem such as using WM, GM and CSF, simple techniques like clustering could do the job at a reasonable speed, but this may not be the case when more than three classes are present. On the other hand, probability-based techniques are more successful, since they are accurate and robust, but can be computationally expensive. Recently, the trend has been to make cortical segmentation systems interactive, which can be accomplished efficiently using 2-D and 3-D morphology-based systems. On the other hand, segmentation techniques could involve knowledge of different structures to provide

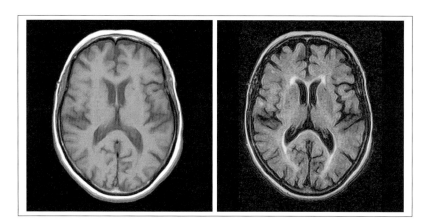

Figure 4.11: **<u>Left</u>**: Spin Echo (SE) T_1-weighted brain image acquired with the following imaging parameters: T_E=16 ms, T_R=451 ms, FoV=22 cm, Matrix Size=220 × 220, NSA=2, Flip Angle=90, Thick=5 mm, Gap=2 mm. **Right**: FSE T_2-weighted FLAIR brain image acquired with the following imaging parameters: T_E=168 ms, T_R=6000 ms, FoV=22 cm, TI=1800 ms, Matrix Size=192 × 192, NSA=1, Flip Angle=90, Thick=5 mm, Gap=2 mm (Courtesy of Marconi Medical Systems, Inc., Cleveland, OH.)

better identification and labeling of the cortex/sub-cortex in image/volume. These are knowledge-based techniques. Thus the goal of this sub-section is to introduce the fundamental features of these segmentation techniques for cortex segmentation and to discuss their pros and cons.

The layout of this sub-section is as follows: Atlas-based and threshold-based techniques are discussed in Sub-section 4.3.1. The Bayesian-based pixel/voxel classification, expectation maximization-based techniques and Markov Random Field-based techniques are discussed in Sub-section 4.3.2. Clustering-based techniques are discussed in Sub-section 4.3.3. Sub-section 4.3.4 presents mathematical morphology-based techniques. The same sub-section also discusses the fusion of mathematical morphology with edge-detectors and region growing. Prior knowledge-based techniques are discussed in Sub-section 4.3.5. Texture-based methods are discussed in Sub-section 4.3.6. Sub-section 4.3.7 presents neural-network based techniques. Regional hyperstack linking-based techniques are discussed in Sub-section 4.3.8. Fusion of probability-based techniques with connectivity and edge-detectors is discussed in Sub-section 4.3.9. We conclude this section by discussing the pros and cons of region-based techniques in Sub-section 4.3.10.

4.3.1   Atlas-Based and Threshold-Based Techniques

Before computation-based methods were developed for estimating the brain boundaries, brain atlas was the guide used for segmentation. The whole idea of using the brain atlas was to provide the *a-prior* knowledge, which can help

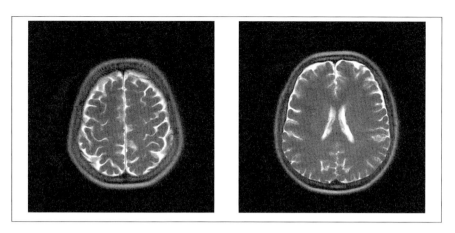

Figure 4.12: T_2-weighted EXPRESS brain images acquired with the following imaging parameters: T_E=120 ms, T_R=2500 ms, FoV=25 cm, Matrix Size=240 × 240, NSA=1, Flip Angle=90, Thick=5 mm, Gap=1 mm (Courtesy of Marconi Medical Systems, Inc., Cleveland, OH.)

in grouping the segments into anatomical structures. This helps in obtaining fully automatic cortical segmentation procedures. The Talairach methodology was one of the earliest ways of dealing with the inter-individual variability of cortical shapes. This method relies on a few landmarks that allows one to define a relatively stable orientation and on a few scale factors. This atlas used an anatomical localization for functional interpretation (see Talairach *et al.* [442], [443], Bohm *et al.* [444], Seitz *et al.* [445], Evans *et al.* [446], Bajcsy *et al.* [447]). They all assumed that there existed a topological in variance among normal subjects. Segmentation was achieved by performing a spatial transformation required to map the atlas data to the MR brain image volume, hence segmentation was actually a registration problem.

Recently, Van Essen *et al.* [448] published work to analyze the functional and structural changes in the human cerebral cortex using surface-based atlas. Recently, Collins *et al.* [449] presented a brain segmented technique that was achieved by identifying the non-linear spatial transformation that best fitted maps corresponding to intensity-based features between a model-image and a new MRI brain volume. When completed, atlas contours defined on the model image were mapped through the same transformation to segment and label individual structures in the new data set. Gibaud, Barillot and their co-workers [450] are also developing an advanced brain atlas for segmentation decisions. In the class of segmentation using a deformable atlas, several authors such as Sandor *et al.* [451], [452] and Ferrant *et al.* [453] did good work. Their work presented a hierarchical multi-object surface-based deformable atlas for the automatic localization, identification and segmentation of brain structures. Since their work focused on sub-cortical structures, it is out of the scope of this chapter. Interested readers can explore these papers and the references therein.

Threshold-based techniques for brain segmentation are those using man-

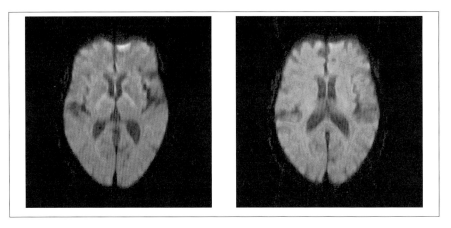

Figure 4.13: Trace diffusion-weighted imaging (DWI) brain maps acquired with the following imaging parameters: T_E=103 ms, T_R=9000 ms, FoV=24 cm, Matrix Size=172 × 172, NSA=1, Flip Angle=90, Thick=5 mm, Gap=1 mm (Courtesy of Marconi Medical Systems, Inc., Cleveland, OH.)

ual and interactive thresholding methods (see Lim *et al.* [454] and Harris *et al.* [455]). These methods are operator biased and are very slow. It is subjective, laborious, tedious, prone to errors and takes almost three to four hours per patient on a volumetric data set. Another class of semi-automatic segmentation algorithms based on thresholding can be seen in Falcao *et al.* [456]. Interested readers may also wish to read about the thresholding techniques by Weszka *et al.* [165]. Threshold has been used as a intermediate stage in 3-D cortical segmentation or is used in conjunction with other techniques. We will see the application of thresholding in two of the major techniques in Sub-section 4.3.4.3 and later in Sub-section 4.4.3.6.

4.3.2 Cortical Segmentation Using Probability-Based Techniques

Here we have three categories of models: (i) one based on the pure Bayesian approach (see Geman *et al.* [457], [259], Lee [201], Sheehan *et al.* [235]), (ii) one based on the expectation maximization algorithm (see Wells *et al.* [458], Grimson *et al.* [383] and Joshi *et al.* [460]) and (iii) one based on the Markov Random Field (see Kapur [463], Li [464] and Held *et al.* [465]).

4.3.2.1 Cortical Segmentation Using Bayesian Pixel/Voxel Classification

In a Bayesian-based approach, the data is assumed to be a multivariate normal distribution with parameters mean and covariance, which are estimated from the training data set. If **X** was the observation vector of length N and c the class which the pixel/voxel is in, then the Bayesian model yielded probability

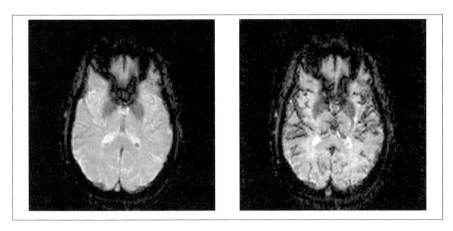

Figure 4.14: Perfusion-weighted brain images based in a $T_2{}^*$-weighted technique acquired with the following imaging parameters: T_E=63 ms, T_R=1500 ms, FoV=24 cm, Matrix Size=120 × 120, NSA=1, Flip Angle=90, Thick=5 mm, Gap=5 mm. **Left**: An early image in the series prior to contrast entering. **Right**: Image at the same spatial location at a later point in time, showing contrast (Courtesy of Marconi Medical Systems, Inc., Cleveland, OH.)

of a class being present when a sample pixel was observed, called *a posterior* probability, $P(c|\mathbf{X})$. This was computed provided we knew: (i) the probability of the sample being observed when a class was present, $P(\mathbf{X}|c)$, (ii) the *a prior* probability of a class, $P(c)$ and (iii) the probability of the sample, $P(\mathbf{X})$. Thus, the Bayesian model for pixel/voxel classification can be mathematically given as:

$$P(c|\mathbf{X}) \;=\; \frac{P(\mathbf{X}|c)P(c)}{P(\mathbf{X})} \;. \tag{4.1}$$

Note that the probability of the sample being observed when a class was present, $P(\mathbf{X}|c)$, was computed from the Gaussian density function, given as:

$$G_{\Sigma(\mathbf{X})} = \frac{1}{(2\pi)^{-\frac{N}{2}}\, \Sigma^{-\frac{1}{2}}}\; exp(-\frac{1}{2}\,\mathbf{X}^T\,\Sigma^{-1}\,\mathbf{X})\,. \tag{4.2}$$

where Σ was the covariance matrix and $\mathbf{X}^T$ was the transpose of the vector $\mathbf{X}$. The *a prior* probability of a class, $P(c)$, was computed using the distribution of different tissue types. Now, the *a posterior* probability was solved and every pixel in the image was assigned a label with the highest *a-posterior* probability (for details, see Geman *et al.* [457], [259], Lee *et al.* [201] and Sheehan *et al.* [235]).

Recently, Zavaljevski *et al.* [323] developed a method for multi-class tissue classification. The algorithm assumed a Gaussian multivariate normal distribution model. The method computed the mean and covariance of the training data set (called model parameters) for the brain MR images. These were called

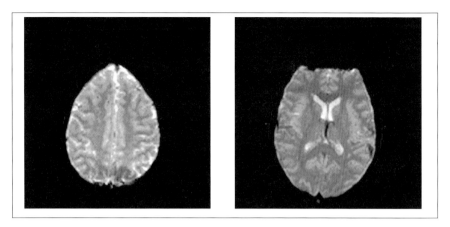

Figure 4.15: fMRI anatomical brain images (based on Single-Shot FE Echo Planar Imaging) acquired with the following imaging parameters: T_E=40 ms, T_R=4000 ms, FoV=24 cm, Matrix Size=128 × 128, NSA=1, Flip Angle=90, Thick=5 mm, Gap=0 mm (Courtesy of Marconi Medical Systems, Inc., Cleveland, OH.)

model signatures. This was then applied to the brain test MR data set which needed to be segmented. So far, the algorithm resembled the standard Bayesian approach. After this, to improve the robustness, accuracy and classification of more than four standard tissue types (WM/ GM/ CSF/ blood), Zavaljevski *et al.* took the neighborhood levels to see if there were any unclassified pixels. If there were, they then relaxed their model parameters and ran the classifier on the test data again for classification and segmentation. Finally, after completing this process, if there were still any unclassified pixels, they then applied the linear unmixing model based on simple Least Squares to estimate the component of the tissue type in the unclassified pixel. Thus the algorithm was adaptive and was able to classify more than 12 classes. The difference between the standard clustering or classification was in the way the algorithm automatically and adaptively determined the number of classes present in the MR images.

Pros and Cons of Zavaljevski's Technique. Although the algorithm was interesting in the sense that it adaptively estimated the classification and segmentation, the way it computed the classification of the mixture zone was not robust. It used a simple thresholding with no constraints on the linear model; as a result, outlier pixels which were composed of noisy points would cause an unreasonable coefficient estimation and would result in mis-classification during the thresholding process. A better methodology would be to put the smoothing constraint on the linear model, where the smoothing constant could improve the accuracy of the segmentation procedure.

Very recently, Shattuck and Leachy [204] presented their cortical surface algorithm which had spherical topology from T_1-weighted MR images. This pipeline consisted of five stages: (**1**) skull-stripping; (**2**) non-uniformity compensation; (**3**) voxel-based tissue classification; (**4**) topological inconsistency removal; and (**5**) tesselation/rendering. We will discuss these stages only briefly, as some of them have been used by other authors and discussed in this chapter. In *stage one*, skull-stripping was done to extract the VOI[30], i.e., the brain. This was accomplished using anisotropic diffusion (see Peronal *et al.* [534]) followed by running the Marr-Hildreth (MH) (see Hildreth [480]) edge detector and a series of morphological operations. *Stage two* was done to compensate for the inhomogeneities in the magnetic field during image acquisitions and susceptibility variations. The compensation was implemented based on Santago *et al.*'s [203] method. Interested readers can refer to that paper. The key idea was the estimation of the bias term which was incorporated in the probability model and later estimated using the mixture model: $p(x_k|b_k) = \sum_{c \in S} p(c) \, p(x_k|c, b_k)$, where c was the tissue class from a set S, $p(x_k|b_k)$ was the probability of a voxel at location x at the kth voxel, given the bias term b_k at voxel k, $p(c)$ was the probability of a voxel present in the class c. Since the algorithm assumed that the bias term varied slowly spatially, thus the bias term was constant in the neighborhood. The output of stage two was the measured values of $p(x_k|b_k)$. *Stage three* was one of the main stages, called the *maximum a posterior probability* (MAP) classifier using a Bayesian-based approach. The goal was to maximize $p(X|c)$ which was given as: $p(X|c) = \frac{p(c|X)p(X)}{p(c)}$. This was a very standard approach for voxel classification and the maximization was done using the ICM[31] algorithm (for details, see Shattuck *et al.* [204]). *Stage four* consisted of topology inconsistency removal. This step was necessary to remove any inconsistent topology of the cerebral cortex. The algorithm used the Topological Constraint Algorithm (TCA), which was an iterative correction procedure that decomposed a volumetric object into a graph representation from which topological equivalence to a sphere was determined. This was done as follows: first, the foreground connected components in each slice were labelled. The connectivity between each of these components was used to form a graph, where each connected component was a vertex in a graph and each connection between a component was represented as a weighted edge between the corresponding vertices. The weight of each edge represented the strength of the connection between two components. The graph captured both topological and geometric information about the object. The process was repeated for the background voxels, creating a second graph. Since the graphs were trees, so the object being analyzed was homomorphic to a sphere. TCA used maximal spanning tree (STA) for finding the pair of desired trees. In this way, the algorithm found the edges that corresponded to the minimum collection of voxels that needed to be removed from the graphs to force them to be trees. These edges corresponded to topological handles or holes. The TCA then removed these holes. The algorithm was applied in all three axes, making the smallest change possible with each iteration. This generated the tesselation topologically equivalent to a sphere, ready for rendering using the marching cubes method.

---

[30]Volume of interest.
[31]Iterated conditional modes.

Pros and Cons of Shattuck's Method.   The algorithm has the following advantages: (**1**) This was the first time that the cerebral cortex algorithm used STA for extracting the correct topology of cortex. This made the method more powerful and accurate. (**2**) The pipeline consisted of stages which were automated and interactive. So, if at any time the user was not satisfied, the settings could be changed. (**3**) The algorithm covered the validation of the brain segmentation system well. The algorithm has the following disadvantages: (**1**) The topological equivalence of the cerebral cortex to a sphere was implemented using the STA algorithm. There was no discussion of how STA improves the accuracy in the convoluted structures of the cerebral cortex. (**2**) The algorithm was a system-based method where the individual stages were a collection of low-level computer vision tools. The pipeline did not use any novel ideas, per se. (**3**) There was no discussion of the estimation of the geometric features of the cortex, even though it was called topological equivalence to a sphere.

4.3.2.2   Expectation Maximization Technique for 2-D and 3-D Cortical Segmentation

In the expectation maximization (EM) approach, Wells *et al.*[458] and Grimson *et al.*[383] presented an adaptive segmentation algorithm for segmenting coronal, sagittal and axial gradient echo T_1-weighted MR brain images to classify the WM/GM/CSF. The system first corrected for MR intensity inhomogeneities due to the RF coil, followed by tissue classification. Wells *et al.* combined the classification (c) and gain field (β) estimation as a non-linear optimization problem using Bayesian's approach. In their model, the bias field and the observed intensities both assumed the Gaussian model, given as:

$$
\begin{cases}
G_{\Sigma_c}(\mathbf{X}) &= \dfrac{1}{(2\pi)^{-\frac{m}{2}} \Sigma^{-\frac{1}{2}}} \, exp\left(-\tfrac{1}{2}\mathbf{X}^T \Sigma_c^{-1} \mathbf{X}\right) \\
G_{\Sigma_\beta}(\mathbf{X}) &= \dfrac{1}{(2\pi)^{-\frac{n}{2}} \Sigma^{-\frac{1}{2}}} \, exp\left(-\tfrac{1}{2}\mathbf{X}^T \Sigma_\beta^{-1} \mathbf{X}\right),
\end{cases}
\tag{4.3}
$$

where $G_{\Sigma_c}(\mathbf{X})$ and $G_{\Sigma_c}(\mathbf{X})$ were the Gaussian distribution of the pixels given a class c and the Gaussian distribution of the bias field. $\Sigma_{c(\mathbf{X})}^{-1}$ and $\Sigma_{\beta(\mathbf{X})}^{-1}$ were the covariances for the class c and bias β. The observed distribution was modelled as:

$$
p(Y_i|C_i,\beta_i) = G_{\Sigma_{c_i}}(Y_i - \mu(c_i) - \beta_i),
\tag{4.4}
$$

where $\mu(c_i)$ was the mean intensity of the tissue class c, at location i and β_i was the bias field at the location i. $p(Y_i|C_i,\beta_i)$ was the probability of an observed pixel at location i, given the class c_i and bias β_i. The goal was to solve the above equation using the maximization of *a-posterior* probability (MAP) to estimate the bias field β (see Wells *et al.*[458] for the complete derivation). The algorithm was implemented using the EM approach, where the E-step consisted of calculating the posterior tissue class probabilities when the bias field was known. The M-step consisted of a MAP estimator of the bias field when the tissue probabilities were known. Wells *et al.* implemented their algorithm over Spin Echo and Fast Spin Echo images. The algorithm used an anisotropic diffusion filter developed by Gerig *et al.*[459]. The results of this algorithm for 3-D gray matter segmentation are shown in Figure 4.26, middle row, left column.

Recently, Joshi *et al.*[460] modeled the brain segmentation problem as a mixture modeling problem, where the histogram of the MR volume was computed and modeled as a mixture model, a superimposition of distributions representing GM and WM. The idea was to construct the first and second order parametric representation of the mixture and solve the model using the EM algorithm (see Dempster *et al.*[461]). Joshi *et al.*'s algorithm consisted of three major steps: the first step consisted of applying the EM algorithm for segmentation of the WM and GM regions. In this method, if the histogram is fitted with M weighted functions, then it could be modeled using the following equation:

$$\Sigma_{m=0}^{m=M-1} \frac{\alpha_m}{\sigma_m} \, \mathcal{P}_m \left(\frac{v - \mu_m}{\sigma_m} \right), \tag{4.5}$$

where v is the neighboring voxel and $\mathcal{P}_m$ is the probability density function of the mth weighted function. $\alpha_m, \mu_m, \sigma_m$ are the area, mean and standard deviation of the mth weighted function, respectively, which was computed using the standard EM algorithm. Step two consisted of using isosurface reconstruction (we will discuss this in Sub-section 4.4.5) and the third step consisted of cortical surface editing. The last step was necessary to bring back the topology of the cortical surface. The results of this technique can be seen in Figures 4.16 and 4.17.

The performance measure of Joshi's technique was based on the normalized variational distance which is defined as: If $\mathcal{M}$, $\mathcal{A}$ and $\mathcal{L}$ are the measures for the manual segmentation, automatic segmentation and the total points in the volume (also called lattice), then the segmentation masks were given as $\mathcal{P}_i^j$, where $j \in \mathcal{A}, \mathcal{M}$ and $i \in \mathcal{L}$. $\mathcal{P}^{\mathcal{M},\mathcal{A}}$ was 1 if the manual (automatic) segmentation was white matter and was 0 if the manual (automatic) segmentation was gray matter. The normalized variational distance $d_{\mathcal{M},\mathcal{A}}$ was defined as:

$$d_{\mathcal{M},\mathcal{A}} = \frac{1}{2} \frac{\Sigma_{i \in \mathcal{L}} \, |\mathcal{P}_i^{\mathcal{M}} - \mathcal{P}_i^{\mathcal{A}}|}{\Sigma_{i \in \mathcal{L}} \, \mathcal{P}_i^{\mathcal{M}}}. \tag{4.6}$$

Kao *et al.*[462] used a probability-based method in conjunction with a vector decomposition method for segmenting the brain images. The theoretical model assumed a simple two class problem and the model assumed the Gaussian distribution.

Pros and Cons of the EM Algorithm and Comparison Between Well's [458] and Joshi's [460] Techniques. Probability-based methods are efficient provided one has good knowledge of prior distribution, and the number of classes is known in advance. This also requires extensive computations and is not very practical for real-time applications. Joshi's algorithm used manual editing as one of the last stages for topology correction. Thus the topology model was not built into it. This method is likely to have errors.

4.3.2.3 Markov's Random Field-Based Technique for 2-D Cortical Segmentation

Kapur [463] recently developed a brain segmentation technique which was an extension to the EM work of Wells *et al.* [458]. The technique added the Gibbs' model to the spatial structure of the tissues in conjunction with a Mean-Field (MF) solution technique, called Markov's Random Field technique (for details on MRF, see Li [464] and Geman *et al.* [457]). Thus it was called the EM-MF technique. By Gibbs' modeling of the homogeneity of the tissue, resistance to thermal noise in the images was obtained. The image data and intensity correction are coupled by an external field to an Ising-like[32] tissue model and the Mean-Field equations are used to obtain posterior estimates of tissue probabilities. This method is more general than the EM-based method and is simple and an inexpensive relaxation-like update. Other work in the area of MRF for brain segmentation can be seen in Held *et al.* [465].

Differences Between Wells' III [458] and Kapur's [463] Techniques. Two novelties and differences between Kapur's and Wells' work are: (**1**) *Addition of Gibbs' Model:* Kapur *et al.* modeled the *a priori* assumptions about the hidden variables as Gibbs' random field. Thus the prior probability was modeled using the following physics-based analogous Gibbs' equation: $P(f) = \frac{1}{Z} exp(-\frac{1}{\kappa T} E(f))$, where $Z = \Sigma_{f'} exp(\frac{-E(f')}{T})$ and $P(f)$ was the probability of the configuration f, T was the temperature of the system, $E(f)$ was energy of the configuration f, $\Sigma_{f'}$ is the standard deviation of the configuration f', κ is the Boltzmann constant and Z is the normalizing constant. (**2**) *Fusion of the Geometric Model in EM-MF Statistical Framework:* Kapur added the *distance-normal model* to the EM-MF tissue classification technique. The idea was to capture a distance-based geometric relationship between the primary and secondary structures and the local surface orientations.

4.3.3 Clustering-Based Cortical Segmentation Techniques

The prominent authors who used clustering-based techniques for brain segmentation were Bezdek *et al.* [466], Hall *et al.* [467] and Pham *et al.* [468], [469]. An interesting paper on adaptive fuzzy C mean (AFCM) was recently published by Pham *et al.* [470]. Usually, the classification algorithm expects one to know how many classes (roughly) the image would have. The number of classes in the image would be the same as the number of tissue types. A pixel could belong to more than one class; therefore, the algorithm uses the fuzzy membership function to associate with each pixel in the image. There are several algorithms used to compute the fuzzy membership functions and one of the most efficient ones is Fuzzy C Mean (FCM). Because of its ease of implementation for spectral data, it is preferred over other pixel classification techniques. Mathematically, the FCM principle is: given the observed pixel intensities in

---

[32]Associated with the author Ising.

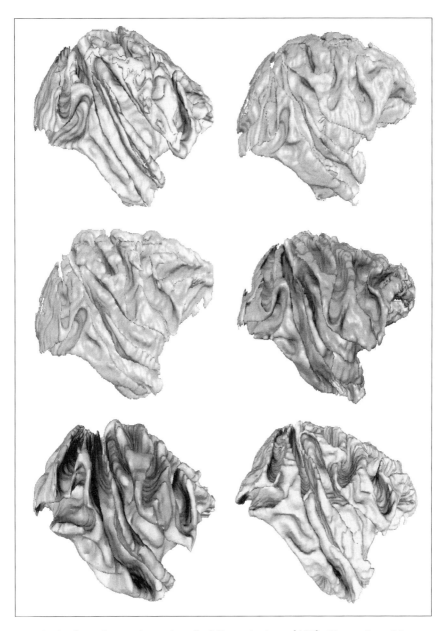

Figure 4.16: Sample results using Joshi's technique [460]. Reproduced by permission of Academic Press from [460]).

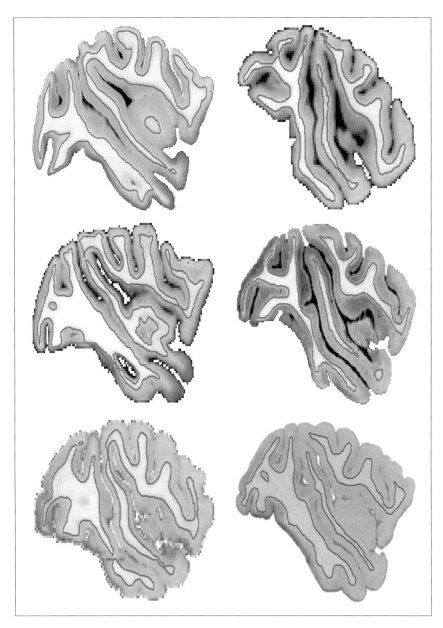

Figure 4.17: Sample results using Joshi's technique [460]. Reproduced by permission of Academic Press from [460].

a multi-spectral image at a pixel location j given as: $\mathbf{y}_j = [y_{j1}\, y_{j2}\, ...,\, y_{jN}]^T$, where j takes the pixel location and N is the total number of pixels in the data set, then the algorithm iterates between computing the *fuzzy membership function* and the centroid of each class. This membership function is the pixel location for each class (tissue type) and the value of the membership function lies between the range of 0 and 1. This membership function actually represents the degree of similarity between the pixel vector at a pixel location and the centroid of the class (tissue type). For example, if the membership function has a value close to 1, then the pixel at the pixel location is close to the centroid of the pixel vector for that particular class. The algorithm can be presented in the following four steps. If $u_{jk}^{(p)}$ is the membership value at location j for class k at iteration p, such that $\Sigma_{k=1}^3 u_{jk} = 1$. As defined before, $\mathbf{y}_j$ is the observed pixel vector at location j and $\mathbf{v}_k^{(p)}$ is the centroid of class k at iteration p, thus, the FCM steps for computing the fuzzy membership values are: (**1**) Choose the number of classes (K) and the error threshold ϵ_{th}, and set the initial guess for centroids $\mathbf{v}_k^{(0)}$, where the iteration number p=0. (**2**) Compute the fuzzy membership function given by the Least Squares Equation:

$$u_{jk}^{(p)} = \frac{||\mathbf{y}_j - \mathbf{v}_k^{(p)}||^{-2}}{\Sigma_{l=1}^K ||\mathbf{y}_j - \mathbf{v}^{(p)}||^{-2}}, \tag{4.7}$$

where $j = 1, ..., M$ and $k = 1, ..., K$. (**3**) Compute the new centroids using the membership function of the previous step as:

$$\mathbf{v}^{(p+1)} = \frac{\Sigma_{j=1}^N (u_{jk}^{(p)})^2\, \mathbf{y}_j}{\Sigma_{j=1}^N (u_{jk}^{(p)})^2}. \tag{4.8}$$

(**4**) Convergence was checked by computing the error between the previous and current centroids $(||\mathbf{v}^{(p+1)} - \mathbf{v}^{(p)}||)$. If the algorithm had converged, an exit would be required; otherwise, one would increment p and return to step (**2**) to compute the fuzzy membership function again. The output of the FCM algorithm was K sets of fuzzy membership functions. Here, one is interested in the membership value at each pixel for each class. Thus, if there were K classes, then there are K number of images and K number of matrices[33] for the membership functions. The results of the pixel-classification and segmentation of the GM, WM and CSF using the fuzzy-clustering are shown in Figure 4.18. This figure shows the four classes segmented. Recently, Ostergaard *et al.* [471] developed a voting technique which takes the best of the three techniques: FCM, k-means (see Duda *et al.* [472] and Rosenfeld *et al.* [473]) and the Bayesian-based approach. Interested readers can explore the voting algorithms for MR brain segmentation. We refer interested readers to an extensive article on data clustering by Jain *et al.* [474] and a book by Kandel [475] and to recent work published by Acton *et al.* [476] on fuzzy clustering applied to SPECT.

---

[33] $M \times K$, each row shows the contribution of each class in each pixel.

Pros and Cons of the Clustering Technique.   The major advantage of the clustering technique lies in the ease of implementation. The major weaknesses of this method are: (**1**) The algorithm is not fast enough to be implemented for real-time applications. (**2**) The performance of the algorithm depends upon a large number of user parameters, such as the error threshold and number of iterations. (**3**) The choice of the initial cluster is important and needs to be carefully selected. (**4**) The algorithm is not very robust to noise, spatial and temporal inhomogeneities.

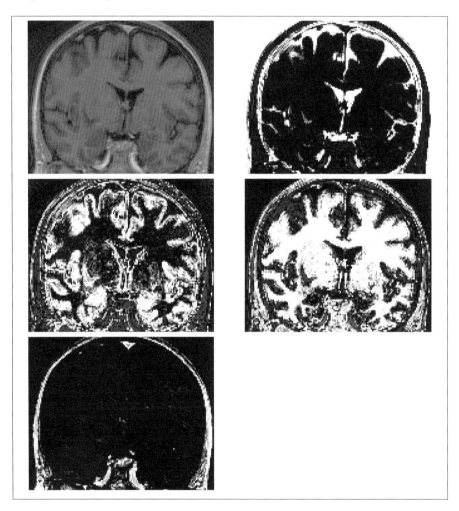

Figure 4.18: Results of the pixel classification algorithm using the Fuzzy Clustering algorithm. **Top Left**: original MR image. **Top Right**: class 0. **Middle Left**: class 1. **Middle Right**: class 2. **Bottom Left**: class 3 (MR Data, Courtesy of Marconi Medical Systems, Inc.).

4.3.4 Mathematical Morphology-Based Cortical Segmentation Techniques

It was Jean Serra (see Serra *et al.* [477]) from France who first performed a massive drive of mathematical morphology and its applications. Following Serra were Sternberg [478], Beucher [196], [197], Vincent *et al.* [198] and Lee *et al.* [187]. This sub-section has three parts: Sub-section 4.3.4.1 discusses 3-D morphology in conjunction with 3-D edge detection for cortical segmentation. Sub-section 4.3.4.2 focuses on morphological filters for cortex segmentation, and finally, Sub-section 4.3.4.3 discusses the fusion of region-growing with 3-D mathematical morphology for cortical segmentation.

4.3.4.1 3-D Morphology in Conjunction with 3-D Edge-Detection

Until 1990, not much was available on the application of 3-D morphology for brain cortical segmentation. Bomans *et al.* [479] applied the morphological filters such as dilation and erosion along with the Marr-Hildreth (MH) operator [34] [480] for 3-D segmentation and reconstruction of the cortex from MRI data sets. The pipeline of the algorithm consisted of the following steps: interpolation, 3-D edge detection, binarization, classification or labeling, 3-D morphologic closing and shading using a voxel model (see Höhne *et al.* [481]). The key idea in this paper was the 3-D Marr-Hildreth edge operator, given as:

$$C(x, y, z) = I(x, y, z, \sigma) * \nabla^2 G(x, y, z, \sigma), \tag{4.9}$$

where I was the original image volume and $\nabla^2 G(x, y, z, \sigma)$ was the LoG operator and defined as:

$$\nabla^2 G(x, y, z, \sigma) = \frac{1}{\sqrt{(2\pi)^3 \sigma^5}} \exp^{-\frac{(x^2+y^2+z^2)}{2\sigma^2}} (3 - \frac{(x^2 + y^2 + z^2)}{\sigma^2}), \tag{4.10}$$

where σ was the standard deviation of the filter or the band-width of the filter, x, y, z are the directions in which the convolutions need to be performed for extracting the edge information. This gave the cortical edge information.

Pros and Cons of the 3-D Morphological Cortical Segmentation Technique with 3-D Edge-Detection. The method of cortex segmentation and shading showed satisfactory results (see Bomans *et al.* [479]) when used in closing, but then there were many issues which could be expected to occur due to the performance of the system. (**1**) The system was too slow (as it took 93 minutes to complete all the steps). (**2**) The system depended on a low-level vision operator such as Marr-Hildreth, which was sensitive to noise and the sensitivity of the filter was a function of σ (band width). Also, the edge detector did not always find the correct contour, especially after the application of the morphological filters and fine details of the objects may be smoothed out.

---

[34]Since this operator works for large neighborhoods and is easily extendable from 2-D to 3-D.

(**3**) The MH operator found edges from the GM to CSF instead of from the WM to GM interface and as a result, they used morphological closing (of size $3 \times 3 \times 3$) to stretch it. Using this method would destroy the topology of the brain sulci and gyri since it is a very convoluted structure. (**4**) Much manual interaction was needed for the 2-D labeling process. (**5**) The pipeline used the connected component analysis in 2-D as one of the steps which loses 3-D connectivity. (**6**) There was no discussion of how the topology of the cortical surface was captured.

4.3.4.2   Interactive 3-D Morphology for Cortex Segmentation

Höhne and Hanson [340] did work in 3-D interactive segmentation for segmenting the cortex using T_1-weighted MR brain images. The system assumed that an object as a region has homogeneous intensity and uses the following tools of mathematical morphology for segmenting the cortex: (**1**) thresholding, (**2**) connected component analysis, (**3**) dilation, (**4**) erosion, (**5**) opening, (**6**) closing, (**7**) region fill and (**8**) boolean operators including AND, OR, NOT and XOR. The mathematical representation of dilation (ORing), erosion (ANDing), closing and opening were given as: $M \oplus S = \bigcup_{x \in S} M_{+x}$; $M \ominus S = \bigcup_{x \in S} M_{+x}$; $M \bullet S = (M \oplus S) \ominus S$; and $M \circ S = (M \ominus S) \oplus S$. The structuring elements used by Höhne and Hanson were a "cross" and a "sphere". The cross was a 7 voxel structure, three voxels in the x, y, z directions on both sides of the common center[35]. The sphere consisted of $27 - 8 = 19$ voxels. The 8 voxels were the voxels of the corners of the $3 \times 3 \times 3$ cube. The result of running the 3-D mathematical morphology for segmentation of the cortex is shown in Figure 4.26 (top row, right column).

Pros and Cons of Interactive 3-D Morphology Cortical Segmentation.   The following are the advantages of such a system: (**1**) Segmentation was independent of the imaging modality and imaging protocol sequence. (**2**) The segmentation algorithm combined the unsurpassed capability of the human visual system (of the user) and the anatomical knowledge of the user. (**3**) At any time, one could tailor the sequence of morphological steps to the segmentation of any occluded organ. It was like a paint program, where one can remove a region or fill in a region as desired to make a 3-D object of interest. A similar morphological approach was developed by Suri *et al.* [482] recently to segment a cell nucleus using 2-D mathematical morphology. This system[36] also does scoring[37] using connected component analysis.

The pitfalls of Höhne *et al.*'s [340] method are as follows: (**1**) the system did not correct for any spatial inhomogeneities and as a result, Höhne *et al.* had to take only the upper half of the entire MR volumetric data set. (**2**) The system needed a recursive human visual system interaction if the structuring element

---

[35] $x_1 x_2 x_3, x_{center} x_4 x_5 x_6$
[36] Developed on NT using Microsoft Foundation Classes.
[37] Counting the total nuclei in the microscopic images.

selected was not of the proper size. (**3**) The morphology pipeline for cortex segmentation was much too dependent on the human user and the filtering sequence would change from user to user, if the user was not knowledgeable about brain anatomy. (**4**) The structuring elements were too simple for the convoluted surface of the brain, hence the topology of the cortical surface would be lost.

Malandain, Bertrand, Robert and their co-workers from INRIA (see Robert *et al.* [483], Malandain *et al.* [484] and Bertrand *et al.* [485]) recently developed techniques for cortical segmentation based on mathematical morphology and topology of the surfaces. Very recently, Lemieux *et al.* [486], [367] also showed 3-D brain segmentation in T_1-weighted brain images, primarily based on mathematical morphology from 2-D slices. Also see the work of Sandor *et al.* [487].

4.3.4.3   Region-Growing with 3-D Mathematical Morphology

Stokking [330] developed a system named CACTUS (Completely Automatic Computer Technique for Unsupervised Segmentation) using a combination of region-growing and mathematical morphology (see Figure 4.19). The critical part in this algorithm was to estimate the final threshold. First, the base volume was extracted given the initial threshold and the seed point. Next, the successive erosions were performed in two steps using a six-voxel structuring element. Then, a region-growing process was initiated given the seed volume which grows one layer of voxels at each iteration. This yielded the region grown volume. The next stage was the peak detection process in discrete stages of one. This threshold and the seed point were fed to the 3-D mathematical morphology.

4.3.5   Prior Knowledge-Based Techniques

The basic principle here is to segment the cortical or sub-cortical structures using anatomical knowledge or guidance. Several authors have implemented the rule-based or knowledge-based system for segmentation of cortex or cortical structures (see Sckolowska *et al.* [488], [489], [490], Sonka *et al.* [491] and Dhawan *et al.* [492]). Knowledge-based systems for segmentation in conjunction with registration were developed by Dhawan *et al.* [493]. The system consisted of the following steps: first, building of the 3-D anatomical computerized model using the human expert and the volumetric scans. This was called global knowledge. Next, a new set of images was taken, normalized and interpolated and then the global knowledge was applied over these images to obtain the labelled cortical/sub-cortical structures. These 3-D labels were the spatial or structural information which was used for 3-D registration with the PET data sets (also called functional information). Thus the segmented MR data became very useful for the quantification of pathology and its changes. This system performed segmentation using knowledge and quantification of pathology using multi-modality fusion.

Saeed [435] also implemented a method for brain segmentation using prior

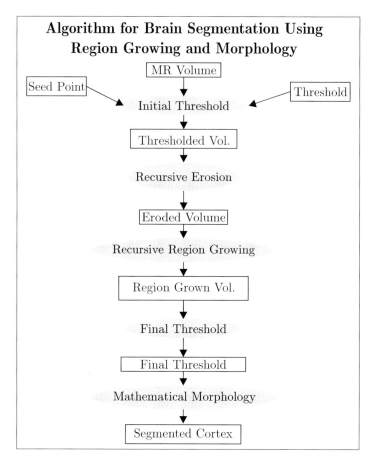

Figure 4.19: Pipeline for segmentation of MR brain using region-growing and mathematical morphology. The pipeline consists of the following steps: (**1**) initial thresholding of the MR volume, given the seed point and the initial threshold; (**2**) successive erosion using a six voxel structuring element; (**3**) recursive region-growing; (**4**) final threshold estimation using peak detection; and (**5**) mathematical morphology (similar to Hoehne's approach).

knowledge. The method formulated a generic shape definition of the brain using the MR brain database to refine the segmented brain region initially estimated using textural features. Very recently, Clark [494] also presented a knowledge-based approach to segment sub-cortical structures in the brain. The application of knowledge-based systems in medical imaging has been available for many years (see Suri *et al.* [495], [496]).

Pros and Cons of Knowledge-Based Techniques. The major advantages are: (**1**) The knowledge-based system helps to identify and label each part of the image for automated diagnostic analysis. (**2**) The knowledge-based systems do a reasonable job in segmentation provided the modeling data does not have much variability. The major disadvantages are: (**1**) The previous techniques do not use domain specific geometrical knowledge or models of anatomical structures to extract the regions. (**2**) The 3-D anatomical computerized model used in knowledge-based interpretation needs an expert's knowledge, which is tedious and time consuming. (**3**) The segmentation methodology using knowledge-based systems involves the registration of data sets, which is likely to incorporate the errors in the final segmentation process.

4.3.6   Texture-Based Techniques

It was in the late 1970s that Haralick *et al.* [497] published an extensive paper on texture, which discussed various measures for analyzing the images. Later, Peleg *et al.* [498] and Cross *et al.* [499] also published work in texture analysis applied to computer vision images. Application of texture in brain segmentation started in the early 1990s when Lachmann *et al.* [500] developed a method for the classification of WM, GM and CSF using texture-based methods. Actually, this technique is a combination of Bayesian classification, texture and k-mean clustering, but we will present the technique in the texture sub-division as this is what it is primarily based on. Lachmann *et al.* used the texture as one of the features for his feature vector generation. The features used were: homogeneity, contrast, differential inverse moment, diagonal moment, maximum of the intensity probability and fractal dimension. The pipeline for segmentation consisted of a cascade of the K-mean clustering algorithm followed by the Bayesian classifier. Clustering was used to obtain homogeneous pixel sets according to their attributes in the multiparametric space. A classifier was used to transform the membership binary decision into probabilities of belonging to different classes. K-mean clustering followed a simple rule of Euclidean distance. The mean vector for cluster k for n-attributes was given as: $\bar{x} = \bar{x}_{1k}, \bar{x}_{2k}, \bar{x}_{3k}, ..., \bar{x}_{nk}$ and $\bar{x}_{ik} = \frac{1}{p_k} \Sigma_{j=1}^{p_k} x_{ij}$, where p_k was the population of the cluster k. The Euclidean distance between the pixel j and the mean vector of the cluster k was defined as: $D_{kj} = \sqrt{\Sigma_{i=1}^{n} (\bar{x}_{ik} - x_{ij})^2}$, where $\bar{x}_{ik}$ was the mean value for the i-th attribute for the pixel set belonging to the cluster k and x_{ij} was the pixel j value for the i-th attribute. The K-mean partition error was defined as: $\epsilon = \Sigma_{j=1}^{M} [D_{k(j)j}]^2$, where M was the total number of pixels and $k(j)$ was the cluster k associated with pixel j. The classification using the relaxation procedure used the Bayesian approach as discussed in Sub-section 4.3.2.1. This technique primarily estimated the probability membership values. The Bayesian classifier used the edge information to make the process more robust, also called the relaxation procedure (interested readers can refer to the work of Eklundh *et al.* [501] on pixel classification). Ehricke [502] also presented work in the area of pixel classification using a polynomial classifier by taking texture as its features.

Pros and Cons of Texture-Based Techniques.   The above technique is certainly a good approach for estimating the WM and GM cortical regions.

This method, however, does not discuss the validation scheme and it is hard, therefore, to judge the performance of such a segmentation algorithm. Besides that, the segmentation system seemed sensitive to the initial textural properties, and no discussion of this was made in the paper.

4.3.7 Neural Network-Based Techniques

Authors who have performed research in brain image segmentation using artifical neural networks are Hall *et al.* [467], Reddick *et al.* [503], Clark [504] and Wang *et al.* [505]. Reddick's techniques used the following principle for segmentation and classification. The algorithm used T_1-, T_2- and PD-weighted MR brain images as an input to the artificial neural network. The system used Kohonen's SOM (self organizing map) to segment MR brain images into regions of similar characteristics. The SOM configuration was a single layer of nine neurons arranged in a three-by-three topology for mapping from input space to output space. The second layer consisted of a multilayer back-propagation neural network which was used for tissue classification. The three-layered feedforward network was trained with error back-propagation utilizing the delta rule for learning. The input layer included three neurons with a linear transfer function, while both the hidden layer and the output layer had seven neurons with sigmoid transfer functions.

Pros and Cons of Neural Network Techniques.   The major disadvantages of neural network-based methods were that: they required three sets of data for cortical segmentation (T_1-, T_2- and PD-weighted, for definitions of these image types, see Chapter 1). The trained neural networks had difficulties segmenting images since from therapy, changes affected the tissue characteristics. Thus this method was not very effective for real-time applications. Clark [494] has used neural network techniques for brain tumor segmentation. Other authors using neural networks and training-based methods are Chiou *et al.* [506] and Suri *et al.* [264].

4.3.8 Regional Hyperstack: Fusion of Edge-Diffusion with Region-Linking

Recently, there has been an attempt to fuse gradient dependent diffusion (GDD)-based edge information with hyperstack-based linking approaches for 3-D cortical segmentation (see the three Ph.D.s from Utrecht University: Koster [507], Vincken [508], Niessen [509] and the four recent papers by Koster *et al.* [510], Vincken *et al.* [511] and Niessen *et al.* [512], [513]). We will summarize their ideas in cortical segmentation. GDD uses the following equation for creating hyperstack images:

$$\frac{\partial L}{\partial t} = \nabla \bullet \left(exp\left(-\frac{||\nabla(L(\sigma))||^2}{k^2}\right) \nabla L \right), \tag{4.11}$$

where $\frac{\partial L}{\partial t}$ represents the new image at time t with the change of scale parameter σ, ∇ was the gradient operator, $L(\sigma)$ was the image at scale σ and k was a constant. Note, $\bullet$ is a dot representing the diverence operator. The algorithm can be summarized as follows: step one consisted of blurring the image volume at different scales using the GDD operator to create the stack of images. Step two consisted of the hyperstack segmentation process which consisted of three sub-steps: linking, root labeling and downward projection. The cumulative effect of this procedure was to break the volume into different structures (similar to the approach of voxel classification). This idea was based on the tree structure (the creation of a parent-child relationship at different levels) and then search for linking the voxel which belonged to the same structure. Step three consisted of region analysis such as cleaning based on mathematical morphology. The last step was user-editing of the brain volume to obtain the segmented WM, GM and CSF volumes followed by volume rendering for display purposes.

Pros and Cons of the Hyperstack Approach. The major advantages of such a system are: (**1**) it is highly accurate. (**2**) It is highly robust. (**3**) There is a minimal amount of user-interaction. (**4**) The system took advantage of lower level vision based on gradient dependent diffusion. The major disadvantages of such a system are: (**1**) the linking process took the maximum amount of time in segmentation. (**2**) The choice of the shape of the structuring elements was not clear. The system did not show any relationship between hyperstack linking and the structuring element. It would be interesting to know if the shape of the structuring element would ever change, or if it would be independent of the pulse sequence parameters of the T_1-weighted MR data sets or changes in the type of weighting.

4.3.9 Fusion of Probability-Based with Edge Detectors, Connectivity and Region-Growing

4.3.9.1 Fusion of Probability with Edge Detectors

Research work has been done where there has been a fusion of low-level vision techniques with probability-based models. In that attempt, Kao *et al.* [462] published work where they used vector decomposition along with probability-based methods. Excellent work has been done by Suri *et al.* [246], where they fuse Haralick's edge detector [184], [185] based on a facet model with a Bayesian probability model for computation of the left ventricle segmentation. Details are available in Chapter 3.

4.3.9.2 Fusion of Probability-Based with Connectivity

Teo *et al.* [514] developed a method for segmenting the WM/GM and CSF to overlay with fMRI measurements collected using rotating wedge and expanding ring stimuli. The segmentation algorithm consisted of four steps: (**1**) White

Matter/Gray Matter/Cerebrospinal Fluid segmentation, (**2**) user interaction of WM cortical segmentation, (**3**) cavity and handle removal and (**4**) GM boundary estimation from the WM segmented from the first step. The main concept in this algorithm was to classify the pixels in the region of WM and CSF first and then propagate the WM boundary towards the CSF to estimate the GM boundary. They used this methodology since the WM hemispheres are constrained in the GM and GM is contained in the outer CSF.

Pros and Cons of Teo's Technique.   Although their attempt was logical, this methodology has major drawbacks, such as: (**1**) the system involves too much user interaction in their four-step pipeline. (**2**) The user has to be totally knowledgeable to tune the mean and standard deviation of the class to adjust the segmentation results. (**3**) The method is only suited to T_1-weighted images. In other words, if the pulse sequence changed, then the algorithm would deviate from its statistical properties and detour from its expectations. (**4**) In step two of the algorithm, Teo *et al.* used the flood fill algorithm which is very sensitive to holes in the images. If the WM boundary is surrounded by a set of GM or a CSF region and a small hole is created, the flood fill needs to be altered or else it would miss the region. No indication was given as to how they handled it. (**5**) One of the major drawbacks of such a system is the hand-editing of the images needed for adjusting the mean and standard deviation of the classification procedure. Lastly, (**6**) Teo *et al.* grew the WM boundary to estimate the GM boundary using the propagation criterion. There was no discussion as to when to stop it and what happens in the layering process when the boundary is highly convoluted and twisted.

4.3.9.3   Fusion of Classification with Region-Growing and Connectivity

Cline *et al.* [515] presented an algorithm to show the 3-D reconstruction of the human brain surface. The algorithm consisted of the following steps: (**1**) *Brain tissue connectivity*: this step consisted of tissue classification using simple thresholding, where the pixel was given a tag equal to one if the gray scale intensity of the pixel was greater than or equal to the manually selected threshold. The next stage in this step was to label all of the pixel points as on the brain surface, inside the brain surface and outside the brain surface depending upon the six neighbors of the given pixel (four neighbors in the same plane and two neighbors corresponding to above and below the current slice). The last stage of the tissue connectivity algorithm was to run the 3-D region growing algorithm by looking at the connected neighbors. Thus the tissue pixels which were connected to the seed pixel were tagged as surface. (**2**) *Brain surface reconstruction*: this step consisted of finding the marked voxels (also called cubic cells, consisting of eight vertices or eight data points) which intersected the tagged surface computed in the previous step. So basically, Cline *et al.* computed those surface patches which passed through the voxel's cubes. The point of intersection of surfaces with the voxel edges was computed using interpolation. Finally, the last stage in this step consisted of finding the number of triangles in this surface patch. (**3**) *Brain rendering*: this step consisted of rendering the surface patches computed in the previous step. The rendering consisted of finding the normals and using the shading using Lambartien's law and later projecting on the screen.

Pros and Cons of Cline's Method. Although the method did estimate the surface of the human brain, it has the following drawbacks: (**1**) The tissue classification was not robust enough and was used manually, hence it was highly susceptible to errors. (**2**) The number of patient studies taken was too small to set up an empirical value of the surface threshold for tissue classification. (**3**) The seed point was inserted manually, hence it was susceptible to errors. (**4**) The accuracy of the system depended upon the number of triangles used in the surface patch, which was inversely proportional to the speed of the brain segmentation system. The greater the accuracy, the slower the system was. (**5**) The region-growing algorithm was totally non-statistical and therefore would miss much of the distant connected tissues.

4.3.10 Summary of Region-Based Techniques: Pros and Cons

The major advantages of classification-based and region-based cortical segmentation techniques are: (**1**) They are more robust compared to plain edge-based techniques. (**2**) They go well with training-based methods or learning-based methods, where one can use the training data sets for shape modeling and apply the estimated parameters to the test data sets. (**3**) These techniques when fused with boundary/surface-based techniques yield very superior results. We will discuss such systems in Sub-section 4.5, but first we will discuss the boundary/surface-based techniques as stand-alone methods.

The major weaknesses of classification-based and region-based cortical segmentation techniques are: (**1**) Due to the partial volume effects and all the reasons discussed previously, the classification and region-based techniques suffer from mis-classification of pixels/voxels and hence, it is difficult to achieve crisp regions. (**2**) Region-based approaches require further processing to group segmented regions into coherent structures. (**3**) This is computationally expensive, if statistical-based methods are used. (**4**) Failure to connect different tissue classes during mathematical morphological operations can occur due to the partial volume averaging.

4.4 Boundary/Surface-Based 2-D and 3-D Cortical Segmentation Techniques: Edge, Reconstruction, Parametric and Geometric Snakes/Surfaces

Boundary/surface-based cortical segmentation techniques are those where one estimates the boundaries of the WM and GM. These techniques help us in understanding medical images. Two-dimensional WM and GM boundary estimation is a difficult problem, as the methodology does not use the neighboring information. It may however be fast, since it does not have to process the whole volumetric MR slices. On the contrary, accurate WM cortical or GM cortical surface segmentation is a difficult problem because it needs a proper connection between the layers of topological cortex and the MR scanning is not in accordance with the topology of the brain. The scanning is rather just in orthogonal directions with a fixed inter-slice distance and slice-thickness.

This sub-section focuses on WM and GM boundary estimation in orthogonal MR slices and WM and GM surface estimation from the MR volumes. For boundary/surface estimation of the WM and GM, the current methods are either based on plain edge detection techniques or deformation-based techniques. The deformation-based techniques could be parametric or geometric.

The layout of this sub-section is as follows: we introduce boundary estimation techniques using the edge detection techniques in Sub-section 4.4.1. Sub-section 4.4.2 presents the 3-D reconstruction of the cortex using 2-D serial cross-sections. Parametric boundary models are discussed in Sub-section 4.4.3. Under this class we will discuss fitting models, ribbon models, topological (T) parametric surfaces and the combination of probability and parametrization. Geometric boundary/surface models are discussed in Sub-section 4.4.4. In Sub-section 4.4.5 we discuss isosurface extraction techniques, which will be used in fusion-based parametric and geometric surfaces cortical segmentation techniques. We conclude the discussion of boundary/surface-based techniques by discussing their pros and cons in Sub-section 4.4.6.

4.4.1 Edge-Based Cortical-Boundary Estimation Techniques

The edge detection field has been active for the last 40 years. Here we will only discuss popular algorithms, such as those by Canny and Deriche with their results applied to MR brain images. Canny edges are estimated by convolution of the MR image with a Gaussian operator. In one dimension, the Gaussian function, its first derivative and its second derivative, are given in Equation

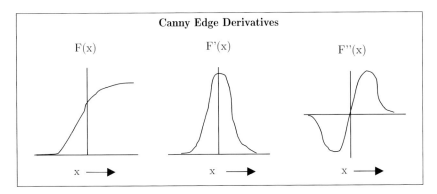

Figure 4.20: Canny derivatives. **Left**: Original signal. **Middle**: First derivative. **Right**: Second derivative.

(4.12) as:

$$\begin{cases} G(x) &= \frac{1}{\sqrt{2\pi}\sigma}\, e^{\frac{-x^2}{2\sigma^2}} \\ G'(x) &= -\frac{1}{\sqrt{2\pi}\sigma^3}\, x\, e^{\frac{-x^2}{2\sigma^2}} \\ G''(x) &= -\frac{1}{\sqrt{2\pi}\sigma^3}\, e^{\frac{-x^2}{2\sigma^2}}\left[1 - \frac{x^2}{\sigma^2}\right]. \end{cases} \tag{4.12}$$

The equivalent 2-D functions are expressed most easily with respect to the polar coordinate system, where the radius r is $\sqrt{x^2 + y^2}$ (see Equation (4.13)). The function is symmetrical and independent of angle θ. The three polar equations, Gaussian function, first derivative and second derivative, are given in Equation (4.13). Figure 4.20 shows the Canny derivatives.

$$\begin{cases} G(r) &= \frac{1}{2\pi\sigma}\, e^{\frac{-r^2}{2\sigma^2}} \\ G'(r) &= -\frac{1}{2\pi\sigma^4}\, r\, e^{\frac{-r^2}{2\sigma^2}} \\ G''(r) &= -\frac{1}{2\pi\sigma^4}\, e^{\frac{-r^2}{2\sigma^2}}\left[1 - \frac{r^2}{\sigma^2}\right] \end{cases} \tag{4.13}$$

Figure 4.21 shows the results of using the Canny edge operator (see Canny [516]) to estimate the boundaries of GM in the coronal slice of the human brain that has a tumor. As one can see, the Canny operator is too sensitive to noise and thus it is likely to estimate false edges.

Deriche *et al.* (see Monga *et al.* [517] and Deriche [518]) gave an optimal operator of width W as $f(x)$ that is defined as:

$$f(x) = a_1\, e^{\alpha x}\, sin(\omega x) + a_2\, e^{\alpha x}\, cos(\omega x) + a_3\, e^{\alpha x}\, sin(\omega x) + a_4\, e^{\alpha x}\, cos(\omega x) + C, \tag{4.14}$$

where α, ω and C are positive reals subjected to boundary conditions $f(0) = 0$, $f(W) = 0$, $f'(0) = S$ and $f'(W) = 0$. Since the shape of this optimal operator was almost equal to the Gaussian, thus the solution could be given as:

$$h(x) = -c\, e^{-\alpha\, |x|}\, sin(\omega x) = -c\, x\, e^{-\alpha\, |x|}. \tag{4.15}$$

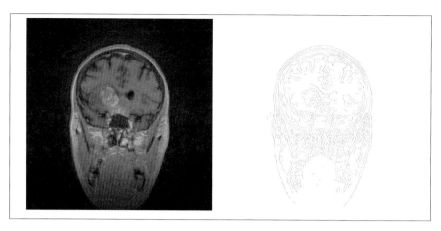

Figure 4.21: **Left**: Original MR coronal slice. **Right**: Results of segmenting the GM boundary in 2-D coronal slices using the Canny operator. Note, the faulty edges are also estimated near the convoluted sulci and gyri (MR Data, Courtesy of Marconi Medical Systems, Inc.).

This optimal filter was realized using two recursive filters moving in opposite directions $y^+(m)$ and $y^-(m)$. Thus $y(m)=a(y^+(m) - y^-(m))$. The results of running Deriche's edge detector can be seen on the right side of Figure 4.22 (for details, see Monga *et al.*[517]). Given this basic mathematical foundation, the 3-D Deriche operator was designed and the algorithm consisted of these three steps: (**1**) three gradient computations in the x, y and z directions; (**2**) computing the zero-crossing of the second derivative, which corresponded to the local maxima of the gradient; and (**3**) hysteresis thresholding (for details, see Monga *et al.*[517]).

Robust edge detectors (see Kennedy *et al.*[519] and Djuric *et al.*[520]) have been used for estimating the boundaries of the WM/GM. Due to the convolutedness and fuzziness in the GM/WM regions and for the reasons discussed in Sub-section 4.1, these edge detection techniques are not robust and are susceptible to errors. Xuan *et al.*[521] then proposed merging the edge-detection and region-growing techniques for segmenting brain images. Application of Haralick's facet model (see Haralick and Shapiro [244] and Zuniga *et al.*[522]) for edge detection in medical imaging has been used extensively by Suri *et al.*[246].

Pros and Cons of Edge-Based Techniques. The major weaknesses of edge-based techniques are: (**1**) they could introduce local gaps in the edge boundaries due to variation in the gradient strengths of the tissue characteristics. (**2**) Variation in edge strength can introduce discontinuities into the boundaries. (**3**) In multispectral MR images, it can introduce false edges. (**4**) These techniques are not very reliable, nor robust and are sensitive to noise.

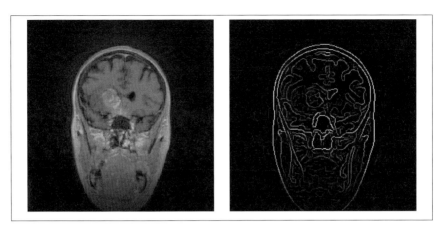

Figure 4.22: **Left**: Original MR coronal slice. **Right**: Results of segmenting the GM boundary in a 2-D coronal slice by running the Deriche operator ([518]). Note, the faulty edges are almost removed (MR Data, Courtesy of Marconi Medical Systems, Inc.).

4.4.2 3-D Cortical Reconstruction From 2-D Serial Cross-Sections (Bourke/Victoria)

In this technique, the brain is acquired in three orientations - coronal, sagittal and transverse and 2-D segmentation is performed using one of the 2-D segmentation techniques discussed previously. The extracted contour is stacked and converted to a triangular mesh using 3-D Delaunay triangulation (see Schroeder *et al.* [556]). This decimated surface is then shaded using rendering algorithms (see Figure 4.26, top row, left column). Boissonnat [557], Geiger [558], Carman *et al.* [559] and Suri [560] all performed reconstruction on medical organs from serial cross-sections, where they stacked the contours, created meshes (patches) and then applied surface rendering.

Pros and Cons of the Cortical Reconstruction Method. As seen from Figure 4.26 (top row, left column), one may try to capture the convoluted surface of the brain geometry to some extent, but the technique loses its topology and is numerically very unstable and problematic. This method is highly dependent upon the accuracy of the segmentation process in the 2-D slices and the accuracy of the decimation process (see Tatsumi *et al.* [561]).

4.4.3 2-D and 3-D Parametric Deformable Models for Cortical Boundary Estimation: Snakes, Fitting, Constrained, Ribbon, T-Surface, Connectedness

Cortical boundary/surface in 2-D/3-D segmentation using parametric deformable models has dominated the CVGIP[38] paradigm and medical imaging field. The layout of this sub-section is as follows: Sub-section 4.4.3.1 presents 2-D classical snakes. Sub-section 4.4.3.2 presents fitting-based models such as super-quadratic and physics-based. Sub-section 4.4.3.3 presents constrained 3-D parametric deformable models. Ribbon modeling for cortical segmentation is discussed in Sub-section 4.4.3.4. Topological adaptive surfaces (T-surfaces) are discussed in Sub-section 4.4.3.5. We conclude this sub-section by discussing cortical segmentation based on a combination of probability and parametrization in Sub-section 4.4.3.6.

4.4.3.1 2-D Classical Snakes

As this concept has already been discussed in Sub-section 3.4.1.1 (in Chapter 3), we will not discuss it further here. Interested readers can explore these techniques further in Wikins *et al.* [523] and Singh *et al.* [210].

Atkins *et al.* [524] presented a brain segmentation technique which used a combination of thresholding, mathematical morphology and parametric active contour. The proton density (PD)-weighted brain MR images were first smoothed using anisotropic diffusion (see Perona *et al.* [534]) followed by thresholding to generate the binary mask. The mis-classification of the mask was removed by the binary morphology of erosion and dilation. This generated a refined mask. Next, the parametric active contour algorithm by Wikins *et al.* [523] was run in this mask to estimate the brain boundary. The method was highly dependent upon the kernel sizes used during the mathematical morphology operation. Besides that, it had a drawback in controlling the elasticity constants. The technique was not robust enough to handle the convolutedness of the brain topology. The algorithm was not fully 3-D and does not work on sagittally acquired T_1-weighted data.

Chalana *et al.* [76] extended Wikins' spatial parametric model in the temporal domain for LV boundary estimation in Ultrasound. For critiques on Chalana's method, see the paper by Suri [139]. Several authors (not listed here) who did work in the area of parametric deformable models such as Fourier snakes applied to cardiac imaging are shown in references [214] to [233]. A discussion on these citations is out of the scope of this chapter since their prime focus was not on convolutedness, like the cortical boundaries. Also, most of these references are focused on non-soft tissues. Some pros and cons of these references are discussed by Suri [139]. In the class of parametric deformable boundary/surfaces, we will not ignore the superquadratic fitting and physics-based models, since they are used directly or indirectly in parametric surfaces.

---

[38]Computer Vision, Graphics and Image Processing.

4.4.3.2 3-D Parametric Deformable Models (Fitting-Based)

Superquadratic Fitting-Based Deformable Models. Here, we will briefly summarize another class of parametric deformable models called superquadratic fitting. Although this has not been dominant in cortical segmentation as much as in cardiac 3-D LV segmentation, we will present a brief summary here. Superquadratic fitting research has been popular at INRIA[39] recently. Bardinet *et al.* [215], [216], Ayache [217] and Staib *et al.* [218] fitted a deformable superquadratic to segment the LV in 3-D cardiac CT and SPECT images. These models were then refined using the volumetric deformation technique known as Free Form Deformations (FFD). The complete algorithm can be summarized as follows: (**1**) extraction of the 3-D data points in the time sequence of slices; (**2**) superellipsoid fitting to find the set of parameters so that the superellipsoid best fits the above 3-D data points. The fitting satisfied the equation $F = 1$, where F was given as:

$$\left\{ \left[\left(\frac{x}{a_1} \right)^{\frac{2}{\epsilon_2}} + \left(\frac{y}{a_2} \right)^{\frac{2}{\epsilon_2}} \right]^{\frac{\epsilon_2}{\epsilon_1}} + \left(\frac{z}{a_3} \right)^{\frac{2}{\epsilon_1}} \right\}^{\frac{\epsilon_1}{2}} , \qquad (4.16)$$

where a_1, a_2 and a_3 were constants. ϵ's are the parameters of shape change. Note the left hand side is the equation of the superellipsoid surface. If we look carefully, $\frac{x}{a_1}$, when squared and added to the squared of the term $\frac{y}{a_2}$, is the equation of the ellipse in a 2-D plane. In the above equation, the power was changed from 2 to $\frac{2}{\epsilon_2}$. Adding the third dimension, we get $\frac{z}{a_3}$ with the power $\frac{2}{\epsilon_1}$. The whole expression was raised to the power of $\frac{\epsilon_1}{2}$. Therefore, the whole idea was to change an ellipse to an ellipsoid, controlling the shape by ϵ's; (**3**) the refinement stage, also called FFD, where Least Squares fitting was performed between the object and the box, was carried out. A good physical analogy for FFD is to consider a parallelopiped of clear, flexible plastic in which is embedded an object, or several objects, which we wish to deform. The object is imagined to be flexible, so that it deforms along with the plastic that surrounds it. Mathematically, the FFD is defined in terms of a tensor product trivariate Bernstein polynomial. If we impose a local coordinate system on a parallelopiped region in three orthogonal directions, any point $\mathbf{X}$ has (s, t, u) coordinates in this system, so that $\mathbf{X} = \mathbf{X}_0 + s\mathbf{S} + t\mathbf{T} + u\mathbf{U}$, where s, t, u can all be computed using linear algebra. On imposing a grid of control points $\mathbf{P}_{ilk}$ on the parallelepiped and letting it form $l + 1$, $m + 1$ and $n + 1$ planes in the $\mathbf{S}, \mathbf{T}, \mathbf{U}$ directions, then these points lie on the lattice and their locations were defined as: $\mathbf{P}_{ijk} = X_0 + \frac{i}{l}\mathbf{S} + \frac{j}{m}\mathbf{T} + \frac{k}{m}\mathbf{U}$. The deformation was specified by moving $\mathbf{P}_{ijk}$ from their undisplaced lattice positions. The deformation function was defined by a trivariate tensor product polynomial. The deformed position $\mathbf{X}_{ffd}$ was thus given as:

$$\mathbf{X}_{ffd} = \sum_i \sum_j \sum_k C_l^i (1-s)^{l-i} s^i \, C_m^j (1-t)^{m-j} t^j \, C_n^k (1-u)^{n-k} u^k \, \mathbf{P}_{ijk} ,$$

$$(4.17)$$

---

[39]Institut National de Recherche en Informatique et Automatique; Research Reports of INRIA can be ftp'ed from: ftp.inria.fr/INRIA/publication/pub-ps-gz/RR.

where $\mathbf{P}_{ijk}$ denoted the volumetric grid of the control points, (s, t, u) denoted by the local coordinates of the object points in a frame defined by the box of control points and (l, m, n) denoted the degrees of the Bernstein polynomials.

Classical Physics-Based Deformable Models. This class of deformable models originated in the early 1990s (also called classical physics-based deformable models, see McInerney *et al.* [228], [229]). Further work was done recently on T-snakes, which will be discussed in Sub-section 4.4.3.5. Classical physics-based deformable models were interesting research since they had distinctive similarities to active contour models and training-based modeling. McInerney's classical algorithm can be summarized in a three step process. Step one consisted of user interaction to gather global shape information, such as the center of the LV and the size collection in each successive slice (just like the Singh's algorithm [210]). In step two, image model construction, which consisted of fitting physics-based deformable models and solving the potential energy terms and dynamic equations, was done. The last step consisted of the refinement stage or smoothing process. McInerney *et al.*'s fitting process used deformable surface models to fit the data. They made the model dynamic as the data was time-varying. This dynamic formulation had the following two advantages: first, the data fitting process was shown as a smoothly animated display, and second, the user was made to interact with the model by applying a constraint force to pull it out of the local minima toward the correct shape. McInerney's deformation model had spatial and temporal components defined as: $x(u, v, t)$. The model was simulated with a mass and damping densities. The deformation energy yielded internal elastic forces, and the potential energy term was minimized when these forces equilibrated against externally applied forces. The model stabilized when the first and second order differentials were set at zero. The fitting process was governed by a second order partial differential equation. This equation followed the law of physics of the pendulum where the first term was a second order term given as $\frac{\partial^2 \mathbf{x}}{\partial t^2}$ pre-multiplied by the mass of the LV. The second term was a single order term given as $\frac{\partial \mathbf{x}}{\partial t}$ pre-multiplied by the damping force γ. The last term represented the elastic forces which resist deformation. All these terms were added and equalized to external forces f_{ext} derived from the image data. Thus, the final equation was given as:

$$\mu \frac{\partial^2 \mathbf{x}}{\partial t^2} + \gamma \frac{\partial \mathbf{x}}{\partial t} + \delta \, \epsilon_p = f_{ext} \, , \qquad (4.18)$$

where ϵ_p was the potential energy term and this energy was the deformation energy of a thin plate under tension. This term consisted of a partial differential equation pre-multiplied by constants. The first and second terms were the first order differential equation in the u-v plane and were given as $|\frac{\partial \mathbf{x}}{\partial u}|$ and $|\frac{\partial \mathbf{x}}{\partial v}|$. The second and third terms were the partial differential equation of the second order, given as $|\frac{\partial^2 \mathbf{x}}{\partial^2 u}|$ and $|\frac{\partial^2 \mathbf{x}}{\partial^2 v}|$. The last term was given as the cross-energy term $|\frac{\partial^2 \mathbf{x}}{\partial u \partial v}|$. Now, by changing these terms to energy by squaring the amplitude and adding them together, we get the final expression of potential energy as:

$$\epsilon_p(\mathbf{x}) = \int\int \alpha_a |\frac{\partial \mathbf{x}}{\partial u}| + \alpha_b |\frac{\partial \mathbf{x}}{\partial v}| + \beta_b |\frac{\partial^2 \mathbf{x}}{\partial^2 u}| + \beta_c |\frac{\partial^2 \mathbf{x}}{\partial u \partial v}| + \beta_d |\frac{\partial^2 \mathbf{x}}{\partial^2 v}|\} \, du \, dv. \quad (4.19)$$

Note that the constants α_a, α_b, β_b and β_c were the terms which caused the stretching, twisting and bending. These terms were very critical in LV modeling, which was used manually by Singh [210]. For details on these parameters, see Samadani [233].

Pros and Cons of Boundary/Surface Parametric Deformable Models.
From the discussion of the work done on the parametric boundary/surfaces model, we conclude that it has the following major drawbacks: (**1**) These snakes need dynamic re-parameterization of active contours in order to maintain a faithful delineation of the object boundary/surface. This increases the algorithm's complexity and computational overhead. (**2**) These snakes fail to adjust to the topology of the structures, i.e., they cannot follow the convolutedness of the shapes. (**3**) They fail to split or merge and thus, splitting and merging of the model parts requires a new topology and construction of a new parameterization. (**4**) The model is non-robust for noisy images. (**5**) Global minimization is always a problem in such a technique.

4.4.3.3   Constrained 3-D Parametric Deformable Models (MacDonald/NMI)

MacDonald *et al.* [562], [563] and [564] presented an iterative algorithm for simultaneous deformation of multiple surfaces with inter-surface proximity constraints and self-intersection avoidance, where the deformation was formulated as a cost function minimization problem. Basically, MacDonald's method was a general polyhedron deformation method, where they fit the model to the *a priori* image data. Such a fitting process was accomplished by solving the weighted objective function. This objective function was the summation of bending, stretching, image (conventional deformation) and self-proximity term, given as:

$$O(S) = \sum_{k=1}^{N_s} w_k \, T_k \,, \quad (4.20)$$

where w_k was the weighting factor, S was the set of N_s deforming polyhedral surface and $\hat{S}$ was the estimated set of N_s model polyhedral surface. The function T_k is basically the weighted signed scalar measure of the derivation from the ideal and was equal to $W(D_k(S))$. The new aspect of this algorithm was the self-proximity term and inter-surface proximity terms which were a function of the distances between the polygons. This means that the objection function in 3-D was doing the equivalent to the first and second differential snakes (from 2-D) plus the error reduction due to self-proximity. In mathematical terms, it was defined by the equation: $T_{sp} = \Sigma_{i=1}^{n_p-1}\Sigma_{j=i+1}^{n_p}[d_{min}(P_i, P_j) - d_{i,j}]^2$. Note that the above equation was valid as long as $d_{min}(P_i, P_j)$ was less than $d_{i,j}$, or else the left hand side was 0. The objective function was solved using a conjugate gradient method, where the derivative direction is computed iteratively. MacDonald *et al.* used the multi-resolution approach to avoid the trapping of the global minima. They demonstrated an interesting application of sulci location deep-seated in the brain using their model. The method was applied to 3-D MR brain data to extract surface models for the skull and the cortical surfaces.

Pros and Cons of MacDonald's Method.   The major advantages of the system are: (**1**) It takes advantage of the information of the interrelationship between the surfaces of interest. (**2**) MacDonald took care of the parametric weights by assigning distances rather than weights in the parametric model. The major drawbacks are the extremely high computational expense (100 hours for segmentation) and the difficulty of tuning weighting factors in the cost function due to the complexity of the problem. Other researchers who did work on the segmentation of the sub-structures of the brain, such as in the corpus callosum using Fourier surfaces, are mentioned in Szekely *et al.* [213].

4.4.3.4   Parametric 2-D and 3-D Ribbon Modeling (Davatzikos/JHU)

Davatzikos *et al.* [565] proposed a ribbon model to capture the cortex from 2-D image slices and later extended the method to 3-D [566]. The cortex is thus represented through a parameterized central layer surface and corresponding maps of depth and curvature. This method starts out by determining a mass function upon which the external image force of the deformable surface for the cortical central layer is derived. This involves two steps: morphological operations to detach brain tissue from non-brain tissue, followed by Markov random field (MRF)-based segmentation to separate cortical Gray Matter from CSF and White Matter. The deformable surface was then deformed under the influence of internal and external forces, to achieve a fit to the center of the mass of cortical Gray Matter while maintaining its smoothness. To yield a representation of the cortical structure that preserves relative distances and angles, a fixed-point algorithm was used to iteratively seek the reparametrization of the deformable surface that is nearly homothetic. A curvature map and a depth map are then derived for further analysis of the cortical shape. This method utilizes knowledge of the cortical anatomy and provides a mathematical representation of the outer cortex. The various shape descriptors, such as curvature map and depth map derived from this representation, can serve as the basis for a number of applications.

Pros and Cons of Ribbon Modeling: The main weakness of this algorithm lies in its difficulty in capturing the deep sulci, which is an intrinsic problem of the conventional snake-type of deformable models. In order to compensate for that, significant human interaction is needed, only to give limited success. Other researchers who did research in active ribbon were Vaillant *et al.* [567] and Goualher *et al.* [411].

4.4.3.5 Parametric Topological-Snakes/Surfaces (McInerney/UT)

McInerney and Terzopoulos developed snakes and surfaces which are topologically adaptive (see McInerney *et al.* [569] and [570]). A topological (T)-surface algorithm was used to segment the cerebral cortex from the MR volume. These models are one step ahead of the classical deformable surface models proposed by Terzopoulos *et al.* [571] and Cohen *et al.* [572]. The base model for the T-surface is given using an equation with spring terms as:

$$\boldsymbol{\gamma}_i\, \dot{\mathbf{X}}_i + \boldsymbol{\alpha}_i + \boldsymbol{\beta}_i = \boldsymbol{\rho}_i + \mathbf{f}_i \,, \tag{4.21}$$

where $\dot{\mathbf{X}}_i$ is the velocity component of the nodal springs in 3-D given as $[x_i(t), y_i(t), z_i(t)]$. $\boldsymbol{\alpha}_i$, $\boldsymbol{\beta}_i$ were the tension and rigidity forces and on the right hand side were the inflation force $\boldsymbol{\rho}_i$ and image force $\mathbf{f}_i$. The framework used to solve this equation is the affine cell decomposition (ACD)-based framework. Using this method, the space is partitioned into cells defined by open simplices, where an n-simplex is the simplest geometrical object of dimension n (a triangle in 2-D and a tetrahedron in 3-D). For a Euclidean space, $\mathcal{R}^n$, the simplest triangulation is the Coxeter-Freudenthal triangulation. This was constructed by dividing the given space using the cubic grids. To obtain the triangulation, the cube was sub-divided into $n!$ simplices. Thus for a 3-D case, one sub-division would be 6 tetrahedrons. The evolution of the T-surface took a similar approach to level set evolution (also called the frame propagation analogy). The steps for cortical segmentation presented by McInerney were: (**1**) Force computation and integration of the motion in Equation (4.21) for updating the node positions. (**2**) Computation of the new grid intersection points for all model triangles. (**3**) Computation of new boundary grid tetrahedra and new model triangles. (**4**) Identification of valid and invalid triangles and continuation to step (**1**). McInerney *et al.* showed appealing results for the cerebral cortex and blood vessel reconstruction.

4.4.3.6 Parametric Surface-Based Cortical Segmentation (Dale/Harvard)

Dale and co-workers (see Fischl *et al.* [328] and [573]) presented a segmentation method which used the assumption that cortical Gray Matter of the brain had a laminar flow. This assumption was based on the fact that the Gray Matter had a finite curvature everywhere, resulting in a locally planar structure where cortical GM meets other tissue types such as WM and CSF. The reasoning behind this technique was that the GM of the cortex was like a sheet, a few millimeters thick and was folded for convenience basically to shorten the cortical connection inside the skull. Dale's algorithm for surface reconstruction can be summarized as follows: step one consisted of RF field inhomogeneity correction of the MR volume. Step two consisted of the removal of the outer skull (skull stripping) in the MR volume using template deformation. Step three consisted of WM/GM segmentation. This step was broken into the following steps: (**1**) pixel classification; (**2**) thresholding or labeling; (**3**) voxel orientation computation; (**4**) order statistics filtering and (**5**) connected component analysis. Step four consisted of cortex surface tessilation and cortex surface smoothing. The skull stripping step was based on a deformable template which deformed the initial ellipsoid to the shape of the brain and eliminated the skull area. The formation process was based on the intensity of the voxels and the normal components of each voxel. The deformation equation was: $\mathbf{X}(t+1) = \mathbf{X}(t) + \mathcal{F}_{sm} + \mathcal{F}_{mri}$, where $\mathbf{X}(t)$ and $\mathbf{X}(t+1)$ were the voxel location at times t and $t+1$, respectively, $\mathcal{F}_{sm}$ was the smoothing force and $\mathcal{F}_{mri}$ is the image force due to the MRI characteristics. These values in terms of normals were defined as: $F_{sm} = \lambda_T (\sum_{j \in N_k} (\mathbf{I} - \mathbf{n}_k \mathbf{n}_k^T) . (\mathbf{x}_j - \mathbf{x}_k)) + \lambda_N ((\sum_{j \in N_k} \mathbf{n} \, \mathbf{n}_k^T) . (\mathbf{x}_j - \mathbf{x}_k)) - \frac{1}{V} \sum_i \sum_{j \in N_i} (\mathbf{n}_i \mathbf{n}_i^T) . (\mathbf{x_j} - \mathbf{x_i})$, where λ_T and λ_N specified the strengths of the tangential and normal components of the smoothness force, $\mathbf{I}$ was 3×3 identity matrix, N_k denoted the set of vertices neightbouring the kth vertex, V was the number of vertices in the template tesselation, $I(\mathbf{x})$ was the MRI value at location $\mathbf{x}$, $\mathbf{n}_k$ and $\mathbf{n}_k^T$ denoted the surface normal at location k and its transpose, respectively. The $\mathcal{F}_{mri}$ force was given in terms of the local intensity as: $\mathcal{F}_{mri} = \lambda_M \, \mathbf{n}_k \prod_{d=1}^{30} \max(0, tanh(\mathbf{I}(\mathbf{x}_k - d \, \mathbf{n}_k) - I_{th}))$, where λ_M specified the strength of the MRI-based force and "tanh" is the trignometric hyperbolic function and d is the index varying from 1 to 30. The values for λ_T, λ_N λ_M and I_{th} were 0.5, 0.1, 1.0 and 40, respectively. Once the skull stripping was performed, the real segmentation took place. If I_o was the skull stripped volume, the three threshold intensities were defined as WM_{low}, WM_{high} and GM_{high}. The labeling process was to assign the voxels a binary value of 1 or 0, depending upon if the skull stripped voxel fell within the intensity range (WM_{low}, WM_{high}) or not. From this labeled volume, further refinement was done to obtain the another smooth volume (A). From this volume (A), the order statistics were computed based on the orientation of each voxel. The last stage in the segmentation process was the connected component analysis whose output was the segmented cortex. In the step of surface tessalation, Dale used "shrink wrapping", a predefined shape driven by intensity values of a T_1-weighted MRI volume. This consisted of the computation of the initial tesselation and the smoothing of the initial surface. The smoothness of the surface was an iterative process based on energy minimization which consisted of three terms, $E_{total} = E_{norm} + E_{tan} + E_{img}$, where the energy components were: $E_{norm} = \frac{1}{2V} [\sum_{i=1}^{V} \sum_{j \in N_1(i)} (n(i).(x_i - x_j))^2]$; $E_{tan} = \frac{1}{2V} [\sum_{i=1}^{V} \sum_{j \in N_1(i)} (e_o(i).(x_i - x_j))^2 + (e_1(i).(x_i - x_j))^2]$; $E_{img} = \frac{1}{2V} [\sum_{i=1}^{V} (T(i) - I(x_i))^2]$. The results of Dale's technique for 2-D and 3-D cortical segmentation can be seen in Figure 4.23 and Figure 4.24.

Pros and Cons of Dale's Technique.   The major advantages are: (**1**) the protocol was run on over 100 human brains; (**2**) the method needed very little human interaction. The disadvantages of this technique are: (**1**) it was slow and took around 1.5 hours for each subject; (**2**) the system used a lot of elas-

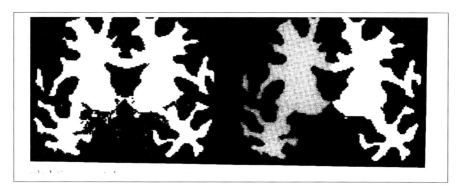

Figure 4.23: 2-D segmented WM/GM regions using Dale's technique. The segmented White Matter is shown in the left image. The segmented White Matter is shown in the right image but the left and right hemispheres are given different colors. Reproduced with permission from [328]. © Academic Press 1999.

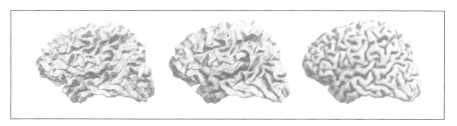

Figure 4.24: 3-D segmented cortex using Dale's technique. **Left**: original. **Middle**: GM/WM surface. **Right**: reconstructed cortex. Reproduced with permission from [328]. © Academic Press 1999.

ticity constants and such methods are very likely to change for pathological brains, hence they could be unstable. This was particularly seen during the labeling process, which was the crux of the segmentation process; (**3**) the algorithm did not prevent self-intersecting topologies, which occurred at opposite banks of a sulcus when extended towards each other; (**4**) it was hard to guarantee that the resulting surface had the topology of a sphere since the method used mathematical morphological filters; (**5**) lastly, Dale's cortical unfolding procedure rearranged these topographical features so that the geometrical features were all contained on a single plane for mapping the neural activity. Dale *et al.* performed work in the area of cortical surface-based analysis. One of the motivations for performing surface area preserving flattening was to ensure "proper" viewing of the functional activity on the cortical surface. By doing that, one could pinpoint activities more accurately on the structural brain surface map. But due to the limitation of the resolution of the functional MR data, it was not clear how much the technique could benefit. Fischl *et al.* [573] also developed a technique based on Dale *et al.*'s work.

4.4.4   2-D and 3-D Geometric Deformable Models

The layout of this sub-section is as follows: Sub-section 4.4.4.1 presents the 2-D geometric level set based methods and the 3-D extensions are discussed in Sub-section 4.4.4.2.

4.4.4.1   2-D Geometric Surface-Based Cortical Segmentation

In 1988 Sethian's Ph.D. thesis [535] brought about another revolution in image segmentation at the same time that Wikins *et al.* [523] published the work on parametric snakes. During the same time, relevant work was also published by Osher and Sethian *et al.* [536] and Rouy *et al.* [537].

The fundamental curve evolution equation of the level set first derived by Sethian was given as:

$$\frac{\partial \phi}{\partial t} = V(\kappa) \, |\nabla \phi| \,, \tag{4.22}$$

where ϕ is the level set function, $V(\kappa)$ is the speed with which the front (or *zero level curve*) propagates and $\nabla \phi$ is the gradient of the level set function[40]. This equation described the time evolution of the level set function (ϕ) in such a way that the *zero level curve* of this evolving function was always identified with the propagating interface. We will use the term "level set function" interchangeably with the term "flow field" during the course of this chapter (for details on level set application to medical imagery, see the article by Suri *et al.* [589]). Using Sethian's approach, Caselles *et al.* [538], Chopp [539] and Rouy *et al.* [537] proposed the geometric active contours followed by Malladi *et al.* [541]. The model of Caselles and Malladi was based on the following equation. If $\phi(\mathbf{x}, t)$ is a 2-D scalar function that embedded the *zero level curve* (ZLC), then the geometric active contour was given by solving:

$$\frac{\partial \phi}{\partial t} = c(\mathbf{x})(\kappa + V_0) \, |\nabla \phi| \,, \tag{4.23}$$

where $\mathbf{x}$ is pixel location (x, y), κ is the level set curvature, V_0 is the constant or propagation force and $c(\mathbf{x})$ was the stopping term or data consistency term based on image gradient and given as:

$$c(\mathbf{x}) = \frac{1}{1 + |\nabla [G_\sigma(\mathbf{x}) * I(\mathbf{x})]|} \,. \tag{4.24}$$

Pros and Cons of the Stand-alone Boundary Geometric Model.   Although Caselles and Malladi's work was able to solve the problem, it has the following weaknesses: (**1**) The stopping term was not robust and hence could not stop the bleeding of the boundaries. (**2**) The pulling back feature was not strong. This meant that if the front propagated and crossed the goal boundary, then it could not come back. Kichenassamy *et al.* [545] and Yezzi *et al.* [546]

---

[40]We will discuss this in more detail in Chapter 8.

tried to solve the above problems by introducing an extra stopping term, called the pull-back term. This was expressed mathematically as:

$$\frac{\partial \phi}{\partial t} = c(\mathbf{x})(\kappa + V_0) \, |\nabla \phi| + \underbrace{(\nabla c.\nabla \, \phi)}_{extra-stopping-term} . \tag{4.25}$$

The above method still suffered from boundary leaking for complex structures as pointed out by Siddiqui *et al.* [547]. Siddiqui *et al.* then changed the above model by adding another extra term to it:

$$\frac{\partial \phi}{\partial t} = c(\mathbf{x})(\kappa + V_0) \, |\nabla \phi| + (\nabla c.\nabla \, \phi) + \underbrace{\frac{V_0}{2} \, (\mathbf{x}.\nabla \, c) \, |\nabla \phi|} . \tag{4.26}$$

We see that Equation (4.26) has an additional term $\frac{V_0}{2} \, (\mathbf{x}.\nabla \, c) \, |\nabla \phi|$ which serves as an extra stopping term and helps in leakage prevention. Although it is possible to tune the value of V_0, this term is sensitive to edge strength variation in general. A weak edge in an image during curve evolution is enough to allow the contour to leak and could yield unpredictable results. Note that the pressure term in the parametric active contours played a similar role to the constant expanding/shrinking term in the geometric active contour model. Several researchers have tried to model the parametric active contour to prevent leaking. It is, however, not very clear how these solutions could help in the geometric active contour framework. Note that the above method was for geometric deformable models as stand-alone methods for WM/GM boundary estimation. We will see the design of four systems in Sub-sections 4.5.3, 4.5.4, 4.5.5 and 4.5.6 and that these geometric deformable models have become among the most powerful cortical segmentation techniques that have existed so far. These techniques are categorized into fusion-based techniques as region-based techniques are fused with boundary/surface-based techniques.

4.4.4.2 3-D Geometric Surface-Based Cortical Segmentation (Malladi/LBL)

The dominance of 3-D shape modeling using Geodesics active surfaces started from the UCLA group (Osher, Sethian, Chopp, see [536], [539]) and then later from the Berkeley Lab (see Malladi and Sethian, [574], [575]). Readers can enjoy a complete discussion on the history of level sets and their applications in a recent paper by Suri *et al.* [576]. Malladi's method was simply an extension from 2-D to 3-D of Equations (4.23) and (4.24) and an additional term, called the gradient of the potential field. Thus, if:

$$\frac{\partial \phi}{\partial t} = c(\mathbf{x})(\kappa + V_0) \, |\nabla \phi| , \tag{4.27}$$

where κ is the level set curvature, V_0 is the constant and $c(\mathbf{x})$ was the stopping term based on image gradient and given as: $c(\mathbf{x}) = \frac{1}{1+|\nabla[G_\sigma(\mathbf{x})*I(\mathbf{x})]|}$, then

Malladi's final equation for cortical segmentation was:

$$\frac{\partial \phi}{\partial t} = \underbrace{c(\mathbf{x})(\kappa + V_0)\,|\nabla \phi|}_{gradient+curvature+stopper} + \underbrace{\beta\,\nabla \mathbf{P}.\nabla \phi}_{attractive-force} \quad , \qquad (4.28)$$

where β was the smoothing constant for the attractive force, $\mathbf{P}$ was the gradient of the potential field given as: $\mathbf{P}(x,y,z) = |(\nabla(G_{sigma} * I(x,y,z)))|$. Note, $G_{sigma} * I(x,y,z)$ is the Gaussian smoothing of the image volume $I(x,y,z)$ "*" represents the convolution operation, ∇ operator is the gradient operator and the parallel bar represents the magnitude of the gradient operator. Note that the term $\nabla \mathbf{P}.\nabla \phi$ denotes the projection of an attractive force on the surface normal. β simply controls the strength of the attractive force. Also note that $V_0 = 1$ and κ was pre-multiplied by ϵ which controlled the mean curvature. The mean curvature κ in 3-D was:

$$\kappa = \frac{1}{(\phi_x^2+\phi_y^2+\phi_z^2)^{3/2}}\left((\phi_{yy}+\phi_{zz})\,\phi_x^2+(\phi_{xx}+\phi_{zz})\,\phi_y^2+(\phi_{xx}+\phi_{yy})\,\phi_z^2-2(\phi_x\,\phi_y\,\phi_{xy}+\right.$$
$$\left.\phi_x\,\phi_z\,\phi_{xz}+\phi_y\,\phi_z\,\phi_{yz})\right) \; .$$

It was not clear from Mallardi's paper [574] how the value of the arrival time T was selected to segment the cortex accurately, but their protocol followed a two-step process. They first reconstructed the arrival time function using the fast marching method (see Sethian [548], [549]). Then, they treated the final $T(x,y,z)$ function as an initial condition to their full model. This meant that they solved Equation (4.27) in a few time steps using the finite difference with $\phi(x,y,z;t=0) = T(x,y,z)$. They however did say that the order of their algorithm was O($\mathcal{N}$ log $\mathcal{N}$), where $\mathcal{N}$ were the total number of points in the space. We will see the modification of this technique in Sub-sections 4.5.4 and 4.5.6, where we will see a new design of the propagation force, step size and introduction of constraints.

4.4.5   A Note on Isosurface Extraction (Lorensen/GE)

All the techniques in Sub-section 4.4 use some kind of surface rendering scheme for the display of the cortical surface. In parametric and geometric deformable models for 3-D cortical segmentation, we use the isosurface extraction process during the evolution process. We will discuss this isosurface extraction process in this sub-section.

Lorensen *et al.* [580] published a method (called marching cubes (MC)) for constructing triangular surfaces fitting the boundary of an object in an image volume without the explicit need for contour extraction (unlike the above mentioned 3-D-surface methods). The algorithm fits a triangulated surface to the boundary of an object in an image volume, using an intensity value at which the surface can be found in the image. Any voxel in the image volume at which the intensity changes from a value below to a value above this boundary value was tiled with triangular facets. Such a surface was therefore referred to as an iso-intensity surface. The algorithm proceeded by constructing the cube whose eight vertices were placed at eight voxel positions in two adjacent slices, with vertices labeled with voxel values from eight voxels in the image. Note, this technique will be used in Sub-section 4.5 as one of the critical steps when dealing with geometric cortical surface extraction techniques.

Pros and Cons of the Marching Cube Method. (**1**) The weakness of the above method was evident in some cases when the eight voxel values labeling the cube vertices did not uniquely determine the topology of the surface path to fit the cube data. To remove the weakness in this algorithm, Cline *et al.* [581] modified the above algorithm. (**2**) Another weakness of the above method was the large number of triangular facets which increased the computational burden. (**3**) Van-Gelder *et al.* [587] also pointed out that the MC algorithm had some inherent ambiguities which could result in surfaces containing holes. Shu *et al.* [582] then resolved the above problems using the adaptive marching cube technique, where the algorithm considered the cube to be of different sizes depending upon the size and curvature of the feature of the surface.

4.4.5.1 Surface Reconstruction by Decomposition of Tetrahedrons and Surface Nets

Guéziec *et al.* [583], [584] presented a triangulated technique similar to the marching cubes method. Instead of tiling the cube directly, the cube was divided into five tetrahedra. This technique forms good topology and correct surfaces, but the number of triangles was two to three times greater than that of the marching cubes technique. A little scheme proposed by Montani *et al.* [585] used an efficient way of computing the number of triangles. Instead of interpolating along the cube edges to calculate the intersection points of the surface facets, this technique places all the intersections at the midpoint of the cube edges. Thus this method is very quick, since the interpolation method is omitted.

Recently, Sarah *et al.* [586] proposed a technique for producing smooth surface models from binary segmented data by avoiding the step artifacts in surfaces generated from binary data using the marching cubes. This method was called "Constrained Elastic Surface Net". The approach taken differed from the marching cubes method in that no triangulated surface was generated until the final stage of the algorithm. This took an input binary segmented image with one or more objects (foreground) and then embedded the image volume (background) in it. Step one consisted of finding the cubes which had a transition from foreground to background. Note that the eight vertices of the cube corresponded to the neighboring slices. Now if at least one of the vertices was labeled with a value different from the other vertices, then the cube would contain the portion of the surface of an object in an image. A surface net was then initialized by placing a node at the center of every surface cube identified, generating links from each surface, not to its neighboring surface nodes. The surface was now relaxed using energy minimization, and finally the relaxed surface was ready for reconstruction.

4.4.6   Summary of Boundary/Surface-Based Techniques: Pros and Cons

The major advantages of boundary/surface-based methods are: (**1**) They are very convenient and can easily adjust to the incorporation of *a priori* models. (**2**) The deformable boundary/surface techniques are very powerful when fused with region-based information, as we will see in Sub-section 4.5. The major disadvantages of boundary/surface-based methods are: (**1**) WM/GM boundary estimation techniques using edge-detection are too sensitive to noise and are not robust. (**2**) Boundary/surface-based techniques are unable to take advantage of neighborhood information, unlike the region-based approach. (**3**) Boundary/surface deformable models do not have a robust stopping mechanism, because they do not use regional or neighborhood-based information. (**4**) Most of the deformable models when used as stand-alone methods are tailored by many elasticity constants and are thus unstable. (**5**) Deformable models do not do as good a job as bi-directional movements, thus deep convolutions are unreachable and shapes like sulci and gyri cannot be detected. Sub-section 4.8.1 will present all the advantages of the geometric deformable models when fused with region-based information.

4.5   Fusion of Boundary/Surface with Region-Based 2-D and 3-D Cortical Segmentation Techniques

Fusing regional statistics into parametric or geometric boundary/surfaces has brought major success in cortical segmentation (see the recent work by Yezzi *et al.* [591], Guo *et al.* [592], Leventon *et al.* [588], Lorigo *et al.* [590] and Suri [614], [615]). The main reason for this is that the system takes advantage of the local and global shape information for pulling and pushing the boundaries/surfaces to capture the topology of the GM and WM cortical areas in the parametric or level set framework based on PDE[41] (for details on PDE-based approaches, see the upcoming paper by Suri [645]). Incorporating such regional-statistics or so-called regularizers makes the overall system more robust and accurate (see Zhu *et al.* [593]).

This sub-section presents six different fusion-based systems: two systems for parametric boundary/surfaces with regions and four systems for geometric boundary/surfaces with regions. The specific layout is as follows: Sub-section 4.5.1 presents the incorporation of the regional-based forces into parametric snakes. Incorporating regional statistics estimated from clustering into parametric surfaces for cortical surfaces estimation is discussed in Sub-section 4.5.2. Sub-section 4.5.3 presents the incorporation of clustering-based region analysis into 2-D geometric snakes or level set curves. Sub-section 4.5.4 presents the fusion of probability-based voxel classification into 3-D level set surfaces for

---

[41]Partial Differential Equations.

cortical segmentation. Sub-section 4.5.5 presents the fusion of shape information into 2-D and 3-D level set boundary/surface. Sub-section 4.5.6 presents
a state-of-the-art system for the fusion of Bayesian-based pixel-classification
into boundary/surface-based 2-D and 3-D level set-based cortical segmentation. Lastly, Sub-section 4.5.7 discusses the similarities and differences between
different cortical segmentation techniques.

4.5.1   2-D/3-D Regional Parametric Boundary: Fusion of Boundary with Classification (Kapur/MIT)

Kapur [594] was one of the original researchers who tried to fuse the region-
based approach with parametric snakes. The technique was a combination of
mathematical morphology, an EM-based algorithm for tissue classification and
parametric snakes. The algorithm consisted of three steps: (**1**) the classification
of tissues using an EM segmenter (see Wells *et al.* [458]); (**2**) the application of
mathematical morphology to disconnect the WM/GM region from the cranium
(based on connectivity and topology). This used the following steps: binarization of the EM segmenter, erosion with a structuring element, largest connected
component (CC) analysis, dilation of the largest CC and conditionally dilated
CC; (**3**) the application of the snakes model of Wikins *et al.* [523] and the balloon force of Cohen [602] to estimate the WM, GM boundaries. Note that
Kapur used a modified version of Cohen's balloon force by introducing a regional directional term called $B(s)$. Thus Cohen's balloon force was changed
from $F = k_1 \mathcal{N}(s) + k \frac{\nabla E_{ext}}{||\nabla E_{ext}||}$ to $F = k B(s)\mathcal{N}(s)$, where k was the amplitude
of the balloon force, $B(s)$ was the regional directional force and $\mathcal{N}(s)$ was the
normal to the contour. Note that the above thesis was converted to a paper
(see Kapur *et al.* [595]).

Pros and Cons of Kapur's Method.   (**1**) This technique was very sensitive to the classical elasticity constants and Kapur was correct in pointing out
[594] that "extraction of the brain did not seem to be an application that best
exploits the strengths of the classical snake model"; (**2**) the above technique
used mathematical morphology for removing the connectedness between the
WM/GM and skull. The approach did not discuss the variability of the SE
size and shape with the change in the brain: variability or subject to subject
variability; (**3**) the balloon force direction vector B was very sensitive and dependent upon the mathematical morphological operation. If the SE was large,
then pixels out of the brain region pixel/voxel would also get a tag of brain
region (which was not correct). As a result of this false tag, the balloon force
would be positive and inflation would take place, though it should have been
deflating. A better solution would have been to make the morphology step
interactive; (**4**) again, the deep convolutions were not identified using Kapur's
technique. Suri [614], [615], [322] recently developed the geometric snake model
for WM/GM boundary estimation which will be discussed in Sub-section 4.5.3,
and which removes all the weaknesses of the above technique.

Other original research was performed by Ivins *et al.* [597], [598]. Along the same lines, Poon *et al.* [599] took the classical energy snake model and added a region analysis term, thereby changing the model as: $E_{snake} = \int E_{int} + \int E_{ext} + \int E_{reg}$. Poon *et al.* chose the Fisher criterion for region analysis because of its simplicity and effectiveness. This gave them the advantage of coupling among contours in a multiple contour image. They defined the region-based energy term as: $E_{reg} = w_r(\frac{S_w^2}{S_b^2})$, where w_r was the weight, S_w^2 was the *between-regions* sum of squares and S_b^2 was the *within-region* sum of squares. They were given as: $S_b^2 = \sum_{i=0}^{N} n_i(\bar{D}_i - \bar{D})^2$ and $S_w^2 = \sum_{i=0}^{N}\sum_{j=0}^{n_i}(\bar{D}_i^j - \bar{D}_i)^2$, respectively, where n_i was the number of image pixels in the ith region, $\bar{D}_i$ was the mean pixel feature parameter of the ith region, $\bar{D}$ was the mean feature parameter of the whole image and D_i^j was the feature parameter of the jth pixel in the ith region.

Ronfard [600] also introduced region-based strategies for parametric snakes. The technique was applied to brain MR images for sub-cortical segmentation such as in the ventricles. We therefore will very briefly present their method. The forces acting on the contour consisting of the parametric curve with parameter "s" was given as:

$$\frac{\partial W}{\partial C} = F(s) = [D(R_{in}, \delta R) - D(R_{out}, \delta R)] \frac{N(s)}{|t(s)|},$$

where D's were the regional ward distances defined as:

$$\begin{cases} D(R_{in}, \delta R) &= W^{reg}(R_{in} + \delta R) - W^{reg}(R_{in}) - W^{reg}(\delta R) \\ D(R_{out}, \delta R) &= W^{reg}(R_{out} + \delta R) - W^{reg}(R_{out}) - W^{reg}(\delta R) \\ W^{reg}(R_k) &= [I\,R_k\,||\triangle I(x,y)||^2\,dx\,dy], \end{cases} \quad (4.29)$$

where R_k was the region number, I was the image (for details, see Ronfard [600]), δR was the deformation, $N(s)$ was the normal to the contour point and $t(s)$ was the amplitude of the normal. The above equation was solved using a "depth-adapting" algorithm which moved from fine to coarse strategy. Before we present their steps, we note that the region considered around a point was like a strip of width L and depth of $2P + 1$. The "depth-adapting" algorithm solved the above equation as: (**1**) Start with the initial B-spline curve, sample it uniformly with the arc-length s as parameter. Choose the depth parameter P. (**2**) Fit all control points in the B-spline basis, compute normals $N(s)$ for every s, move all control points from $M(s)$ to $M(s) + tN(s)$ according to the sign of the dissipated energy. This was the work done and given by the above equation. (**3**) Increment P and compare the energy levels obtained in step (**2**) with those of the increased neighborhoods, allowing lower energies at a coarser scale. Note that all points with increasing energies were made inactive. (**4**) Repeat steps (**2**) and (**3**) until no more control points are active. Ronfard also presented the "Adaptive Diffusion Algorithm (ADA)" which performed better than the "depth-adapting" algorithm. ADA was based on the concept of the retinex scheme (see Land [601]), where the scheme computed lightness or color using path integrals away from the boundaries. This in terms of active contours meant the "filling-in" took place away from the object boundaries and acted like a diffusion barrier. The algorithm's performance was based on the diffusion-coefficient which was similar in concept to line-process energy (see Geman *et al.* [259]).

Pros and Cons of Fusion of Regional Statistics into Parametric Snakes. (**1**) Although the incorporation of the regional statistics into the parametric snakes improved the performance of the cortical boundary estimation, all these methods were still subjected to the elasticity constants which brought instability in the boundary estimation process. (**2**) Besides that, the deep convolution shapes of the ventricles could not be reached accurately (see Figure 11 in Ronfard [600]). (**3**) Above all, the techniques had too many parameters to be computed which were very unstable, these being: normals, width of window L and depth of window $2P + 1$, sign of the energy, total number of sampled points on the contour and standard deviation σ used to estimate smooth normals along the curve. (**4**) The technique was too sensitive to the constant contrast around the objects in the image. (**5**) Separate contours were needed for separate objects and needed to be optimized separately.

One of the recent improvements to stabilize the parametric curve was by Xu *et al.* [604], who presented work on the computation of external forces by solving the image forces using the diffusion method, the so-called gradient vector flow (GVF) method. The GVF model was first presented by Prince *et al.* [603], where the external force field was replaced by a new force field. Thus, the classical energy model equation: $\alpha \mathbf{X}''(s) - \beta \mathbf{X}'''(s) - \nabla E_{ext} = 0$, was changed to $\alpha \mathbf{X}''(s) - \beta \mathbf{X}'''(s) - f_t = 0$, where f_t was given as a combination of solenoidal fields as $\zeta f_g + (1 - \zeta) f_s$ and ζ fell in the range of 0 to 1. This model was used in conjunction with 3-D fuzzy clustering for cortical segmentation. We will discuss this model and the superiority of GVF in the next sub-section.

4.5.2 Regional Parametric Surfaces: Fusion of Surface with Clustering (Xu/JHU)

An application of 3-D fuzzy clustering segmentation as a regularizer in parametric surfaces for cortical segmentation was shown by Xu *et al.* [605], [606]. This algorithm reconstructed the central layer of the cortex given the T_1-weighted MR brain scans of the human brain. This layer is the middle layer of the Gray Matter thickness. The algorithm consisted of four steps. Step one was called pre-processing, which extracted the cerebrum (that is, removed the skin, bone, fat and non-cerebral tissue) followed by trilinear interpolation. Step two consisted of adaptive fuzzy segmentation of the WM, GM and CSF, which was necessary to generate the WM membership function, a necessary step for the next stage. This third stage was called initial surface generation and consisted of two steps. The first step was called median filtering and the second step was called isosurface extraction. This stage was very critical for preserving the topology of the cortex. The isosurface extraction consisted of manually removing the hippocampus and filling the ventricles and putamen using region-growing. This was an iterative process and was terminated when the Euler characteristics were less than or equal to the number two. The final stage consisted of running the deformable surface using the generalized GVF (gradient vector flow) method (see Prince *et al.* [603] and Xu *et al.* [604]) for the final surface extraction or reconstruction of the cortex. If $\mathbf{x}(\mathbf{u}) = [x(\mathbf{u}), y(\mathbf{u}), z(\mathbf{u})]^T$, $\mathbf{u} = (u^1, u^2) \in [0,1] \times [0,1]$, then the the steady-state dynamic equation of deformable model was given as:

$$
\mathbf{x}_t = \underbrace{w_1 \left(\frac{\partial^2 x}{(\partial u^1)^2} + \frac{\partial^2 x}{(\partial u^2)^2} \right)}_{Smoothness-Term} - \underbrace{w_2 \nabla_u^2 \left(\frac{\partial^2 x}{(\partial u^1)^2} + \frac{\partial^2 x}{(\partial u^2)^2} \right)}_{Rigidity-Term} - \underbrace{\nabla E_{ext}(x)}_{Image-Energy-Term} \quad ,
$$

(4.30)

where $\mathbf{x}_t$ was the deformable dynamic surface w_1 and w_2 were the weights of the internal energy terms which controlled the smoothness and rigidity of the surface, while ∇E was the external energy of the surface that pushed and pulled the deforming surface to fit to the central layer of the cortex. The symbol ∇_u^2 was the Laplacian operator defined in parameter space as:

$$
\nabla_u^2 = \frac{\partial^2 x}{(\partial u^1)^2} + \frac{\partial^2 x}{(\partial u^2)^2} \; .
$$

(4.31)

The key idea on surface reconstruction was the adaptive FCM (AFCM), which brought the initial surface topology to its correct place and captured the central layer of the GM cortex. Authors who use Xu's technique in their paper are Angenent *et al.* [610] and Haker *et al.* [611], [612].

Pros and Cons of 3-D Clustering Fused in Parametric Surfaces.   This technique was definitely a good way of integrating the AFCM, isosurface and deformable surface, but there are certain issues which still need to be addressed to resolve these issues, such as: (**1**) the speed of computing the brain surface, since it takes around 3 hours alone to do the deformation from the initial surface and one hour to perform the AFCM. (**2**) There was too much manual interaction in cleaning the first step the so-called cerebrum extraction and cubic interpolation. They used human interacted region-growing to remove the skin, bone, fat and non-cerebral tissues. (**3**) This method showed in two out of six cases where the superior temporal gyrus did not correctly identify the GM/WM interface. (**4**) This method expected the initial surface to always be placed inside the cortex rather than placing it outside (so-called shrink wrapping). If the initial surface was placed on the inside, the error was in the range of 1-2 mm, while if the surface was placed on the outside, the error was from 4 to 10 mm. (**5**) Another issue was the convergence of the deformable surface, how robust it was and when to stop the convergence to obtain to the central layer of cortex. The method used by Zeng *et al.* [327] resolved some of the above issues, which we will discuss in Sub-section 4.5.4. Another author who also worked in preserving the topology of the brain structures and segmenting the brain was Mangin *et al.* [609]. This method is a combination of deformable models and Markovian segmentation and interested readers can explore this method.

4.5.3 2-D Regional Geometric Boundary: Fusion of Boundary with Clustering for Cortical Boundary Estimation (Suri/Marconi)

Fusing the pixel-classification approach in the form of clustering was attempted by Suri [614], [615] and [322]. Since we will discuss this in detail in Chapter 8, we will only present this very briefly here. To start with, the standard dynamic classical energy model as given by Wikins *et al.* [523] was:

$$\gamma \frac{\partial \mathbf{X}}{\partial t} = \underbrace{\frac{\partial}{\partial s}(\alpha \frac{\partial \mathbf{X}}{\partial s}) - \frac{\partial^2}{\partial s^2}(\beta \frac{\partial^2 \mathbf{X}}{\partial s^2})}_{internal-energy} + \underbrace{F_{ext}(\mathbf{X})}_{external-energy} \,, \qquad (4.32)$$

where $\mathbf{X}$ is the parametric contour along the parameter, s, α, β were the smoothing constants and γ was the damping coefficient. The final equation obtained in the form of the partial differential equation (PDE) is given as:

$$\frac{\partial \phi}{\partial t} = (\epsilon \kappa + V_p)|\nabla \phi| - V_{ext}.\nabla \phi \,. \qquad (4.33)$$

Note, V_p can be considered as a regional force term and and can be expressed mathematically as a combination of the inside-outside regional area of the propagating curve. This can be defined as $\frac{w_R}{\gamma R}$, where w_R was the regional weight constant and R was the region indicator term that fell in the range between 0 and 1. An example of such a region indicator could come from a membership function of a fuzzy classifier (see Bezdek *et al.* [466]). Thus, we see that regional information was one of the factors which controlled the speed of the geometric snake or propagating curve in the level set framework. A framework in which a snake propagated by capturing the topology of the WM/GM, navigated by the regional, curvature, edge and gradient forces was called geometric snakes. Also note that Equation (4.33) has three terms: $(\epsilon \kappa)$, V_p and V_{ext}. These three terms were the speed functions which controlled the propagation of the curve. These three speed functions were known as curvature, regional and gradient speed functions, respectively, as they contributed towards the three kinds of forces occurring during the curve propagation. The results of the application of the above model for GM boundary estimation are given in Figure 4.25[42].

Pros and Cons of Geometric Boundary Fused with Clustering. The above system is the latest in the state-of-the-art with the following advantages: (**1**) The fuzzy clustering acted as a regularizer for navigating the geometric geodesic snake. Since it is a pixel-classification procedure, one can estimate boundaries for different structures in the brain MRI data. (**2**) The key characteristic of this system is that it is based on region, so the local noise or edge would not distract the growth process. (**3**) The technique was non-local and thus the local noise could not distract the final placement of the contour or the diffusion growth process. (**4**) The technique is very suitable for medical organ

---

[42]We will discuss this system in detail in Chapter 8.

segmentation since it can handle any of the cavities, concavities, convoluted-ness, splitting or merging. (**5**) The technique was extendable to multi-phase, which means that if there are multiple level set functions, then they automat-ically merged and splitted during the course of the segmentation process. The major weakness of such a system lies in the computational expense of the fuzzy membership computation, however it is compensated for by the fast level sets implementations (see Suri [322]). Besides that, although the system has a min-imal number of coefficients when compared to parametric snakes, they are not totally independent of image characteristics.

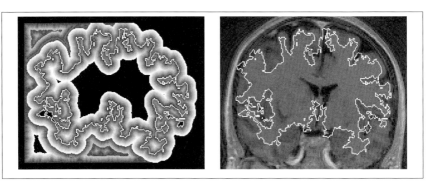

Figure 4.25: **Left**: Results of the superimposition of the ZLC and its Level Set Function using the "fast marching method" in the narrow band (NB). Tube reconstruction. **Right**: Segmented GM boundary (results courtesy of Marconi Medical Systems, Inc. For details, see the articles by Suri *et al.* [614], [615]).

4.5.4   3-D Regional Geometric Surfaces: Fusion of Geometric Surface with Probability-Based Voxel Classification (Zeng/Yale)

Zeng *et al.* [616], [327] presented an approach to coupled-surfaces propagation with level set methods for the segmentation of the cerebral cortex and the mea-surement of cortex thickness from T_1-weighted MR images. Modeling the cere-bral cortex as a volumetric layer bounded by the inner (WM/GM boundary) and outer (CSF/GM boundary) cortical surfaces, Zeng's method was motivated by the nearly constant thickness of the cortical mantle and takes this tight cou-pling as an important constraint. The algorithm started with two embedded surfaces in the form of concentric sphere sets. The inner and outer surfaces are then evolved, driven by their own image-derived information, respectively, while maintaining the coupling inbetween through a thickness constraint. Thus a final representation of the cortical bounding surfaces and an automatic seg-mentation of the cortical volume was achieved (see Figure 4.26, bottom row, left column). The image-derived information is obtained by using a local oper-ator based on gray-level information rather than image gradient alone, which gave the algorithm the ability to capture the homogeneity of the tissue inside the volumetric layer. The algorithm was implemented using a level set method. Instead of evolving the two surfaces directly, two level functions ψ_{in} and ψ_{out} whose *zero level set* corresponding to the cortical bounding surfaces were calculated and given as:

$$\begin{cases} \psi_{in} + V_{in} |\nabla \psi_{in}| &= 0 \\ \psi_{out} + V_{out} |\nabla \psi_{out}| &= 0, \end{cases} \quad (4.34)$$

where V_{out} and V_{in} are the speed terms for the outer and inner surfaces. The coupling between the two surfaces was realized through the propagation speed terms V_{out} and V_{in}. While the distance between the two surfaces is within the normal range, the inner and outer cortical surfaces propagated according to their own image features. When the distance started to fall out of the normal range, the propagation slowed down and finally stopped when the distance was outside the normal range, or the image feature (gradient information) was strong enough. The speed terms were computed using the two functions g and h which controlled the speed of the propagation. The function g was a function of the local operator and h was a penalization function. Thus they were defined as:

$$\begin{cases} V_{in} = g(p_{GW})\,h(\psi_{out}) \\ V_{out} = g(p_{CG})\,h(\psi_{in}). \end{cases}$$

Note, G stands for "Gray Matter" and W stands for "White Matter" and C stands for "CSF". p_{GW} and p_{CG} are the local operators, given as:

$$p_{GW} = \prod_{g \in G} \frac{1}{\sqrt{2\pi}\sigma_G} e^{-\frac{(I_g - \mu_G)^2}{\sigma_G^2}} \prod_{w \in W} \frac{1}{\sqrt{2\pi}\sigma_W} e^{-\frac{(I_w - \mu_W)^2}{\sigma_W^2}}, \quad (4.36)$$

where W and G were the WM and GM regions, μ_W and μ_G were mean values of the WM and GM regions. σ_W^2 and σ_G^2 were standard deviations of the WM and GM regions, I_w and I_g were the WM and GM pixel intensities. Note, the output of the GM-WM likelihood function was the image which had edge information about the boundary of the GM-WM. Similarly, the WM-CSF likelihood function was an image which had the WM-CSF edge or gradient information. A coupled narrow band algorithm was customized for the coupled-surfaces propagation. The correspondence between points on the two bounding surfaces falls out automatically during the narrow band rebuilding, which was required for surface propagation at each iteration. This shortest distance-based correspondence was essential in imposing the coupling between the two bounding surfaces through the thickness constraint (see Plate 5 for results).

Pros and Cons of Geometric Surfaces Fused with Classification. The coupled-surfaces propagation with the level set implementation offered the advantages of easy initialization, computational efficiency (one hour), the ability to handle complex sulcal folds, simultaneous "skull-stripping" (delineation of non-brain tissues) and GM/WM segmentation, as well as the ready evaluation of several characteristics of the cortex, such as surface curvature and a

cortical thickness map (see Zeng [616]). This work integrated the efficiency
and flexibility of level set methods with the power of shape constraint. It had
shown promise in brain segmentation through extensive experiments on both
simulated brain images and real data. Other work following this line included
that of Gomes *et al.* [617]. The strong points of the coupled surface method
were its ability to handle complex geometry, high computational efficiency and
the natural correspondence between the boundary surfaces. The major weaknesses are: (**1**) The method did not include a model that deals with image
inhomogeneity. (**2**) The technique imposed no constraint to preserve the cortical surface topology, however it did take advantage of the topological flexibility
of the level set methods. (**3**) The resulting surface may not produce a two
dimensional manifold.

4.5.5   2-D/3-D Regional Geometric Surface: Fusion of Geometric Boundary/Surface with Global Shape Information (Leventon/MIT)

Another application of the fusion of Bayesian statistics to model shape and
fusing that with the geometric boundary/surface-based technique was done
recently by Leventon *et al.* [588]. This technique did not show the segmentation
of the cortex, rather it focused on the segmentation of the sub-cortical area such
as the corpus callosum, and was a good example of the fusion of the boundary
and region-based techniques. Leventon *et al.* derived the shape information
using *maximum a posterior probability* (MAP) and fused that with gradient
and curvature driven boundary/surface in the level set framework. This MAP
mode of shape used *priors* in the Bayesian framework from the training data
set (analogous to Cootes *et al.*'s [227] technique). Using Equation (4.25) (from
Sub-section 4.4.4.1), the level set curve/surface evolution is given as:

$$\frac{\partial \phi}{\partial t} = c(\mathbf{x})(\kappa + V_0)\,|\nabla \phi| + \underbrace{(\nabla c . \nabla \phi)}_{extra-stopping-term} \quad , \qquad (4.37)$$

where the symbols have the same meaning as discussed in Sub-section 4.4.4.1.
Note that this equation is exactly the same as Equation (8) used by Leventon
et al. in [588], whose solution using finite difference was:

$$\phi(t+1) = \phi(t) + \lambda_1 [c(\mathbf{x})(\kappa + V_0)\,|\nabla \phi| + (\nabla c . \nabla \phi)] . \qquad (4.38)$$

If $[\phi^*(t) - \phi(t)]$ represented the optimized shape information at time t, then
Leventon *et al.* added this term to the above equation to yield the final evolution
equation in the level set framework as:

$$\phi(t+1) = \phi(t) + \lambda_1 [\underbrace{c(\mathbf{x})(\kappa + V_0)\,|\nabla \phi|}_{Gradient+Curvature-Forces} + \underbrace{(\nabla c . \nabla \phi)}_{Image-Force}] + \underbrace{\lambda_2 [\phi^*(t) - \phi(t)]}_{Global-Shape-Force} .$$
$$\qquad (4.39)$$

The key to the above model was the extraction of the shape information from
the training data (called global shape information) and fusing with the local

information (gradient and curvature) in the level set framework based on partial differential equations. If α and β represent the shape and pose parameters, then the optimized ϕ^*_{MAP} would be given as the *argmax* of $P(\phi^*|\phi, \nabla I)$. This model using Bayes' rule can be broken down as: $\frac{P(\phi|\alpha,\beta) \, P(\nabla I|\alpha,\beta,\phi) \, P(\alpha) \, P(\beta)}{P(\phi,\nabla I)}$, where $P(\alpha)$ and $P(\beta)$ are the shape and pose priors. To understand the computation of $P(\alpha)$, we take, say, n-curves, each sampled N times and each surface is represented by ϕ_i, then the training set $\tau = \{\phi_i, ... \phi_n\}$. This mean shape can be computed as $\mu = \frac{1}{n}\Sigma\phi_i$ and the mean offset map is $\hat{\phi}_i = (\phi_i - \mu)$. Each of these is a column vector of a matrix $(N \times n)$. If r, c represent the rows and columns of the matrix M, then $M = [\phi_{r,c}]$, where $1 \leq r \leq N$ and $1 \leq c \leq n$. Now this matrix M undergoes SVD[43] to decompose to $U\Sigma V^T$. Taking the k-principal components, that is k-rows and k-columns, gives the new matrix $\bar{\Sigma}$. Thus the shape coefficients α are computed as: $\alpha = U_k^T(\phi - \mu)$. Using the Gaussian distribution, the priors shape model can be computed as:

$$P(\alpha) = \frac{1}{\sqrt{(2\pi)^k|\bar{\Sigma}|}} \, exp(\frac{1}{2} \, \alpha^t \, \bar{\Sigma}^{-1} \, \alpha) \, . \tag{4.40}$$

This equation is used in the computation of optimized ϕ^*. The pose prior is from uniform distribution.

Pros and Cons of Shape Information Fused in Geometric Boundary/Surface. The major advantages of this system are: (**1**) Robustness and successful capture of topology based on Bayesian shape information. (**2**) The shape and pose parameters converged on the shape to be segmented. The major disadvantages of such a system are: (**1**) The time taken for such a system was six minutes (for vertebra segmentation), which was relatively long for spinal navigation real-time applications. (**2**) Besides that, the system would need the training data sets which had to be collected off-line. (**3**) No results were shown for cortical segmentation which had deep convolutions, large twists and bends. (**4**) The performance of systems which had coefficients estimated from training data off-line and the application of these estimated coefficients on-line, was dependent upon the training data and test data sets. The above system is like the first layer of a neural network (see Suri *et al.* [250]) whose performance is governed by the shapes of the training data and tuning parameters of the Gaussian model (see Lee [201]).

4.5.6   2-D/3-D Regional Geometric Surface: Fusion of Boundary/Surface with Bayesian-Based Pixel Classification (Barillot/IRISA)

Baillot and his co-workers (see Baillard *et al.* [619] [621]) recently designed a brain segmentation system based on fusion of region into boundary/surface estimation. This algorithm is quite similar in approach to Suri's method which was

---

[43]Singular Value Decomposition.

discussed previously in Sub-section 4.5.3. This algorithm is another instance where the propagation force V_0 in the fundamental level set segmentation equation $\frac{\partial \phi}{\partial t} = c(\mathbf{x})(\kappa + V_0) \, |\nabla \phi|$, was changed into a regional force. There were in all three changes by Barillot and his co-workers. First in the propagation force V_0, second in the data consistency term or stopping term $c(\mathbf{x})$ and third in the step size δt. We will briefly discuss these equations and their interpretation. The key idea is to utilize the probability density function inside and outside the structure to be segmented. The pixel/voxel in the neighborhood of the segmenting structure was responsible for creating a pull/push force on the propagating front. This was expressed in the form of the probability density function to be estimated inside the structure $p_i(u)$, the probability density function to be estimated outside the structure $p_e(u)$ and the prior probability for a voxel to be inside the structure. Note, here u is the intensity value of a voxel at location (x, y, z). Using the above concept, the bi-directional propagation force was estimated as:

$$V_0 = sgn\{\alpha_i \, p_i(u) - (1 - \alpha_i)p_e(u)\}, \qquad (4.41)$$

where $sgn(x)$ was 1 if $x \geq 0$ and was -1 if $x < 0$. The second modification to the data consistency term was changing the gradient term into an extended gradient term[44] was changed from $c(\mathbf{x}) = \frac{1}{1+|\nabla[G_\sigma(\mathbf{x})*I(\mathbf{x})]|}$ to a term which was based on the transitional probability of going from inside to outside the object to be segmented. This was given mathematically as: $c(\mathbf{x}) = g[p_T(x|I,c)]$, where $g(x)$ was $1 - 4x^3$ if $x < 0.5$ and was $4(1-x)^3$, if $x \geq 0.5$. The term p_T was computed based on these three parameters: α_i, $p_i(u)$ and $p_e(u)$, and estimated mathematically if the probability of a pixel/voxel class c belonged to a set of inside and outside the object. If the c was inside the region, then p_T was given as $\frac{(1-\alpha_i)\,p_e(I(x))}{\alpha_i\,p_i(I(x))+(1-\alpha_i)\,p_e(I(x))}$, while it was $\frac{(\alpha_i)\,p_i(I(x))}{\alpha_i\,p_i(I(x))+(1-\alpha_i)\,p_e(I(x))}$ if c was outside.

Pros and Cons of Baillard/Barillot's Technique. The merits of this technique are: (**1**) The paper was an excellent example of the fusion of region-based information into the boundary/surface. It is the state-of-the-art algorithm for cortical segmentation. (**2**) The results are very impressive, however, it would have been useful to see the enlarged version of the results. (**3**) The algorithm is adaptive since the data consistency term ($c(\mathbf{x})$) and step size (δt) are estimated adaptively in every iteration of the front propagation. This provides a good trade-off between convergence speed and stability. (**4**) This method uses stochastic-EM (SEM) instead of EM[45], which is a more robust and accurate method for estimation of probability density function parameters. (**5**) It has been applied to various brain structures and to various imaging modalities such as ultrasound. (**6**) The algorithm hardly needs any tuning parameters and thus

---

[44]In the equation $c(\mathbf{x}) = \frac{1}{1+|\nabla[G_\sigma(\mathbf{x})*I(\mathbf{x})]|}$, $|\nabla[G_\sigma(\mathbf{x})*I(\mathbf{x})]|$ was nothing but the convolution of image I by the Gaussian operator G with known σ, then taking the gradient in x and y directions and finally taking the magnitude of the gradient.

[45]Expectation Maximization.

is very efficient. Note that this algorithm is in parallel to the algorithm discussed in Sub-section 4.5.3. The difference lies in the approach for estimating the propagation force. Both methods (Suri's and Baillard's) are designed to control the propagation force using the regional-based analysis. Suri's method uses regional force computed using pixel-classification based on clustering, while Baillard's method uses pixel-classification based on Bayesian-statistics.

4.5.7 Similarities/Differences Between Different Cortical Segmentation Techniques

This sub-section briefly summarizes the 3-D cortical segmentation techniques in the class of deformable models (parametric and geometric). The following points can be considered for comparison: (**1**) *Parametric Vs. Geometric Framework*: Malladi and Zeng's methods were based on geometric surfaces (level sets). Xu's method was based on parametric surfaces (classical snakes in 3-D), as were Dale's method and MacDonald's. McInerney's method was based on a parametric deformable model. (**2**) *Preservation of Cortical Topology*[46]: Malladi, Dale, Xu and MacDonald's methods do preserve the topology of the cerebral cortex. Zeng and McInerney's methods did not preserve the topology. (**3**) *Usage of Cortical Structure Information*: Malladi's method did not use any special structural information. Zeng and MacDonald used the structural information of cortical thickness and integrated it into their deformable models, while Xu's and Dale's methods did not. Davatzikos's ribbon model used cortical structural information, and Xu further improved that method. McInerney's method did not use cortical structure information on segmenting the cerebral cortex. (**4**) *Computation Time for Cortical Segmentation*: Malladi's method claims to be the fastest. Zeng's method is faster than Dale's, MacDonald's and Xu's methods, since Zeng's method did not take time in preserving the topology of the brain cortex. MacDonald's method is very slow, due to terms forcing the surface into deep sulci and preventing the surface from crossing over itself. McInerney's method was fast enough but not as fast as Zeng's method. (**5**) *Purpose Behind the Segmentation (Application)*: Malladi's method was purely for the 3-D display of Gray/White Matter. MacDonald's technique was applied for the location of sulci. Xu's and Dale's methods used this for displaying 3-D Gray Matter. Zeng's method was for the display of 3-D Gray Matter, but more importantly, for quantitative measurements. McInerney's method was totally geared towards display. (**6**) *Human Interaction During the Segmentation Process*: Malladi's method used the initialization of 3-D seeds as starting surfaces. The amount of user interaction was heavy in Xu's method. MacDonald used initialization of an ellipsoid around the brain. Zeng did initialization of bubbles in White Matter, which was minimal. McInerney's method did not require any user interaction. (**7**) *Overall Pipeline for 3-D Segmentation*: Malladi's method used the standard surface evolution equation by

---

[46]This topic is still very debatable and is out of the scope of this chapter. Niessen *et al.* [513] point out that "No 3-D geometric flow is known which preserves the topology of arbitrary isosurfaces."

Sethian navigated by the gradient, curvature and image potential terms. Malladi's method does use the isosurface extractor algorithm for capturing of the cortical topology in each iteration in time when they solve the PDE using finite difference. Zeng's technique uses a combination of probability-based voxel classification (based on Gaussian distribution) and they implemented their method using surface evolution in the level set framework. This method used coupled surfaces with the cortical thickness as a constraint. Dale's method for the segmentation of WM/GM consisted of pixel-classification, and labeling based on intensity values, thresholding and connected component analysis. They used parametric deformation for skull-stripping and surface tesselation for cortical surface smoothing. Xu's method of adaptive fuzzy segmentation of WM, GM and CSF, which was necessary to generate the WM membership function, was a necessary step for the next stage. This method was based on running the deformable surface using generalized gradient vector flow. The topology was extracted using the isosurface extraction. McInerney's method was based on a physics-based deformable model. The framework used to solve this equation was the affine cell decomposition (ACD)-based framework. Using this method, the space is partitioned into cells defined by open simplices, where an n-simplex is the simplest geometrical object of dimension n (a triangle in 2-D and a tetrahedron in 3-D). MacDonald's method used an iterative algorithm for the simultaneous deformation of multiple surfaces with inter-surface proximity constraints and self-intersection avoidance, where the deformation was formulated as a cost function minimization problem. Basically, MacDonald's method was a general polyhedron deformation method, where they fit the model to the *a priori* image data. Such a fitting process was accomplished by solving the weighted objective function.

4.6   3-D Visualization Using Volume Rendering and Texture Mapping

4.6.1   Volume Rendering Algorithm for Brain Segmentation

Volume rendering (VR) is basically a method of displaying volumetric data as a 2-D image. A typical volume rendering (VR) pipeline is shown in Figure 4.31. It consists of the following steps: (1) Segmentation, (2) Gradient Computation, (3) Resampling, (4) Classification, (5) Shading and (6) Composition. Segmentation is the most difficult process (as we have seen in the previous sub-sections) and once this process is completed, the voxels are labeled as fat, air, tissue, bone and skin. These labeled voxels are used in the classification stage of the VR pipeline. The gradient computation step involves finding the boundaries and edges of the voxels where the tissue type changes the intensity values. A good source of gradient estimation in volume rendering is discussed

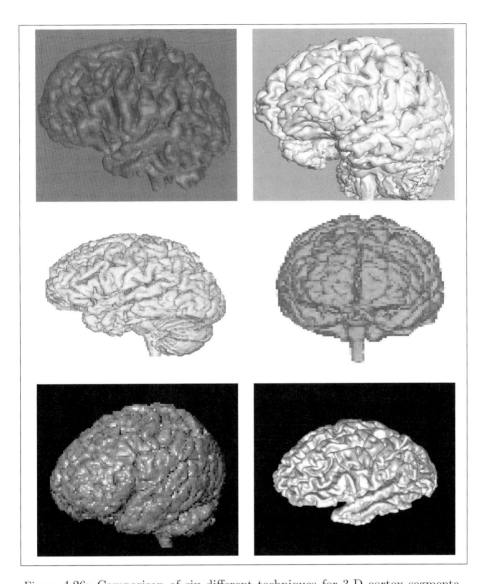

Figure 4.26: Comparison of six different techniques for 3-D cortex segmentation. **Top Left**: Using 2-D serial cross-sections (Courtesy of Paul Bourke, Astrophysics and Supercomputing, Victoria, Australia). **Top Right**: Using 3-D mathematical morphology (Reproduced with permission from [340]. © Lippincott, Williams and Wilkins 1992). **Middle Left**: Using EM Segmenter, 3-D GM surface (Reprinted with permission from [458]. © 1992 IEEE). **Middle Right**: Using 3-D level sets with propagation force estimated using Bayesian statistics (Courtesy of Christian Barillot, IRISA, Rennes Cedex, France). **Bottom Left**: Using 3-D level sets (Courtesy of Xiaolan Zeng, R2 Technology, Inc., Los Altos, CA). **Bottom Right**: Using 3-D parametric deformable model with GVF (Reprinted with permission from [606]. © 1999 IEEE).

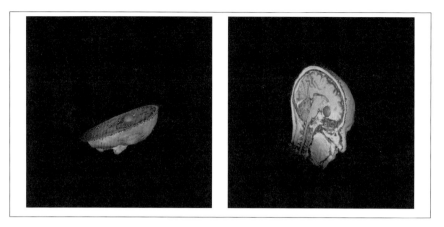

Figure 4.27: Results of texture map on the cut sections of the MR brain data. Finally segmenting the tumor and embedding the tumor into the 3D volume. VTK and tcl/tk tool kit was used for design of the textured slices. **Left**: Head cut into two halves and tumor seen (top view). **Right**: Head cut into two halves and tumor seen (sagittal view). (MR data, Courtesy of Marconi Medical Systems, Inc., Cleveland, OH.)

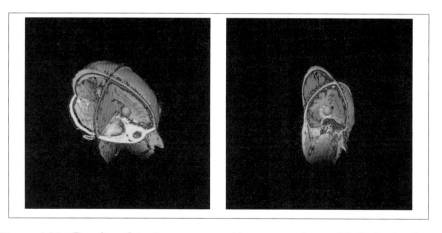

Figure 4.28: Results of texture map on the cut sections of MR brain data. Finally segmenting the tumor and embedding the tumor into the 3D volume. **Left**: Head cut into four halves and tumor seen (sagittal view). **Right**: Head cut into eight halves and tumor seen (side view). VTK and tcl/tk tool kit were used for design of the textured slices. (MR data-Courtesy of Marconi Medical Systems, Inc., Cleveland, OH.)

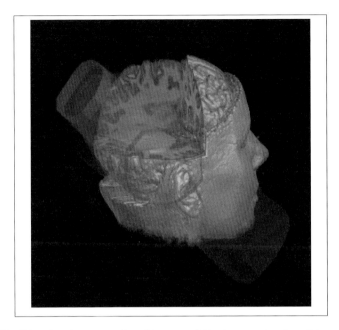

Figure 4.29: Direct volume rendered image of the human brain with cut sections (Courtesy of Marc Levoy, Stanford University, Stanford, CA).

by Bentum *et al.* [666]. In the classification step, we opacify values[47] and color values to the labeled voxels. For example, one can give a gray color to the skin, green color to tissue, etc. The resampling step involves interpolation of the voxels along the ray. It generates new values for samples that lie between the actual voxels. Next, shading is used to highlight parts of the brain (such as a tumor, etc.) using an illumination model. The last stage is the compositing (also called blending), which consists of estimating the final color value at a pixel point on the 2-D image when the casted ray goes through the volume of data, which is given by the formula:

$$I(x,y) = \int_x^y g(s)\, e^{-\int_x^s \tau(z)dz}\, ds\,, \qquad (4.42)$$

where $\tau(z)$ is the opacity or transparency of the voxel and tells how much of the light gets occluded per unit length due to scattering and $g(s)$ is the intensity of the voxel. This is also called a transfer function. Usually, the Riemann's sum is used to change the above integral to a discrete form. There are two kinds of basic compositing algorithms; front to back (FB) and back to front (BF). The equation for front to back volume rendering is given as:

$$I(x,y) = \Sigma_{i=0}^n I_i \prod_{j=0}^{i-1} (1 - \alpha_j)\,. \qquad (4.43)$$

---

[47]Giving opacity to the voxels.

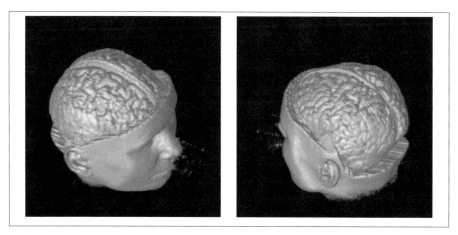

Figure 4.30: Volume rendered image of the human brain with cut sections. **Left**: Front to back. **Right**: Back to front (Courtesy of Yun-Mo Koo, Seoul National University, Seoul, Korea).

We will not go into detail on any of the methods in the pipeline but rather point out the reference papers which present excellent brain volume rendering. A good source on volume rendering is found in the book by Lichtenbelt *et al.* [667], which has around 273 references. We refer to this source for learning volume rendering and rendering organs of the human body. We also refer to a good survey on volume rendering architectures by Kaufman *et al.* [668]. Most work in volume rendering began in 1990. Some of the work most commonly referred to is by Levoy [671], [670], [669] (see Figure 4.29). Fast volume rendering was also done by Lacroute *et al.* [673]. Guo [674] also showed brain volume rendering. There is some very recent work also by Koo *et al.* [672] (see Figure 4.30).

Bottleneck of Volume Rendering: One of the major weaknesses of volume rendering is the speed at which the final rendered 2-D image of the 3-D volume is computed. Udupa's paper [675] compares surface vs. volume rendering in great detail.

4.6.2 Texture Mapping Algorithm for Segmented Brain Visualization

In this type of approach, one can render the 3-D skull surface and texture map in the segmented MR brain slices to show the visualization of the human brain (see Figures 4.27 and 4.28). We will not discuss texture mapping any further here. Interested readers can refer to the survey article by Heckbert [676], [677] and a two part texture mapping procedure by Bier *et al.* [678]. Texture mapping is very important for fMRI applications, especially when used in mapping 3-D cortical surfaces to unit spheres. This can then be used for overlaying the fMRI information on these spheres. Very recently, Angenent and his co-workers [355] presented work in which they texture mapped the cortical 3-D surface onto a

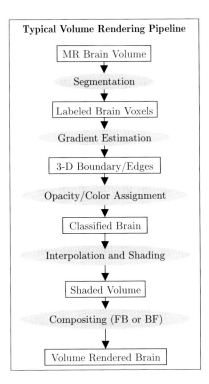

Figure 4.31: Typical volume rendering pipeline for the human brain. The major steps are: image segmentation, gradient computation, classification, resampling, shading and composition.

unit sphere. They used the finite element formulation. Since the algorithm is critical for our fMRI applications, we will discuss that next.

Texture Mapping Algorithm for 3-D Cortical Surface Projection.
The pipeline for mapping the 3-D cortical surface onto the sphere is shown in Figure 4.32. The pipeline consists of 3-D cortex segmentation, followed by 3-D mesh generation and texture mapping. If the input used was 2-D brain slices, then the steps consist of 2-D cortex segmentation, followed by mesh generation and texture mapping. The texture mapping method is based on conformal mapping of a surface on the unit sphere. The mapping is implemented using the finite element method (see Hughes [679]) whose solution lies in solving the partial differential equation:

$$\delta z = \left(\frac{\partial}{\partial u} - \frac{\partial}{\partial v} \right) \delta_p , \qquad (4.44)$$

where z is the mapped surface and u and v are the conformal coordinates.

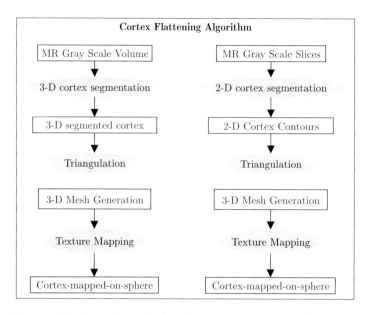

Figure 4.32: Typical cortical surface mapping to a unit sphere.

4.7 A Note on fMRI: Algorithmic Approach for Establishing the Relationship Between Cognitive Functions and Brain Cortical Anatomy

This sub-section briefly introduces the relationship between fMRI analysis and the 2-D and 3-D brain segmentation techniques covered in detail in Sub-sections 4.3, 4.4 and 4.5.

What is fMRI? fMRI is a technique for estimating which parts of the brain are activated by different kinds of activities, such as vision, finger movements, touch, taste and smell, color, texture, sound, speech, language, pain, pleasure, etc. Basically during the activation process, the MRI scan captures the increased blood flow in the cortical zones of the brain.

How is fMRI data collected? Two types of images are collected for the brain. One is a high resolution scan and the other is a low resolution scan. The high resolution scan is taken using a conventional scan, say T_1-weighted. The low resolution scan is taken when the subject is undergoing functional activity, such as, say, wearing special eye glasses (for the creation of the stimulus). This scan can be taken every 5 seconds in a lap of about 150 seconds. During this time, the stimulus is given to the subject/patient. This constitutes two kinds of low resolution scans, the case in which there is no activation and the case in which there is an activation. They can then be compared to find which parts of the brain became activated. We can also overlay this functional information over the reconstructed anatomy from the high resolution scan.

Functional mapping of the human visual cortex by MRI was first done by Belliveau *et al.* [683]. Recently, Raichle [684] published an excellent paper on the latest developments on fMRI. We also recommend readers to the survey works on fMRI by Friston [685], Kim *et al.* [686] (102 references) and Salle *et al.* [325] (126 references).

4.7.1 Superiority of fMRI over PET/SPECT Imaging

PET and SPECT also give functional information, but fMRI has several advantages over PET/SPECT. They are as follows:

1. *Spatial resolution*: fMRI offers higher spatial resolution compared to PET/SPECT image data.

2. *Temporal resolution*: fMRI offers higher temporal resolution than PET/ SPECT image data.

3. *Non-invasiveness*: fMRI procedures are completely non-invasive.

4. *Exposure to ionization*: in fMRI, there is no danger of exposure to ionizing radiation and as a result, one can do many repetitive studies.

5. *Functional and anatomical acquisitions*: since one can acquire the functional and anatomical images at the same time, we can thus compare the functional maps to the anatomical images without much registration complexity.

6. *Interface with other medical devices*: it is easy to interface and incorporate medical devices with an MRI system to collect functional information for neuropathology and neuro-functions.

The remainder of this section has the following layout: Sub-section 4.7.2 covers the applications of fMRI covered to-date. Sub-section 4.7.3 presents the application of cortex reconstruction in the fMRI analysis. Next, we discuss time course analysis of fMRI data in Sub-section 4.7.4. Finally, Sub-section 4.7.5 discusses the measure of cortex geometry.

4.7.2 Applications of fMRI

Several research groups have attempted to study different functions of the brain. Here, we will summarize the list of functions covered so far from the years 1990 to 2000. The following is the list of applications of fMRI in the clinical world.

1. *Touch and finger movements*:
   Research in the area of touch and figure movements has been done extensively. For details, see Rao *et al.* [710] and Schlaug *et al.* [711].

2. *Vision*:
   Goebel *et al.* [691], [693] and Poldrack *et al.* [692] performed experiments on fMRI to study the projection of the retina on the visual cortex (known as retinotropy).

3. *Color analysis*:
   Recently, Howard *et al.* [708] showed results of color experiments.

4. *Texture analysis*:
   Beason-Held *et al.* [709] performed experiments on texture perception.

5. *Speech and language analysis*:
   It has been recently shown that the dorso lateral prefrontal cortex becomes activated during linguistic experiments (see Gabrieli *et al.* [699]). Work has also been done in the area of word generation, word semantics, word reading and listening to words (see Friedman *et al.* [700], Chee *et al.* [707], Fiez *et al.* [701], Neville *et al.* [702] and Schlosser *et al.* [703]).

6. *Fetal brain development*:
   Recently, researchers have tried to study the brain development of the fetus (see Hykin *et al.* [704] and Wakai *et al.* [705]). It is important to learn how the fetal brain grows and responds to different kinds of activities, such as listening to music. Images acquired during these fMRI experiments can be analyzed in a similar way to other fMRI experiments.

7. *Taste/Pleasure*:
   Very recently, Francis studied the effect of taste over the cortical areas (see Francis *et al.* [706]).

8. *Emotions*:
   It would be interesting to know which part of the cortex is activated when a person smiles, cries, laughs, or is under stress.

4.7.3   Algorithm for Superimposition of Functional and Anatomical Cortex

Goebel *et al.* [695] gave a good presentation on cortical segmentation in relation to fMRI. The typical algorithm for analyzing an fMRI data set is shown in Figure 4.33. An EPI pulse sequence is used for collecting the fMRI data set under one of the fMRI experiment protocols for studying one of the functions in the list in Sub-section 4.7.2. Correspondingly, we collect the MR data set using the T_1-weighted protocol. Once both the data sets are collected, we perform post-processing on both these data sets. The fMRI data undergoes two types of registration or alignment. This is done first by taking the T_1-weighted images and second, by the alignment of fMRI data between the first and the subsequent scans. Next, the fMRI data undergoes statistical analysis to generate the canonical images (called score images). On the side pipeline, we have the 3-D reconstruction of the GM surface, its inflation and then its flattening

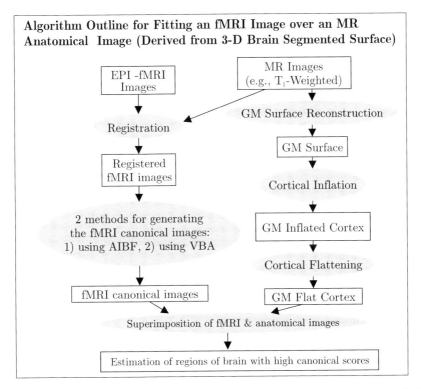

Figure 4.33: Typical application of fMRI using brain segmentation. Note, AFIB and VBA stand for Automatically Informed Basis Functions and Voxel-Based Approach, respectively (For details, see Kiebel *et al.* [326]).

so that it is like a 2-D sheet (see Angenent's method in Sub-section 4.6.2). (See Plate 4.) Finally, the 2-D information from both pipelines is superimposed to estimate the regions of the brain which have high canonical scores. Those regions correspond to the activation zones of the functional information. Figure 4.34, right, shows the results produced by such an algorithm.

4.7.3.1　3-D Mapping Vs. Surface-Based Technique

The surface-based technique offers the advantages of speed, data reduction and high statistical sensitivity compared to the direct 3-D mapping technique. Since the localization of the signal can be easily included in the cortical sheet, hence one saves much disk space and improves speed and sensitivity.

4.7.4　A Short Note on fMRI Time Course Data Analysis

This sub-section is divided into two parts: Sub-section 4.7.4.1 briefly talks about the history of BOLD processing and Sub-section 4.7.4.2 and Sub-section 4.7.4.3 discuss the algorithm for fMRI data analysis.

4.7.4.1 Brief History of BOLD

Although we will cover a brief history of the Blood Oxygen Level Dependent (BOLD) invention in this sub-section, readers are encouraged to refer to the good book on functional brain imaging by Orrison *et al.* [989]. Until the late 1980s, the decay of signal associated with local magnetic field inhomogeneities, called T_2^* relaxation, was considered a nuisance and represented a limitation in MR imaging. To mitigate this, either the "spin-echo" technique was used[48], in which a second "refocusing" RF pulse following the initial excitation pulse removed the effects of dephasing, or the time between the RF excitation pulse[49] and the acquisition of the signal was reduced as much as possible, as in the FLASH[50] technique. It was only then that it was realized that the presence of a paramagnetic substance in the blood stream acted as a vascular marker, giving useful contrast, and that sequences without a refocusing pulse, with a relatively long time between the excitation pulse and data acquisition, began to be used. Initially, the paramagnetic contrast agent was exogenous, a nontoxic compound of Gadolinium (Gad) introduced into the bloodstream via a leg vein. A fraction of a millimole of contrast agent per kg of body weight was sufficient to result in a loss of signal from tissue surrounding the cerebral blood vessels as perhaps a 40% bolus of contrast agent passed through. The group at MGH[51] pioneered the application of this approach to brain perfusion, using the Central Volume Theorem to obtain local cerebral blood flow as the ratio of blood volume to mean transit time. In a landmark paper published in 1991, Belliveau and collaborators [988] finally applied this technique to functional activation studies in humans. The subjects were given a visual stimulation while a bolus of contrast agent was injected into a leg vein. Then, single slice images of the brain in the plane of the clacarine fissue were acquired at 0.75 sec intervals to monitor the bolus passage. By integrating the time course of image intensity, estimates of relative blood volume were obtained and compared (by image subtraction) with those obtained when the subjects were at rest in darkness. Consistent increases of blood volume in primary VI visual cortex were observed.

Subsequent developments rapidly overtook this pioneering work. Ogawa *et al.* [991] and Turner *et al.* [992] working independently had shown in laboratory animals that similar changes of MRI image contrast extending around the blood vessels could be obtained, simply by changing the oxygenation state of the blood. This observation arose from the fact (noted by Faraday, measured by Pauling and Coryell [990]) that deoxyhemoglobin was more paramagnetic then oxyhemoglobin, which itself had almost exactly the same magnetic susceptibility as tissue. Thus the deoxyhemoglobin was seen as nature's own contrast agent. Interventions to the state of the brain which created an imbalance between oxygen uptake and blood flow inevitably caused a change of MRI signal around the cortical vessels, if MR imaging sequences were used which were

---

[48]See Chapter 1.
[49]See Chapter 1.
[50]Fast Low Angle Shot Imaging.
[51]Massachusetts General Hospital, Boston, MA.

sensitive to magnetic field inhomogenity.

This development culminated in the work of Kwong *et al.* [993] and Ogawa *et al.* [999]. They succeeded in showing that the change in the deoxyhemoglobin in the human visual cortex while the subject viewed a bright light was sufficient to cause measurable changes in the gradient-echo MRI images of a slice passing through the calcarine fissue. The techniques was dubbed "Blood Oxygenation Level Dependent (BOLD) Contrast". Thus the way was opened to functional mapping studies of the human brain without the use of a contrast agent, without a radiation dose and with high spatial resolution of MRI.

It was significant that a rise in signal was observed during visual stimulus, indicating a relative decrease in the concentration of paramagnetic deoxyhemoglobin. This confirmed earlier work using PET (see Fox *et al.* [994]) in which the measured rise in the oxygen uptake rate during visual stimulus was found to be much smaller than the rise in blood flow. Earlier observation during open skull surgery (see Penfield [995]) had also demonstrated that the blood leaving the active cortical regions was a brighter red, i.e., more oxygenated, than normal, as a result of this mismatch between demand and supply. In theory, the change of signal was affected by changes in blood arterial oxygenation, blood volume, blood flow, hematocrit, tissue oxygen uptake and possibly blood velocity. This effect increased with field strength (see Turner *et al.* [997]). Changes in blood flow apparently dominated, via dilution of deoxyhemoglobin, but detailed modeling and experimental investigation are in still in progress (see Fisel *et al.* [996], Ogawa *et al.* [999], Weisskoff *et al.* [1000] and Kennan *et al.* [1001]). Recently, a number of studies (see Boxerman *et al.* [1002] and Menon *et al.* [1003]) have shown that a significant fraction of the water molecules responsible for the change in signal observed in BOLD contrast are in fact inside unresolvable venules or veins draining the active cortex. This represents a limitation on the spatial resolution. This discussion is out of the scope of this book.

BOLD methods for functional brain mapping suffered from certain problems which could give false positive results, or obscure the effect altogether. It must be understood that the signal changes of interest were usually not much larger that the thermal and physiological noise which inevitably accompanied MR images of living tissues. But other issues have been the subject of controversy in the literature. These are related to the precision and localization for neural activity and to artifactual image differences associated with subject motion. These will not be discussed here. Having discussed the brief history of BOLD, we now present the algorithm that was used for the time series analysis of the BOLD data set using the Anatomically Informed Basis Functions (AIBF) technique.

4.7.4.2 AIBF Method for Time Series Analysis

There are two approaches for analyzing fMRI data sets: (**1**) Voxel-based approach and (**2**) Anatomically Informed Basis Function (AIBF)-based method. For details, see Friston *et al.* [680], [681], [682] and [689]. Very recently, Kiebel,

Goebel and Friston [326] came up with a method for performing fMRI data analysis. This sub-section presents the state-of-the-art method applied today for fMRI data analysis. Figure 4.33 shows the use of AIBF in relation to spatial MR data sets. The following are the main features of AIBF: (**1**) It incorporates prior knowledge. (**2**) It can be represented as a set of basis functions. AIBF makes the two following assumptions: (**1**) BOLD effects are on the cortical surface. (**2**) BOLD can be represented by a smooth distribution on the cortical surface. AIBF has the following features: (**1**) It does not use any additional 3-D spatial low pass filtering but directly operates on realigned unsmoothed data. (**2**) It provides superior resolution. (**3**) It can be used to differentiate among underlying signal sources. (**4**) AIBF can be used to implement an anatomical Least Squares deconvolution to remove the point spread function (PSF) effects. Having presented the assumptions on AIBF and its key features, we now briefly present the mathematical model for performing the temporal data analysis (for details, see Kiebel, Goebel and Friston [326]).   Let $\mathbf{A}$ be a matrix of $N_k \times N_p$ and b_Y^j be the basis function in voxel space, then $Y = \mathbf{A}\beta + \epsilon$, where β is the coefficient vector or parameter vector. ϵ was the residual error vector. Using Least Squares, the parameter vector $\hat{\beta}$ was given as:

$$\hat{\boldsymbol{\beta}} = (\mathbf{A}'\mathbf{A} + \lambda\mathbf{I})^{-1}\,\mathbf{A}'\mathbf{Y}\,, \qquad (4.45)$$

where λ was the regularization factor and $\mathbf{I}$ was the identity matrix. A acceptable value of λ was given as: $\frac{trace(\mathbf{A}'\mathbf{A})}{N_p}$ [52]. Thus β was the spatial distribution of activity for one time point. If the adjacent basis functions do not have any overlap or only a small overlap, the regularization factor λ turned out to be zero and the Equation (4.45) reduced to the plain Least Squares equation, given as:

$$\hat{\boldsymbol{\beta}} = (\mathbf{A}'\mathbf{A})^{-1}\,\mathbf{A}'\mathbf{Y} \qquad (4.46)$$

Voxel-Space to Vertex-Space.   Given a series of functional observations $Y_1, ... Y_{N_Y}$, Kiebel estimated for each Y_l a coefficient vector $\hat{\beta}_l$ which was estimated using Equation (4.45) to assemble a $N_Y \times N_p$ estimated parameter matrix $\mathbf{B}^T$, given as:

$$\mathbf{B}^T = [\hat{\beta}_1 | \hat{\beta}_2 | ... | \hat{\beta}_{N_Y}]\,, \qquad (4.47)$$

which represented the estimated functional observations, projected into the space of anatomically informed basis functions. The estimated signal in voxel-space was given as:

$$\mathbf{B}^T_{voxel-space} = \mathbf{A}\mathbf{B}^T\,. \qquad (4.48)$$

If the columns of the matrix $\mathbf{A}_{vertex}$ were the folded basis functions in the vertex-space b_G^j, then the estimated signal in the vertex-space was given by: $\mathbf{B}^T_{vertex} = \mathbf{A}_{vertex}\mathbf{B}^T$.

---

[52]A trace of a square matrix is the sum of squares of all the diagonal elements of that square matrix.

4.7.4.3   An Example of Temporal Data Analysis Using SVD

Let the temporal basis functions be $T = [T_1|T_2]^{53}$, where T was a $N_Y \times N_T$ matrix, N_T was the number of temporal basis functions, T_1 and T_2 are $N_Y \times N_{T_1}$, T_1 and T_2 are orthogonal to each other. $N_T = N_{T_1} + N_{T_2}$. T_1 contains the covariates of interest and T_2 the covariates of no interest. Using singular value decomposition (SVD), the effects of no interest were given as: $B_c = B - T_2(T_2'T_2)^{-1}T_2'B$. The SVD of the corrected parameter matrix B_c was given as: UWV', where U and V were orthogonal matrices and W was the diagonal matrix. Let $B_P = U_J W_J$, a $N_Y \times N_J$ matrix, where the columns of B_P contain the temporal expansion of the first N_J spatial models over observations. N_J was found by thresholding the associated singular values contained in the W as discussed in Friston *et al.* [689], and U_J and W_J were the reduced versions of U and W. Thus the temporal model was given as: $B_P = T_1\gamma + \epsilon_T$, where γ was a $N_{T_1} \times N_J$ matrix and ϵ_T a $N_Y \times N_J$ matrix. Using the Least Squares method, the $\hat{\gamma}$ was given as: $\hat{\gamma} = (T_1'T_1)^{-1}T_1'B_P$. Thus the sum of the squares and products due to error are: $R_E = (B_P - T_1\hat{\gamma})'(B_P - T_1\hat{\gamma})$. The sum of the squares and products due to the effects of interest are: $H = (T_1\hat{\gamma})'(T_1\hat{\gamma})$ and the sum of squares and products under the null hypothesis (that the effect due to T_1 do not exist) are $R_0 = B_P'B_P$. The significance of the effects of interest can be tested with Wilk's Lambda as: $\frac{R_E}{R_0}$ (see Chatfield and Colins [998]). The characterization of the significant effects employs CVA, i.e, finding the matrix of canonical images $\mathbf{C} = [\mathbf{c_1}, ..., \mathbf{c_J}]$ such that the variance ratio $(\frac{\mathbf{c}'H\mathbf{c_m}}{\mathbf{c}'R_E\mathbf{c_m}})$ was maximized successively for $m = 1, ..., J$, under the condition that $cov(\mathbf{c_m}, \mathbf{c_n}) = \mathbf{0}$ for any m and n, with $1 \leq m, n \leq J$ and m not equal to n. These canonical modes can be visualized in the voxel-space (in functional space) or in vertex-space (folded, inflated and flattened surfaces). So, we see how the functional information is analyzed and superimposed over the structural information (see Figure 4.33).

4.7.5   Measure of Cortex Geometry

Van Essen *et al.* [448] showed two methods for measuring the overall surface geometry of the cortex. We will briefly present the methods here:

1. Intrinsic curvature index (ICI):

$$ICI = \frac{1}{4\pi} \int \int k_{max} \, k_{min} \, dA, \tag{4.49}$$

   where k_{max} and k_{min} are the maximum and minimum curvature values, respectively.

2. Folding index (FI):

$$FI = \frac{1}{4\pi} \int \int k_{max} \, (k_{max} - k_{min}) \, dA. \tag{4.50}$$

---

[53] Not to be confused with T_1- and T_2-weighted MR images.

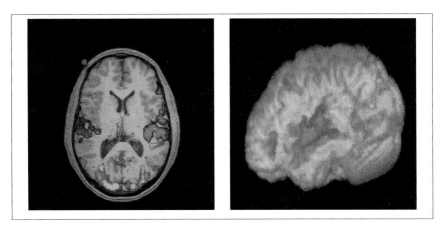

Figure 4.34: **Left**: fMRI data superimposed over the spatial transverse slice of the brain. **Right**: fMRI data superimposed over the 3-D rendered brain (Courtesy of Steve Smith, FMRIB Centre, John Radcliffe Hospital, Headington, Oxford, UK).

4.8 Discussions: Advantages, Validation and New Challenges in 2-D and 3-D Cortical Segmentation Techniques

This sub-section summarizes the salient features of the most successful approaches to cortical 2-D and 3-D segmentation. This includes the advantages of the regional-based geometric boundary/surfaces cortical segmentation, which are discussed in Sub-section 4.8.1. A discussion on the validation of cortical segmentation algorithms is presented in Sub-section 4.8.2. The challenges in 2-D and 3-D cortical segmentation are discussed in Sub-section 4.8.3.

4.8.1 Advantages of Regional Geometric Boundary/Surfaces

We have seen that in both 2-D and 3-D segmentation schemes, the dominant techniques have been the deformable models integrated with regularization terms, classification terms and terms which handle the knowledge and *a-priori* information, i.e., regional level sets/volumetric level sets. Here we will summarize the key features and advantages of the deformable models based on the level sets. Overall, the following are the key advantages of the geometric-based techniques fused with region/volumes: (**1**) The greatest advantage of this technique is that this algorithm increases the "capture range" of the field flow and thereby increases the robustness of the initial contour placement. Anywhere that the contour/surface is placed in the image/volume, it will find the object to segment itself. (**2**) The key characteristic of this system is that it is based on region, so the local noise or edge will not distract the growth process. (**3**) The technique is non-local and thus the local noise cannot distract the final placement of the contour or the diffusion growth process. (**4**) It is not controlled by the elasticity coefficients, unlike parametric contour methods. There is no need to fit the tangents to the curves and compute the normals at each vertex. In such a system, the normals are embedded in the system using the divergence of the field flow. (**5**) The technique is very suitable for medical organ segmentation since it can handle any of the cavities, concavities, convolutedness, splitting or merging. (**6**) There is no problem finding the local minima or global minima, unlike the optimization techniques of parametric snakes. (**7**) This technique is less prone to normal computational error which is very easily incorporated in the classical balloon force snakes for segmentation. (**8**) It is very easy to extend this model from semi-automatic to completely automatic because the region is determined on the basis of prior information. (**9**) This technique is based on the propagation of curves (just like the propagation of ripples in a tank or the propagation of flames in a fire) utilizing the region statistics. (**10**) This method adjusts to the topological changes of the given shape. Diffusion propagation methods are a very natural framework for handling topological changes (the joining and breaking of the curves). (**11**) The technique can be applied to unimodal, bimodal and multi-modal imagery, which means it can have multiple gray level values in it. (**12**) It implements the fast marching method in the narrow band for solving the Eikonal Equation for computing the signed distances. (**13**) One can segment any part of the brain depending upon the membership function in fuzzy clustering. (**14**) It is easily extendable to higher dimensions. (**15**) It can easily incorporate other features for controlling the speed of the curve. This is done by adding an extra term to the region, gradient and curvature speed terms. (**16**) The system takes care of the corners easily unlike the parametric curves, where special handling is needed at the corners of the boundary. (**17**) The technique is extendable to multi-scale resolutions, which means that at lower resolutions, one can compute regional segmentations. These segmented results can then be used for higher resolutions. (**18**) This technique is extendable to multi-phase, which means that if there are multiple level set functions, then they automatically merge and split during the course of the segmentation process.

4.8.2 Validation of 2-D and 3-D Cortical Segmentation Algorithms

Segmentation methods are often measured through their accuracy, efficiency and repeatability. Depending on the particular application, one objective may outweigh the others. While accuracy is the first priority for the quantitative measurement of brain structures, image visualization applications require efficiency as the most desired feature. Efficiency of brain segmentation algorithms can be measured objectively, however, accuracy and repeatability are more a subjective matter due to the lack of ground truth. There are two approaches that are often taken to provide surrogate ground truth: simulation through a brain phantom and the use of a manual tracing result. An example of generating the brain phantom is generating the metasphere, which is a 3-D surface model that has convolutedness similar to a *true cortex*. An example of a metasphere is shown in the work by Yu *et al.* [626]. Notable work has been done by the McConnell Brain Imaging Center at the Montreal Neurological Institute on the simulation of image data from a brain phantom [653]. The Center for Morphometric Analysis at the Massachusetts General Hospital has taken the trouble to assemble a repository of brain images and corresponding manual segmentations by experts [654]. Such work permits a standardized mechanism for the evaluation of segmentation methods and encourages their new development and application. Very recently, Grabowski *et al.* [628] published a paper on the validation of tissue segmentation of single-channel MRI of the brain. This paper discusses the validation scheme on local statistical mixture modeling for segmenting T_1-weighted MRI images of the brain. A detailed discussion of the cortical segmentation techniques is out of the scope of this chapter. Interested readers can refer to the previously mentioned articles.

4.8.3 Challenges in 2-D and 3-D Cortical Segmentation Algorithms

Even though as of today we have a number of computer graphics, vision and image processing (CGVIP) techniques, we still have not established a gold standard as to which technique is best for a particular application. For example, in 2-D segmentation, fused deformable models are becoming the most successful and dominant method. In 3-D segmentation, active surface fused with clustering and constrained active surface are becoming more successful and efficient. The question still remains if we can develop fast and intelligent cortical segmentation techniques which can become the abstract method fulfilling the majority of clinical needs. Some of the challenges being investigated are discussed below (for details, see the challenge and requirement chapter by Ayache *et al.* in [629], articles by Haacke *et al.* [630], and Turner *et al.* [631], and the book by Kaufman *et al.* [632]). (**1**) *MRI System and Scanning:* it is a challenge to produce images of high spatial resolution while also keeping the temporal resolution high. Besides that, it will be a more of a challenge to build compact MRI machines which are dedicated to certain applications. (**2**) *Inhomogeneity Correction:* the quality of segmentation largely depends upon the spatial resolution of the MR data volume produced by the scanner. One of the challenges which image processing researchers are facing is the intensity non-homogeneity correction (see Vokurka *et al.* [633] and Volker *et al.* [640]). (**3**) *Improving the Signal to Noise (S/N) Ratio:* one of the requirements in segmentation is to have high S/N ratio images (see Alexander *et al.* [663]) to work with. The image segmentation pipeline is highly dependent on the quality of smoothing one uses. Both 2-D and 3-D segmentation (surface reconstruction and volume rendering) are affected by the quality of smoothing one uses. If the smoothing is very good, the pixel classification in 2-D is robust (see page 180, Bomans *et al.* [479]), thus the performance of the morphological filters is optimal. Similarly, the voxel classification in volume rendering is better if the initial images are noise free.

(**4**) *Initialization of the Curves and Surfaces in Deformable Models:* initial placements of the curves/surfaces for cortical boundary/surface estimation is also one of the challenges (see Neuenschwander *et al.* [635]). Even though level sets have proved to be robust and have a large capture range for curve/surface estimation, the initial symmetry could become a challenging task (see Kimia *et al.* [636], Siddiqi *et al.* [637], Stoll *et al.* [638] and Tek *et al.* [639]). (**5**) *Quantification of Cortical Topography:* Robust quantification tools for studying the cortical topography is another area where challenge lies. This involves finding the deeply buried sulci and gyri and estimating the skeletons (see Malandain *et al.* [641]) and curvatures (see Zeng [616]). Besides these, we have to measure the sub-cortical structures (see the work by Brady and his co-workers [642], [643]). (**6**) *General and Robust Segmentation for Varying System and Tissue Parameters:* efficiently computing key features of the brain and then using them as an *a-priori* information to improve the robustness of the overall brain segmentation system. Effort is still needed where one can efficiently handle the large variability of the data sets (with anatomy, pathology) using this kind of information. (**7**) *Validation:* another set of challenges is in the validation of the image processing and graphics techniques developed for MR brain data segmentation. This is especially necessary when more than four classes of tissue types exist in complex brain pathology and have different kinds of neurological disorders. This becomes even more necessary when the functional information gathered from fMRI has started to be investigated (see Suri *et al.* [247], Zwehl *et al.* [248], Aboutanous *et al.* [623] and Vannier *et al.* [624]). (**8**) *Integrating Fast 3-D Segmentation in Daily Therapy in Real-Time:* interventional MR techniques require fast and robust 3-D segmentation, which is still a challenge to be conquered. Superimposition of the complex vasculature in real-time along with the 3-D reconstruction of the brain helps neuro-surgeons to perform successful surgery, which is still a challenge. An attempt has been made by Osher and Sethian [536], Suri [322] and Vemuri *et al.* [362] to speed up model fitting and brain segmentation methods.

4.8.4   Challenges in fMRI

With the growth in technology in fMRI and medical devices, there are still many issues which need to be resolved. Some of them are: (**1**) reduction of the acoustic scanner noise during fMRI data collection; (**2**) spatial smoothing of the fMRI data; (**3**) alignment of the fMRI images with the anatomical images due to head movements; (**4**) robust development of the canonical images using the time course fMRI data; (**5**) real-time 3-D reconstruction of the brain anatomy to superimpose the functional information; (**6**) developing a fusion of functional tasks such as size, color and motion; (**7**) exploration of BOLD fMRI for pre-surgical planning and treatment; (**8**) fusion of fMRI with EEG and MEG data sets for studying brain pathology and physiology; (**9**) fusion of fMRI with brain perfusion imaging for understanding the blood flow during the actions of complex functions; (**10**) analyzation of the experimental data, also called time series data; (**11**) finding how much functional information (stimulus) is disintegrated into different cortical regions of the brain. A very powerful approach for estimating this would be to use the pixel classification approach to classify the fMRI data corresponding to each functionality independently.

4.9   Conclusions and the Future

State-of-the-art brain segmentation techniques in 2-D and 3-D were first presented, given the nature of the MRI brain images and the objective behind the brain segmentation. The major thrust of this chapter was on three kinds of segmentation techniques: region-based, boundary/surface-based and the fusion of region and boundary/surface-based. We saw that the fusion-based techniques are the most powerful, robust and accurate. Fusion-based techniques using geometric deformable models turned out to be the most successful in grabbing the topology of the brain, both in 2-D and 3-D. This chapter presented these fusion algorithms/systems which are the state-of-the-art in cortical segmentation and concluded with a discussion of the salient features of such fusion techniques, the validation of cortical segmentation algorithms and challenges in cortical segmentation.

The Future: Mathematical Techniques, Clinical Applications and Therapy. We have started to see the use of pixel classification merged with deformable models for cortical segmentation in 2-D and 3-D deformable models fused with clustering approaches in cortical segmentation. With time, we will see the use of cortical segmentation in the functional aspect of brain segmentation. We hope to see more clinical applications of the reconstructed brain from deformable models to deform to a flat surface or sphere which can be overlaid on the functional MRI data to study neurological disorders. We will also see more growth in mathematical techniques for parametric deformation models (see Xu *et al.* [644]) and geometric deformable models (see Suri [645]) since they offer an attractive approach to medical image segmentation. We hope to see more sophisticated tools for the extraction of human cortical topography (see Rettmann *et al.* [646], [647] and Lohmann *et al.* [648], [649]). We also hope to see the application of unification of low level vision techniques in the parametric domain (see Liang *et al.* [650], [651]) or in the geometric domain (see Paragios *et al.* [652]).

We will see more web sites like the ones from McConnell Brain Imaging Center, Montreal Neurological Institute, McGill University [653] and Massachusetts General Hospital [654] coming up and making generic systems for everyone to compare and share their algorithms for cortical segmentation. As we have seen the use of brain segmentation is starting to become a daily part of any therapy system, neurosurgeons, oncologists, neuroradiologists, internists, and psychiatrists have already started to use brain segmentation systems to a large extent to evaluate the patient's conditions during and after surgery, and during and after therapy. We do, however, need more monitoring of brain changes over time in patients with disease. In the future, we hope to see that brain segmentation will become one of the critical components as the role of fMRI increases, the MR system moves into the operating room and dedicated and more compact MRI systems are developed (see Jolesz *et al.* [655], [656]).

4.9.1 Acknowledgements

The first author expresses special thanks to Elaine Keeler and John Patrick, both with Marconi Medical Systems, Inc., for their encouragements. Thanks go to Marconi Medical Systems, Inc., for the MR data sets. Our thanks go to Springer Verlag, Academic Press, and IEEE Press for permission to reproduce material from their respective journals. Thanks are also due to Anthony Goreham, Oxford, UK, for clarifying some of the LaTeX issues.

Chapter 5

Segmentation Techniques in the Quantification of Multiple Sclerosis Lesions in MRI

Rakesh Sharma, Jasjit S. Suri, Ponnada A. Narayana

5.1 Introduction

Volumetry of the brain can provide fundamental information about the development and function of the normal human brain and can yield important clues for pathology in patients suffering from neurological brain disorders (see Jernigan *et al.* [713]). Valuable information has been gained about the pathological processes in epilepsy (see Stone *et al.* [714]) and Alzheimer's disease (see Tanabe *et al.* [715]) from the volume measurements of various brain structures. Brain tissue in Alzheimer's disease was compared with elderly control volunteers by using an MR-based computerized segmentation program. Semi-automated segmentation of MR brain images revealed significant brain atrophy with significant white matter hyperintensities. In many focal diseases such as Multiple Sclerosis (MS) and cancer, the total lesion volume is indicative of the overall disease burden and may be useful in the quantification and objective evaluation of therapeutic intervention in disease (see Dastidar *et al.* [716] and Fillippi *et al.* [717]). These investigators demonstrated that MRI images provide excellent quantitative MRI tissue volume measurement. Different tissues can be identified on the images, either manually or by computer-assisted means for computing the volumes. The process of identifying and isolating a given tissue is generally referred to as segmentation. Segmentation allows color-coding of different tissues for improved delineation and makes for easier visual identification of pathology. Segmentation is evaluated as being useful in radiation therapy (see Vaidyanathan *et al.* [718]) and for simulating sensitive procedures for interventional neurosurgery (see Dickson *et al.* [719]). Evaluation of a semi-Supervised Fuzzy C-Means (SFCM) clustering method was used for monitoring brain tumor volume changes. This method's results were compared with others: a) a k-Nearest Neighbor (k-NN); b) gray level thresholding and the Iterative Seed Growing (ISG-SG) method; c) manual pixel labeling by Ground Truth (GT). The SFCM and k-NN methods were applied to multi-spectral, contrast-enhanced T_1-weighted, proton density weighted, T_2-weighted

318

MR images whereas the ISG-SG and GT methods were applied to contrast enhanced T_1-weighted images. These approaches were compared with manually labeled ground truth estimations that exhibited limited agreement between these methods for absolute tumor volume with less than 10% intra-observer reproducibility. However, multi-spectral k-NN and SFCM methods were preferred over the seed growing method. In another study, the authors emphasized simulating the brain evaluation of brain tumors such as acoustic neuroma from head MR images. These tumors could be detected by a neural network, a multi-layer perceptron (MLP), to classify images at the pixel level to achieve the target of segmentation by using gray levels of square of pixels. This method was combined with edge region based segmentation and morphological operation. This produced a cluster of adjacent regions considered to be tumor regions. Each possible combination of these regions allows feature identification and tumor interpretation. This approach is significant for figuring false positive errors in these images.

Segmentation is a critical step in tissue volumetry and quantification. Accurate segmentation and quantification of a given tissue volume depends on the contrast-to-noise ratio in an image. The introduction of magnetic resonance imaging (MRI) into the clinical arena increased interest in tissue segmentation for at least two reasons. Firstly MRI provides superb soft tissue contrast which allows clear identification and segmentation of different soft tissues, such as Gray Matter (GM), White Matter (WM), and Cerebrospinal Fluid (CSF) in brain MRI. Second, MRI provides a multi-parametric modality in the sense that simply changing the scan parameters or pulse sequences can alter tissue contrast. This multi-parametric nature of MRI plays an important role in image segmentation. The main focus of this chapter is on the quantification of MS lesions in the brain. Multiple Sclerosis is the most common demyelinating disease in humans (see Kikinis *et al.* [720]). MR examinations were segmented into four tissue image types using a self-adaptive statistical algorithm. Partial Volume-based misclassification could be corrected by a combination of morphological operators and connectivity criteria. The reproducibility of the system was superior to supervised segmentation, evidenced by the coefficient of variation. Computerized procedures allowed routine quantitative analysis of large serial MRI data sets. MS is a complex disease with a relapsing remitting course (see Udupa [721]). 3-D operation is classified under four basic headings: reprocessing, visualization, manipulation and analysis. There are many challenges involving the matters of precision, accuracy and efficiency in 3-D imaging, which is an exciting technology. This promises to offer an expanding number and variety of applications. MRI is the radioimaging modality of choice for the non-invasive visualization of lesions and the clinical follow-up of MS patients. Recent studies suggest that MRI is capable of detecting the sub-clinical activity of neuronal tissue (see Guttman *et al.* [722]) and that MRI-defined lesion burden(or lesion volume) may provide an objective measure of the disease's severity. Therefore, there is considerable interest in using MRI-estimated quantitative lesion load as a valuable measure in clinical trials (see O'Riordan *et al.* [723], Molyneux *et al.* [724], Vinitski *et al.* [725]). Such an outcome measure may considerably reduce the cost of conducting clinical trials, since fewer patients are required to achieve statistical significance. This is particularly relevant in view of the large number of ongoing clinical trials for treating MS patients.

5.2   Segmentation Techniques

Segmentation includes the classification of tissues in images. It can be performed using a variety of techniques that have been recently reviewed (see Magnotta *et al.* [726], Joshi *et al.* [727], Karayiannis *et al.* [728], Velthuizen *et al.* [729], Harris *et al.* [731], Dale *et al.* [732], Pachai *et al.* [733], van Waesberghe *et al.* [734], Manousakas *et al.* [735], Glass *et al.* [736], Lee *et al.* [737], Heinonen *et al.* [738], Clark *et al.* [739], Atkins *et al.* [740]). Several new MR image segmentation methods are covered in the above-mentioned works, along with assessment of their advantages and limitations. Among these methods are the use of Artificial Neural Networks to measure brain structures in two- and three-dimensional applications (ANNs are capable of measuring distinct structures accurately); the use of fuzzy algorithms for learning vector quantification in brain segmentation; MRI segmentation based on feature extraction of the brain tissue (where the features represent well-defined boundaries); a new Locally Excitatory Globally Inhibitory Oscillator Network (LEGION) segmentation method for medical images (this method still needs further evaluation); and a 3-D multi-spectral discriminant analysis method with automated training class selection which has resulted in improved tissue classification in MRI. This method involves three White Matter segmentation methods and the generation of the cortical surfaces using: local parametric modeling and Bayesian segmentation, surface generation, local quadratic co-ordinate fitting and surface editing. Results for macaque brains were automated and compared for surface generation.

A segmentation method was recently proposed (see Bedell *et al.* [741]) based on dual echo MR images and described as being prone to classifying false MS lesions. It used: (1) improved lesion-tissue contrast on MR images using a fast spin echo sequence involving both CSF signal attenuation and magnetization transfer contrast, and (2) information from MR flow images. This dual approach to tissue segmentation was enough to reduce 87% of the false lesion classifications. One of the authors (see Bedell *et al.* [32]) reported automatic detection and quantification of contrast enhanced lesions in MRI in MS disease staging with the mention of blood-brain-barrier complications. This method was designed based on stationary and marching saturation bands and gradient dephasing for suppressing the enhancements within the cerebral vasculature. A postprocessing technique based on automatic image segmentation was implemented to identify and eliminate enhancing structures such as the choroid plexus and to identify areas with minimal or no false lesions.

Segmentation based on the fuzzy algorithm was used for learning vector quantification by updating all prototypes of a competitive network by the unsupervised learning process. The experiments evaluated a variety of Fuzzy Algorithms for Learning Vector Quantitation (FALVQ) in terms of the ability to identify different abnormal tissues as distinct from normal tissue. Cortical surface-based analysis for segmentation and surface reconstruction was used routinely in functional brain MR imaging. A pyramidal approach to the automatic segmentation of multiple sclerosis lesions in the brain MRI was proposed for quantitative assessment of the lesion load. The systematic pyramidal decomposition in the frequency domain provided a robust and flexible low level tool for MR image analysis. The best MR correlations using surface-based thresholding segmentation techniques to obtain the $\frac{T_1}{T_2}$ ratio and magnetization transfer ratio for lesion parameters were evaluated. The split and merge segmentation technique for magnetic resonance images was analyzed for performance evaluation and extension into three dimensions. Hybrid artificial neural network segmentation and classification of dynamic contrast-enhanced MR imaging (DEMRI) for osteosarcoma was reported as non-invasive visualization of necrotic and viable tumors without inter- and intra-operator errors between methods or operator bias. Comparison of pre- versus post-contrast loads and of manual versus semi-automated threshold techniques for lesion segmentation demonstrated T_1 hypointense lesion load in secondary progressive multiple sclerosis. An algorithm for automated unsupervised connectivity-based thresholding segmentation of mid-sagittal brain MR images was evaluated for developing a robust method. A semi-automatic window-based image processing method using a graphic interface enabled a combination of different segmentation methods. Automatic tumor segmentation using multispectral analysis by knowledge-based segmentation provided separation of intracranial region extraction along cluster centers for each class. A fully robust automatic brain MRI using anisotropic filters and the "snake contour" technique with an *a priori* knowledge-based method was evaluated for multi-stage refining of the brain outline. Of all these techniques, three methods have been predominantly employed for the segmentation of MS lesions (see Bedell *et al.* [748]). These methods are: (1) manual tracing, (2) intensity-based single image segmentation, and (3) multi-spectral methods. Both manual tracing and thresholding are simple to use and required relatively little additional software development in our lab. However, these techniques were prone to operator bias, were time consuming, and impractical for analyzing a large number of images. The accuracy of these techniques depends on well-maintained quality control over the method.

5.2.1 Multi-Spectral Techniques

A unique feature of MRI is the ability to alter the relative contrast of tissues simply by manipulating the pulse sequences and/or sequence parameters. For instance, both MS lesions and CSF appear bright on T_2-weighted spin echo images. On the other hand, MS lesions appear bright on proton density-weighted images while CSF appears somewhat isointense with the rest of the brain parenchyma. In T_1-weighted images, MS lesions generally appear isointense with the parenchyma and CSF appears hypointense. Multi-spectral segmentation techniques based on multiple image sets exploit the powerful multi-parametric nature of MRI. In contrast, both manual tracing and thresholding techniques are performed using a single set of images. Multi-spectral segmentation techniques are generally more robust since they combine information from multiple image sets with different contrasts for tissue classification. The concept of multiple-spectral segmentation was originally developed for the classification of the earth's surface based on images acquired with a Land Remote Sensing Satellite (LANDSAT). LANDSAT was the name used by NASA for satellites designed for monitoring the earth's resources. The sensors of LANDSAT acquired images at different spectral wavelengths. Each frame of LANDSAT imagery consists of four images of the same scene acquired in the red, green and two infrared spectral channels. Combining information from all four images then generates the segmented image. Similar multi-spectral techniques can be applied by combining data from multiple MR images with different contrasts to classify an image into different tissue classes (see Mohamed *et al.* [742]). The input images used for tissue classification are referred to as "features". The pixel intensities of the basic set of images are generally referred to as "feature vectors". Therefore, if two sets of images are utilized, their respective sets of intensities ($a1$ and $a2$) form the feature vector $a=a1,a2$.

Multiple-spectral segmentation can be performed either by "feature space-based" or by "non-feature space-based" methods. Non-feature space-based techniques such as Artificial Neural Network-based techniques (see Lee *et al.* [737]), adaptive segmentation (see Burghart *et al.* [743]), the model-based techniques (see Summers *et al.* [744]), and unsupervised automated multispectral relaxometric methods (see Alfano *et al.* [745]) have recently been proposed. These authors addressed the problem of the variability of the individual anatomy and different characteristics of the scanning systems. They developed an anatomy knowledge-based system to improve the recognition of structures in CT or MRI scans. During the last decade, the quality of MR angiograms has risen substantially and their clinical utility has been demonstrated progressively based upon the model-based segmentation technique, which was proven to be effective for multi-resolution data structure for recursive decision-making. This allowed for more efficient data handling in subsequent processing and visualization of the connected graph model of the vascular regions. The above-mentioned authors extracted vascular morphology and local flow parameters from phase contrast MR angiograms (PC-MRA). They developed a multi-spectral segmentation method based on two spin echo sequences and used unsupervised, automated segmentation of the tissue voxels in a 3-D spectrum of the brain to automatically segment the GM, WM and CSF and to measure the tissue volumes. They tested the reproducibility and accuracy of three measurements by using a three brain compartment phantom. In the feature-space based, multi-spectral segmentation technique, the feature vector is typically plotted in an n-dimensional space, referred to as the "feature space", where n is the order of the vector. In a two dimensional (2-D) feature space, for example, the abscissa corresponds to the pixel intensities in one image, while the ordinate corresponds to intensities in a second image. For instance, $n=2$, if dual echo images are used for segmentation. Pixels comprising an image can be plotted in feature space to generate the "scatter plot". Plate 7 shows feature maps for Attenuation of Fluid by Fast Inversion Recovery with Magnetization Transfer Imaging with Variable Echoes (AFFIRMATIVE), an MR image set showing points plotted in 2-D feature space for three tissue classes: WM, GM and CSF. In an ideal case, one can see clearly clustering of different tissues in the feature space. Based upon these clusters, it is possible to classify different tissues and calculate the individual volumes by using a Magnetic Resonance Image Automated Processing (MRIAP) program. Each tissue is assigned an arbitrary, but unique, color for the visual inspection of the images. In fact, considerable overlap exists between these clusters, resulting in some ambiguity in tissue classification due to limited tissue contrast and image noise.

5.2.2 Feature Space Classification

The pixels from different tissues often form "clusters" in feature space, arising from the differences in signal intensities among the tissues. As the contrast between the tissue increases, the clusters become further separated. Due to considerable overlap between different tissues in the feature space, it is essential to utilize statistical techniques for partitioning the feature space into different tissue classes. This can be accomplished using a "feature space classifier" which can be either supervised or unsupervised. Supervised multi-spectral segmentation techniques are our main focus and will be described here. Unsupervised techniques, such as those based on fuzzy logic and fuzzy connectivity (see Jackson *et al.* [746]) are not described here. Semi-automated segmentation of dual contrast MR images was used for measuring the total brain volume of GM, WM, and CSF. The results showed intra-observer and inter-observer reproducibility. Supervised methods permit the operator to select representative points from the WM, GM and CSF, each of the different tissue types, to generate "training data sets" of data, while the unsupervised methods automatically find the structure in the scatter plot. In the supervised segmentation technique, the partitioned feature space is generally referred to as the "feature map". The feature map is essentially used as a "look-up table" to classify each pixel in the image into the appropriate tissue classes and, thereby, generate the segmented image.

5.2.3 Supervised Segmentation

Supervised segmentation techniques require the operator to select representative points from each of the different tissue types. The training data set is collected by sampling 30 to 40 points from the segmented image data set. These points are plotted in the feature space and a feature classifier is invoked. This partitions the feature space based upon this training set data (see Jackson *et al.* [746]). This feature space classifier can be either of the following: (i) parametric Maximum Likelihood Method (MLM); (ii) non-parametric k-

Nearest Neighbors (*k*-NN); and (iii) Parzen window. These points are plotted in the feature space and a feature space classifier is invoked which partitions the feature space based on this training data set. The space classifier is generally a statistical technique, which can be either parametric (Maximum Likelihood Method (MLM)) or nonparametric (*k*-nearest neighbors and Parzen window). The maximum likelihood method assumes a particular distribution of the features, usually a multi-variate Gaussian distribution. For each of the tissues, the means and covariance matrices are estimated from the training set. Each pixel in the image is then classified by determining the likelihood for each possible tissue class and assigning the one with the maximum likelihood. The MLM method is based on the Bayes decision function, $d(x)$, for a tissue class (j) which has the form:

$$d_j(x) = p(x|j) \, \mathbf{P}(j) \qquad (5.1)$$

where x is the feature vector, η is the arbitrary constant whose value is 3.1. $p(x|j)$ is the probability density function (PDF) and $\mathbf{P}(j)$ is the *a priori* probability for class (j). In the n-dimensional case, the PDF is given by the Gaussian function:

$$p(x|j) \;\; = \;\; \frac{1}{(2\eta)^{\frac{n}{2}} \, |C_j|^{\frac{1}{2}}} \; \exp\{\frac{-1}{2}(x - m_j)^T \, C_j^{-1} \, (x - m_j)\} \qquad (5.2)$$

where m_j is the mean vector and C_j is the covariance matrix, both of which were determined from the training set. The classification process typically assumes that *a priori* probabilities of the tissue classes are equal. For each point in feature space, then, the PDF for each tissue class is calculated and the point is assigned to the tissue class with the highest decision function, i.e. the maximum likelihood.

Clarke *et al.*[747] have recently compared parametric and non-parametric techniques and reported that the *k*-NN technique is optimum both in terms of accuracy and stability. The *k*-NN method does not assume a particular distribution of the data, rather it uses the actual distribution of the training data itself (i.e., it is non-parametric). The *k*-NN algorithm basically classifies each point in feature space into tissue classes based on its proximity to the training points. The "nearest" training points are determined using a distance measure, usually the Euclidean distance. Therefore, the k (a value selected by the operator) neighbors with the smallest distances from a point in feature space, x_j, become the k nearest neighbors and form the neighborhood about x_j. The total distance x_i includes assigned neighboring points. The point x_j is labeled by determining the tissue class, which is most frequently represented by the k nearest neighbors. Suppose the operator selects $k = 7$ nearest neighbors within a circular neighborhood, which surround the point x_j, three neighbors should belong to class A, two to class B, and two to class C. The point x_j is assigned to class A. This process is repeated over all the points in feature space to generate the appropriate tissue classifications based on the *k*-NN method.

The Parzen technique falls in the same category as the *k*-NN technique and is more appropriate for low dimensional feature space. A Parzen technique is a supervised technique as an operator input is required to generate a training set and also assures convergence for a smaller sample size. In it, the neighborhood about a feature space point x_j is determined by a window function, rather than by the k-nearest neighbors. The Parzen window about x_j can be defined as:

$$p_n(x) = \frac{1}{n} \Sigma \frac{1}{h_n} \phi(u) \tag{5.3}$$

where h_n and $\phi(u)$ are given as:

$$h_n = \frac{h_i}{\sqrt{n}} \tag{5.4}$$

$$\phi(u) = \frac{1}{\sqrt{2\eta}} \exp \frac{-1}{2} u^2 , \tag{5.5}$$

where u is given as:

$$u = \frac{x_i - x_j}{h_n} \tag{5.6}$$

In the above equations, the value of the parameter h_n controls the relative size of the Parzen window and is selected by the operator. The choice of h_n can affect the location of the border between two tissue classes and therefore alters the feature space classification. Once an appropriate value of h_i has been selected, each point in feature space is classified by determining the class with the greatest number of training points contained within the Parzen window. Repeating this process again generates the feature map for all points in the feature space.

5.2.4 Unsupervised Segmentation

Unsupervised segmentation does not require any training data for feature map generation. Feature space classification is achieved by the automatic determination of the inherent structure in the scatter plot. Two similar techniques are capable of providing unsupervised feature space classification, namely the k-means and the fuzzy c-means techniques. Although unsupervised algorithms perform automatic classification, the operator still must assign a particular tissue class to each classified region of feature space.

5.2.4.1 k-Means Algorithm

The k-means method is an iterative procedure, which identifies compact tissue clusters. The algorithm iteratively minimizes the object function:

$$J(x, v) = \sum_{i=1}^{n} \sum_{j=1}^{k} ||x_i - v_j||^2 \tag{5.7}$$

where x_i is a point in feature space, v_j is the cluster center of class j, and k is the number of tissue classes. Essentially, the algorithm minimizes the distance between the cluster centers in order to determine the most compact clusters. In the Fuzzy C-Means algorithm (FCM) the membership value of a pixel essentially serves as a weighting factor in the objective function J. The fuzzy nature of the FCM method, therefore, takes into account the apparent overlapping intensities of different tissues which can arise, for example, due to the partial volume averaging effect present in MR images. A single "master" feature map for segmentation of all the images may be performed by using the intensity normalization on all the data sets which allows the automatic segmentation of MR images, eliminating the operator bias in less time for segmentation.

Non-feature space techniques: these perform multi-spectral image segmentation without the use of feature space by nonstatistical classifier techniques. The prototypical non feature space-based technique is the Artificial Neural Network (ANN). This method is based upon Artificial Intelligence (AI) and basically uses the feature vector as an input, makes various decisions based upon this input, and then directly generates the segmented images. The ANN is modeled on the manner in which neurons in the brain are thought to interconnect. Therefore, a structure of individual units (neurons or nodes), usually comprised of multiple parallel layers, is designed with connections between the individual units. Each node receives input data, performs various operations, and then outputs the resulting data via a single or multiple connections to other nodes. The training or "learning" process occurs by altering the strength of each connection.

Most neural networks designed for image segmentation use a feed-forward architecture where all data proceeds in a forward direction, i.e. from input to output nodes, without any data being fed in the reverse direction. Providing an input set of data and a typical desired output data set generally performs the training. The weights of each node are then adjusted by feeding the data in a backward direction, and performing error analysis and corrections at each stage. The procedure is referred to as "back-propagation". Essentially, back-propagation minimizes the error between the output of the network and the training data by iteratively varying the strength of the connections between the various nodes. The ANN is considered a supervised technique, since it requires the operator to generate training data. Multi-spectral segmentation techniques mostly utilize the non-parametric supervised methods (k-NN, Parzen window) as they are the most stable. They are semi-automatic techniques which use dual echo images (such as proton density-weighted and T_2-weighted images) as input images (see Reddick *et al.* [503]). An operator is needed to generate a training set.

Input images such as T_1-weighted and Magnetization Transfer Contrast (MTC) images are used for accurate classifications of GM, WM, and CSF, although this generates a large number of false positive and false negative lesion classifications, mainly due to the limited Lesion-to-Tissue Contrast (LTC). Therefore, accurate lesion segmentation requires manual intervention which introduces significant operator bias and increases the analysis time. Hence, segmentation techniques based on conventional MR images offer lesion quantification with limited success. Moreover, using intensity normalization on all the data sets, it is possible to utilize a single "master" feature map for segmentation. This master map allows the automatic segmentation of MR images and reduces operator bias and the time requirement.

5.2.5 Automatic Segmentation

To avoid more time consumption, the AFFIRMATIVE algorithm is used to perform automatic lesion enhancement into two discrete components: one to identify all contrast enhancements, and the other to identify and eliminate non-lesion enhancements based on a search for pixels in post-contrast images by a predetermined threshold. The pre-contrast and post-contrast image sets are co-registered using the 3-D algorithm. After spatial registration of the pre-contrast and post-contrast images, the average intensity and standard deviation over all slice locations in the pre-contrast image set are computed. Next, the difference in pixel intensity between pixel(i,j) in the pre-contrast image and the corresponding pixel in the post-contrast image is computed for all the pixels. Pixel (i,j) would be considered to exhibit possible contrast enhancement only if $(i > 2)$. Pixel by pixel, post-contrast and pre-contrast images are compared to identify contrast enhancements. This procedure is susceptible to false classifications from a number of sources. These false classifications can be eliminated completely or minimized for robust image segmentation as shown in Plate 8. Through the use of this algorithm, false classification from regions of flow ghosts can be identified based on pixel intensities outside the region of the head. Thus the combination of intensity thresholding and flow ghost identification minimizes a large number of false classifications of the contrast enhancements, leaving only the problem of discriminating lesion enhancements from the other remaining contrast enhancements.

5.3 AFFIRMATIVE Images

It was observed that the quality of MS lesion quantification, irrespective of the segmentation technique used, depends on the Lesion-to-Tissue Contrast (LTC). Lesions appear in the peri-ventricular regions mostly and experience considerable partial volume averaging with the CSF, which degrades the LTC; on the other hand, the LTC is improved by suppressing the CSF without lesion suppression. Moreover, the FLAIR (Fluid Attenuation by Inversion Recovery) method improves the LTC significantly by suppressing the CSF. Multiple Sclerosis lesions mostly occur in the White Matter around the ventricles, which needs be to suppressed to visualize lesions without their signal intensity being lost. This could be done to some extent by exploiting the Magnetization Transfer Ratios (MTR) between the WM and the lesions because of the higher MTR of the WM. This introduction of MTR and CSF suppression into a single imaging sequence improves the LTC. In this pursuit, an imaging sequence AFFIRMATIVE (Attenuation of Fluid by Fast Recovery with Magnetization Transfer Imaging with Variable Echoes) was designed (see Bedell *et al.* [748]),

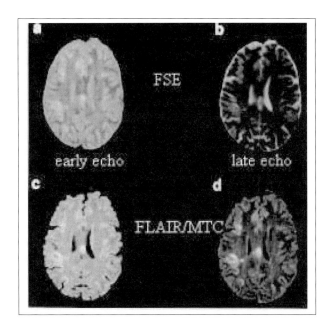

Figure 5.1: Axial MR images of a patient with MS using FSE and AFFIRMA-
TIVE pulse sequences. Lesions can be seen clearly in the early- and late-echo
FLAIR/MTC images (c and d), as compared to the FSE images (a and b).
Reproduced by permission of John Wiley & Sons Inc. from [748]. © 1997.

generating four images per slice. These correspond to early and late echo Fast
Spin Echo (FSE) images and early echo and late echo images which incorporate both MTC and FLAIR (FLAIR/MTC images). Figure 5.1 shows improved
LTC in the late echo FLAIR/MTC (d), compared to the FSE images (a and
b) which can be easily seen. In the cortical and sub-cortical areas, lesions not
visible in FSE images can be clearly seen in FLAIR/MTC images. Visualization of cortical and sub-cortical MS lesions appears to be an important aspect
in diagnosing MS patients.

5.4 Image Pre-Processing

Prior to lesion quantification, MS pathology rich tissue composition and selective brain image pre-processing are required for better lesion visualization. For
instance, MS lesion quantification is performed in a series of image processing
techniques including the following: image anisotropic diffusion filtration for
better Signal-to-Noise Ratio (SNR); correction of Radio-Frequency (RF) inhomogeneity; removal of extrameningeal tissues from images; image stripping;
segmentation of images and flow correction.

Anisotropic diffusion filter: in a clinical setting, image anisotropic diffusion
filtration is a pre-requisite without image blur and information loss. The filter

is modeled as a diffusion process, which is attenuated at the edges by adaptively modifying the diffusion strength. This automatic process allows optimal selection and avoids over- or under-smoothing. The number of iterations also characterizes the filter. From experience, three iterations seem to be highly effective while keeping the processing time for a typical MR data set to under 15 minutes. The effect of an anisotropic filter can be appreciated by noise reduction without concomitant blurring in the filtered images. The increased SNR in the images following the application of this filter produces tighter clustering of the sampled pixels in feature space and results in both improved classification of the pixels and a higher degree of reproducibility for lesion volumes. Normally, application of the anisotropic filter reduces low frequency noise without image edge blurring and enhances SNR in images by a factor of approximately 2.2. Accurate image quantification requires the signal intensities in the images to originate from the inherent tissue contrast mechanisms. Inhomogeneous RF fields and images' non-uniformity pose significant limitations on MR data. Modern RF coils with highly homogeneous RF fields have played an important role in RF correction, which results in clusters in feature space showing up as undistorted high quality segmentation. RF inhomogeneity correction allows for the use of a single master feature map, thus an automatic setting-up of the parameters characterizing the filter from the image becomes easier (see Stoll *et al.* [749]).

5.4.1   RF Inhomogeneity Correction

In multiple sclerosis image segmentation, image intensity variations due to RF inhomogeneity in low frequency components allow for the determination of in-plane RF inhomogeneity and image smoothing. This smoothing introduces ringing artifacts around the regions with sweep intensity gradients, such as those encountered near the ventricles and at the edge of the brain. Therefore, pixels with intensities greater or less than one standard deviation away from the mean intensity of the parenchyma were set as the parenchyma intensity. Of course, using a standard deviation of one or less eliminates ringing artifacts without reducing the effectiveness of the RF inhomogeneity correction. The resulting images usually are filtered with a 25×25 averaging filter. So, RF inhomogeneity modulates the image intensity, which deteriorates the segmentation of the images, for example, having a deleterious effect on multi-spectral segmentation. Modern RF coils like the birdcage resonator are often used to produce homogeneous RF fields throughout the image volume, even though some RF field inhomogeneity is not completely minimized. This RF field inhomogeneity is responsible for the observed scan to scan and inter-observer variation in the segmentation. A number of techniques have been proposed for RF inhomogeneity correction. A simple algorithm was proposed (see Narayana *et al.* [751]), similar to that proposed earlier (see Harris *et al.* [750]), to correct RF inhomogeneity and its effect on segmentation. This algorithm was based on the fact that RF inhomogeneity contains only low frequency spatial components that can be filtered out. The smoothed image, following filtration,

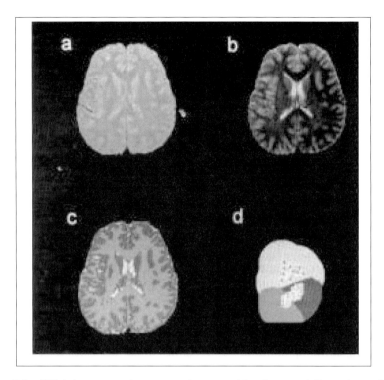

Figure 5.2: RF inhomogeneity correction provides better delineation of Gray Matter. (a) An early-echo FSE image before RF inhomogeneity correction, (b) the smoothed image, and (c) the early-echo FSE image following RF inhomogeneity correction. (d) tight clustering of the feature map. Reproduced by permission of John Wiley & Sons Inc. from [751]. © 1995.

contains information about the in-plane RF inhomogeneity with steep intensity gradients, such as those encountered near the ventricles and the edge of the brain. The very first step to overcome this problem is to identify the pixels which deviate from the mean parenchymal intensity by one standard deviation or more using a histogram analysis. In the next step, these pixels are replaced by the mean intensity of the brain parenchyma. The resulting images are smoothed with for example a 25×25 averaging filter, reflecting an in-plane RF profile. The anisotropically filtered images are divided by this RF profile to obtain the corrected image. All the corrected images are normalized based on the average CSF pixel intensities from a representative data set as shown in Figure 5.2 representing (a) an early-echo FSE image before RF inhomogeneity correction, (b) the smoothed image, (c) the early-echo FSE image following RF inhomogeneity correction and (d) the tight clustering of feature map.

Earlier segmentation methods without RF correction were underestimating the cortical GM and overestimating the WM and the application of RF correction reduced both scan-to-scan and intersubject variability. The important aspect for RF inhomogeneity correction and intensity normalization of images was that a single feature map could be used for tissue segmentation for all subjects/scans and RF correction converts a semiautomatic technique to an automatic one. RF correction is very important for automatic lesion quantification despite the RF field variation along the slice selective direction. To correct for RF inhomogeneity in all dimensions requires a complicated algorithm.

5.4.2   Image Stripping

Many of the Extra-Meningial Tissue (EMT) structures that surround the brain have high signal intensities close to the MS lesions. In multi-spectral segmentation, extra-meningeal tissues are a major source of false positives. So, removal or stripping of the extrameningeal tissues from the images is required prior to segmentation. Automatic removal of the extrameningeal tissue is a nontrivial problem. Traditionally, the removal of extrameningeal tissue is carried out using a variety of semiautomatic techniques and automatic removal of extrameningeal tissue based on one or two echo images. The relatively poor contrast seen on the images could be improved by a number of heuristics, not always valid, resulting in a significant error in extrameningeal tissue removal. Recently, an algorithm has been proposed for automatic removal of extrameningeal tissues based upon a multi-spectral segmentation technique using four AFFIRMATIVE images, which exhibits excellent parenchyma-to-extrameningeal tissue contrast, as the input data is located in very difficult regions to reach such as the vertex, optic nerve and inferior temporal gyri (see Bedell *et al.* [752]). Briefly, 30 to 40 points are sampled from three tissue classes – White Matter and Gray Matter, CSF, with other low-intensity EMT (generally bony structures), and high-intensity EMT(including scalp and bone marrow). Points are plotted in 3 different feature spaces with various combinations of pixel intensities from the four AFFIRMATIVE images comprising the x and y axes. The axes can be optimized to generate the most accurate tissue classifications. Following the appropriate segmentation of the AFFIRMATIVE and flow image sets, a simple algorithm for the removal of EMT from both image sets initially reclassifies all pixels segmented as low- or high-intensity EMT as background, leaving only the true brain pixels. The remaining EMT pixels are usually eliminated(reclassified as background) by an "exclusive" 2-D connectivity algorithm. In exclusive connectivity, a single object is identified in the image, and all pixels disconnected from the object are eliminated. Such an exclusive connectivity algorithm identifies the largest connected "island", considers it to be the brain and then removes all the pixels lying outside this structure. There are difficult regions, such as: a) close to the vertex, in which the hemispheres often appear to be separated due to the extensive nature of falx cerebri in this region, b) near the orbits and optic nerve, c), in the inferior temporal gyri. The EMT is removed from these slices by an alternative "masking" algorithm. It assumes that the brain size slowly decreases if one moves out in either direction from the center of the brain mass. Each successive slice should be completely within the borders of the previous slice. This explains how the algorithm uses the third slice as the center in the image set, in which EMT is already eliminated by the connectivity algorithm, as an image mask. Both hemispheres are retained, and EMT is removed in the slice immediately superior to this mask image by keeping only those pixels classified as brain contained within the borders of the mask image. This slice serves as a mask image for the slice immediately superior to it (the top slice). Other less visible regions are the orbits near the optic nerve, and the inferior temporal gyri. The exclusive connectivity algorithm does not eliminate this. On the other hand, the inferior temporal gyri being a part of the brain, appear as disconnected islands in the axial slices. Usually they are removed by the exclusive connectivity procedure. The automatic identification of these ventral structures could be simplified by the "graphic prescription" method into the algorithm, whereby the operator prescribes a left-right line in both the orbital and temporal lobe regions. This line does not cut the brain, however it cuts the optic nerve. By selecting the "temporal lobe line", the brain area of interest is isolated and EMT is removed. The procedure eliminates all small, isolated islands, background islands and non-parenchymal regions.

5.4.3   Three Dimensional MR Image Registration

The correction of spatial orientation due to positional variation needs 3-D image registration based on the Inter-hemispheric Fissure(IF). The registration algorithm requires manual identification of the end points of the Inter-hemispheric Fissure in all axial slices for fitting a plane to these points. One linear and two angular offsets can be determined from this plane. The other offsets can be determined by manually aligning the sagittal MR slices. Thus, the 3-D problem is reduced to a 2-D problem. The automated robust registration of the MR image algorithm registers two sets of axial MR images of the human brain, i.e., a standard set and a shifted set. Registration requires the determination of three angular and three linear offsets between the two image sets. The algorithm uses the plane containing the Inter-hemispheric Fissure to determine two rotations and one translation as shown in Figures 5.3 and 5.4, whereas the remaining offsets are found from a sagittal slice that has been reconstructed parallel to the IF. By convention, the x-, y- and z-axes correspond to the patient's left-right, ventral-dorsal, and superior-inferior axes, respectively. The Inter-hemispheric Fissure plane is based on the automatic identification of the two end points – ventral and dorsal – in about 20 axial slices. First, the center of mass (x, y) of each axial image is determined. Then, the edge points of the image are defined by scanning, first across rows and then down columns, for points with non-zero intensity. The point bordering five consecutive pixels with zero intensity is the edge point. After the edge points are identified, a "search window" containing 15 pixels on each side of the center mass is defined, within which the algorithm will find the end points of the fissure by detecting the edge point with the most dorsal y-coordinates on the ventral surface and the edge point with the most ventral y-coordinates on the dorsal surface. Later, about 40 end points are fitted to a plane by the least square method to determine the approximate IFP. After this, the shifted image data set rotation along the x- and y-axes relative

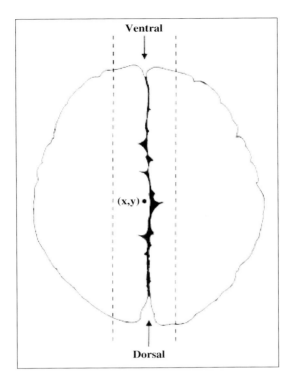

Figure 5.3: An axial section drawing with the center of mass and x, y search area for interhemispheric fissure (IF). Reproduced by permission of John Wiley & Sons Inc. from [755]. © 1996.

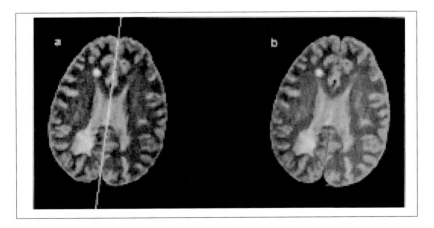

Figure 5.4: Axial MR images of the brain with calculated IFP superimposed (a) and IFP unsuperimposed (b). Reproduced by permission of John Wiley & Sons Inc from [755]. © 1996.

to the standard image set is determined from the direction angles between the
normal and the IFP for the two sets of images. Determination of the rotation
about the x-axis and the linear offsets from the reconstructed sagittal plane,
needs a 3-D center of mass for each image set as the y- and z-coordinates, while
the x-coordinate is calculated by substituting the y- and z-coordinates into the
equation for the IFP and solving for x. The linear offsets are then calculated
as the difference between the 3-D center of mass of the standard image set
and the 3-D center of mass of the shifted image set. After getting three angular and three linear offsets for the shifted image set, a spatial transformation
is computed for transforming each coordinate (x,y,z) in the shifted image set
onto the standard image set coordinates (x',y',z'). The spatial transformation
applied to all points in the shifted image set produces the registered images.

5.4.4   Segmentation

After the pre-processing steps are completed, the AFFIRMATIVE images are
segmented for determining the MS lesion load. The AFFIRMATIVE sequence
generates four images per slice. It is possible to generate a 4-D feature map
for segmentation. However, segmentation based on a 4-D feature space needs
powerful computers. Stated another way, it is more efficient to perform segmentation based on multiple 2-D feature maps with various image combinations.
Initial segmentation was performed using the early echo and late echo FSE
images in order to evaluate the improvement in the quality of segmentation
by incorporating the FLAIR and MTC techniques. Segmentation can be performed using early echo and late echo FLAIR/MTC along with the input images
at the level of the lateral ventricles. FSE-based segmentation produces a large
number of false positive and false negative lesion quantifications. The number of false classifications was decreased in the FLAIR/MTC-based segmented
images (see Rovaris *et al.* [753]).

5.4.5   Flow Correction

Segmentation based on FLAIR/MTC images does well for the regions superior
to the lateral ventricles, however, a large number of false positives occur in
regions with substantial vascularity and CSF flow. These rich regions such as
insula, posterior fossa, and cerebellum. It is possible to automatically identify
both vascular flow (coherent flow) and CSF flow (incoherent flow) on 3-D phase
contrast images. Incorporation of the flow information into the segmentation
process reduces the number of false positives, even in less visible brain regions
such as the posterior fossa. Despite the incorporation of flow information into
segmentation, the segmented images still show a few false positives arising from
flow ghost artifacts, as they can mimic lesions. Such ghosts can be identified
automatically and eliminated. An improvement in the segmentation follows
this correction for the flow ghosts. With this technique, the generation of a
single master map is adequate for segmenting all images generated on different
patients showing FLAIR/MTC images.

5.4.6 Evaluation and Validation

Quantitative evaluation of any segmentation technique is a non-trivial issue. The quality of segmentation is evaluated in terms of stability (i.e. inter- and intra-operator variability) and methodical accuracy. Multi-spectral segmentation based on AFFIRMATIVE images is fully automatic except for the initial generation of the master feature map. Therefore, the intra- and inter-operator variabilities are minimal. However, evaluation of the accuracy of any lesion quantification is much more difficult because the true lesion volumes are not known, due to the difficulty in getting autopsy lesion bearing tissue, and the fact that the estimation of lesion accuracy depends on using an experimental phantom. It is common practice for the evaluation of the accuracy of segmentation techniques to be done by comparing the segmentation results with those generated manually by an experienced expert. In this area, the largest study of this kind has been performed for validating the segmentation technique (see Fillipi *et al.* [754]).

5.5 Quantification of Enhancing Multiple Sclerosis Lesions

MS lesions lead to perivenous inflammation and an associated disruption of the regional blood-brain barrier. This loss of local blood-brain barrier can be visualized as an enhancement on T_1-weighted MRI images following the administration of a paramagnetic contrast agent, such as gadopentate dimeglumine (Gd). Some of these enhancing lesions are clinically symptomatic and Gd enhancement is used as a surrogate marker for evaluating the therapeutic efficacy. The correlation between active lesions, determined by histopathology and contrast enhancement, is well documented and demonstrable. It is important to determine the volume and number of enhancing lesions either manually or by computer-assisted means. This can be done automatically by an automatic technique. The cerebral vasculature and choroid plexus, where no blood-brain barrier is present, make visual identification and lesion volumetric analysis of enhancing lesions difficult because they mimic lesions. By using an automatic technique based on fuzzy connectivity, these false lesions are discarded by the operator. Bedell and Narayana proposed a new pulse sequence and post-processing technique for image generation and automatic detection of lesion enhancement (see Bedell *et al.* [32]). The pulse sequence is based on a spin echo sequence incorporating both stationary and marching saturation bands and gradient dephasing for suppressing enhancements within the cerebral vasculature. The post-processing technique automatically identifies other non-enhancing structures such as the choroid plexus leaving truly enhancing lesions in the final segmented images for quantification, as shown in Figure 5.5. Despite this, automatic techniques show few false positive enhancements smaller than 3 pixels. Sometimes they do appear but these contribute little to the estimated total enhancing volume of the lesion.

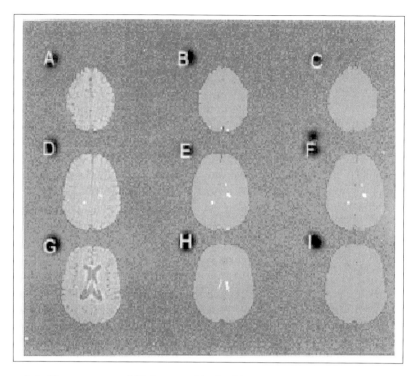

Figure 5.5: Post-contrast MR images (A, D, G), showing segmented images with white lesions (B, E, H), and images (C, F, I) with minimal false classification. Reproduced by permission of John Wiley & Sons Inc. from [32]. © 1998.

5.6 Quadruple Contrast Imaging

Partial Volume Averaging (PVA) which plagues most of the segmentation techniques in MRI results from the acquisition of relatively thick slices (greater than 3 mm). Consequently, the signal arising from each voxel is the average of the signals from each individual tissue type such as WM, GM and CSF where, because GM and CSF are often in close physical proximity, many voxels yield a signal intensity as a combination of GM and CSF signals. Most segmentation methods do not account for this effect and such a binary operation classifies "pure" GM or CSF in inaccurate tissue volumes. Alternatively, PVA between different tissues resulting from both false positive and false negative lesion classifications can be reduced by acquiring thinner slices with smaller pixels or by suppression of the CSF signal through the use of the fluid-attenuated inversion recovery (FLAIR) method. This is achieved by prolonging the acquisition time where the resolution is limited by the available signal to noise ratio. Recently, a new FSE-based pulse sequence, the Quadruple Contrast sequence (QC) has been implemented, which has reduced Partial Volume Averaging by simultaneously suppressing CSF and either GM or WM in the image (see Bedell *et al.* [32]). This pulse sequence is based on the double inversion recovery concept for a conventional spin-echo sequence. It allows for the acquisition of an image set that is suitable for a robust fractional volume analysis of WM, GM and CSF. The QC sequence employs the time-multiplexing concept and produces four images for each slice. These are: WM/CSF-suppressed (GM visible); GM/CSF-suppressed (WM visible); CSF-suppressed (FLAIR); and conventional proton density-weighted images. The sequence is based on a fast spin-echo (FSE) acquisition scheme to reduce the scan time, permitting the acquisition of contiguous slices from the entire brain in less time. An algorithm fit is applied on these QC images to generate fractional volumes of tissues of interest within the voxel reduces PVA contribution significantly to tissue quantification. Briefly, a diffusion filter is used to reduce noise, extrameningeal tissue is removed by four neighbor connectivity, a RF inhomogeneity correction is applied before fractional volume analysis of the brain. This is complicated because each tissue-contrast type is acquired from a different image sequence with different times, resulting in differential T_1-weighting into each type of contrast with different intensity scales. This is normalized by taking the T_1-weighting difference into account while describing the signal intensity. GM-visible and WM-visible images have only one type of tissue. These images are normalized to either FLAIR or FSE images after dividing the signal intensity of the WM- or GM-visible image by their total image signal intensity. In other words, "synthetic FLAIR" images are generated by summing the normalized GM-visible and WM-visible images to evaluate the accuracy of the normalization process. The synthetic FLAIR images are subtracted from the actual FLAIR images for a determination of the accuracy of the T_1 correction and intensity normalization, whereas a quantitative measure can be performed by knowing the average error over all the pixels. The FLAIR images are utilized for assessing the accuracy and validity of the methods for the determination of the fractional voxel volumes. After each tissue fraction for each voxel is known, intensity maps can be generated for each tissue to visualize the tissue contribution of the voxel volume. These maps provide information about PVA rich regions by comparing the total tissue volumes (fractional methods) with volumes (non fractional methods). Total tissue volumes can be calculated by summing fractions of each tissue over all the voxels in the image set and multiplying this by the in-plane resolution and slice thickness. Furthermore, potentials of this QC imaging method have been shown to allow for the accurate and robust determination of the brain constituent volumes at conventional slice thickness. It serves as a potentially powerful method to quantify MS lesions which appear bright in WM-suppressed ventricular regions. This is shown in Figure 5.6 where the lesions appear hyperintense and more conspicuous in the CSF/WM suppressed images compared to the FLAIR/MTC images. The same lesions appear hypointense on the CSF/GM suppressed images. This different appearance of the lesions on different images is expected to generate tight clusters in the feature space and lead to an accurate segmentation. Images generated with this sequence have been used for quantifying GM, WM, CSF and lesions in MS patients along with normal volunteers by using spectroscopic images and lo-

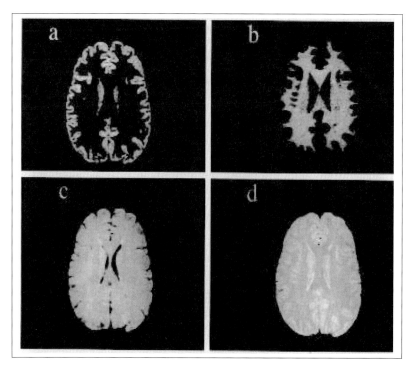

Figure 5.6: Axial T_1-weighted MR images using Quadruple Contrast pulse sequence images are: (a) GM visible (b) WM visible, (c) FLAIR, and (d) FSE images. CSF suppression is shown in image (a). Reproduced by permission of John Wiley & Sons Inc. from [748]. © 1997.

calized MR metabolite spectral analysis. This combined information from QC contrast CSF/WM-suppressed image segmentation with chemical shift imaging and metabolite maps provides quantitative patho-chemical information in Multiple Sclerosis.

5.7   Discussion

This chapter has focused on segmentation methods and the need for segmentation with emphasis on the automatic lesion quantification of MS lesions in a clinical set-up.

The brain is made up of WM, GM and CSF. All of these tissue fractions show individual true signal intensity but some effects, like Partial Volume Averaging (PVA) and poor contrast to noise ratio, deteriorate the demarcation of the tissue edges. Improved pulse sequences are needed to increase the lesion-to-tissue contrast and robust automation in lesion volume measurement and quantification of brain tissue components. This offers tissue composition information and better visualization of WM, GM and CSF features where distinct, well-defined tissue pathology is absent, such as in Alzheimer's Disease and Multiple Sclerosis. Segementation provides various features for different tissue components by color coding them with individual signal intensity. Several segmentation techniques are now available, although no single technique is perfect. These are: 1) manual tracing, 2) intensity-based single image segmentation, and 3)multi-spectral methods. The accuracy of these techniques depends on the well-maintained quality control over the method. Multiple-spectral segmentation techniques exploit the powerful multi-parametric nature of MRI. In contrast, both manual tracing and thresholding techniques are performed using a single set of images. Multi-spectral segmentation techniques are generally more robust, since they combine information from multiple images sets with different contrast for tissue classification. Multiple-spectral segmentation can be performed either by "feature space-based" or by "non-feature space-based" methods. Non-feature space-based techniques such as artificial neural network-based techniques, adaptive segmentation and model-based techniques, unsupervised automated multi-spectral relaxometric methods, have been recently proposed as effective methods. The feature space-based, multi-spectral segmentation technique to generate the "scatter plot" appears promising.

In this chapter, AFFIRMATIVE, quadruple contrast imaging, feature map-based segmentation and manual tracing-based segmentation were highlighted to delineate MS lesion rich regions. We discussed how FSE and FLAIR methods provide information on tissue fractions and visualize the minimization of false lesion classification to calculate the individual volumes by using the MRIAP program. Each tissue is assigned an arbitrary, but unique, color for visual inspection of the images. In fact, considerable overlap and ambiguity exists between these clusters, resulting in ambiguous tissue classification due to the limited tissue contrast and image noise. Supervised segmentation techniques can classify space as either parametric (maximum likelihood method) or non-parametric (k-nearest neighbors and Parzen window). These methods have long been in use and are promising. In recent years, the main focus has been on diverted "Automatic Segmentation" methods, minimizing flow ghosts, improved lesion-tissue contrast by Fast Spin-Echo (FSE) and FLAIR (Fluid Attenuation by Inversion Recovery), and Magnetization Transfer methods. Other important aspects of segmentation are: fast image processing methods involving RF correction, stripping of EMT, 3-D image registration, flow correction and validation. The ultimate goal of segmented images lies in good pathology identification, characterization and quantification. AFFIRMATIVE and Quadruple Contrast pulse sequences generate good images with bright MS lesions without false classification. These segmented images offer high potential to speculate metabolic screening in a clinical set-up and characterization of biochemical abnormalities in serial studies over several months. Still, several problems remain unsolved and demand careful development and the evaluation of newer, faster robust automated techniques. With the advent of supercomputers and effective programs, segmentation will hopefully be improved further for tissue composition and characterization with metabolite absolute concentrations for on-line information.

5.7.1   Acknowledgements

The authors express their thanks to Professor Ponnada A. Narayana, Radiology Department, University of Texas Medical School, Houston, TX for the MR data set. This project was funded by NIH grants to Professor Ponnada A. Narayana.

Chapter 6

Finite Mixture Models[1]

Sanjay S. Gopal

6.1 Introduction

Image segmentation can be considered to be essentially a process of classifying the pixels in a two-dimensional (2D) image into different subsets of classes. If the number of classes is known or can be estimated then we can associate a numeric label with each class. Pixel labeling then consists of assigning a numeric label to each pixel. Various different metrics can be used for arriving at a distinct label configuration for the pixels in an image. These include simple grey level thresholding, color, or local property values such as those which measure texture or region homogeneity.

Simple gray level thresholding typically provides acceptable results only in the absence of statistical noise and partial volume effects. One widely used technique for improving an initial label configuration is an iterative scheme termed relaxation labeling [756], [757]. This is primarily meant to be used for pixel labeling of images corrupted by noise. Here, label assignments for all pixels are initially formed based upon the observed image. Then this initial labeling is iteratively changed to maximize a particular function that models user defined relationships between neighboring pixel labels. Linear relaxation converges to a solution that depends only upon the user defined relationships, but upon neither the observed image nor the initial labeling. Nonlinear relaxation labeling provides a solution that depends upon the initial labeling and is typically a reasonable improvement. However, its convergence properties have not been established. Both linear and nonlinear relaxation labeling suffer from a common drawback in that these methods make little or no use of the observed image, except perhaps to initialize the label configuration for the iterative algorithm. Relaxation labeling remains a somewhat *ad hoc* technique that often provides an improvement of labels that have been assigned using some other labeling method.

More recently, finite mixture models have attracted considerable interest

---

[1]This chapter is based on material published in the *IEEE Transactions on Image Processing*. © 1998 IEEE. Reprinted with permission from [766].

for pixel labeling. The application of these models to labeling is based on the assumption that the intensity (gray scale or color) value of each pixel in the observed image is a sample from a finite mixture distribution. Upon estimating the parameters of this distribution a suitable labeling rule is applied to assign labels to the pixels of an image. Finite mixture models can also be used with other appropriate models for partial volume effect for optimal pixel labeling.

In this chapter a basic introduction of finite mixture models is provided. The classical mixture model and its application to image segmentation is explained. We also review a recent extension to finite mixture models which permits true Bayesian pixel classification. The material in this chapter is provided to fully understand: (i) the advantages and limitations of using mixture models for image segmentation, and (ii) the critical issues involved in estimating parameters of mixture densities.

A word on notation: bold lowercase letters are used to denote vectors and bold uppercase letters are used to denote matrices. The matrix $\mathbf{I}$ is used exclusively to denote the identity matrix, while the vector $\vec{\mathbf{1}}$ denotes the vector of all ones. Superscripts on a vector or matrix denote a particular vector or matrix from among a set of a vectors or matrices. Subscripts on a vector or a matrix denote a particular element of the vector or matrix.

6.2   Pixel Labeling Using the Classical Mixture Model

The classical mixture model (CMM) [758] defines the density function of the observation $\vec{\mathbf{x}}_i$ as

$$f(\vec{\mathbf{x}}_i) = \sum_{j=1}^{L} \vec{\pi}_j f_j(\vec{\mathbf{x}}_i | \vec{\theta}^j) \ , \tag{6.1}$$

with $0 \leq \vec{\pi}_j \leq 1$ and $f_j(.) \geq 0$, for $1 \leq j \leq L$. Here $\vec{\mathbf{x}}_i, 1 \leq i \leq N$ denotes the observation at the ith pixel of an image having N pixels. These observations are modeled as independent and identically distributed (*i.i.d.*) random variables. The elements of vector $\vec{\pi}$ are termed the *mixing weights* and they satisfy two constraints: $\vec{\pi}_j \geq 0 \ \forall j$ and $\sum_{j=1}^{L} \vec{\pi}_j = 1$. The set $\{f_j(\vec{\mathbf{x}}_i | \vec{\theta}^j)\}$ denotes L density functions termed *component densities*. The $\vec{\theta}^j$'s denote a vector of parameters that describe each of the L individual component densities. Equation (6.1) defines a *finite mixture density function* and the random variable describing the observation $\vec{\mathbf{x}}_i$ is deemed to have a *finite mixture distribution*. The vector $\vec{\mathbf{x}}$ is used to denote N observations from such a finite mixture distribution. Equation (6.1) is the classical mixture density model as described by Titterington *et al.* in [758]. This model has frequently been used to address the problem in which the observations $\vec{\mathbf{x}}_i$ are assumed to be independent. With this assumption the joint conditional density of the observations is given by:

$$f_x(\vec{\mathbf{x}}|\vec{\pi}, \vec{\theta}^{\,1}..\vec{\theta}^{\,L}) = \prod_{i=1}^{N} \sum_{j=1}^{L} \vec{\pi}_j f_j(\vec{\mathbf{x}}_i|\vec{\theta}^{\,j}) \ . \tag{6.2}$$

In the context of pixel labeling these observations are assumed to be the pixel intensities or gray scale values. Given a set of N such observations, the goal is to estimate the unknown mixing weights $\vec{\pi}$ and parameters $\{\vec{\theta}^{\,j}\}$. Depending on the application, these parameters can be estimated using graphical methods, the method of moments, or via Maximum Likelihood (ML) estimation.

A commonly used technique for ML estimation is the Expectation Maximization (EM) algorithm [759]. Let us assume that $f_j(\vec{\mathbf{x}}_i|\vec{\theta}^{\,j})$ are all univariate Gaussian and that the measurements $\vec{\mathbf{x}}$ are independent and identically distributed. Let vectors $\vec{\mu}$ and $\vec{\sigma}$ contain, respectively, the unknown means and standard deviations so that:

$$f_j(\vec{\mathbf{x}}_i|\vec{\theta}^{\,j}) = f_j(\vec{\mathbf{x}}_i|\vec{\mu}_j, \vec{\sigma}_j) = \frac{1}{\sqrt{2\pi}\vec{\sigma}_j} \exp\left[\frac{-(\vec{\mathbf{x}}_i - \vec{\mu}_j)^2}{2(\vec{\sigma}_j)^2}\right] \ . \tag{6.3}$$

Then, Equation (6.2) can be written as

$$f_x(\vec{\mathbf{x}} \mid \vec{\pi}, \vec{\mu}, \vec{\sigma}) = \prod_{i=1}^{N} \sum_{j=1}^{L} \vec{\pi}_j \frac{1}{\sqrt{2\pi}\vec{\sigma}_j} \exp\left[\frac{-(\vec{\mathbf{x}}_i - \vec{\mu}_j)^2}{2(\vec{\sigma}_j)^2}\right] \ . \tag{6.4}$$

Now we can apply the EM algorithm to obtain ML estimates of the parameters $\vec{\mu}$ and $\{(\vec{\sigma}_j)^2\}$. At each iteration of the EM algorithm we estimate these parameters using the following equations:

$$\vec{\mathbf{w}}_j^{i\,(k)} \equiv E[\vec{\mathbf{z}}_j^i|\vec{\mu}^{(k)}, \vec{\sigma}_j^{(k)}] = \frac{\vec{\pi}_j^{(k)} \, f_j(\vec{\mathbf{x}}_i|\vec{\mu}_j^{(k)}, \vec{\sigma}_j^{(k)})}{\sum_{l=1}^{L} \vec{\pi}_l^{(k)} f_l(\vec{\mathbf{x}}_i|\vec{\mu}_l^{(k)}, \vec{\sigma}_l^{(k)})} \ , \tag{6.5}$$

$$\vec{\pi}_j^{(k+1)} = \frac{1}{N} \sum_{i=1}^{N} \vec{\mathbf{w}}_j^{i\,(k)} \ , \tag{6.6}$$

$$\vec{\mu}_j^{(k+1)} = \frac{1}{\sum_{i=1}^{N} \vec{\mathbf{w}}_j^{i\,(k)}} \sum_{i=1}^{N} \vec{\mathbf{w}}_j^{i\,(k)} \vec{\mathbf{x}}_i \ , \tag{6.7}$$

and

$$[(\vec{\sigma}_j)^2]^{(k+1)} = \frac{1}{\sum_{i=1}^{N} \vec{\mathbf{w}}_j^{i\,(k)}} \sum_{i=1}^{N} \vec{\mathbf{w}}_j^{i\,(k)} [\vec{\mathbf{x}}_i - \vec{\mu}_j^{(k+1)}]^2 \ . \tag{6.8}$$

The closed form expression of Equation (6.6) results when the constraint $\sum_j \vec{\pi}_j = 1$ is enforced in the maximization step. At convergence we obtain the ML estimates for $\vec{\mu}$ and $\{(\vec{\sigma}_j)^2\}$. However, it is to be noted that the likelihood function of Equation (6.2) exhibits several local maxima. The EM algorithm converges to one of these local maxima. This is sufficient for most practical purposes.

The astute reader will have noted that so far we have just estimated the parameters $\vec{\pi}$, $\vec{\mu}$, and $\vec{\sigma}$. However, these only describe the global properties of the measurements $\vec{x}$. They tell nothing about how to assign labels to the pixels. So how then do we label the pixels? To solve this problem, note that the classical mixture model incorporates classes in the following manner. Let there be N pixels, each of which belongs to one of L classes. Let vectors $\{\vec{p}^i\}$ contain the pixel labels such that $\mathbf{p}_j^i = 1$ if the ith pixel belongs to the jth class, and $\mathbf{p}_j^i = 0$ otherwise. Let the probability of any pixel belonging to the jth class be denoted by $\vec{\pi}_j$, so that $\mathrm{Prob}(\mathbf{p}_j^i = 1) = \vec{\pi}_j$ for all i. Associated with each class is a component density $f_j(\vec{x}_i|\vec{\theta}^{\,j})$. If $\mathbf{p}_j^i = 1$, then the corresponding pixel value $\vec{x}_i$ is generated from the component density $f_j(\vec{x}_i|\vec{\theta}^{\,j})$, i.e.,

$$f(\vec{x}_i|\mathbf{p}_j^i = 1, \vec{\theta}^{\,j}) = f_j(\vec{x}_i|\vec{\theta}^{\,j}) \ . \tag{6.9}$$

Bayes' rule gives:

$$\mathrm{Prob}(\vec{p}_j^i = 1|\vec{x}_i, \vec{\theta}^{\,j}) = \frac{\vec{\pi}_j \, f_j(\vec{x}_i|\vec{\theta}^{\,j})}{f(\vec{x}_i|\vec{\theta}^{\,1}..\vec{\theta}^{\,L})} \ , \tag{6.10}$$

where:

$$f(\vec{x}_i|\vec{\theta}^{\,1}..\vec{\theta}^{\,L}) = \sum_{j=1}^{L} \vec{\pi}_j f_j(\vec{x}_i|\vec{\theta}^{\,j}) \tag{6.11}$$

is simply some constant value dependent upon measurement $\vec{x}_i$. In general, $\vec{x}_i$ can be used to estimate $\vec{p}^i$ through Equation (6.10) if the parameters $\{\vec{\theta}^{\,j}\}$ of the component densities are known. Now, to assign labels to the pixels, if the parameters $\{\vec{\theta}^{\,j}\}$ were known, the Bayes' classifier could be used to assign a label to pixel i by solution of:

$$\max_{j} \ \mathrm{Prob}(\vec{p}_j^i = 1|\vec{x}_i, \vec{\theta}^{\,j}) \ . \tag{6.12}$$

Since the component density parameters are not known, the common approach is to use ML estimates of parameters in place of the parameters themselves in the Bayes' classifier. In the case of univariate Gaussian component densities, this entails the use of ML estimates $\vec{\pi}^{ML}$, $\vec{\mu}^{ML}$, and $\vec{\sigma}^{2\,ML}$ from the EM algorithm in the Bayes' classifier of Equations (6.10-6.12). For more detailed discussion of the CMM, ML estimation of the model parameters, and application of the CMM to pixel labeling, see [203], [758] and [760]–[765].

6.3 Pixel Labeling Using the Spatially Variant Mixture Model

Although the use of the CMM and Bayes' rule as described provides acceptable estimates of the pixel labels, it is not an optimal approach. This is because the labels computed on the basis of ML estimates for $\vec{\pi}$ and $\{\vec{\theta}^{\,j}\}$ are not themselves ML estimates. Maximum likelihood estimation of the labels requires the likelihood function $f(\vec{x}|\vec{\pi}, \vec{p}^1..\vec{p}^N, \vec{\theta}^{\,1}..\vec{\theta}^{\,L})$. A more severe limitation of applying the classical mixture model to pixel labeling is the independence assumption on the elements of $\vec{x}$ in Equation (6.2). This implies that elements $\vec{x}_i$ are uncorrelated. The classical mixture model, therefore, prohibits the existence of spatial correlation between the observations at neighboring pixels. In most applications, measurements at neighboring pixels are spatially correlated. One can reintroduce spatial correlation into the labeling process using the classical mixture model by imposing dependence structures in the form of Markov chains and 2-D MRF models on the complete data of the EM algorithm, but, again, this is a non-optimal approach and the resulting algorithms have been found to be considerably complicated and computationally intractable.

To overcome these limitations we need a better, more flexible model for pixel labeling. One such model is the *Spatially Variant finite Mixture Model* (SVMM). To define the SVMM, let $\vec{p}_j^i$ denote the probability of the ith pixel belonging to the jth class with $0 \leq \vec{p}_j^i \leq 1$ and $\sum_j \vec{p}_j^i = 1 \;\; \forall i$. As in the classical mixture model, $\vec{x}_i$ denotes the observation at the ith pixel of an image, with $\vec{x}_i$ modeled as *i.i.d.*. Again, $\{f_j(\vec{x}_i|\vec{\theta}^{\,j})\}$ is a set of L density functions, each having its own vector of parameters $\vec{\theta}^{\,j}$. The SVMM defines the density function of the observation $\vec{x}_i$ as:

$$f(\vec{x}_i|\vec{\theta}^{\,1}..\vec{\theta}^{\,L}) = \sum_{j=1}^{L} \vec{p}_j^i f_j(\vec{x}_i|\vec{\theta}^{\,j}) \, , \qquad (6.13)$$

with the joint conditional density $f_x(\vec{x}|\; \vec{p}^1..\vec{p}^N, \vec{\theta}^{\,1}..\vec{\theta}^{\,L})$ of the observations formed as

$$f_x(\vec{x}|\vec{p}^1..\vec{p}^N, \vec{\theta}^{\,1}..\vec{\theta}^{\,L}) = \prod_{i=1}^{N} \sum_{j=1}^{L} \vec{p}_j^i f_j(\vec{x}_i|\vec{\theta}^{\,j}) \, . \qquad (6.14)$$

The SVMM presents several distinct advantages for pixel labeling compared with the CMM:

(1) It lends itself easily to direct ML estimation of the pixel labeling information $\vec{p}_j^i$ through specification of the likelihood function in Equation (6.14).

(2) The $\vec{\pi}_j$s of Equation (6.1) in the classical mixture model can be thought of as the "global probability" of occurrence of label j in the entire image. For the pixel labeling problem it seems reasonable to desire $\vec{p}_j^i, j = 1, 2, ..., L; i = 1, 2, ..., N$, the "local probability" of occurrence of label j

at pixel i. The spatially variant mixture model provides a means for capturing this "local probability" of label occurrence.

(3) It facilitates the modeling of spatial correlations directly on the label information $\{\vec{\mathbf{p}}^i\}$ through specification of prior densities $f(\vec{\mathbf{p}}^1..\vec{\mathbf{p}}^N)$. Algorithms using the classical mixture model impose dependence structures such as Markov chains or Markov Random Fields (MRFs) on the complete data rather than on the labels. The resulting algorithms are, therefore, not truly Bayesian. Use of the spatially variant model permits imposing dependence structures on the label parameters themselves.

(4) Even when dependence structures are imposed on the complete data, the resulting algorithms using the classical mixture model are considerably complicated and numerically involved. Estimation of the parameters of the mixture and the Bayesian hyperparameter are virtually impossible if a hidden MRF is imposed on the complete data. This leads to the search for simpler numerical optimization techniques for implementing pseudo-Bayesian parameter estimation using the CMM. On the other hand, elegant, computationally tractable Bayesian algorithms can be derived based on the SVMM.

(5) The CMM is a special case of the SVMM wherein $\vec{\mathbf{p}}^i_j = \vec{\pi}_j \ \forall i$. Hence, the spatially variant model can also be applied to data that conform to the CMM.

(6) In the case of ML estimation, the label probabilities $\vec{\mathbf{p}}^i_j$ all converge to 0 or 1, so that labeling is unambiguous.

We can easily derive an EM algorithm for ML estimation of both the pixel label probabilities $\{\vec{\mathbf{p}}^i\}$ and the parameter vectors $\{\vec{\theta}^{\,j}\}$ using the joint conditional density of Equation (6.14). As we did for the CMM, let us assume that the component densities $\{f_j(\vec{\mathbf{x}}_i|\vec{\theta}^{\,j})\}$ are univariate Gaussian. Based on this assumption, the following closed form expressions can be derived for estimating the various model parameters:

$$\vec{\mathbf{w}}^{i\,(k)}_j = \frac{\vec{\mathbf{p}}^{i\,(k)}_j \dfrac{1}{\sqrt{2\pi\vec{\sigma}^{2\,(k)}_j}} \exp\left[-\dfrac{\left(\vec{\mathbf{x}}_i - \vec{\mu}^{(k)}_j\right)^2}{2\vec{\sigma}^{2\,(k)}_j} \right]}{\displaystyle\sum_{l=1}^{L} \vec{\mathbf{p}}^{i\,(k)}_l \dfrac{1}{\sqrt{2\pi\vec{\sigma}^{2\,(k)}_l}} \exp\left[-\dfrac{\left(\vec{\mathbf{x}}_i - \vec{\mu}^{(k)}_l\right)^2}{2\vec{\sigma}^{2\,(k)}_l} \right]} , \tag{6.15}$$

$$\vec{\mathbf{p}}^{i\,(k+1)}_j = \frac{\vec{\mathbf{w}}^{i\,(k)}_j}{\displaystyle\sum_{l=1}^{L} \vec{\mathbf{w}}^{i\,(k)}_l} = \vec{\mathbf{w}}^{i\,(k)}_j , \tag{6.16}$$

$$\vec{\mu}^{(k+1)}_j = \frac{1}{\displaystyle\sum_{i=1}^{N} \vec{\mathbf{w}}^{i\,(k)}_j} \sum_{i=1}^{N} \vec{\mathbf{w}}^{i\,(k)}_j \vec{\mathbf{x}}_i , \tag{6.17}$$

and

$$[(\vec{\sigma}_j)^2]^{(k+1)} = \frac{1}{\sum_{i=1}^{N} \vec{w}_j^{i\,(k)}} \sum_{i=1}^{N} \vec{w}_j^{i\,(k)} \left[\vec{x}_i - \vec{\mu}_j^{(k+1)}\right]^2 \,. \tag{6.18}$$

Here, use has been made of the fact that $\sum_{j=1}^{L} \vec{w}_j^{i\,(k)} = 1 \; \forall i, k$. This EM algorithm, defined by Equations (6.15)–(6.18), yields ML estimates for the pixel label parameters $\vec{p}_j^i$, as well as the parameters $\vec{\mu}$ and $\vec{\sigma}$. Having obtained these ML estimates we use the Bayes' classifier of Equations (6.10)–(6.12) as in the case of labeling using the CMM. A nice feature of the SVMM is that pixel labeling is unambiguous because the ML estimates of the class probabilities converge to ones and zeros. For a detailed proof of this the interested reader is referred to [766].

6.4 Comparison of CMM and SVMM for Pixel Labeling

Figures 6.1–6.4 show the results of a detailed performance analysis of applying the CMM and SVMM for pixel labeling. The EM algorithms incorporating the CMM and SVMM are referred to as the EM-CMM and ML-SVMM algorithms respectively. We examine their performance with respect to the mixing weights $\vec{\pi}$, the mean value of each class $\vec{\mu}$, the variances in each class $\vec{\sigma}^2$, and the number of classes L in the image. Shown in the figures are the results from an extensive Monte Carlo simulation to compare these two algorithms from the point of view of classification or labeling error. The classification error is defined as the percentage of the total number of pixels in the image that are incorrectly labeled.

We can infer a few general results from Figures 6.1–6.4. For instance, the percentage labeling error of the EM algorithm using the SVMM compares very well with that of the EM algorithm using the CMM. This is expected and is an acceptable result. The SVMM-based EM algorithm does no worse than the CMM-based EM algorithm. However as can be seen from the above plots, the SVMM-based EM algorithm has a significantly smaller error variance than the CMM-based EM algorithm. The SVMM-based algorithm performs well when the class memberships are approximately equal. Also if the number of labels in the image is large, then the SVMM-based algorithm results in lower labeling error than the CMM-based algorithm. Two properties are apparent from Figure 6.1:

(1) When an image does not have roughly the same number of pixels in each class, the EM-CMM classifier performs better than the ML-SVMM classifier.

(2) The variance in the EM-CMM classifier is much larger than that in the ML-SVMM classifier.

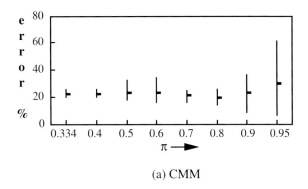

(a) CMM

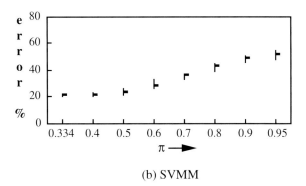

(b) SVMM

Figure 6.1: Effect of mixing weights: percentage labeling error as $\vec{\pi}_1 = \pi$ is varied from 0.334 to 0.95 with $\vec{\mu} = (100, 140, 180)$, and $\vec{\sigma} = (20, 20, 20)$ for (a) EM algorithm based upon the classical mixture model (EM-CMM), and (b) ML EM algorithm based upon the spatially variant mixture model (ML-SVMM). Shown are the errors obtained for ten noise realizations and the mean error for these ten realizations.

   As one would anticipate, the classification error increases for both algorithms as the separation between adjacent class means $\vec{\mu}_1$ and $\vec{\mu}_2$ is decreased. Again, we observe that the variance in the EM-CMM classifier is much larger than that in the ML-SVMM classifier. Also, the classification error from both algorithms increases as the ratio $\frac{\vec{\sigma}_3}{\Delta\mu}$ increases. Comparable mean classification error rates are observed, but once again the variance in classification error is considerably larger for the EM-CMM algorithm than for the ML-SVMM algorithm. As can be seen, the classification error for EM-CMM remains fairly constant as the number of labels is increased. However, the classification error increases for ML-SVMM. This is attributed to the fact that as the number of labels increases, ML-SVMM must estimate proportionally more parameters than EM-CMM, while the number of samples from each class is reduced.
   One advantage of the ML-SVMM algorithm is that it eliminates the need

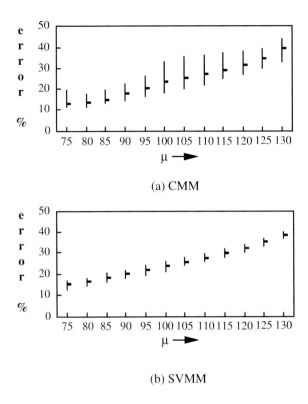

(a) CMM

(b) SVMM

Figure 6.2: Effect of the separation of class means: percentage classification error with $\vec{\mu}_1 = \mu$ being varied from 75.0 to 130.0, with $\vec{\mu}_2 = 140$, $\vec{\mu}_3 = 180$, $\vec{\pi} = (0.5, 0.25, 0.25)$, and $\vec{\sigma} = (20, 20, 20)$ for (a) EM-CMM algorithm, and (b) ML-SVMM algorithm. Shown are the errors obtained for ten noise realizations and the mean error for these ten realizations.

for a Bayes' classifier. This implies reduced computational requirements, especially when labeling a large image. However, the utility of the SVMM is in its application for the Bayesian estimation of the parameters of the mixture density. Incorporation of dependence structures on label configurations is straightforward if the SVMM is used for labeling. Dependence structures such as MRFs have been used along with the CMM for Bayesian estimation of the mixture parameters [765]. Such MRFs have been imposed on the complete data, which is a confusing and awkward way to incorporate dependence structures. This results in computationally intensive algorithms and does not represent Bayesian estimation of label parameters in the strictest sense. The SVMM, on the other hand, allows the easy incorporation of prior densities on the pixel label parameters $\{\vec{p}^i\}$. Bayesian estimation of the pixel labels is made simple and the algorithms for their implementation are computationally less intensive. We discuss one such algorithm in the next section. As we shall observe, Bayesian estimation of the label parameters results in considerably lower

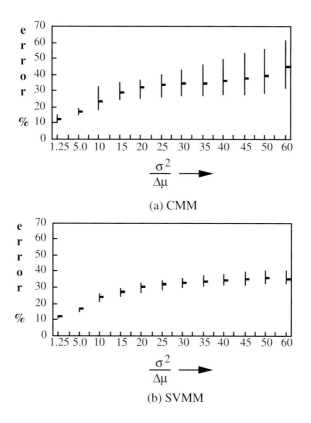

Figure 6.3: Effect of class variances: percentage labeling error variation as $\vec{\sigma}_3^2 = \sigma^2$ is varied from 50 to 2400, with $\vec{\sigma}_1 = \vec{\sigma}_2 = 20$ and $\vec{\pi} = (0.25, 0.25, 0.5)$ for (a) EM-CMM algorithm, and (b) ML-SVMM algorithm. Shown are the errors obtained for ten noise realizations and the mean error for these ten realizations.

labeling error.

All of these advantages of the SVMM do not come without a cost. The introduction of the SVMM does indeed over-parameterize the estimation problem. Such over-parameterization perhaps necessitates the use of a Bayesian estimation technique for meaningful results. This is acceptable as the author is primarily interested in Bayesian pixel labeling. It has been widely accepted that images in general exhibit local spatial correlation. What is interesting, however, is the fact that the EM algorithm incorporating the SVMM performs as well as the EM algorithm using the CMM inspite of this over-parameterization.

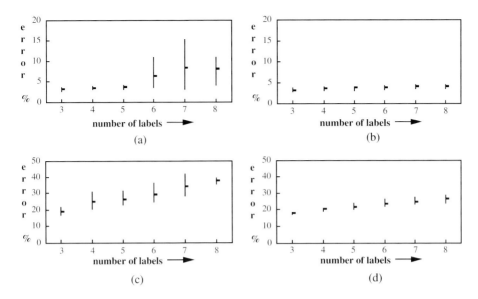

Figure 6.4: Effect of the number of classes L: percentage classification error as L is varied from $L = 3$ to $L = 8$, with $\vec{\pi}_j = 1/L \; \forall j$, and $\vec{\mu}_j = j*100$ for $j = 1,..,L$ for (a) EM-CMM algorithm with $\vec{\sigma}_j{}^2 = 625 \; \forall j$, (b) ML-SVMM algorithm with $\vec{\sigma}_j{}^2 = 625 \; \forall j$, (c) EM-SVMM algorithm with $\vec{\sigma}_j{}^2 = 2000 \; \forall j$, and (d) ML-SVMM algorithm with $\vec{\sigma}_j{}^2 = 2000 \; \forall j$. Shown are the errors obtained for ten noise realizations and the mean error for these ten realizations.

6.5   Bayesian Pixel Labeling Using the SVMM

In the previous section we have discussed only ML pixel labeling using the EM algorithm. This EM algorithm has several positive features with respect to computational speed, convergence and labeling errors. However, it basically yields ML estimates and has no mechanism for incorporation of any prior information on possible labels. Failure to use prior information can lead to results which range from being sub-optimal or inferior to even absurd [767]. Pixel labeling and image segmentation is a classical example of a case where prior information could be put to very effective use to yield meaningful results. As we shall see shortly, there is a compelling need for the incorporation of *a priori* information in labeling. It is envisioned that such information could lead to really superior performance in terms of labeling errors.

   In this section we look at a fast algorithm for the Bayesian estimation of the pixel labels. We shall then investigate *a priori* densities for pixel labeling and examine the results of a rigorous quantitative analysis of this new algorithm by means of computer simulations. In the next section we shall look at a comparison of the performance of this Bayesian algorithm with the EM algorithm using the classical mixture model as well as the ML pixel labeling algorithm derived earlier. We shall also see a few examples of the application of this algorithm to the segmentation of magnetic resonance images. Finally, in Section 6.7, we comment on certain practical aspects of all three algorithms and discuss issues such as convergence, initializations of mixture weights, class means and variances, and optimal choices for the prior parameter β for the Bayesian algorithm.

The spatially variant mixture model, when applied to ML estimation of pixel labels, results in simple closed form expressions for the M-step of the EM algorithm. However, it should be noted that given an NxN image, this algorithm estimates a large number of parameters: (i) N^2 label parameter vectors $\{\vec{\mathbf{p}}^i\}$ each of length L, (ii) a L-element vector $\vec{\mu}$ of means, and (iii) a L-element vector $\vec{\sigma}$ of standard deviations. Here, the number of data values is less than the number of parameters being estimated, so that the ML estimates themselves have large variances. As a result of these variances, in a region wherein all pixels are of the same class, the estimated pixel labels will consist of a random arrangement of different labels. When these estimated pixel labels are viewed as an image, the variances of these estimates obscure some of the underlying spatial correlation within the labeled image. This is not surprising, because the likelihood function does not incorporate local correlations between the neighboring label parameters $\vec{\mathbf{p}}^i$. Local correlation can be incorporated in the estimation process through application of a suitable prior density function $f(\vec{\mathbf{p}}^1..\vec{\mathbf{p}}^N, \vec{\theta}^1..\vec{\theta}^L)$ that models this local correlation. Given this prior density, the *a posteriori* density function can be formed and maximized for maximum *a posteriori* (MAP) estimation of the label parameters $\{\vec{\mathbf{p}}^i\}$ and the component density parameters $\{\vec{\theta}^j\}$.

The general form of this *a posteriori* density function for the case of univariate Gaussian component densities is:

$$f(\vec{\mathbf{p}}^1..\vec{\mathbf{p}}^N, \vec{\mu}, \vec{\sigma}|\vec{\mathbf{x}}) = f_x(\vec{\mathbf{x}}|\vec{\mathbf{p}}^1..\vec{\mathbf{p}}^N, \vec{\mu}, \vec{\sigma})f(\vec{\mathbf{p}}^1..\vec{\mathbf{p}}^N, \vec{\mu}, \vec{\sigma}) , \qquad (6.19)$$

with $f_x(\cdot)$ defined in Equation (6.14). Here we have omitted $f(\vec{\mathbf{x}})$ in the denominator as it is a constant which does not affect the maximization. The prior density $f(\vec{\mathbf{p}}^1..\vec{\mathbf{p}}^N, \vec{\mu}, \vec{\sigma}|\vec{\mathbf{x}})$ is used to incorporate the investigator's insight about the underlying classes in the image, possible pixel label configurations, any relevant structure present in the image which may be obscured by noise, and in general, any information which would be useful in obtaining meaningful segmentations. A powerful model for the parameters $\{\vec{\mathbf{p}}^i\}$ that incorporates local correlation is given by the MRF model [768] defined through the Gibbs density function [457], [769] given by:

$$f(\vec{\mathbf{p}}^1..\vec{\mathbf{p}}^N) = \frac{1}{K_\beta}\exp\left[-U(\vec{\mathbf{p}}^1..\vec{\mathbf{p}}^N)\right] , \qquad (6.20)$$

where:

$$U(\vec{\mathbf{p}}^1..\vec{\mathbf{p}}^N) = \frac{1}{\beta}\sum_{c\in\mathcal{C}}V_c(\vec{\mathbf{p}}^1..\vec{\mathbf{p}}^N) . \qquad (6.21)$$

Here $V_c(\vec{\mathbf{p}}^1..\vec{\mathbf{p}}^N)$ is potential function associated with each clique[2] c, and $\mathcal{C}$ de-

---

[2]See Geman *et al.* [259].

notes the set of all cliques within the image. The set of clique types is specified by the order of the neighborhood assigned to the model. The joint density should assign higher probability to sets of label vectors $\{\vec{\mathbf{p}}^i\}$ wherein neighboring $\vec{\mathbf{p}}^i$'s are similar and lower probability otherwise. Let $\{\vec{\mathbf{p}}^i\}$ be modeled as being described by two-pixel cliques with associated clique potential function $V(\vec{\mathbf{p}}^i, \vec{\mathbf{p}}^m)$ such that:

$$\sum_{c \in \mathcal{C}} V_c(\vec{\mathbf{p}}^1..\vec{\mathbf{p}}^N) = \sum_{(i,m) \in \mathcal{C}} \sum_{j=1}^{L} \left(\mathbf{p}_j^i - \mathbf{p}_j^m\right)^2 , \qquad (6.22)$$

where pixels i and m are nearest neighbors. Then, we have:

$$f(\vec{\mathbf{p}}^1..\vec{\mathbf{p}}^N, \vec{\mu}, \vec{\sigma}) = \frac{1}{K_\beta} \exp\left[\frac{-1}{\beta} \sum_{(i,m) \in \mathcal{C}} \sum_{j=1}^{L} \left(\mathbf{p}_j^i - \mathbf{p}_j^m\right)^2 \right] f(\vec{\mu}) f(\vec{\sigma}) , \quad (6.23)$$

where K_β is a constant and parameter vectors $\vec{\mu}$ and $\vec{\sigma}$ are modeled as independent from each other and from $\{\vec{\mathbf{p}}^i\}$ by specifying prior density functions $f(\vec{\mu})$ and $f(\vec{\sigma})$ as uniformly distributed over the corresponding feasible parameter spaces. Equation (6.23) defines the sum-squared-error prior and assigns maximum probability to pixel label probability configurations with identical label probability vector assigned to all neighbors. The sum-squared error prior has a continuous first partial derivative given by:

$$\frac{\partial f(\vec{\mathbf{p}}^1..\vec{\mathbf{p}}^N, \vec{\mu}, \vec{\sigma})}{\partial \vec{\mathbf{p}}_j^i} \equiv \sum_{m \in \eta_i} (\mathbf{p}_j^m - \mathbf{p}_j^i) , \qquad (6.24)$$

which enables its easy use in the MAP-SVMM algorithm described later. For other useful priors please refer to [766].

To derive an EM algorithm for MAP estimation of the parameters $\{\vec{\mathbf{p}}^i\}$, $\vec{\mu}$ and $\vec{\sigma}$ we use the complete data $\vec{\mathbf{y}} = (\vec{\mathbf{x}}, \{\vec{\mathbf{z}}^i\})$ where $\vec{\mathbf{z}}^i$ denotes an indicator vector with:

$$\mathbf{z}_j^i = \begin{cases} 1 & \text{if the true label of pixel } i \text{ is } j \\ 0 & \text{otherwise.} \end{cases}$$

The E-step for the EM MAP algorithm consists of forming:

$$Q'(\Psi|\Psi^{(k)}) \equiv E_{\vec{\mathbf{y}}} \left\{ \mathrm{Ln}\left[f_y(\vec{\mathbf{y}}|\Psi)\right] | \vec{\mathbf{x}}, \Psi^{(k)} \right\} + \mathrm{Ln}\{ f(\vec{\mathbf{p}}^1..\vec{\mathbf{p}}^N, \vec{\mu}, \vec{\sigma}) \} , \qquad (6.25)$$

where the parameter sets Ψ and $\Psi^{(k)}$ are defined as:

$$\Psi \equiv (\vec{\mathbf{p}}^1..\vec{\mathbf{p}}^N, \vec{\theta}^1..\vec{\theta}^L) \qquad (6.26)$$

and

$$\Psi^{(k)} \equiv (\vec{\mathbf{p}}^{1(k)}..\vec{\mathbf{p}}^{N(k)}, \vec{\theta}^{1(k)}..\vec{\theta}^{L(k)}) , \qquad (6.27)$$

with $\{\vec{\theta}^{\,j}\} = (\vec{\mu}, \vec{\sigma})$ for univariate Gaussian component densities. The complete data likelihood function $f_y(\vec{y}|\Psi)$ is defined as:

$$f_y(\vec{y}|\Psi) = \prod_{i=1}^{N}\prod_{j=1}^{L}\left[\vec{\mathbf{p}}_j^i f_j(\vec{\mathbf{x}}_i|\vec{\theta}^{\,j})\right]^{\vec{\mathbf{z}}_j^i}. \tag{6.28}$$

Using Equations (6.20) and (6.21), the E-step of Equation (6.25) for the case of Gaussian component densities is given by:

$$
\begin{aligned}
Q'(\Psi|\Psi^{(k)}) =\;& \sum_{i=1}^{N}\sum_{j=1}^{L} E\{\vec{\mathbf{z}}_j^i|\vec{\mathbf{x}}_i, \Psi^{(k)}\}\left[\mathrm{Ln}(\vec{\mathbf{p}}_j^i) - \frac{1}{2}\mathrm{Ln}(2\pi\vec{\sigma}_j^2) - \frac{(\vec{\mathbf{x}}_i - \vec{\mu}_j)^2}{2\vec{\sigma}_j^2}\right] \\
& -\frac{1}{\beta}\sum_{c\in\mathcal{C}} V_c(\vec{\mathbf{p}}^1..\vec{\mathbf{p}}^N) + \mathrm{Ln}(K_\beta) + \mathrm{Ln}f(\vec{\mu}) + \mathrm{Ln}f(\vec{\sigma}),
\end{aligned} \tag{6.29}
$$

with $E\{\vec{\mathbf{z}}_j^i|\vec{\mathbf{x}}_i, \Psi^{(k)}\} = \vec{\mathbf{w}}_j^{i\,(k)}$ given by Equation (6.15). Scalars $\mathrm{Ln}(f(\vec{\mu}))$, $\mathrm{Ln}(f(\vec{\sigma}))$ and $\mathrm{Ln}(K_\beta)$ will not affect the result from the subsequent M-step, so that these terms can be dropped from $Q'(\Psi|\Psi^{(k)})$.

The M-step of the EM algorithm requires the maximization of $Q'(\Psi|\Psi^{(k)})$ at each iteration subject to the two constraints:

$$0 \le \vec{\mathbf{p}}_j^i \le 1.0 \quad \text{and} \quad \sum_{j=1}^{L}\vec{\mathbf{p}}_j^i = 1.0, \tag{6.30}$$

for $1 \le i \le N$ and $1 \le j \le L$. Note that $Q'(\Psi|\Psi^{(k)})$ is the same as $Q(\Psi|\Psi^{(k)})$ except for the addition of the prior terms. These terms preclude the existence of a closed-form expression for the maximum in the M-step, so that an iterative optimization technique for maximizing $Q'(\Psi|\Psi^{(k)})$ would be required. Rather than maximizing $Q'(\Psi|\Psi^{(k)})$ at each iteration M-step, simply finding a $\Psi^{(k+1)}$ at each iteration, such that:

$$Q'(\Psi^{(k+1)}|\Psi^{(k)}) > Q'(\Psi^{(k)}|\Psi^{(k)}), \tag{6.31}$$

results in a generalized EM (GEM) algorithm [759, 769] for MAP estimation of the label probabilities.

Gradient projection [770] is an established technique for constrained optimization. Here, at each iteration the updated parameters always lie within the hyperplane wherein the constraints are satisfied. Updated parameters are found by adding a component along the direction defined by projecting the gradient of the function being optimized onto that hyperplane. Note that MAP estimation could be implemented through gradient projection applied to the conditional likelihood defined in Equation (6.14). However, a better updating structure is obtained by applying it within the framework of the EM algorithm, because the M-step of the algorithm allows independent maximization of $Q'(\Psi|\Psi^{(k)})$ with respect to the parameters sets $\{\vec{\mathbf{p}}^i\}$, $\vec{\mu}$, and $\vec{\sigma}$.

Let the vector $\vec{\mathbf{q}}^i$ denote the gradient of $Q'(\Psi|\Psi^{(k)})$ with respect to the label probability vector $\vec{\mathbf{p}}^i$ so that:

$$\vec{\mathbf{q}}_j^i \equiv \frac{\partial Q'}{\partial \vec{\mathbf{p}}_j^i} = \frac{\vec{\mathbf{w}}_j^{i\,(k)}}{\vec{\mathbf{p}}_j^i} - \frac{1}{\beta}\sum_{c\in\mathcal{C}}\frac{\partial V_c(\vec{\mathbf{p}}^1..\vec{\mathbf{p}}^N)}{\partial \vec{\mathbf{p}}_j^i}. \tag{6.32}$$

Furthermore, let $\vec{\mathbf{q}}^{i\,(k)}$ denote the evaluation of $\vec{\mathbf{q}}^i$ at $\vec{\mathbf{p}}^i = \mathbf{p}^{i\,(k)}$. Projecting $\vec{\mathbf{q}}^{i\,(k)}$ onto the plane of the constraints consists of multiplying by a matrix $\mathbf{R}^{i,k}$ to obtain:

$$\vec{\mathbf{d}}^{i\,(k)} = \mathbf{R}^{i,k}\vec{\mathbf{q}}^{i\,(k)} , \tag{6.33}$$

where $R^{i,k}$ denotes a $L \times L$ projection matrix defined by:

$$\mathbf{R}^{i,k}_{j,l} = \begin{cases} 0 & \text{if condition}(\vec{\mathbf{p}}^i_j{}^{(k)}, \vec{\mathbf{q}}^i_j{}^{(k)}) \text{ or condition}(\vec{\mathbf{p}}^i_l{}^{(k)}, \vec{\mathbf{q}}^i_l{}^{(k)}) \text{ holds} \\ \frac{K-1}{K} & \text{if } j = l \text{ and condition}(\vec{\mathbf{p}}^i_j{}^{(k)}, \vec{\mathbf{q}}^i_j{}^{(k)}) \text{ does not hold} \\ -\frac{1}{K} & \text{otherwise.} \end{cases}$$
$$\tag{6.34}$$

Here $K = L-$ number of elements in $\vec{\mathbf{p}}^{i\,(k)}$ satisfying condition $(\vec{\mathbf{p}}^i_j{}^{(k)}, \vec{\mathbf{q}}^i_j{}^{(k)})$[3]. The generalized EM algorithm for simultaneous MAP estimation of label parameter vectors $\{\vec{\mathbf{p}}^i\}$ and parameter vectors $(\vec{\mu}, \vec{\sigma}^2)$ can now be described [766] as consisting of three steps:

Step 1:
For $i = 1, 2, ..., N$ and $j = 1, 2, ..., L$ compute:

$$\vec{\mathbf{w}}^i_j{}^{(k)} = \frac{\vec{\mathbf{p}}^i_j{}^{(k)} f_j(\vec{\mathbf{x}}_i | \vec{\mu}_j{}^{(k)}, \vec{\sigma}_j{}^{(k)})}{\sum_{l=1}^{L} \vec{\mathbf{p}}^i_l{}^{(k)} f_l(\vec{\mathbf{x}}_i | \vec{\mu}_l{}^{(k)}, \vec{\sigma}_l{}^{(k)})} , \tag{6.35}$$

where

$$f_j(\vec{\mathbf{x}}_i | \vec{\mu}_j{}^{(k)}, \vec{\sigma}_j{}^{(k)}) = \frac{1}{\sqrt{2\pi}\vec{\sigma}_j{}^{(k)}} \exp\left[\frac{-\left(\vec{\mathbf{x}}_i - \vec{\mu}_j{}^{(k)}\right)^2}{2\vec{\sigma}_j^{2(k)}}\right] . \tag{6.36}$$

Step 2: Sequentially visit all N pixels.
Step 2a: At each pixel site i compute:

$$c_1 = \sum_{j=1}^{L} \vec{\mathbf{w}}^i_j{}^{(k)} \mathrm{Ln}\vec{\mathbf{p}}^i_j{}^{(k)} - \frac{1}{\beta} \sum_{m\in\eta_i} V_m(\vec{\mathbf{p}}^{i\,(k)}, \vec{\mathbf{p}}^m) ,$$

and

$$\vec{\mathbf{q}}^i_j{}^{(k)} = \frac{f_j(\vec{\mathbf{x}}_i | \vec{\mu}_j^{(k)}, \vec{\sigma}_j^{(k)})}{\sum_{l=1}^{L} \vec{\mathbf{p}}^i_l{}^{(k)} f_l(\vec{\mathbf{x}}_i | \vec{\mu}_l^{(k)}, \vec{\sigma}_l^{(k)})} - \frac{1}{\beta} \sum_{m\in\eta_i} \left[\frac{\partial V_m(\vec{\mathbf{p}}^i, \vec{\mathbf{p}}^m)}{\partial \vec{\mathbf{p}}^i_j}\right]_{\vec{\mathbf{p}}^i = \vec{\mathbf{p}}^{i\,(k)}} .$$

Note η is the neighborhood, m is the clique potential and j represents the element. *Step 2b:* Determine the active constraints on $\vec{\mathbf{p}}^{i\,(k)}$ and form projection matrix $\mathbf{R}^{i,k}$ using Equation (6.34). Project the gradient vector $\vec{\mathbf{q}}^{i\,(k)}$ onto the plane of active constraints to obtain:

$$\vec{\mathbf{d}}^{i\,(k)} = \mathbf{R}^{i,k}\vec{\mathbf{q}}^{i\,(k)} .$$

---

[3]Condition $(\vec{\mathbf{p}}^i_j{}^{(k)}, \vec{\mathbf{q}}^i_j{}^{(k)}) = [\vec{\mathbf{p}}^i_j{}^{(k)} = 0 \& \vec{\mathbf{q}}^i_j{}^{(k)} < 0]$

Set $\alpha = 1.0$.

Step 2c: Compute:

$$\vec{\mathbf{p}}^{i\,(k+1)} = \vec{\mathbf{p}}^{i\,(k)} + \alpha * \vec{\mathbf{d}}^{i\,(k)}\,.$$

Step 2d: Compute:

$$c_2 = \sum_{j=1}^{L} \vec{\mathbf{w}}_j^{i\,(k)} \mathrm{Ln}\vec{\mathbf{p}}_j^{i\,(k+1)} - \frac{1}{\beta}\sum_{m \in \eta_i} V_m(\vec{\mathbf{p}}^{i\,(k+1)}, \vec{\mathbf{p}}^m)\,.$$

Step 2e: If $c_2 < c_1$ multiply α by 0.5 and go to step 2c. Otherwise go to the next pixel and perform steps 2a-e.

Step 3:

Compute:

$$\vec{\mu}_j^{(k+1)} = \frac{1}{\sum_{i=1}^{N} \vec{\mathbf{w}}_j^{i\,(k)}} \sum_{i=1}^{N} \vec{\mathbf{w}}_j^{i\,(k)} \vec{\mathbf{x}}_i\,,$$

and

$$[(\vec{\sigma}_j)^2]^{(k+1)} = \frac{1}{\sum_{i=1}^{N} \vec{\mathbf{w}}_j^{i\,(k)}} \sum_{i=1}^{N} \vec{\mathbf{w}}_j^{i\,(k)} [\vec{\mathbf{x}}_i - \vec{\mu}_j^{(k+1)}]^2\,.$$

Go to step 1.

In step 2, $V_m(\vec{\mathbf{p}}^i, \vec{\mathbf{p}}^m)$ is the potential function of the Gibbs distribution associated with the two-pixel cliques. The iteration number has been omitted from $\vec{\mathbf{p}}^m$ as the neighborhood set η_i could include pixels with updated label parameter vectors as well as pixels with label parameter vectors yet to be updated. Step 2c essentially implements coordinate ascent with the direction of movement determined by the projection of the gradient onto the plane of working constraints. Step 2e ensures that the function $Q'(\Psi|\Psi^{(k)})$ does not decrease along the direction of movement. Note that since $Q'(\Psi|\Psi^{(k)})$, as given by Equation (6.29), contains separate terms involving $\vec{\mathbf{p}}^i$ and $\{\vec{\mu}, \vec{\sigma}^2\}$, we can independently maximize for $\vec{\mathbf{p}}^i$ and $\{\vec{\mu}, \vec{\sigma}^2\}$. Step 3 is the same as in ML estimation discussed earlier, due to the assumption of a uniform prior on $\vec{\mu}$ and $\vec{\sigma}$.

6.6 Segmentation Results

We shall now examine a quantitative and qualitative analysis of the Bayesian algorithm for MAP estimation of pixel labeling. We shall compare the MAP-SVMM algorithm with the EM-CMM and ML-SVMM algorithms described in the previous sections. The quantitative analysis is based on computer simulations while the qualitative analysis is based on the segmentation of MRI brain images. For the simulations, noisy sample images were generated using a realistic label image.

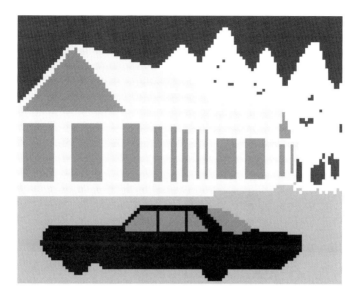

Figure 6.5: A spatially correlated image containing six classes.

6.6.1   Computer Simulations

The EM-CMM and ML-SVMM algorithms are derived using the inherent assumption that the image pixels are statistically independent. Such images contain no structure and therefore represent uninteresting examples for the labeling problem. Most real world images involve a high degree of local spatial correlation. It is this correlation that is modeled within the *a priori* Gibbs distribution. With this in mind, let us compare these algorithms using a spatially correlated image containing six classes shown in Figure 6.5. We shall see how the algorithms perform on noisy images generated from this base image. For a detailed description of the Monte Carlo analysis the interested reader is referred to [766]. The labeling error obtained using these images is plotted in Figure 6.6 as a function of $\frac{\vec{\sigma}}{\Delta\mu}$. As can be seen from Figure 6.6, EM-CMM and ML-SVMM yield more or less the same percentage labeling error. The MAP-SVMM algorithm consistently yields lower labeling error as the class variances are increased. Figure 6.7 shows a noisy data image from Figure 6.5 and the corresponding labeled images pixels using the EM-CMM, ML-SVMM and MAP-SVMM algorithms. The EM-CMM and ML-SVMM algorithms yield comparable results in this example. The labeling errors are spread evenly throughout the image. The MAP-SVMM algorithm yields considerably lower labeling error, with each class comprising more homogeneous regions. The benefits from the *a priori* model are more pronounced at high noise levels.

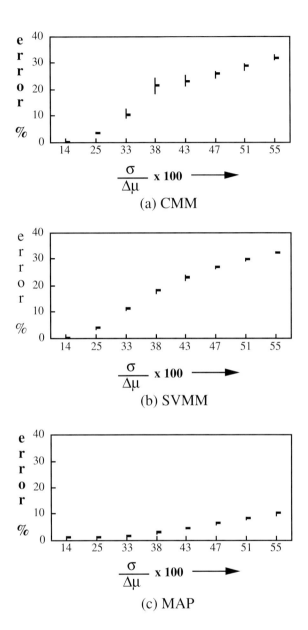

(a) CMM

(b) SVMM

(c) MAP

Figure 6.6: Sensitivity to class variances within an image with local spatial correlation (using the segmented image in Figure 6.5): percentage labeling error as all class variances $\vec{\sigma}_j$ are varied from 200 to 3000 with $\vec{\mu}_j = j\Delta\mu \ \forall j$ where $\Delta\mu = 100$ for (a) EM-CMM algorithm, (b) ML-SVMM algorithm, and (c) MAP-SVMM algorithm with $\beta = 0.01$. Shown are the errors obtained for ten noise realizations and the mean error for these ten realizations.

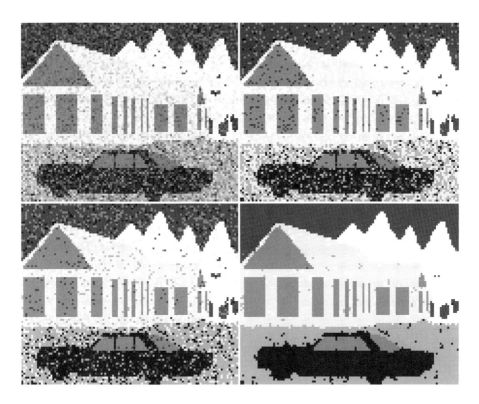

Figure 6.7: A spatially correlated images containing six classes (car, wind, grass, house, tree and sky): noisy image generated using the "true" label image with $\vec{\sigma}_j{}^2 = 2000 \ \forall j$ (top left), the labeling from the EM-CMM algorithm (top right), the labeling from the ML-SVMM algorithm (bottom left), and the labeling from the MAP-SVMM algorithm using $\beta = 0.01$ (bottom right).

6.6.2 Application to Magnetic Resonance Images

In this section we present results from applying the EM-CMM, ML-SVMM and the MAP-SVMM algorithms for segmenting magnetic resonance images[4] of the adult brain. Plate 6 shows a T_2-weighted MRI slice of the brain of a 28-year old normal male subject. T_2-weighted MRI images differentiate between three classes of tissue (bone marrow, White Matter, Grey Matter/cerebro-spinal fluid) plus a class for air. Also shown are the labels estimated using the EM-CMM and ML-SVMM algorithms. The MAP-SVMM algorithm was applied with a sum-squared error prior and empirically determined β (note β is a constant) values of $1.0, 10.0$ and 1000.0. The resulting labeled images are also shown in Plate 6. Close examination of the resulting images leads to the following observations:

(1) EM-CMM and ML-SVMM algorithms tend to yield erroneous labels along

---

[4]MRI studies obtained from Methodist Hospital, Houston, TX.

the boundaries of the Gray Matter/csf and the White Matter.

(2) The MAP-SVMM algorithm gives acceptable labeling results over a wide range of β values (1-1000). This can be more easily minimized by a judicious choice of β values in the MAP-SVMM algorithm.

(3) The MAP-SVMM algorithm yields more homogeneous class regions separated by a crisper boundary. Note the clear delineation of the space between skull and surface of the brain in the MAP-SVMM labeled images.

6.7 Practical Aspects

There are several practical issues in implementing the labeling algorithms presented here. The first issue is how these algorithms should be initialized. The likelihood functions for both the classical mixture model and the spatially variant mixture model have multiple local maxima. These local maxima can generally be avoided by following several simple rules for initializing the parameters to be estimated.

(1) **Initializing the mixture weights.** The best method for initializing the mixture weights for the classical mixture model $\vec{\pi}$ or the probability vectors for the spatially variant mixture model $\{\vec{\mathbf{p}}^i\}$ is also the simplest method. Set all mixture weights to $\vec{\pi}_j = 1/L$ or set all elements of $\vec{\mathbf{p}}^i$ to $\vec{\mathbf{p}}^i_j = 1/L$ where L is the number of classes. There appears to be no advantage in any more complicated method.

(2) **Initializing the class means.** In considering how to initialize the class means, note that the classes are anticipated as having means that are separated from one another. Therefore, it seems reasonable to initialize the class means at some non-zero separation. It is not advised to initialize all class means to values at or near the peak value in the histogram of the data image, as this seems to often lead to convergence to an undesirable local maxima wherein one of the classes is estimated as having a large mixture weight and a large class variance. To initialize the means, the minimum and maximum values in the data, respectively *xmin* and *xmax*, are helpful. One method that works well is to form a coarse histogram of $4L$ quantization levels over the range of data values, *xmin* to *xmax*. Then initialize the L means to the L peaks in the coarse histogram. This ensures that the initial means are separated by at least $(xmax\text{-}xmin)/(4L)$. Other simpler methods may work equally well, as long as the class variances are initialized as follows.

(3) **Initializing the class variances.** Initialize the variances within each class to very large values. The algorithms will require more iteration to converge, but large initial variances tend to help these algorithms avoid local maxima. How large is large enough? Again, the range of the data is helpful. Find the minimum and maximum values in the data, respectively

xmin and *xmax*. Where there are three or more classes in the data, set the initial variances to $\sigma = 0.1 \ (xmin - xmax)^2$.

On the question of how many iterations of each algorithm should be run on a given application, about 500 iterations of the EM-CMM and ML-SVMM algorithms yields parameter estimates that were converged to at least 4-5 significant digits. The pixel labels typically do not change after 300-400 iterations. Approximately 150 iterations are enough for similar convergence of the MAP-SVMM algorithm, but each iteration may require approximately three to four times more computation. Finally, at this time it is recommended that the β value in the MAP-SVMM algorithm be chosen through trial and error. Several statistical measures to determine acceptable convergence and to determine β can be found in the literature [771]–[774].

6.8 Summary

We analyzed the use of mixture models for pixel labeling and discussed the drawbacks of the classical mixture model when applied to pixel labeling. We have examined a spatially variant finite mixture model to overcome these drawbacks and an EM algorithm for ML estimation of pixel labels. Images in general involve spatial correlation to a reasonable degree. To incorporate such spatial correlation *a priori* density functions can be used to model spatial relationships between image pixels and the SVMM can be uncorporated into a Bayesian algorithm for segmentation. The only requirement of this algorithm is that the prior term have a continuous first partial derivative. As seen above this algorithm yields quantitatively accurate and visually appealing segmentation results.

6.9 Acknowledgements

The algorithm described in this chapter was developed by the author and published in the *IEEE Transactions on Image Processing*, July 1998. The author is grateful to the IEEE for permission to use portions of this material and the figures in this publication.

Chapter 7

Application of Segmentation in Localized MR Chemical Shift Imaging and MR Spectroscopy

Rakesh Sharma

7.1 Introduction

Since the discovery of NMR (Nuclear Magnetic Resonance) half a century ago, biophysical NMR approaches to brain imaging have shifted to non-invasive methods. Mainly brain segmentation, metabolic mapping and steady-state biochemical approaches are now being explored for normal and developmental neurochemistry with an exposure to common disorders of brain functions. Basically, NMR detects frequency dependent signals from individual odd numbered atomic nuclei. MRI (Magnetic Resonance Imaging) detects signals from populations of these nuclei at different locations in the tissues. Major advancements have been made in non-invasive MR imaging in two directions. Spatial information with good resolution in different tissue locations was achieved primarily by segmentation. Spatial information of metabolites and the peak sensitivity of metabolites were achieved by Chemical Shift Imaging (CSI). There exists a trade-off between these two informations. The highest quality of spatial chemical information by the MR technique is affected by the trade-off due to several physical and chemical factors. Localized MR Spectroscopy still remains a powerful tool to identify neuro-chemicals and metabolite concentrations precisely in relative or absolute terms in different locations in the brain. The latest major emphasis was concentrated on neurochemicals and their spectral peaks referenced with abundant tissue water at very short intervals. MR Spectroscopy (MRS) and MR Spectroscopic Imaging (MRSI) methods are used to define regional differences of peaks within the tissue. Moreover, their capability depends upon high spatial and temporal resolution and subtle MR properties such as T_1, T_2, $T_2{}^*$, proton density weighting of water and fat as well as CSF components in the brain.

To achieve such spatial resolution, the segmentation of images is mandatory. The reason is that the variation of the brain tissue composition inside of a Magnetic Resonance Spectroscopic Imaging voxel can mimic with changes of metabolite peak intensities in different locations of the voxel. The major focus to improve segmentation was concentrated on identifying partial volume artifacts. Partial volume average artifacts originate along with peak intensity changes due to the presence of different metabolites in the brain. These artifacts can be minimized through using co-registration, tissue composition analysis and segmentation techniques. Co-registration is a method used to align the subsequent images. Segmentation is a method used to distinguish the constituents of various tissue components such as Gray Matter, White Matter and CSF in the brain. For example, the observed Choline (Cho) or N-Acetyl Aspartate (NAA) resonances are obtained from Gray Matter and White Matter, not from CSF or outside the brain region. In such a case, each Magnetic Resonance Spectroscopic Imaging (MRSI) small voxel can be defined by the tissue content as: Proton Density = (Gray Matter + White Matter) and an index for Gray Matter, f = Gray Matter/(Gray Matter + White Matter). The corrected metabolite intensity for tissue volume is known as Metabolite (corrected) = Metabolite (observed)/proton density. As mentioned above, the index f is also useful to account for variations in Gray and White Matter voxel composition.

In this direction, automated segmentation techniques have been recently described using: a neural network system (see Magnotta *et al.* [726]); intensity corrected multi-spectral MRI with stochastic relaxation method utilizing partial volume analysis of each brain voxel (see Rusinek *et al.* [777]); and multi-spectral feature space classification methods (see Udupa [721]) as shown in Figures 7.1, 7.2 and Plate 9. Current attempts are in progress, focusing on fast and automated segmentation methods to analyze the brain tissue composition and neurochemical distribution. Popular methods used are integrated Magnetic Resonance Imaging and Spectroscopy (MRI/MRS). Several popular segmentation algorithms and automated methods are described in Sub-section 5.2. Our segmentation technique could emphasize the tissue and metabolite composition of Gray Matter, White Matter and Multiple Sclerosis lesions as shown in Plates 7 and 8.

Segmentation methods require using extensive pre-processing and post-processing on MR images. The pre-processing step involves obtaining image quality enhancement. The post-processing step involves obtaining the application of threshold techniques to develop a mask image from the area of interest, such as Multiple Sclerosis lesions in White Matter (see Dastidar *et al.* [716]). A mask image is obtained for a region of interest (ROI) from segmented images. Individual neuro-chemical images can be generated by using an automated selection of chemical shifts from spectra for each metabolite with reference to the tissue water signal in the mask image. In the brain spectra, chemical shifts of N-Acetyl Aspartate (NAA) show up at 2.01 ppm, Creatine (Cr) at 3.0 ppm, Choline (Cho) at 3.2 ppm, myo-Inositol(MI) at 3.6 ppm, Lactate(Lac) at 1.33 ppm and Lipids(Lp) at 0.88 ppm, with traces at 1.2 ppm, 1.4 ppm, 1.6 ppm as the main MR visible neurochemicals. Simultaneously, chemical shift images are fingerprinted by individual voxel spectra which overall represent the location and distribution of metabolite concentrations in different locations in the brain. Information on metabolites and the contribution of Gray Matter, White Matter and CSF from different columns and raw images in the region of interest may provide significant information on morphological and neuro-functional dynamics.

Using this approach of "chemical shift imaging and segmentation" answers two questions: (1) what are the normal brain neurochemicals and tissue composition, and (2) how do these neurochemicals and tissue composition differ in neurological or neurodegenerative disease? It also describes the perturbations encountered in such diseases as shown in Figure 7.3. Magnetic Resonance Imaging (MRI) and Magnetic Resonance Spectroscopy (MRS) are used in evaluating the brain patho-chemical neurodegeneration of diseases such as Multiple Sclerosis (MS) and Alzheimer's Disease (AD). In Multiple Sclerosis, MRI shows lesions in the White Matter around the ventricles. In Alzheimer's Disease, a general loss of cortical tissue is associated with neurofibrillar tangles and cortical plaques with hippocampal volume reductions (see Schuff *et al.* [778]). In these neurodegenerative diseases, anatomical changes and volume measurements by MRI reflect neuronal loss and neuron cell body shrinkage. Proton Magnetic Resonance Spectroscopic Imaging performs a metabolite distribution and measurement in the cerebrum. Mainly N-Acetyl Aspartate (NAA), Creatine (Cr), Choline (Cho), myo-Inositol (MI) and lipids are visible using Magnetic Resonance Spectroscopic Imaging (MRSI). With reference to the brain water, Cr is considered approximately constant and NAA as a neuronal marker of neuronal integrity in the brain. The origin of these metabolites is described in Sub-section 7.6.1.

The layout of this chapter is as follows: Section 7.2 describes the purpose and effectiveness of MR techniques in metabolite distribution and tissue composition for anatomical and patho-chemical details for better neuro- diagnosis. Further emphasis is placed on the continued efforts to improve the methodology of segmentation, neuro-chemical distribution analysis focused on longitudinal tissue atrophy in Alzheimer's Disease and lesion volumetry in Multiple Sclerosis. In Section 7.3, basic concepts of patient preparation, types of data acquired, a brief introduction to localization, shimming, and different scan parameters are discussed. Our experiences in achieving MRSI data with good segmentation are described. The unique importance of inhomogeneity minimization, water suppression in the volume of interest region and lipid saturation around the scalp by using image pre-processing are described in Section 7.4. Later, image post-processing steps will be described for possible good image co-registration and flow correction to get better tissue neuro-chemical details.

Section 7.4 introduces the concept of combining information from segmentation and spectral analysis to obtain integrated anatomical and metabolic information of enhancing MS lesions in a time dependent manner. Emphasis will be placed on distinguishing the Normal Appearing White Matter (NAWM) abnormal metabolite peaks associated with MS and visualizing MS lesions. The capability of identifying abnormal metabolite peaks in classifying MS and the nature of demyelination are described, as is the role of MR-visible lipids in MS lesion progression. Section 7.5 describes using similar concepts of data acquisition as described for Multiple Sclerosis. For Alzheimer's Disease, different scan settings are used with similar principles to Single Voxel Spectroscopy. Resolved

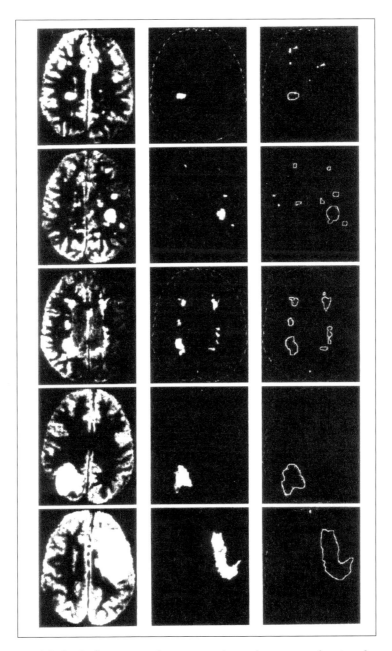

Figure 7.1: Method of automated segmentation using a neural network system. This figure shows spin density-weighted images (left column) with extracted lesions (center column) and lesion edges (right column) obtained by an automated edge detection method using a search algorithm. Raw images 1 to 3 show sclerosis is plaques, while raw images 4 and 5 show tumor and idiopathic lesion. The artificial neural network extracts very small lesions without operator bias. Reproduced with permission from Raff *et al.* [775]. © 1992 AAPM.

Spectroscopy (PRESS) for composite single spectrum, and Chemical Shift Selective Saturation (CHESS) for specific metabolite saturation will be emphasized. Section 7.6 describes the interpretation of segmentation and metabolite variations in the characterization and classification process for dementia and Multiple Sclerosis. Specific examples of metabolites and the potential of MRSI in tissue classification are considered. Section 7.7 describes the benefits of using a combined approach of segmentation by MRI and spectral imaging with its use in MS lesion and plaque in AD in an automated, robust manner. Several possibilities of rare metabolites are presumed, based on our laboratory experiments. The current problems of shimming, spatial resolution, contrast enhancement, and tissue classification are discussed. The limitations of segmentation are described along with the latest reported technique improvements used by other authors. Section 7.8 focuses on the capability of combining segmentation and spectroscopy techniques. Its prediction power is highlighted for disease prognosis, as well as for better interpretation of anatomical and metabolic events in clinical and therapeutic monitoring.

7.2 A Short History of Neurospectroscopic Imaging and Segmentation in Alzheimer's Disease and Multiple Sclerosis

Both of these neuro-degenerative brain diseases have been widely reported as being considerable frontline health hazards. The mechanism of neuro-degeneration in Alzheimer's Disease and MS lesions remains unsolved. The complexity of neuronal loss, shrinkage of neuron cell bodies and glial loss with brain volume measurements are less specific indicators of neuronal integrity. MR Spectroscopic Imaging measures the regional distribution of important cerebral metabolites at a much coarser spatial spectral resolution. The main metabolites in the brain are amino acid N-Acetyl Aspartate (NAA), Choline (Cho) and Creatine (Cr) in neurons, glial cells. MR Imaging and localized proton MR spectroscopy (H-1 MRS) have been used to characterize these diseases. Cortical tissue loss, reduced hippocampus volumes, regional metabolites with related signal hyperintensities in Alzheimer's Disease are commonly seen. Multiple Sclerosis is shown as enhancing lesions based on the distribution of these metabolites. MRI and MR Spectroscopic Imaging have both been accepted as effective tools in demonstrating Alzheimer's Disease from the point of view of: (1) having statistically significant regional metabolite variations; (2) H-1 metabolite levels in White Matter Signal Hyperintensities relative to contralateral Normal Appearing White Matter (NAWM) regions; (3) comparison of different metabolite levels in Alzheimer's Disease with a control normal group; (4) White Matter Signal Hyperintensities (WMSH) and metabolite concentration based on the classification of Alzheimer's Disease and other dementia types in the brain for improved visualization. Later, emphasis was placed on designing improved pulse sequences, automation in MR Spectroscopic Imag-

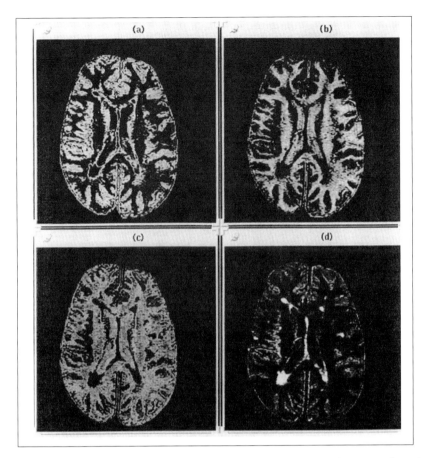

Figure 7.2: Intensity-corrected multi-spectral MRI, stochastic relaxation method utilizing the partial volume analysis classification method. Note images (a), (b) before image intensity correction is applied and images (c), (d) after intensity correction is applied, now showing better tissue differentiation. © IEEE. Reprinted with permission from [776].

ing and spectral analysis methods, comparison of left versus right hemisphere metabolites and MR signal intensities for better disease interpretation.

MRSI is a superior technique for MS lesion diagnosis. Studies using Gadolinium (Gd) enhancement, dating of MS plaques and correlating acute lesion activity with neurological activity are not encouraging due to poor contrast resolution. Improvements are urgently needed before effective therapies can be introduced into clinical trials. Larger MS plaques are easier to study for single voxel spectroscopic characterization due to easier localization and Region-of-Interest (ROI) setting. Other unsolved problems are: (1) the need for an internal reference for the calibration of metabolite absolute concentration, (2) the identification of important neuro-chemically active lesion metabolites (lipids, lactate, myo- Inositol, alanine and acetate), (3) metabolite bleed-through, (4)

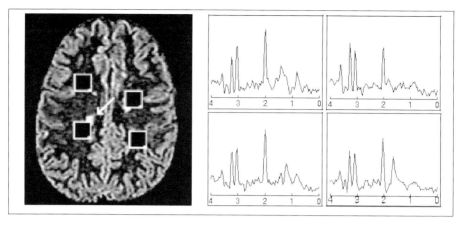

Figure 7.3: The image shows four square regions of interest in the representative quadrupule contrast image with dark White Matter. Two of the square ROI's are in the MS lesions (the bottom square in the left hemisphere and the upper square in the right hemisphere). The other two ROI's are in normal appearing White Matter locations. Also shown in the figure are the four Metabolite peaks (left to right, top to bottom) of spectroscopic volumes of interest (VOI) in the segmented brain image. Note the altered peak amplitudes in the fitted spectra are shown for specific chemical characteristic of these lesion rich regions. The imaging parameters used were: Time of Echo [TE = 10 ms]; Repetition Time [TR = 10,000 ms]; slice thickness = 3 mm (MRSI Data, Courtesy of MR Lab., University of Texas Medical School, Houston, TX.)

Partial Volume Averaging (PVA) effects, (5) the false classification of MS lesions. Strong evidence is available for the presence of regressed acute neurological symptoms associated with MS lesion history. White Matter Signal Hyperintensities (WMSH) and chemical shift imaging provide significant information along with single voxel lesion MR Spectroscopy information. This further emphasizes the need for having an integrated routine MRI-MRSI to improve MS lesion activity assessment. This can be accomplished by improving the quality of clinical trials for the use of newer therapeutic agents.

Recently, this author has focused upon several issues related to the quantitative analysis of tissue composition and metabolite screening by Magnetic Resonance Spectroscopic Imaging. The main goal has been to use these on MS serial studies for: (1) neuro-chemical characterization of MS lesions; (2) absolute concentration measurement of metabolites; (3) chemical shift imaging; (4) critical evaluation of lesion bearing single voxel spectral analysis of metabolites; (5) validation of enhancing lesion bearing single voxel metabolite abnormalities; and (6) Promiscol drug trial for MS lesions as part of a research study. In the next sub-section, the purpose and urgency of Point Resolved Spectroscopy in plaque metabolites are introduced with combined information on tissue composition and possible localized atrophy in the brain. Some of the currently accepted controversies that are relevant to segmentation and metabo-

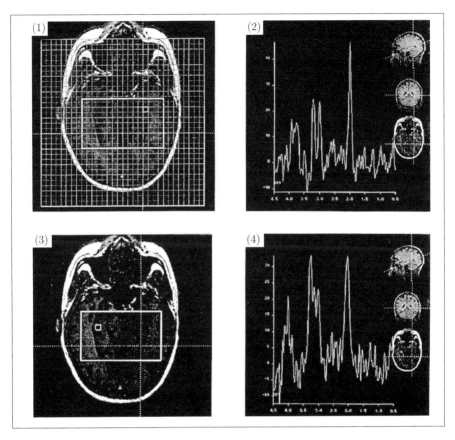

Figure 7.4: Metabolite changes in Alzheimer's Disease with low NAA and high choline. The images seen in (1) and (3) represent the position of the VOI box with a grid and area of interest on both sides of the hippocampus for spectra seen in (2) and (4). Note that the metabolite changes in (4). Note also the changes in the Cho peak in spectrum (4). The imaging parameters used were: TE/TR=35/5000 ms (MRSI Data, Courtesy of MR Lab., University of California, San Francisco, CA.)

lite imaging are also introduced.

7.2.1 Alzheimer's Disease

The application of MR Imaging segmentation methods in Alzheimer's Disease (AD) reveals that the VOI tissue type may not contribute to metabolite alterations, such as in NAA/Cr and Cho/Cr differences. These differences are mainly due to out-of-plane spatial shifts of Point Resolved Spectroscopy (PRESS) volumes for chemically shifted metabolites. Segmentation methods are shown to be of great importance in characterizing Gray Matter, White Matter and CSF regional composition and their contribution in AD. For example,

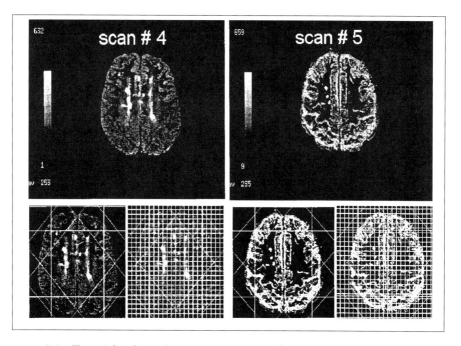

Figure 7.5: T_1-weighted axial segmented FLAIR/MTC (AFFIRMATIVE pulse sequence acquired image) using TE/TR=30/1000 ms shown on the left; and T_1-weighted axial CSF suppressed (Quadruple Contrast pulse sequence acquired image) using TE/TR 10/3000 ms on the right, with bright MS lesions seen in the White Matter regions. On the bottom row, images are shown the position of Octagonal Saturation Bands (OVS) (on the lower left side images) and with a grid (on the lower right side images). Note the improved clarity of the MS lesions in WM in the CSF suppressed images on the top right. (MRSI Data, Courtesy of MR Lab., University of Texas Medical School, Houston, TX.)

patients with AD and control subjects can be distinguished by the difference in posterior mesial Gray Matter NAA/Cho ratio. Moreover, the proton spectrum seen for Alzheimer's Disease is different from the spectrum seen for the normal brain, as is indicated by the elevated myo-Inositol(MI) with MI/Cr ratio and reduced NAA/Cr ratio (see Figure 7.4). The useful MRSI capability of screening Alzheimer's Disease is still not established. Proton spectra in AD differ from normal elderly persons with elevated MI/Cr and reduced NAA/Cr (see Mackay *et al.* [779]), while AD differs from other dementia types by MI/Cr. However, increased MI in cerebral gliosis is associated with AD. Proton spectroscopy with MR imaging is being used in current practice as an integration of MRI and metabolites. This integration method is robust and accurate (see Soher *et al.* [780]). The biochemical cause of AD happens to be due to β-amyloid abnormal protein as a neuro-toxic, and it develops neurofibrillary plaques and tangles. Cholinergic neuron loss is associated with altered membrane phosphorylcholine lipids. Cholinergic receptors in the central nervous system act

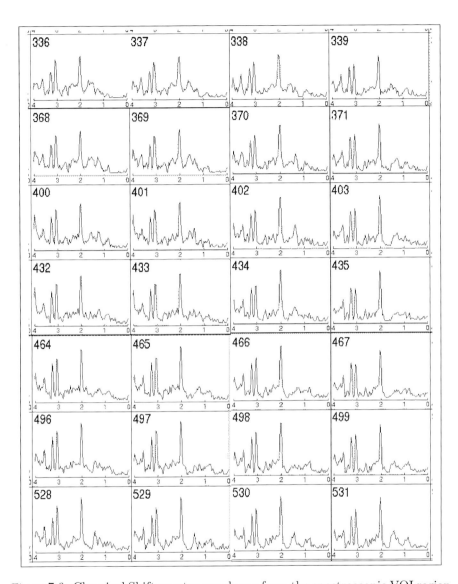

Figure 7.6: Chemical Shift spectra are shown from the spectroscopic VOI region of a segmented brain image rich with MS lesions (see Figure 7.5, scan number 4). Each small voxel is shown with 4 spectral peaks for NAA at 2.01 ppm (middle), Creatine at 3.0 ppm, Choline at 3.2 ppm (left) and lipids at 0.8-1.2 ppm (right). The rightmost single and double lipid peaks at 0.8-1.2 ppm may be due to true-bulky and mobile-derived lipids, respectively. (MRSI Data, Courtesy of MR Lab., University of Texas Medical School, Houston, TX.)

through the phosphoinositol pathway. Moreover, apolipoprotein E-ϵ4 identifies a gene responsible for the increased risk of AD in the general population. These biochemical changes in AD need better proton MR spectroscopic images and peaks as shown in Plate 9. Having discussed Alzheimer's Disease, in the following sub-section, the logic of MS lesion enhancement and blood-brain barrier will be highlighted with possible regional differences in metabolite distribution, brain tissue components, and volumetric analysis of brain tissue. Metabolite absolute concentrations, lesion frequency and their regional location show the possibility of lesion characteristics. The importance of segmentation analysis is described to suggest some insights into the biological nature of demyelination in lesions by the use of feature maps, tissue-lesion contrast and patterns of NAA, Creatine and Choline.

7.2.2 Multiple Sclerosis

MS is the most common demyelinating disease in humans. The presence of perivenous inflammatory change is usually associated with locally altered blood-brain barrier dysfunction. It is believed to be an early event in the evolution of MS plaques. It is, however, not known if it is an obligatory event for demyelination. In serial MRI and single voxel magnetic resonance spectroscopy, studies observed that demyelination is frequently associated with local alterations of the blood-brain-barrier. Serial studies by Proton Magnetic Resonance Spectroscopic Imaging in patients with MS have confirmed these observations. Active demyelination has been observed in the areas of the brain showing no evidence of an altered blood-brain barrier and/or MRI-observed lesions. This observation provides fundamental information about the pathological evolution of MS lesions. Two distinct processes affect myelin integrity and/or stability of MS in the brain. One process is associated with regional inflammation and locally altered the blood-brain-barrier permeability. The second process is independent of blood-brain-barrier change and inflammation.

Serial MRI and MRSI patients with MS allow us to distinguish between these two processes. To achieve this, better lesion to noise contrast is obtained by using CSF suppression and magnetization transfer contrast. The AFFIRMATIVE pulse sequence with improved visualization of contrast enhancement is used by serial MRI for pre-contrast and post-Gd contrast agent administration. Associated with these lesions, MR Spectroscopic Imaging offers improvement over MRI and Single Voxel Spectroscopy. This provides images of the regional metabolite distribution with increased spatial resolution in the single voxel size up to 1 cc. MRSI is analogous to conventional MRI except that the signal intensity in each voxel is based on the proton signal from metabolites, rather than on the signals from water. The concentration of metabolites is 1000 times less than that of water. So, the resolution and signal-to-noise ratio of metabolite images are much lower than that of water-based images. In this direction, low NAA/Cr, high Cho/Cr ratio with or without lipids and lactate have been evaluated by other authors as MRSI metabolite indicators of MS lesion and Normal Appearing White Matter (NAWM) in Multiple Sclerosis (see Nagatomo *et al.* [781], Rooney *et al.* [782], Arnold *et al.* [783], Pouwels *et al.* [785], Hennig *et al.* [784], Sarchielli *et al.* [786]). Characteristically, these MS lesions take up the contrast agent Gadolinium-Dithylene-Triamine-Penta-Acetate (Gd-DTPA), indicating a compromised blood-brain-barrier contrast enhancement associated with clinically active MS lesions (see Shareef *et al.* [730], O'Riordan *et al.* [723], Hirsch *et al.* [810]).

MS is a complex disease with a relapsing and remitting course. MRI has rapidly become the modality of choice for studying patients with MS. MRI has been an important clinical modality in diagnostic approaches to MS. It defines the natural history of the disease process, providing new parameters that predict the disease's course. It is generally recognized that the extent of the disease seen on MRI is more severe than the actual clinical disability. This indicates that not all the plaques are active or contribute to the clinical symptoms and lesions. These plaques appear homogeneous in conventional MRI. They are pathologically heterogeneous. The ability to distinguish active plaques from inactive ones may help in our understanding of the pathophysiology of the disease. Being able to perform a non-invasive characterization of plaques is significant in the objective evaluation of the efficacy of the treatment. This is particularly relevant in view of a large number of ongoing clinical trials for MS. An active MS plaque exhibits perivenous inflammatory changes usually associated with local blood-brain-barrier breakdown. This can be detected as an enhancement following the administration of an appropriate contrast agent. Studies using the paramagnetic contrast agent Gadolinium-Dithylene-Triamine-Penta-Acetate (Gd-DTPA) have shown the enhancement associated with active lesions, some of which are clinically symptomatic. Furthermore, unenhanced lesions have been observed through post-contrast MRI before they become clinically symptomatic. Serial studies of patients with MS have demonstrated that the value of MRI segmented images can be significantly extended when combined with *in vivo* MRS (see Narayana *et al.* [787]).

The proton spectrum of the normal brain exhibits peaks mainly arising from NAA, Cr and Cho. The relative concentrations of various metabolites are altered in MS plaques, depending on the regional pathology. Increased Cho in acute plaques from increased concentrations of choline, phosphorylcholine and other products are associated with cellular inflammation and consistent with active blood-brain-barrier disruption as reflected by Gd enhancement. A reduction in the concentration of NAA is observed in chronic plaques and transient reduction of NAA occurs with acutely evolving lesions. Reduced NAA may reflect the axonal loss known to occur in more severely demyelinated plaques. This assumption is based in part on the restriction of NAA to nerve cells and their processes. NAA is not produced by astrocytes. Due to the high degree of structural organization of lipids in myelin and cellular membranes in the brain, mobile lipids appear in the 0.8-1.5 ppm region of the spectrum in some MS lesions. Lipids are seen as broader and shorter peaks. These reflect the presence of mobile lipids (which may also include possible contributions from cytosolic proteins and thymosin $\beta 4$) in the spectra from some lesions that have been interpreted as arising from the myelin breakdown products. Mobile lipids are consistently seen in about 20-40% of the regions selected for MRS study based on the presence of MRI-defined lesions. Regions selected based on the appearance of post-Gd contrast enhancement or a newly MRI-defined lesion are more likely to show metabolite signals attributable to the presence of myelin breakdown.

Metabolite changes are very informative and reinforce early pathological observations in MS, based on biopsy and autopsy studies. However, observations of lipid signals in several patients from different regions of the brain remain unassociated either with Gd enhancement or MRI-defined lesions, which later develop into new lesions on MRI. MRSI evidence of lipid release in the absence of MRI- defined pathology is sometimes possibly due to: (1) irregular sampling interval, (2) failure to capture a brief enhancing event in these regions, (3) persistent enhancement of lipids over months. Most of the lesion enhancements are associated with MRI-defined lesions on spin density and T_2-weighted MRI images. MRSI is an extremely sensitive method to image the lipid release and is capable of detecting activity in lesions well within the limits of the spatial resolution of MRI. Coupling more sensitive MRI techniques such as FLuid Attenuated Inversion Recovery (FLAIR) and Magnetization Transfer Contrast (MTC) to our MRSI/MRI strategy strengthens this ability.

The acquisition of MRSI data of MS in the brain may provide significant information of myelin integrity and/or the myelin stability. Gadolinium enhancement and increased regional Cho suggest the classical model of T-cell mediated, macrophage-associated stripping of myelin from axons. The other process possibly reflects a primary oligodendrogliopathy, and may be independent of inflammation or blood brain-barrier changes. The acquisition of MRSI data from a large region of a brain with MS is required to increase the chances of sampling areas of the brain which appear "normal" on MRI but active in terms of lipid release. Lesion quantification allows us to probe the relationship between metabolic changes and lesion burden. These relationships require robust and accurate lesion quantification. Magnetization Transfer Contrast (MTC) and diffusion imaging show great promise for lesion characterization. MTC depends on the interaction between mobile tissue water and macromolecular protons. Myelin is the main macromolecular matrix in the brain. Therefore, the value of MTC or Magnetization Transfer Ratio (MTR) depends on the integrity of the myelin structure. Water diffusion in tissues exhibits directional dependence. Diffusion anisotropy depends on the extent of myelin damage. The average value of diffusion or the Apparent Diffusion Coefficient (ADC) depends on the pathology of the plaque, i.e., the loss in anisotropy in lesions. This indicates a loss of the myelin barrier to water motion, subsequently developing a lesion on MRI after pathological evolution and patho-physiological changes are seen in evolving MS plaques.

MRSI and lesion quantification techniques provide highly useful surrogate markers important in therapeutic treatment and clinical efficacy. The biochemical basis for the cause of MS happens to be inflammatory demyelination of the central nervous system. It is manifested as focal lesions distinguished by their contents of activated macrophages and T cells, edema and axonal transection associated with high serum E-selectin protein. Recently, lipids and cytosolic proteins with β-thymosin formation were hypothesized as being associated with MS.

7.3 Data Acquisition and Image Segmentation

One of the prime goals of clinical MR data acquisition is to obtain the required information in the minimum amount of time. Scan time is affected by several factors: (1) metabolite concentration, (2) fast Fourier noise and interference, (3) spin-lattice relaxation time T_1, (4) flip angle and delay between successive pulses or TR. The simplest data-acquisition method consists of a brief RF transmitter pulse followed by Free Induction Decay (FID) digitization and then an inter-pulse delay. The operator should attempt to reduce these scan parameters for the lowest possible scan time before data collection. The signal strength depends on two acquisition parameters: the flip angle and the pulse repetition time. A large flip angle and a short TR show small signals. Faster pulses allow signal recovery even at smaller flip angles. Furthermore, the use of surface coils improves the signal significantly from a smaller volume element. Additionally, the sensitivity of the magnetic field gradient becomes uniform over the volume under the surface coil. The signal also depends upon the spatial distribution of protons in the brain tissue and metabolites of interest. At the beginning of the data collection, the nuclei are fully relaxed and saturation builds up over a few pulses until an equilibrium or steady-state is reached. Later FID from these pulses contribute to signal build up. The effects of pulse distortions are avoided by transmitter-pulse and receiver phase cycles increasing by 90° for each successive pulse. Spectrum-baseline distortions by using k-filters are reduced by using the correct setting of the switch-on times for the receiver and digitizer after the RF transmitter pulse. Other important aspects of data acquisition are avoiding unwanted signal from the outer scalp, selection of a defined brain shape, image size, and brain tissue Volume of Interest (VOI) location with its sharp boundaries. This is achieved using localization techniques. MR Spectroscopic Imaging mainly depends on spatial localization accuracy.

Our MR studies were done on a 1.5 T MR scanner (GE, Milwaukee, WI) equipped with a shielded gradient coil system and using software version 5.6 at Hermann Hospital, Houston, TX. A quadrature birdcage resonator head coil is generally used for Radio Frequency (RF) transmission and signal reception. Initially, spin-echo sagittal scout images were obtained using an Echo Time [TE=16 msec]; Repetition Time [TR=600 msec]; slice thickness 3 mm contiguous and interleaved slices; the Number of Excitations [NEX=0.5] followed by the acquisition of AFFIRMATIVE [Attenuated Fluid Fast Inversion Recovery Magnetization Transfer Imaging with Variable Echoes] using [TE=30 msec; TR= 1000 msec]. Quadruple Contrast using double inversion recovery method to suppress CSF or WM/GM was based on a fast spin-echo pulse sequence for axial images. In both these pulse sequences, the scan parameters were set as:

[TE=10 msec; TR = 3000 msec], NEX = 0.5. The acquisition matrix was set as 256 × 192 and later zero-filled to 256 × 256 for the acquisition of contiguous (interleaved), 3 mm thick axial images, extending from the vertex to the foramen magnum of the brain. These axial images are necessary for locating and quantifying the lesion volumes and localizing the VOI for MRSI studies.

Immediately after the acquisition of these axial images, two dimensional 2-D MRSI scanning was performed on the VOI. The axial images were used for localization of the VOI by using the stimulated echo sequence. The pre-localization reduces lipid contamination from the extrameningeal tissues and minimizes the susceptibility effects for improved magnetic field homogeneity over the VOI. The size of the VOI chosen is typically 0.75 × 0.75 × 1.5 cc and is contained within a large area of White Matter of the centrum semiovale. Mostly MS lesions show up in this region. This is an unbiased selection of un-enhanced and enhanced lesions for the longitudinal studies. Spectral changes in this region with no MRI-defined lesions are also included. Another more advanced technique, two-dimensional 2-D MRSI, was performed with an additional 32 ×32 phase encoding steps introduced at a relatively short echo time [TE = 30 msec] for detecting resonance with short T_2, such as those of lipids. These appear in the spectra after the suppressed tissue-water peak. The other sequence parameters used were TR = 1000 msec, Mixing Time [TM = 11.3 msec], number of complex points = 256, spectral width = 1000 Hz and number of averages = 2. The nominal spectroscopy voxel size is 0.75 × 0.75 × 1.5 cc, although the actual voxel volume is larger because of the effects of the "point spread function" and filtration. All of these procedures are modified GE protocols. MRI images and VOI spectra are shown in Figures 7.5 and 7.6.

It is important for the VOI localization to be placed over a segmented image. MRSI data were acquired without water suppression followed by water suppression for automatic spectral processing and analysis of the longitudinal changes in metabolite concentrations. The tissue-water peak was suppressed for visualizing the relatively weak metabolites by using three chemically selective Shinnar-Le-Roux (SLR) pulses. It was performed by using the above-mentioned parameters but the acquisition time was reduced by using the Number of Excitations [NEX = 1] and 16 × 16 phase encoding steps. By acquiring MRSI data before the post Gd MRI studies, any possible effect of Gd on spectral data is eliminated, as shown in Figure 7.3. After the acquisition of MRSI data, T_1- weighted [TR = 800 msec], [TE = 20 msec], contiguous, interleaved, 3 mm thick pre-contrast axial images were acquired before administering Gd (Magnevist, Berlex Laboratories, Wayne, NJ). Ten minutes after the administration of the contrast agent (0.2 ml/kg body weight, followed by the normal saline flush), post-contrast T_1-weighted images were acquired with the identical scan parameters used for the pre-contrast scan (see Figure 7.7). The total scan time is about 1.5 hours per session.

For longitudinal studies, visual inspection for consistent repositioning is done by the aid of scanner-alignment lights using the nasal bridge as a landmark every time. After the initial positioning, all imaging planes for all axial images are aligned parallel to the orbital ridge by a custom neck support for

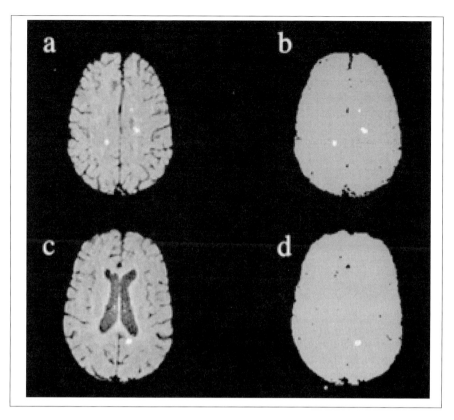

Figure 7.7: T_1-weighted axial post Gd contrast segmented images (b) and (d) showing bright MS lesion without false classification. Corresponding flow- suppressed high resolution images (a) and (c) show MS lesion enhancements in the supraventricular and ventricular regions. The imaging parameters used were: TE/TR= 25 msec /800 msec. Reproduced by permission of John Wiley & Sons Inc. from [741]. © 1998.

each patient. This is identified in the mid sagittal scout image. The consistent positioning of the VOI is fixed by careful visual examination of the lesion position, sulcus and vascular pattern and cortical junctions. Magnetic Resonance Image Analysis Package (MRIAP), a locally developed software, is used for all of the following image post-processing methods. Having described the data acquisition methods, in the following sub-section pre-segmentation methods for segmentation will be described along with the concept of image artifacts such as RF inhomogeneity and extrameningial tissue. Furthermore, the meaning of robust and automation will be correlated with minimization of these artifacts. Some of our current lab experiences in fractional volume analysis, Magnetization-Transfer Contrast and inversion recovery pulses will be briefly described.

7.3.1   Image Pre-Processing for Segmentation

Segmentation requires a number of pre-processing steps, which must be automated, faster, robust and accurate for classifying different brain tissue types. The two main pre-processing steps are: (1) Radio Frequency (RF) inhomogeneity correction, (2) removal of Extra-Meningeal Tissues (EMT). These are described with reference to the algorithms developed at MR Laboratory, University of Texas Medical School, Houston as described in this sub-section. Measuring the MRI-defined lesion burden requires a segmentation technique that is robust and automatic. In supervised (semi-automatic) segmentation techniques, the multi-spectral methods based on non-parametric analysis appear quite robust with the feature space analysis. This is based on the Parzen window technique, a non-parametric method, for brain images of normal and patients with MS using a dual spin-echo sequence. Recently, fractional volume analysis of Quadruple Contrast and AFFIRMATIVE images was adopted (see Figure 7.5). This involved using several steps: (1) anisotropy diffusion filter, (2) introduction of differential T_1 weighting into each contrast type to provide different signal intensities, (3) corrected T_1 with intensity normalization by subtracted synthetic FLAIR from actual FLAIR images. This gives an FSE image with a weighted combination of GM, WM and CSF signals. Total tissue volumes were obtained as the sum of tissue fractions over all of the voxels in the image set multiplied by the in-plane resolution and slice thickness. In the following sub-section, the need for image smoothing and use of averaging filters are described to correct in-plane RF inhomogeneity. The use of histogram analysis is defined with the focus on RF correction of Fast Spin-Echo images in Multiple Sclerosis.

7.3.1.1   RF Inhomogeneity Correction

In Multiple Sclerosis image segmentation, image intensity variation due to RF inhomogeneity low frequency components allows determination of in-plane RF inhomogeneity and image smoothing. This smoothing introduces ringing artifacts around the regions with steep intensity gradients, such as those encountered near the ventricles and at the edge of the brain. Therefore, pixels with intensities greater or less than one standard deviation away from the mean intensity of parenchyma are set to the mean parenchymal intensity. Standard deviation of one or less eliminates ringing artifacts without reducing the effectiveness of the RF inhomogeneity correction. The resulting images are usually filtered with a pixel averaging filter. So, RF inhomogeneity modulates the image intensity, which deteriorates the segmentation of the images. It causes a deleterious effect on multi-spectral segmentation. Modern RF coils such as the birdcage resonator are often used to produce a homogeneous RF field throughout the image volume. However, RF field inhomogeneity is not completely minimized. This RF field inhomogeneity is responsible for the observed scan to scan and interobserver variation in the segmentation.

A number of techniques have been proposed for RF inhomogeneity correction. At the MRI Laboratory at the University of Texas Medical School,

Houston, a simple algorithm was proposed to correct for RF inhomogeneity and its effect on segmentation. This algorithm was based on the fact that RF inhomogeneity contains only low frequency spatial components that can be filtered out. The smooth image after filtration contains information about the in-plane RF inhomogeneity. However, it introduced ringing artifacts around the regions in the images with steep intensity gradients, such as those encountered near the ventricles and the edge of the brain. The very first step to overcome this problem was to identify the pixels which deviate from the mean parenchymal intensity by one standard deviation or more using a histogram analysis. In the next step, these pixels were replaced by the mean intensity of brain parenchyma. The resulting images were smoothed with a 25×25 pixel averaging filter, reflecting the in-plane RF profile. The anisotropy filtered images were divided by this RF profile to obtain a corrected image. All of the corrected images were normalized based on the average CSF pixel intensities from a representative data set as shown in Figure 5.2 which represents (a) an early-echo FSE image before RF inhomogeneity correction, (b) the smoothed image, and (c) the early-echo FSE image following RF inhomogeneity correction. The elimination of operator bias at a 95% confidence level is expected for the application of RF inhomogeneity correction by robust and reproducible image segmentation. In the following sub-section the common appearance of extrameningeal tissues belonging to the scalp as a major artifact in metabolite analysis is described. The logic to eliminate this by the use of fat-saturation pulses is demonstrated in Multiple Sclerosis images to achieve MRSI spectroscopic Volume of Interest.

7.3.1.2   Removal of Extra Meningial Tissues

Many of the Extra Meningial Tissue (EMT) structures that surround the brain have high signal intensities close to that of MS lesions. In multispectral segmentation, extrameningeal tissues are a major source of false positives. So, the removal or stripping of extrameningeal tissues from the images is required prior to segmentation. Automatic removal of the extrameningeal tissue is a nontrivial problem. Semi-automatic techniques perform removal of extrameningeal tissue based on one or two echo images. The relatively poor contrast observed on images can be improved using a number of heuristics. However, this introduces a significant error in extrameningeal tissue removal. An algorithm has been used in the MR Laboratory, University of Texas Medical School, Houston, for the automatic removal of extrameningeal tissue based upon a multi-spectral segmentation technique using four AFFIRMATIVE images. These images exhibit excellent parenchyma-to-extrameningeal tissue contrast for the input data in very difficult regions, such as the vertex, optic nerve and inferior temporal gyri. Briefly, 30 to 40 points were sampled from three main tissue classes: White Matter, Gray Matter and CSF. These also include low-intensity extrameningeal tissues, generally bony structures, and high-intensity EMT, such as the scalp and bone marrow. Points were plotted in three different feature spaces with various combinations of pixel intensities from four AFFIRMATIVE images comprising the x and y axes. These axes can be optimized to generate the most accurate tissue classifications.

After the pre-segmentation of the AFFIRMATIVE and flow image sets, a simple algorithm was used for the removal of EMT from both image sets. It initially reclassifies all pixels segmented as low-intensity or high-intensity EMT as background. This leaves only true brain pixels. The remaining EMT pixels were usually eliminated for reclassification as background by the use of an "exclusive" 2-D connectivity algorithm. In exclusive connectivity, a single object was identified in the image, and all pixels disconnected to the object were eliminated. Such an exclusive connectivity algorithm identifies the largest connected "island", considers it to be the brain and then removes all the pixels lying outside of this structure. There are regions where this is difficult to perform, such as: (a) the flax cerebri and hemispheres around the vertex, (b) the orbits and optic nerve, (c) the inferior temporal gyri. The EMT are removed from these slices by use of an alternative "masking" algorithm. This assumes that the brain size slowly decreases if one moves out in either direction from the center of the brain mass. Each successive slice should be pre-processed completely within the borders of the previous slice.

For EMT removal, a masking algorithm uses a third slice in the image set as an image mask. EMT is eliminated by the connectivity algorithm in this mask image. Both hemispheres are retained and EMT is removed. The remaining pixels are classified as the brain contained within the borders of the mask image. This slice serves as a mask image for the slice immediately superior to it. The exclusive connectivity algorithm is not capable of eliminating these. On the other hand, the inferior temporal gyri, being a part of the brain, appear as disconnected islands in the axial slices. Usually they are removed by using the exclusive connectivity algorithm. The automatic identification of these ventral structures could be simplified by including the "graphic prescription" method into the algorithm. In this method, the operator prescribes a left-right line in both orbital and temporal lobe regions. This line does not cut the brain but cuts the optic nerve. By selecting the "temporal lobe line", the brain area of interest is isolated and EMT is removed. The procedure eliminates all small, isolated islands, background islands and non-parenchymal regions.

The removal of EMT minimizes false lesion classifications and is a part of many segmentation techniques. It has traditionally been accomplished by variations of semi-automatic techniques. These techniques are: multi-spectral, non-parametric based Parzen window techniques. They are applied to three feature maps, based on various combinations of the four AFFIRMATIVE images per slice location. Images prior to and following the removal of EMT are shown in Figure 7.8. The removal of the EMT minimizes false lesion classifications by removal of EMT based AFFIRMATIVE images. Having discussed image pre-processing, the next sub-section introduces concepts of segmentation for post-processing by automation, image registration, alignment of contiguous images and tissue composition and/or volumetry with minimum operator bias.

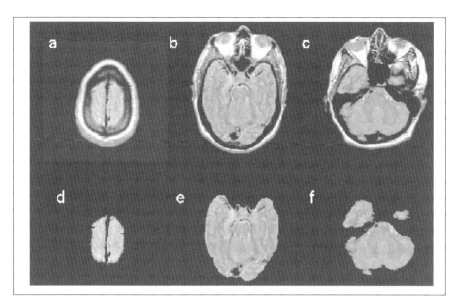

Figure 7.8: Removal of extrameningeal tissue. Note the axial MR brain images (3 mm thick) near the vertex (a),(d), in the region of the orbits (b),(e) and in the region of the temporal lobes (c),(f). The upper row of images (a),(b),(c) are surrounded by the skull. This is stripped off after the extrameningeal tissue is removed as is shown in the lower row of images (d),(e),(f) from superior (left most column) to inferior (right most column) (Courtesy of Professor Narayana, P. A., University of Texas Medical School, Houston, TX.)

7.3.2 Image Post-Processing for Segmentation

Complete automated segmentation and elimination of operator bias in MS lesion quantification are the major objectives of this technique. Segmentation involves a number of pre-processing steps which must be automated for postprocessing. The three main post-processing steps are: (1) image registration, (2) aligning the flow images with the MRI slices, and (3) image segmentation analysis. After the removal of the extrameningeal tissue, the registration of images is described in Sub-section 7.3.2.1 by the use of a search window in locating the plane of the Interhemispheric Fissure.

7.3.2.1 Image Registration

The correction of spatial orientation due to positional variation needs 3-D image registration based on the Interhemispheric Fissure (IF). An algorithm for this purpose requires manual identification of the end points of the IF in all the axial slices for fitting a plane to these points. One linear and two angular offsets can be determined from this plane. The other offsets can be determined by manually aligning the sagittal MR slices. Thus the 3-D problem is reduced to a 2-D problem. So, the automated robust registration of an MR image algorithm registers two sets of axial MR images of the human brain, i.e., a standard set and a shifted set. The registration requires the determination of three angular and three linear offsets between the two image sets. An algorithm was developed at the MR Laboratory, University of Texas Medical School, Houston, which used the plane containing the Interhemispheric Fissure to determine two rotations. The remaining offsets were found from a sagittal slice that had been reconstructed parallel to the IF. By convention, the x-, y- and z- axes correspond to the patient's left-right, ventral-dorsal, and superior-inferior axes, respectively.

The Interhemispheric Fissure Plane (IFP) is based on the automatic identification of the two end points, the ventral and the dorsal, in about 20 axial slices (see Figure 5.3). First, the center of mass (x,y) of each axial image is determined. Then, the edge points of the image are identified by scanning, first across the rows and then down the columns, for points with non-zero intensity. The point bordering five consecutive pixels with a zero intensity is an edge point. After the edge points are identified, a "search window" containing 15 pixels on each side of the center of mass is defined. Within the search window algorithm, this will find the end points of the fissure by detecting the edge point with the most dorsal y-coordinates on the ventral surface and the edge point with the most ventral y-coordinates on the dorsal surface. Later, about 40 end points are fitted to a plane by the least square method to determine the approximate Interhemispheric Fissure Plane. After this has been done, the shifted image data set shows a rotation along the x- and y-axes relative to the standard image set. This is determined from the direction angles between the normal to the IFP for the two sets of images. Determination of the rotation about the x-axis and the linear offsets from the reconstructed sagittal plane needs the 3-D center of mass for each image set as y- and z-coordinates, while the x-coordinate is calculated by substituting y- and z-coordinates into the equation for the IFP and solving for x. The linear offsets are then calculated as the difference between the 3-D center of mass of the standard image set and the 3-D center of mass of the shifted image set. Upon getting three angular and three linear offsets for the shifted image set, a spatial transformation is computed for transforming each coordinate (x, y, z) in the shifted image set onto the standard image set coordinates (x', y', z'). The spatial transformation is applied to all points in the shifted image set, which produces registered images. Image registration allows precise pixel-by-pixel comparison among images of the same set or different sets of images. This is an important method for comparing several longitudinal images at the same slice level with exact pixel-by-pixel correspondence. Now that the registration of images has been covered, in the next sub-section the importance of flow correction in phase contrast images will be highlighted by the estimation of angular and linear offsets. Briefly, segmentation will be described for flow correction in Multiple Sclerosis Fluid Attenuated and Inversion Recovery/Magnetization Transfer (FLAIR/MTC) images.

7.3.2.2 Flow Correction

Segmentation based on FLAIR/MTC images is an excellent method for the regions superior to the lateral ventricles. The prevalence of false positives in the vascular regions and CSF flow, insula, posterior fossa, and cerebellum is a common problem. Automatic identification of both vascular flow due to coherent flow and CSF flow due to incoherent flow can be performed using 3-D phase contrast images. Flow analysis performed in the segmentation process reduces the number of false positives in troublesome areas, such as the posterior fossa and other tissues. Flow ghost artifacts can also mimic lesions. Such ghosts can be identified automatically and can be eliminated. The improvement in the segmentation follows the correction for the flow ghosts. With this technique, a single master map is generated which is adequate for segmenting all images generated on different patients that had been acquired with FLAIR/MTC images. An automatic three-dimensional image registration technique is used to determine its accuracy to predict the angular and linear offsets achieved by rotating and translating a set of images by a known amount. This algorithm estimates angular offsets to within 0.50 of a degree and linear offsets within one pixel, prior to repositioning, on a pixel-by-pixel basis.

Finally, in Sub-section 7.3.2.3, segmentation analysis is briefly discussed using supervised, validated or unsupervised methods. This description is focused on current concepts of segmentation methods. Use of 4-D feature maps with the introduction of multi-spectral, non-parametric and Parzen window methods are described in the segmentation analysis of Multiple Sclerosis images. Readers are encouraged to read Sub-section 5.2 for coverage of these concepts in greater detail.

7.3.2.3 Image Segmentation Analysis

After the pre-processing and post-processing steps are completed, AFFIRMATIVE images are segmented to determine the extent of MS lesion development or "lesion load" in the brain. The AFFIRMATIVE sequence generates four images per slice. It is possible to generate a 4-D feature map for segmentation. However, segmentation based on a 4-D feature space needs powerful computers. Stated in another way, it is more efficient to perform segmentation based on multiple 2-D feature maps with various image combinations. Initial segmentation is performed using the early-echo and late-echo FSE images. In order to evaluate the improvement in the quality of segmentation by incorporating the FLAIR and MTC images, multi-spectral feature map techniques for segmentation are applied with AFFIRMATIVE images used as the input. Segmentation quality improves considerably thereafter.

After visual inspection of a large number of segmented MR images, false lesions appear near regions of CSF flow such as in the third and fourth ventricles. Information from the two images sets is combined into a single set of images as flow images. These are spatially registered to the AFFIRMATIVE images by an automatic 3-D image registration algorithm. This minimizes the number of false lesions. Segmentation can be performed using early-echo and late-echo

FLAIR/MTC images along with the input images at the level of the lateral ventricles. FSE-based segmentation produces a large number of false positive and false negative lesions. The number of false classifications decreased in the FLAIR/MTC-based segmented images.

Flow information in segmentation is incorporated in a two-step process. Each step requires the generation of individual feature maps. The feature maps for both steps are generated using a multi-spectral, non-parametric, Parzen window technique. The first step involves the segmentation of MS lesions based on the flow and the late-echo FLAIR/MTC images. In the second step, those pixels not classified as lesions are subdivided into GM, WM and CSF, based on the second feature map generated from the early-echo and late-echo FSE images. The final result is a set of segmented images with lesions; GM, WM and CSF are classified. These segmented images are used for proton Magnetic Resonance Spectroscopic Imaging (MRSI).

7.4 Proton Magnetic Resonance Spectroscopic Imaging and Segmentation in Multiple Sclerosis

Chemical Shift Imaging (CSI) and MRSI have been popular methods over the last ten years to achieve separate images from water or fat protons from different brain tissue voxels. These combine imaging and spectral information from adjacent voxels covering a large volume of interest in one measurement. It may be either 1-D, 2-D or 3-D chemical shift imaging, depending upon the spatial localization in one, two and three directions of slices, columns and voxels, respectively. For example, in a well-known 2-D Echo-CSI spectroscopic sequence, slice selective excitation or volume selective excitation is applied, and the read out gradient is not applied during data collection. This results in tissue slice selection by a slice selective RF pulse in one direction. Phase encoding gradients define the other direction. Different spectra are achieved by multi-dimensional Fourier transformations as metabolite spectral maps appearing as gray scale images. In other words, spatial Fourier transformation and time-Fourier transformations provide spatial distribution and chemical shift details. Spatial resolution is achieved by phase encoding steps. This spatial resolution can be distributed as fractions of the field of view, i.e., in the x, y and z directions for 3-D CSI. Thus, the measurement time depends on the product of three parameters: repetition time (TR), the number of acquisitions and the phase encoding steps. So, there is a trade-off between the measurement time and the volume of interest.

Other important factors are the point-spread function due to contamination from the neighboring voxels. Voxel shifting or grid shifting also contaminate multi-voxel CSI data from different tissue sources and tissue types. In our study at the University of Texas Medical School, Houston, an Octagonal Volume Selective (OVS) excitation by 2-D CSI was commonly used over a confined octagon volume or selective spins, i.e., avoiding signals from the skull's sub-cutaneous fat. For this, a Point Resolved Spectroscopy (PRESS) sequence is used with two-phase encoding tables. Three RF excitation selective pulses are used. High amplitude phase encoding was performed by the z gradient with a slice thickness of 3.0 mm in the z direction, while lower amplitude thick slices are phase encoded by the x and y gradients. Phase encoding in a field-of-view larger than the excited VOI avoids aliasing of the lipid signals. The echo is generated so there is no delay between excitation and signal collection. This offers good spectra baseline. For example, long echo delay times (TE = 50-250 ms with PRESS) and short T_2 lipid signals cause baseline flattening. So, a short TE sequence with lipid suppression allows for short T_2, j-coupled[1] proton rich multiple metabolite resonance peaks. Such water and fat suppression is achieved by an amplitude adjustment of Gaussian narrow bandwidth Chemical Shift Selective Saturation (CHESS) pulses before the final MR spectrum peak amplitudes measurement. This needs high quality shimming to be performed by using adiabatic RF pulses. This multiple-slice 2-D CSI method is good for peripheral Gray Matter examination. It uses a 90°–180° spin-echo sequence or a gradient echo sequence with CHESS water suppression pulses or outer volume saturation by fat suppression. This allows measurements for several slices using sequential excitation and phase encoding in two dimensions.

Let us now explain the power of MRSI and segmentation in MS lesion characterization. For MS lesion identification and characterization, proton MR Spectroscopic Imaging has proven to be a very powerful automated tool based on metabolite concentrations. MRI has been valuable only in understanding the *in-vivo* natural history of MS. More than 5% of MRI examinations can not suggest early MS lesions. Recent attempts at the MR Laboratory, University of Texas Medical School, Houston, were focused on the evaluation of the biochemical characterization of localized/regional heterogeneity of lesions and their temporal evolution associated with spectroscopic changes with the histological state of lesions: inflammation, myelin breakdown, neuronal loss and gliosis. This may improve the histopathological specificity of T_2-weighted MR Imaging changes in MS. It can distinguish between MS lesions and Normal Appearing White Matter (NAWM) in primary progressive (PPMS) and relapsing remitting (RRMS) Multiple Sclerosis. This technique provides a good opportunity to compare metabolite levels in lesion rich voxels, Normal Appearing White Matter (NAWM) with normal brain regions in serial MS studies. On the other hand, this leaves some difficulties, such as ring-like appearance, NAA black holes, contaminated metabolite spectral peaks and lesion metabolite heterogeneity. MR Spectroscopic Imaging is performed along with the routine basic MRI protocol involving: a sagittal scout; axial AFFIRMATIVE or Quadruple Contrast imaging; MR Spectroscopic Imaging; MRA imaging; Pre-and Post-Gd MRI imaging.

In the following sub-section, the features of an automated locally designed Magnetic Resonance Image Analysis Package (MRIAP) are introduced. The unique capabilities of this program are highlighted, such as minimal operator

---

[1]J-coupling means two neighbouring protons with diferent eigen functions.

bias, automation in brain tissue and lesion anatomical/neurochemical analysis.

7.4.1   Automatic MRSI Segmentation and Image Processing Algorithm

One of the goals of proton MRSI in MS is to quantify metabolite changes in the brain with time as a means of characterizing and following the evolution of lesions. Data processing is very significant in interpreting the MRSI results. Most published MRSI processing techniques appear to require operator intervention and show significant operator bias. A robust algorithm automatically processes MRSI data and generates quantitative metabolic maps and spectroscopic images. Metabolic maps are generated using the fitted peak areas of phased metabolic resonances with the Levenberg-Marquardt algorithm. These images are normalized to tissue water to evaluate quantitative metabolite changes. Ideally, the algorithm should accommodate any user-defined line shape function. A unique feature of the algorithm is that it can align spectra from different voxels in terms of frequency and phase. The algorithm should calculate the concentrations of metabolites relative to the tissue water. Automatic phasing of the spectra remains a major hurdle to be overcome. Another unique feature of the algorithm is its ability to superimpose metabolic maps onto high-resolution images for anatomic-metabolic correlation.

Algorithms developed at the MR Laboratory, University of Texas, Houston, allowed image operations which were useful in visualizing longitudinal changes in the concentrations of metabolites. Current improvements in the segmentation algorithms allow faster, automatic, supervised, interactive analysis of molar concentration. These perform an analysis of tissue fractions in any desired part of the brain and water suppression in diffusion-weighted and functional images. In brief, the MRIAP package performs: (1) Manual segmentation by paintbrush, seed growing, editing, erasing methods; (2) Supervised segmentation by single- and multiple-feature map methods; (3) Automatic segmentation by fractional volume analysis of the brain; (4) Contrast enhancement analysis. 3-D interactive analysis and 3-D automatic lesion analysis have been of specific interest.

For MRSI post-processing, an automatic method was reported using locally developed Automated Processing of Spectroscopic Imaging Program (APSIP) (see Doyle *et al.* [788]). The following sub-section introduces current experience in tissue composition and relative metabolites analysis in Multiple Sclerosis, with an emphasis on obtaining a better interpretation of the disease.

7.4.2   Relative Metabolite Concentrations and Contribution of Gray Matter and White Matter in the Normal Human Brain

The nominal spectroscopy voxels are generally large, of the order of 0.8 cc, due to the relatively weak metabolite concentrations. The relatively large spectroscopic voxels have metabolite contributions both from Gray Matter and White

Matter. CSF has very low concentrations of NAA, Cr, and Cho resonances as seen on MRS. Both metabolite and tissue composition are essential to determine the relative concentrations of the MRS-visible neuro-chemicals in GM and WM. These determine the contributions of GM and WM to an individual spectroscopic voxel. This metabolite segmentation method utilizes the maximum information from high resolution MRI by deconvolution or attenuating the contributions of metabolites in GM, WM, and CSF to a given spectroscopic voxel. It has been observed that both NAA and Cr are about 20% higher in GM than in WM in normal subjects (data not shown). Choline concentration appears to be fairly similar in both GM and WM. It is believed these results are of fundamental importance for the correct interpretation of the MRSI data. In the next sub-section, the possibility of evolving MS lesions by use of paramagnetic Gadolinium will be described with anatomical, neurochemical and lesion volumetry correlation for better interpretation of the disease.

7.4.3 MRSI and Gadolinium-Enhanced (Gd) MRI

The MRSI data is acquired after the acquisition of dual echo or AFFIRMA-TIVE images for lesion quantification prior to the administration of Gadolinium-Dithylene-Triamine-Penta-Actetate (Gd-DTPA). In our studies these MRI imaging sessions were performed on a GE 1.5 T scanner equipped with a shielded gradient coil system. Two-dimensional MRSI imaging was performed with 32 × 32 phase encoding steps on a predetermined Volume of Interest (VOI) localized using the stimulated echo sequence. The VOI was always contained within a large White Matter area of the centrum semiovale, whether or not any lesions were present in this area. This introduced an unbiased selection of unenhanced and enhanced lesions in the longitudinal studies based on the spectral changes, even in regions with no MR-defined lesions.

As indicated below, this strategy allowed us to make some unique observations about the MS disease process. The size of the VOI used was typically a $0.9 \times 0.9 \times 1.5 \text{ cm}^3$ volume, with a nominal spectroscopy voxel size of 1.2 cm^3. The MRSI data was acquired with an echo time of 30 ms to enable detection of resonances with short T_2, such as in lipids. Following the acquisition of MRSI data, T_1-weighted [TE = 20 ms], [TR = 800 ms], contiguous, interleaved, 3 mm thick axial images were acquired prior to administering Gadolinium-Dithylene-Triamine-Penta-Acetate (Gd-DTPA) (Magnevist, Berlex). Ten minutes after the administration of the contrast agent (0.2 ml/kg), post-contrast T_1-weighted images were acquired with the identical parameters. By acquiring the MRSI data prior to the administration of Gd-DTPA, any possible effect of Gd on the spectral data was eliminated. The MRSI data was analyzed by self-designed APSIP using the automatic processing algorithm. The pre-contrast and post-contrast images were processed using an anisotropy diffusion filter for improved signal-to-noise ratio. In the longitudinal studies, great care was exercised in consistently positioning for slice registration and spatial localization. This usually varies from scan to scan in a longitudinal study. This method is described in detail elsewhere (see Samarasekera *et al.* [789]). In the following sub-section the concept of segmentation analysis is introduced. Segmentation analysis was used to analyze the heterogeneous variations of neuro-chemicals and for interpretation of the MS lesion heterogeneity. This is useful in studying the morphological description and biochemical nature of lesion progression in MS.

7.4.4   Lesion Load and Metabolite Concentrations by Segmentation and MRSI

In the present ongoing study at the Departments of Radiology and Neurology, University of Texas Medical School, Houston, more than 200 MRSI sessions have been completed in this MS patient serial study on clinical metabolite MR screening. The MRSI quantitative analysis of MS patients' data showed stable NAA and Cr concentrations, while the Cho enhanced in these patients. Normal subject and most of the MS volunteers showed stable NAA, Cr and Cho peaks over several serial MRI sessions. In some patients, a regional increase in the Cho concentration, mostly in the mid-fissure, was usually observed preceding any of the MRI-defined lesions. In addition, Cho was observed to increase between 20–80% in the enhancing lesions. This increase typically lasted for a period of about six to eight weeks. Other characteristically reversible and regionally depressed NAA levels were also observed as strongly associative with the acute lesions evolved in a time-dependent manner. These well-developed and stable MRI-defined lesions can be associated with the locally diminished Cho and NAA concentrations when these lesion-rich voxels were compared with the normal White Matter voxels within the metabolic map. Lipid peaks were occasionally observed in this MS patient series (see Doyle *et al.* [788]).

The observed lipids were frequently associated the lesion enhancement. These lipid peaks were also observed with stable MRI-defined lesions over time intervals of 4–16 weeks. These lipid peaks presumably exceeded the usual interval of MS plaque enhancement. The representative temporal change in the lipid maps is shown in Plates 10 and 11. Different lipid resonance maps are shown in the different serial scan sessions from a non-enhancing lesion (lesion number 2) in the left hemisphere as shown in Plate 11. At this lesion location initially on session 1, the NAA and Cr maps appeared relatively homogeneous, while a slight increase in the Cho around this lesion was noticed. On session 2 (day 35), lesion number 1 still exhibited the enhancement. In addition, lesion number 2 was also enhanced, and a decrease in both the lipid spatial resolution and the intensity of the different lipid signals was observed. In general, a decrease in the NAA and Cr levels was also observed but less frequently seen in this patient series. During the third session (day 77), no further lesion enhancement was observed. However, the lipid resonances persisted from both lesions number 1 and 2. The levels of the NAA, Cr and Cho later recovered in due course. A continued decrease in the lipid levels was observed on day 105 (session 4). On day 203 (session 6), strong lipid signals were observed at the region slightly superior to the lesion 1 location, but not from lesion 1. A dramatic decrease in the Cho is also observed as shown in Figure 7.9. It was difficult to completely understand these observations, demonstrating the dynamic and

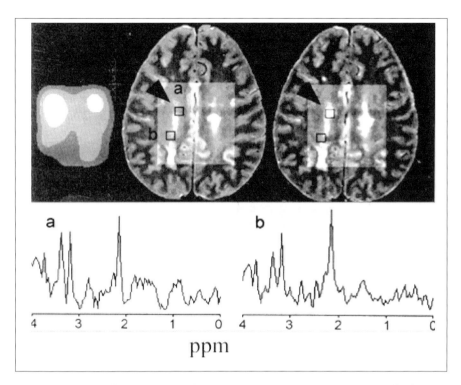

Figure 7.9: The Choline spatial distribution in a patient with MS showing serial changes in the MRI-defined lesion at (a) and (b) locations in a 3 mm thick axial image. Note the increased Cho levels on the left and in spectrum (a), but without the lesion appearance at location (a) in the left image. Note the appearance of an MRI defined lesion (arrowhead in the right image) after 10 weeks. Reproduced by permission of John Wiley & Sons Inc. from [787]. © 1998.

complex metabolic changes that occurred in MS brain White Matter and Gray Matter.

The correlation analysis between the MRI-defined lesion load and the concentrations of different metabolites based on the MRSI are summarized in Figure 7.10. The NAA concentration was inversely correlated with the lesion load ($p = 0.001$; $r^2 = -0.54$). This implies that neuronal/axonal damage increases with the increase in the MRI-defined lesion load. A weak positive correlation between the lipids and the MS lesion load was also observed ($p = 0.04$; $r^2 = 0.3$). However, this observed weak correlation, based on a relatively small number of patients, needs to be explored further. The temporal time-dependent variation is shown in Plate 10 for the concentrations of the NAA, Cho, Cr and lipids, with the volume of an acute lesion as determined by the Gd enhancement. The concentrations of all the metabolites, with the exception of the lipids, reached a minimum when the lesion volume reached its maximum. At maximum lesion volume, the concentrations of all three of the metabolites

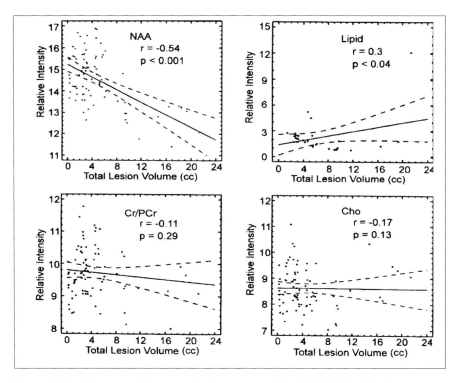

Figure 7.10: The correlation analysis between the MRI-defined lesion volume (in cc) and the concentrations of metabolites with reference to internal water is shown based on MRSI. The average concentration of NAA, Lipids, Creatine and Choline as relative intensities are shown with lesion volumes measured at different time points over all voxels. Solid lines show the regression lines and dashed lines show a ± 2 standard deviation for different metabolites. Reproduced by permission of John Wiley & Sons Inc. from [787]. © 1998.

increased further towards a steady value. This type of variation suggested decreased concentrations of metabolites due to the fluid accumulation leading to edema associated with acute lesions or due to altered metabolism. These observations suggested the possibility of two distinct biological processes in MS. These MR visible metabolites speculate the myelin integrity and/or myelin stability in the brain with MS. One process is associated with the inflammation and blood-brain-barrier disruption, while the other process is associated with an oligodendrogliopathy. With this assumption, MRSI has tremendous potential for understanding the MS etiology of the disease and the treatment of MS. Having discussed the serial changes in metabolites of a lesion, the need for a VOI selection as a pre-requisite will now be highlighted by localization techniques to obtain better neurochemical information for matched segmentation analysis. The use of specific RF pulses and gradients is described for MRS and MRSI techniques which are in common use at the moment.

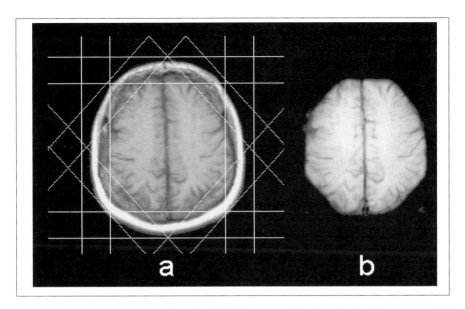

Figure 7.11: The position of eight lipid suppression bands is shown as solid and orthogonal lines applied over the skull region of a corresponding brain AFFIRMATIVE axial image (a). Note the MRSI octagonal VOI shown as a selected region (b) for data analysis by Chemical Shift Imaging and MR Spectroscopy (MRSI Data, Courtesy of MR Lab., University of Texas Medical School, Houston, TX.)

7.4.5 MR Spectroscopic Imaging and Localization for Segmentation

The *in vivo* MR approach of spatial localization is defined as an accurate assignment of a detected MR signal from a specific volume of the brain. A clinically acceptable MR Spectroscopy localization method can produce the localized spectra from a VOI with a minimum contribution to the signal from outside of the defined VOI volume. The spectra must have good Signal-Noise-Ratio (SNR) with well-resolved narrow peaks and a relatively clean baseline to allow for accurate metabolite quantification. This acquisition method should be fast and easy to use. Most of these methods are based on spatial selectivity with B_0 gradients, using slice selection gradients and phase encoding gradients. The main spatial localization concepts are: (1) elimination of signals from outside of a volume of interest by using spatial saturation bands; (2) application of slice gradients such as: Stimulated Echo Acquisition Method (STEAM), Point Resolved Spectroscopy (PRESS) and Depth Resolved Spectroscopy (DRESS); (3) phase encoding gradients for Chemical Shift Imaging (CSI). Current spatial localization procedures confine the signals from smaller brain volumes compared to the total sensitive volume of a surface coil. These localization techniques are characterized as single-volume or multi-volume methods based upon selective excitation pulses to localize the signal from a small tissue volume or the tissue columns in many spatial encoding dimensions. These dimension-based methods may be 1-D, 2-D or 3-D localization techniques depending upon different linear magnetization positions. In the 1-D method, the MR signal originates from an excited volume, which is a tissue column, divided into slices by a gradient or RF encoding. In the 2-D method, the signal comes from the plane that is further sliced into two dimensions by the spatially encoding gradient pulses, e.g. 2-D Chemical Shift Imaging allows a spatial resolution of 1 cc for H-1 spectra by the use of standard quadrature head coils. The three-dimensional localization method excites a large volume and encodes it into a 3-D grid of many smaller voxels by using a gradient or RF pulses.

The very first step in spatial localization by an MR Imaging sequence consists of slice-excitation to a tissue slice with a frequency selective RF pulse. The pulse is applied simultaneously with a linear field gradient, perpendicular to the plane of the slice. The position of the slice is determined by the center frequency of the applied RF pulse. The tissue slice thickness is defined as the function of gradient amplitude and frequency bandwidth of the RF pulse. However, within the slice, a linear field gradient in one direction causes a linear variation in proton precessing frequencies along one dimension, called "frequency-encoding gradient". Another linear field gradient, perpendicular to the frequency-encoding gradient and to the slice selection gradient, introduces the spatially dependent phase shifts to the precessional motion of the proton spins. This gradient is referred to as the "phase-encoding gradient". This phase information along with the recorded frequencies are translated into the corresponding spatial distribution in the form of a 2-D image.

A detailed description of the spectroscopic imaging sequence is beyond the scope of this chapter. Briefly, a spin-echo sequence uses a slice selection gradient "on" along with the frequency-selective RF pulses, followed by the dephased refocused spins (negative lobe) during the application of long RF pulses. The next frequency encoding gradient is applied during the echo-sampling. Thereafter, the additional gradient preceding the data sampling refocuses the center of the echo at the center of the Analog-to-Digital Conversion (ADC) window. This gradient following the data sampling period spoils or dephases any of the remaining transverse magnetization. As a result, it prevents the formation of unwanted echoes in later sampling periods. Various methods for MS lesion localization are in current use for "Proton MR Spectroscopic Imaging".

Point Resolved Spectroscopy (PRESS) is a 1-D technique used for localization in three dimensions. For better results in proton MR spectroscopy, initial Chemical Shift Selective Saturation (CHESS) pulses are needed to suppress the water signal. Thereafter, slice-selective RF pulses excite the proton spins in the three intersecting orthogonal planes. Finally, all three RF pulses excite the spins at the intersection of the two slice columns in the direction perpendicular to each other. Their net magnetization generates the second echo soon after TE/2 echo time applied second 180° pulse, which is sampled and processed further. The second G_x gradient is applied for reversing the dephasing that occurred during the excitation period. The Gradients G_z and G_y behave similarly to 180° applied pulses, to refocus the echo. This echo is then measured.

Stimulated Echo Acquisition Mode (STEAM) is another spectroscopic imaging method. The three slice-selective 90° RF pulses are applied with the slice-selection gradients in three orthogonal directions of x, y, z. The second 90° pulse returns the magnetization to the longitudinal direction after a time delay of Mixing Time [TM = 11.3 msec]. The three 90° pulses produce the four echoes after the last RF pulse applied. The gradients in the sequence optimize the stimulated echo and suppress the other echoes and the Free Induction Decay (FID) from the last RF pulse. In other words, only the stimulated echo is sampled during total acquisition time. The water suppression can be observed by the CHESS pulses at the beginning of the sequence.

In the Image Selected *in vivo* Spectroscopy (ISIS) method, a series of measurements are performed for the preparation of the magnetization. This includes the selective 180° inversion pulses that are applied in different combinations. In the next phase of applying a non-selective 90° pulse, an FID is collected. Finally, signals from outside the ROI are cancelled and the algebraic sum of the MR signals from all the measurements is produced based on 1-D, 2-D or 3-D spatial selectivity. In this direction, localized brain single voxel spectroscopy is widely used.

Single Voxel Spectroscopy (SVS) produces one spectrum from the single localized volume. The one measurement depends on the single voxel volume size, the sequence applied and the corresponding scan parameters. This method appears simple, i.e., it is easy to obtain one spectrum and magnet shimming is easier for a small voxel area. Single voxel spectroscopy has become a popular technique and is also clinically acceptable.

MRSI data from a pre-localized volume using a stimulated echo sequence minimizes the problems of spectral bleed-through from the lipids coming from the EMT. It also minimizes the tissue susceptibility-induced magnetic field inhomogeneities. However, the pre-localization prevents the acquisition of MRSI data from the whole slice due to the applied fat-suppression bands as shown in Plate 10. The other problem with MRSI is the long acquisition time required. It takes approximately 34 minutes to acquire metabolic maps from a pre-localized volume. The MRSI acquisition echo-CSI sequence is applied which alleviates these two problems and allows acquisition of the MRSI data at a short echo time of 21 msec. After application of this sequence, the lipids from EMT are suppressed by using eight spatial fat saturation pulses. The implementation of a variable repetition time (TR) also reduces the scan time. Application of the variable TR exploits the fact that the signal intensity is high in the central part of the k-space. Noisy outer k-space contributes less to the resolution enhancement. Thus at a low TR value, the signal can be acquired from the center part of the k-space towards outer k-space without significantly affecting the signal-to-noise ratio. Using this technique, one can acquire the MRSI data from all of the brain slices in 11 minutes. The echo-CSI MR Spectroscopy sequence is currently used for our human studies. This application of an MRSI sequence is used on T_1-axial images (AFFIRMATIVE or Quadruple Contrast). A localized image is generated first, followed by Chemical Shift Imaging by modifying a few control variables (CV). These include the application of eight outer volume suppression (OVS) fat saturation bands and three CHESS pulses for water suppression. The position and the size of the rectangular box defines the positions of OVS bands from a 15 mm thick volume comprised of five slices, each 3 mm thick. For this, AFFIRMATIVE or Quadruple Contrast images are used (see Figure 7.11). These user control variables are described for understanding the MRI scanning parameter settings used which were strictly set as follows: spectral width = 2000; right-left resolution = 32; anterior-posterior resolution = 32; superior-inferior resolution = 1. For the CSI imaging, the scan parameters were set at: [TE = 30 ms; TR = 1000 ms] at scan set-up for Auto Center frequency of water at 4.76 ppm; slab thickness = 15 mm; scan location as superior/inferior; data acquisition time 45 min; frequency matrix of 256; phase matrix of 128; frequency direction anterior/posterior. This set of CV's including AX, R1, R2, region of interest (ROI) size and ROI location allows image data processing for MS lesion quantification. These details can be seen in GE scan version 5.6 protocols.

In the next sub-section we will describe our current experiences in MS lesion quantification by use of supervised or seed growing automated segmentation methods.

7.4.6   Lesion Segmentation and Quantification

Before MS lesion quantification can be performed, all of the axial T_1-weighted MR images are post-processed for segmentation by using a self designed Magnetic Resonance Image Analysis Package (MRIAP). For this image processing, an anisotropy diffusion filter is used to improve the signal-to-noise (SNR) ratio considerably with no MR image blurring. This filter is characterized by the diffusion constant K = 7 and the number of iterations = 3 for each of these image sets from the image background noise as described elsewhere (see Gawne-Cain *et al.* [790]). These images are corrected for Radio Frequency (RF) inhomogeneity and these intensities are normalized. Later, the lesion volumes are quantified by using a modified "supervised" or "seed growing" segmentation method (see Rovaris *et al.* [791], Jackson *et al.* [792]).

Other segmentation methods for lesion analysis and volumetry are: (1) an iterated sequence of spatially varying classification and nonlinear registration; (2) a probabilistic neural net performing segmentation into four tissue classes after supervised training; (3) a Fuzzy C-Means (FCM) algorithm; (4) standardizing the MR intensity; (5) combining precise rigid registration of three-dimensional (3-D) (volumetric) medical images; (6) non-rigid deformation computation, and flow-field analysis; (7) four-dimensional (4D) feature maps; (8) a pyramidal approach for automatic segmentation; (9) dual-echo MRI segmentation using vector decomposition and probability techniques. More details can be seen in Sub-section 5.2. In the following sub-section it is presumed that readers are aware of the concepts described in Sub-section 5.2. Basic steps of spectral analysis are not described in detail, such as the parametric description of data, *a priori* information, Fourier Transform NMR including Deconvolution, Zero-filling, Apodization, High or Low-pass filters, Baseline and Phase correction, Peak reference, Autoregression and Curve fitting for comparable data. We describe our experiences at the MR Laboratory in using these concepts to obtain segmentation and Chemical Shift Imaging analysis in Multiple Sclerosis. Emphasis is placed on tissue water suppression, metabolite peak resolution and specificity of MS lesions in Gray Matter or White Matter.

7.4.7 Magnetic Resonance Spectroscopic Imaging and Segmentation Data Processing

MRSI data-processing is described using the self designed software Automatic Processing of Spectroscopic Imaging Program (APSIP), as described by Doyle *et al.* [788]. The post-processing includes using several settings, such as: (1) DC baseline correction; (2) spatial apodization using a Fermi filter (cutoff = 12, width = 4); (3) 2-D spatial Fourier transformation (FT); (4) spatial alignment with the axial images; (5) using unsuppressed water data as the reference; (6) post-acquisition water suppression by low frequency filtering; (7) baseline offset by a deconvolution difference technique using the exponential spectral filter with 50 Hz line broadening; (8) time axis apodization with 1 Hz exponential resolution enhancement and 6 Hz Gaussian line broadening; (9) zero filling of complex points, and 1D FT. In the next step, the unsuppressed water data are processed by using the same procedure after the zero filling to a level of 32×32 by adding more points in the spectrum. The water-suppressed data are fitted with Gaussian line shapes and the unsuppressed data with the Lorentzian line shapes. These line shapes provide the best fit to the observed spectra. Careful resolution is mandatory for the Cr and Cho peaks with metabolite line widths of less than 4.5 Hz, which are achieved in the voxel at the level of the water suppression for more than 300 fold with proper zero order and first order phasing. The internal reference is obtained with a water peak at 4.76 ppm.

The use of the above-mentioned parameters and data derived from the fitted line shapes produced metabolic maps. A self-designed APSIP program produced these metabolic maps. In these lipid maps, lipid peaks were visible in the range of 0.8–1.5 ppm region. It exhibited poorly defined line shapes. So, their maps were generated based on the digital integration of the spectra in this region. Identification of these lipid peaks was based on a signal-to-noise ratio of 3.0 in the VOI inside the center and 6.0 at the outer edge of the VOI for lipids (see Narayana *et al.* [787]). All of these metabolite concentrations were expressed as peak integration values, which represent the proton density, relative to the average tissue water contained within the spectroscopic VOI. Thereafter, these peak values were multiplied by a numerical constant. This procedure minimizes the effect of water fluctuations within a given voxel due to the changing tissue pathology.

All of the MR imaging segmentation is performed by using a self designed MRIAP in the manner described in previous sub-sections. The operator is always blinded to the MR data collection. All of these data are processed at the earliest convenient time on a SPARC station 10 (Sun Microsystems, Mountain

View, CA) equipped with 32 megabytes of RAM and a 2-gigabyte hard disk.

In Sub-section 7.4.8, the power of statistical analysis generated by automated MRIAP and APSIP programs is highlighted to compare the composite post-segmentation images and spectroscopic data of patients with MS.

7.4.8   Statistical Analysis

The temporal stability of metabolite MRSI data in normal volunteers and patients is evaluated by a procedure described earlier (see Jackson *et al.* [792]). Currently, intra-subject and inter-acquisition variations in the NAA, Cr, and Cho levels are evaluated using multivariate analysis. A commercial statistical analysis package (SAS) is used for the on-going study of tissue composition and metabolites along with lipids in MS. These lipids are rarely seen in the normal brain, so the temporal stability is not needed on lipids in normal volunteers. Linear regression analysis is performed to determine the correlation between the total lesion volume and the metabolite levels.

The next section focuses on techniques used for evaluating Alzheimer's Disease.

7.5   Proton Magnetic Resonance Spectroscopic Imaging and Segmentation of Alzheimer's Disease

For acquiring MRSI data in patients with Alzheimer's Disease (AD), a similar segmentation approach to that previously described for MS is used with optimized experimental scan parameter settings. For studying AD, a 1.5 T Magnetom VISION (Siemens Erlangen MRI scanner) system set with a standard circularly polarized head coil, is good to use to acquire T_2- and T_1-weighted MRI images for the later segmentation of these images. CHESS pulses are used first, followed by PRESS pulses applied on a Region of Interest (ROI), chosen over 100 mm from left to right, and 70 mm anterior to posterior, with a slice thickness of 15 mm, spatial in-plane resolution of 9.0×9.0 mm^2 using a spin-echo 2-D MRSI sequence at TR/TE $= 1800/135$ ms. This selected region mainly covers hippocampi and the surrounding mesial temporal lobes as described by MacKay *et al.* [793]. The total acquisition time was 13 minutes. For the multi-slice H-1 MRSI and spatial in-plane resolution of 8.0×8.0 mm^2, the images are acquired by using a spin-echo sequence at TR/TE $= 1800/135$ ms, data sampling at the sweep width $= 1000$ Hz with a total acquisition time of 30 minutes.

Next, Sub-section 7.5.1 introduces the need for using Point Resolved Spectroscopy (PRESS) and Chemical Shift Selective Spectroscopic (CHESS) techniques and the difficulties in segmentation which we encountered at the MR Laboratory with regard to scan parameter settings.

7.5.1 MRSI Data Acquisition Methods

Brain H-1 MRSI was performed to estimate the MR visible metabolites from the entire brain area in the form of multi-voxel spectral peaks for Chemical Shift Imaging. More accurately, spectral peaks were visualized by single voxel spectroscopy where only one voxel or one Region of Interest was described to obtain a single spectrum. Alzheimer's Disease is a heterogeneous pathological disease, so H-1 MRSI best explains its spectral characteristics. Moreover, segmentation analysis of GM, WM and CSF metabolites in the brain with AD seems less promising in metabolites distribution. This method is based upon using spatial phase encoding gradients along with the acquisition of a strong MR signal. This requires a highly homogeneous magnetic field by tuning the gradients for obtaining the best shimming. This produces a chemical shift spectral image of all metabolites with low sensitivity in a long acquisition time. Thus, the H-1 MRSI method uses data sampling to the limited phase encoding steps. Short VOI or truncated sampling results in poor spatial resolution with contamination of the brain spectra. This shows MR visible alanine, lipid or other spectral peaks originating from outside of the brain VOI. The application of lipid saturation bands is widely reported to avoid such contamination (see Saunders *et al.* [794]). The metabolite images of the NAA, Cr, Cho, MI were generated by applying the STEAM sequence (see Frahm *et al.* [795]) and applying the PRESS sequence method (see Hennig *et al.* [784]) along with the corresponding MRI images for anatomical orientation. Moreover, in PRESS method, one is limited to acquisition of one voxel at a time. Hence, data collection is performed at one time from the whole voxel in the slice. So, multi-slice H-1 MRSI provides good coverage of the cortex. It uses localized lipid saturation pulses to avoid lipids from the skull. Naturally, these saturated pulses affect the metabolite quantification. Such lipid saturated pulses could be avoided by reducing intense lipid resonances after data post-processing (see Tanabe *et al.* [715]). This spectral data is Fourier transformed for each of the spectral peaks to generate an image. These spectral images can be co-registered with MRI (see Nelson *et al.* [796]).

At present, the Single Voxel Spectroscopy (SVS) technique is preferred over CSI, as this acquires a spectrum from a small volume of tissue defined by the intersection of the three orthogonal planes. Moreover, it also provides more chemical information from the selected tissue volume than any other existing technique. Two approaches are commonly used for brain VOI definition. In the first approach, only the VOI is excited with frequency selective RF pulses. The second approach involves the excitation and the subsequent subtraction of all the unwanted signals. The first approach is used in the Stimulated Echo Acquisition Mode (STEAM) and Point Resolved Spectroscopy (PRESS) techniques. Both of these PRESS and STEAM techniques contain a series of three selective RF pulses. These two methods differ from each other in many respects, such as the flip angles used, the sequence timing, and the sequence of applied spoiled gradient pulses. The second approach is utilized in the Image Selective *in vivo* Spectroscopy (ISIS) technique. It is worth discussing the limitations and the disadvantages of this single voxel spectroscopy technique in clinical brain applications. It produces a single spectrum over in a long time (6 minutes) with an optimized volume size, sequence and corresponding scan parameters. This requires the repetition of measurement several times for the different volumes in different areas of the brain. Hence, this method is less efficient. However, it is simple, easily implemented with fast shimming and it provides a simple, interpretable spectrum.

Having discussed data acquisition methods for Alzheimer's Disease, next, Subsection 7.5.2 describes different approaches to spectroscopic imaging to obtain MRI and MSIS or MRS data with analysis. The utility of Single Voxel Spectroscopy is highlighted in the detailed analysis of the metabolites in Alzheimer's Disease.

7.5.2   H-1 MR Spectra Analysis

Metabolite spectra from MR Spectroscopy (SVS) are traditionally analyzed with commercial software packages such as NMR1 and NMR2, where the phasing and the spectral fitting are done manually for the resonance peaks. These methods suffer from low processing speed and operator-induced bias. Later, automated spectral methods of post-processing algorithms were used and developed for spectral fitting programs. These methods were based upon a parametric model which combines *a priori* information with iterative wavelet-based non-parametric baseline characteristics. Based on these concepts, recently, a spectral simulation procedure using chemical shift and spin coupling parameters for each metabolite was evaluated (see Maudsley *et al.* [797], Young [798]).

An automated spectral analysis procedure was applied to MR CSI data over all the VOI voxels to provide the metabolite image. Based on these individual MRSI voxels, a manually selected method could be used for metabolite changes expressed as NAA/Cr, Cho/Cr and NAA/Cho. This used anatomical MR images as a guide. These metabolite peak ratios do not involve partial volume effects. Furthermore, time-domain smoothing was done by the application of the following steps to analyze these peak ratio calculations: Gaussian apodization filtering, Fourier Transformation, phase correction, baseline correction, peak assignment, reference peak selection and curve fitting for NAA, Cr, Cho resonance lines. With reference to an internal standard peak, the relative metabolite concentrations can be measured. The next sub-section will discuss applications of MRSI and segmentation.

7.6   Applications of Magnetic Resonance Spectroscopic Imaging and Segmentation

The main focus in recent years has been on localized MR spectroscopic metabolite screening and interpretation of spectra in the MS brain. Some of the abnormalities are identified as: reduced NAA as a neuronal marker; elevated creatine as a gliosis marker; elevated metabolites such as choline, lactate, acetate, alanine, questionable glutamate and glutamine screened in the different regions of acute MS, Primary Progressive Multiple Sclerosis (PPMS), Recurrent Regressive Multiple Sclerosis (RRMS) lesions and Normal Appearing White Matter (NAWM) brain areas. These metabolites were determined to confirm the regional metabolite changes. Metabolites were associated with the activated macrophages, T cells, edema, demyelination and axonal transection. To make a comparison of these metabolites in the MS lesions and in the NAWM of PPMS, RRMS and control White Matter requires a specific *a priori* knowledge-based hypothesis, such as: Cr is increased in PPMS-NAWM and the lesions for the possible gliosis in PPMS; the NAA decreased in PPMS-NAWM and in the lesions for neuron loss in PPMS. Such issues raise questions about the validity of the MRSI examination in MS. The possibility of using MR spectroscopic imaging can be extended for drug trials and routine clinical MS examination, however this still remains to be established.

On the other hand, segmentation analysis in Alzheimer's Disease is complicated for the evaluation of Ventricular CSF, Sulcus CSF and CSF in mid-line fissure. CSF segmentation is difficult to achieve on the lowest axial sections especially in images from the regions of the frontal, temporal and occipital lobes. Difficulty arises as these regions appear contiguously between the superior aspect of the temporal lobes and the inferior aspect of the temporal lobes. These remain visible in the apical section to contain 50% or more tissue with clear sulci and gyrate features representing supra-ventricular and superior brain volume. Segmentation analysis of hippocami in Alzheimer's Disease is of further benefit for utilizing the MRSI capabilities as demonstrated in Figure 7.3.

Sub-section 7.6.1 describes various aspects of segmentation analysis for metabolite MR visibility, along with some of its limitations. Several difficulties are highlighted for spectral peak analysis, peak patterns of MS lesion, serial follow-up metabolites and tissue composition of MS lesions. However, several questions are still unanswered such as the issues of Gray Matter and Normal Appearing Gray Matter (NAGM)-seated MS lesions and lesion heterogeneity. Other segmentation limitations are shown, such as mixed GM/WM composition in either the GM or WM of the fronto-parietal lobe.

7.6.1 Multiple Sclerosis Lesion Metabolite Characteristics and Serial Changes

In our studies the spectral quality and temporal stability in MS patients was usually observed at the average observed water line width within the entire VOI at water peak width at half height = 7 Hz. The water spectral width within a voxel is a good measure to use. The mean number of voxels within a VOI normally depends upon the ROI dimensions in the superior/inferior/anterior/posterior directions. The application of fat saturation bands causes artifact. Some of the voxels at the corners of all 8 edges may not be acceptable for spectral quality. This causes lipid and alanine bleed-through, resulting in enhanced single metabolite throughout the corners of the VOI. Hence, such voxels need to be excluded from the spectral analysis. On an average, 132 out of 832 voxels of image VOI were acquired by the AFFIRMATIVE sequence or by the Quadruple Contrast sequence. These were sufficient to map the whole brain metabolites. Several times the MRSI examinations were not taken, due to the following reasons: a lack of patient cooperation, inadequate shimming or other technical reasons of spectral file acquisition. In these MRSI examination for MS, a composite image was obtained as a combination of five 3 mm thick images as part of the VOI representing the area of the centrum semiovale composed mainly of the ventricles. The MR spectra from this VOI clearly showed well-resolved peaks of the NAA, Cr, and Cho and MI. Other metabolites such as lipids, acetate, alanine and lactate were also visible in these MS patients. Occasional low intensity of lipid peaks in the 0.8 to 1.5 ppm region were observed in all MS subjects. These signify spectral contamination from extrameningeal tissue lipids. The temporal stability of metabolites was best analyzed by multivariate analysis (see Doyle *et al.* [788]). Another problem was registration errors in the identification of the MS lesion location. Different scan studies of the same patient suffer from registration errors. Longitudinal studies require the co-registered and superimposed position of the VOI for all of the subsequent patient examinations. This is fully dependent on a visual inspection for consistent patient repositioning. The metabolite changes in these MS patients are conventionally expressed as metabolite peaks. They are optimized metabolite integrated peak areas after the CSF corrected values. The serial study of MS patients provides *in vivo* metabolite and tissue composition information from subsequent follow-up scans of a patient undergoing therapy.

Next, Sub-section 7.6.1.1 describes N-Acetyl Aspartate (NAA) as a marker of neuronal loss in MS and possibly in Alzheimer's Disease. NAA is highlighted as a major factor with possible Creatine and Choline and myo-Inositol changes in serial follow-up studies in MS patients.

7.6.1.1   N-Acetyl Aspartate

The origin of the NAA in the brain is still not established. The depressed NAA level is a less common feature in the acute MS lesions that evolve in MS patients based upon Gd enhancement. In these MS enhancing lesions, the decrease in the NAA level was mostly relative to the steady-state values after the enhancement. The assessment of the lesion recovery to a steady-state becomes very difficult because of the irregular patient scan frequency. The recovery time of the NAA seems to be around 120 days in MS patients. Other authors have also defined the NAA and resembling NAAG possibility in MS (see Pouwels *et al.* [800]). A typical example of the MS lesion site and NAA holes in the NAA map is shown in Figure 7.12 and Figure 7.13. The MS lesion and NAA hole disappeared after subsequent MS recovery. This low NAA image intensity at a MS lesion site is shown perhaps for the first time in Figures 7.12 and 7.13. During recovery, choline was simultaneously normalized. Fully grown, stable, MRI-defined lesion sites showed up with the reduced NAA levels. These were locally comparable with those of the NAA in NAWM. The total lesion volume and the total lesion load in the brain exhibited the inverse relationship with

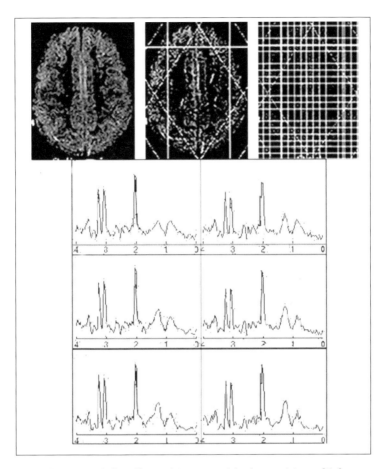

Figure 7.12: The upper left collapsed image, with the position of 8 fat-saturation bands (the octagon in the middle) and the grid (on the right) show the localization of MS lesions as bright areas in the White Matter background. (MRSI Data, Courtesy of MR Lab., University of Texas Medical School, Houston, TX.)

the averaged NAA over all of the scans and all of the voxels within the VOI in each patient. The low NAA was normally associated with a high choline, occasionally with high lipids (visible at 0.8 ppm, 1.6 ppm and 1.4 ppm), other lipid derivatives at 1.2 ppm but rarely with the acetate and lactate peaks.

Next, Sub-section 7.6.1.2 demonstrates the capability of Choline distribution in VOI with tissue composition by the segmentation of images. Choline perhaps highlights the role of Choline products such as phosphatidyl- and/or Glycero-phosphocholines in disease development and early intervention.

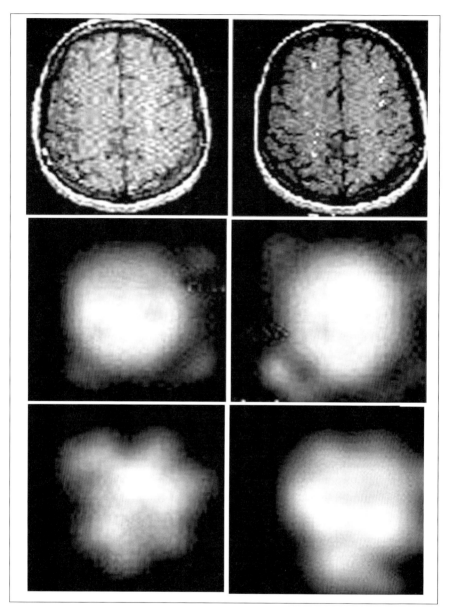

Figure 7.13: The lower left figure shows the acute lesion rich region and its spectra with corresponding voxel numbers. On the right, a typical example is shown for the low NAA intensity (holes in image in the left column) and subsequent NAA recovery (loss of hole in the image in the right column) with choline peak normalization after two months. Metabolites (octagonal) NAA and lipid images are shown in the left column before, and in the right column, after the MS recovery (MRSI Data, Courtesy of MR Lab., University of Texas Medical School, Houston, TX.)

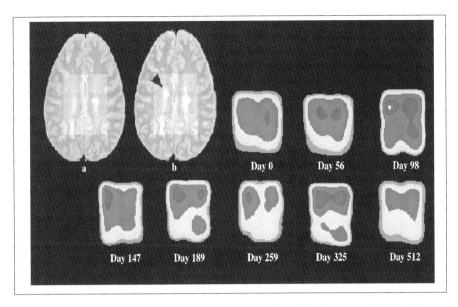

Figure 7.14: Temporal changes are shown in Cho levels in serial MS lesions obtained from all MRSI scan sessions, shown in the number of days at the bottom of each of the Choline images. The left image is a collapsed 15 mm composite image (a). In the right image, a spectroscopic VOI is highlighted on a 3 mm thick MR image with an arrowhead pointing at the lesion for better visualization (b). Time dependent changes in the Cho maps indicate the heterogeneous nature of Choline intensities in the entire VOI and the total lesion volume in the brain is shown. Note the enhanced Choline intensity after day 56 and day 259 (MRSI Data, Courtesy of MR Lab., University of Texas Medical School, Houston, TX.)

7.6.1.2 Choline

The origin of Choline is ascribed to the glycero-phosphocholine and the phosphocholine as the main phospholipid metabolite constituents or choline demyelination. The enhanced MS lesions appear to be associated with the increased Cho levels relative to the steady-state values attained within 6–9 weeks of the MS lesion enhancement. Stable lesions were associated with the reduced Cho levels in MS lesions compared with the choline levels in the NAWM. The average Cho levels in the lesion-containing voxels were mostly significantly high in comparison with those in the NAWM. In MS patients, the regional Cho increase was seen more than the Cho in the NAWM. Initially, Cho increased at the MRI-invisible lesion regions. Later, these developed as lesions, as shown in Figure 7.14. This highlighted the importance of high Cho sensitivity to MRI-invisible early MS lesions. Moreover, Cho levels were increased in a confined MS lesion and other adjacent voxels as shown in the Figure 7.14. The dependence of the Cho levels in the entire VOI and the total lesion volume in the brain are shown in Figure 7.9. High choline concentration in the lesion was associated with those of low NAA, higher acetate, lactate, alanine and lipid concentrations (data unpublished).

Next Sub-section 7.6.1.3 highlights the current issues on the role of Creatine in Glioma as an additional factor in the MS disease and its possible ability to classify Primary Progressive or Recurrent Regressive Multiple Sclerosis (PPMS and RRMS).

7.6.1.3   Creatine/Phosphocreatine

The origin of Creatine is mainly from the phosphocreatine abundant in the neuronal or glial cells. The average Cr level at the MS lesion rich voxels and in the NAWM remains almost the same. The Cr level may be increased or decreased in NAWM. Due to the small number of such changes in the NAWM, the correlation between the total lesion volume and the total Cr concentration in the VOI seems insignificant. The Cr levels increase mainly in the midline fissure or in the NAWM usually associated with the lipids.

Next, Sub-section 7.6.1.4 focuses on several lipid products. These are possibly visible by MRI and MRSI or MRS. The possible major role of lipids in MS disease prognosis and therapeutic decision-making is highlighted with the strong possibility of MS lipids as major representatives of MS lesions to predict the evolution history of the lesion.

7.6.1.4   Lipids

Lipids are observed in a wide range of values between 0.8 ppm to 1.2 ppm as a weaker and broader or a sharp, single peak. These are mainly contributed by the $-CH_3$ (0.8 ppm), $-CH_2COO$ (1.2 ppm) and $-CH_2CH_2$ (1.6 ppm) active groups of different fatty acids and lipids. Often, lipid peak areas vary in MS lesion or NAWM voxels. The distortions in the baseline further make lipid peak identification difficult in the region. In MS patients, the maximum SNR around and average SNR inside the VOI are other factors of poor lipid peaks. At an SNR of more than 6.0, most of the MS patients do not show any lipid peaks due to the less prominent broader lipid peaks. The association of the lipid appearance with the lesion and the lipid enhancement is common in the VOI of these MS patients (data unpublished). Moreover, the lipids represent the variable relationship with the lesion enhancement, acute lesions and NAWM tissues. These lipid rich NAWM tissues appear without MRI defined pathology. However, the lipid patterns appear the same in both the defined lesions and the NAWM. The voxels representing strong lipids in MS lesions are shown in Figures 7.15, 7.16, 7.17, 7.18, 7.19.

Recently, lipid rich regions which were presumed to be MS lesions in GM and Normal Appearing Gray Matter (NAGM) were analyzed by segmentation and metabolites. These lesions were more common in the parietal lobes. However, we need a further analysis of lipid rich MS lesions in NAWM.

The qualitative association could be analyzed between lipids, acetate, alanine and lactate peaks in spectrum and the image intensities in these metabolite maps. These showed a weaker correlation between metabolite maps and the

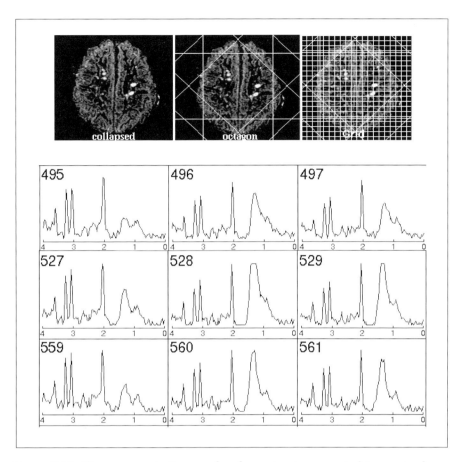

Figure 7.15: The representative quadruple contrast segmented image is shown with bright MS lesions in the White Matter dark background. On the left, a collapsed (15 mm) image is shown with octagonal fat-saturation bands (center) and the grid on the image (right) is shown for the VOI localization. Note that the lesion voxels rich in lipids are shown on the bottom with voxel numbers reported at the upper left corner (MRSI Data, Courtesy of MR Lab., University of Texas Medical School, Houston, TX.)

lesion load, i.e., for those of lactate and alanine. The correlation of lipids for other metabolites was apparent as shown in Figures 7.16 and 7.17. In the next sub-section, one of our MS examples is described to show the serial metabolite changes and MS lesion volumes over several weeks. Some of the rare possibilities are introduced for MRS visible metabolites. These are good predictors for unresolved controversies like amino acids and energy metabolites.

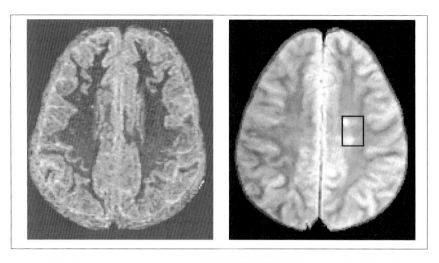

Figure 7.16: A representative normal AFFIRMATIVE image (left) and an image showing the MS lesion area in White Matter (right) are shown. Imaging parameters used: TE/TR=30 ms/1000 ms, slice thickness=3 mm. (Courtesy of Professor Narayana, P. A., University of Texas Medical School, Houston, TX.)

7.6.1.5   Temporal Changes

In our MS example, the temporal changes of all metabolites were analyzed to get stable data from all these metabolites. The average concentrations of the NAA, Cho, Cr, MI, lactate, acetate, alanine and lipids remained constant within the entire spectroscopic VOI, with no significant variations with time. Lactate, acetate, alanine and lipid levels within the voxels varied with time. Plate 10 shows that most of the metabolites except lipids reached a minimum. The lesion load was at a maximum after approximately 10 weeks, followed by the steady-state. Other important features were observed as the regional appearance of lipids, high choline, acetate, and alanine resonances from the voxels without lesion enhancement or other MRI-defined abnormalities, as shown in Figure 7.20, which later developed into an MS lesion.

Let us discuss longitudinal MRSI follow-up lesion load estimation and contrast-enhanced MRSI practical problems for MS patients. These patients had mild to modest clinical disability with extensive lesion loads and significant pathology in the NAWM. These studies enabled us to probe the assessment of evolving new MS plaques. Serial absolute concentration of all these metabolites could be measured by MRS in the lesions. This did not seem to be feasible initially because most of the data available uses the peak ratios as an indicator of the disease status. Interpretation of the metabolite concentrations relative to the tissue water minimized the problems, despite the tissue water changes in pathologic states. In that way, the relative metabolite concentrations in the CSF seem to be a good control reference as CSF is quite stable.

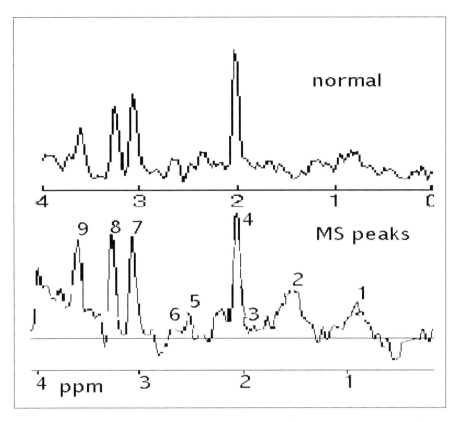

Figure 7.17: Representative spectra shown are after post-processing a brain image voxel. In the normal brain spectrum (top), only three peaks for the metabolites NAA, Cr and Choline are seen. Note the strong peaks of the lipids (1), lactate (2), Acetate (3), NAA (4), Glu/Gln (5), possible taurine (between the Glu/Gln and Creatine peak), Creatine (7), Choline(8), Myo-inositol (9) with suppressed water (4.76 ppm) peak in the MS lesion area (bottom spectrum). (MRSI Data, Courtesy of MR Lab., University of Texas Medical School, Houston, TX.)

In our MS study, the VOI was located superior to the ventricles, so the CSF estimation could not be made due to the long time needed for extending the patient examination. It was presumed that the tissue water and T_1 do not change with MS pathology changes in the individual voxels. So, the metabolite concentrations were measured in the spectroscopic VOI with [TR = 1000 msec] in a shorter time of acquisition. Both the tissue water and the metabolite resonances remained unaffected, as if the saturation factor of both of these was time-invariant. The T_1 value of tissue water from the VOI remains relatively stable with time. For this unsuppressed tissue-water data from the VOI 24 × 24 phase encoding steps are applied to extract tissue-water suppressed data with amplified metabolite resonances. Metabolite signals were normalized relative

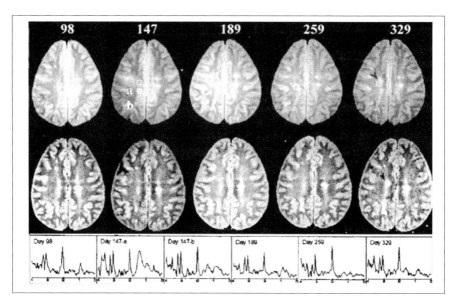

Figure 7.18: Serial T_1-weighted MR images with corresponding spectra from a voxel near to new MS lesions are shown. The 15 mm thick images at the top row and the 3 mm thick images in the bottom row are shown for time dependent lipid changes. Note the strong lipid peaks on the day 147 (top row) image (voxel 147-a) from the MS lesion area (a), before the appearance of a new lesion on the day 329 image (shown by an arrowhead) on upper rightmost image. For comparison, a control spectrum (voxel 147-b) from the normal area (b) is shown, just below voxel 147-a (shown by a white circle) in image 147 (top row). The amplitude of the lipid peaks was decreased by day 259. Reproduced by permission of John Wiley & Sons Inc. from [787]. © 1998.

to the water signal from the whole VOI. After that, different phase-encoding steps could be used for the tissue-water suppressed and the tissue-water unsuppressed data. These phase encoding steps should have a relatively small effect on the estimated metabolite levels.

This section now describes the spatial resolution of the MRSI. This is limited by the relatively low concentration of the metabolites causing the partial volume averaging between the lesions and the surrounding tissues. This may be the reason for the low metabolites measurement in the lesion regions of the VOI. This effect becomes more severe in smaller lesions. The spatial high resolution of MRI detects the new lesions or the post-Gd MS lesion enhancements better. The voxels are statistically independent of each other. This may not be true if lesions are scattered and cover more voxels, which is quite common.

The regional changes of the metabolites in MS seem to be quite dynamic and reversible. Metabolite concentrations are usually at a minimum when the maximum lesion volume is followed by the steady-state lesion values. There are other factors accounting for variation, such as edema, a smaller number

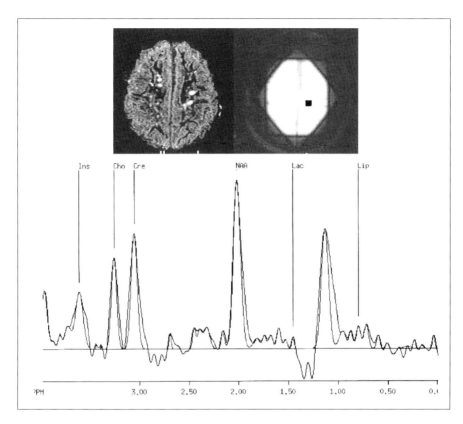

Figure 7.19: **Top**: A representative MS lesion rich image (left) and Region of Interest image showing the position of the lesion (right). **Bottom**: The post-processed spectrum is shown, with the dotted lines showing the automatic curve fitting by the APSIP image processing program. Note that the lipid derivatives appear at 1.2 ppm (MRSI Data, Courtesy of MR Lab., University of Texas Medical School, Houston, TX.)

of lesions, different insensitive pathology microenvironment to metabolic alterations. The NAA is believed to be restricted to the nerve cells and the nerve processes. It is not produced by astrocytes. So, the reduced NAA due to the neuronal loss and the axonal damage acts as an indicator of chronic or acute plaque development. Transient changes in the NAA may be misleading, based upon the limited MRSI sessions. The reversible depressed NAA in chronic plaques is well understood. The inverse relation of the NAA and the lesion volume in Relapsing Remitting MS has been supported (see Matthews *et al.* [801]).

Let us discuss the nature of the increased MRI-defined lesion burden in the brain. It is associated with the reduced density of axons and the axonal injury. The reduced NAA and the total lesion burden both measure the extent of the disease. Non-depressed NAA levels in the MRI defined lesions suggest that

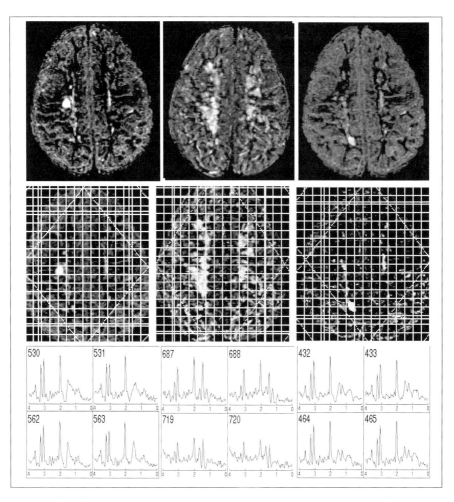

Figure 7.20: Serial T_1-weighted axial images were taken during different sessions over a two month interval with the following imaging parameters used: TE/TR=10/3000 ms, slice thickness=3 mm. **Top Left**: This shows the composite image (15 mm) having a fully developed MS lesion. **Top Middle**: This shows how the lesion became larger in the surrounding regions. **Top Right**: This shows the lesion frequency was reduced after four months. **Middle Row**: This row shows the the position of the octagonal grids. **Bottom Row**: This shows spectra from three different images. Note the enhancing lipids (doublet peaks at 0.8-1.2 PPM) in the MS lesion rich voxels as shown in **Bottom Row and Middle Column** (MRSI Data, Courtesy of MR Lab., University of Texas Medical School, Houston, TX.)

the lesion is not always associated with the axonal metabolism. However, the poor correlation of NAA with the lesion load in a VOI is not clear. Several deficiencies can be thus explained such as the neuronal loss, edema and atrophy in the lesion area by segmentation. The choline increase in acute plaques before the appearance of the MRI defined lesion is implied by the increased concentrations of the choline, phosphorylcholine and glycerophosphorylcholine associated with the markers not essentially related with the demyelination. A robust segmentation or the administration of a double dose of Gd can show Cho rich lesion areas as MRI-visible. Present assumptions suggest using the demonstrated blood-brain barrier breakdown after the Gd has been injected in standard T_1-weighted imaging.

In the brain, observations of lipid signals from the MS brain regions appear not to be associated with Gd enhancement or MRI-defined lesions. Segmented tissues such as the NAWM and GM are shown as probable sites for evolving new lesions in MRI scans. Sometimes, important lipid information is skipped, due to: (1) MRS and MRSI, which are done at long echo times, resulting in short T_2 times. As a result the sensitive lipids are unaccountable; (2) displaced VOI due to patient movement; (3) voxel bleed through due to the finite sampling of k-space; (4) increasing SNR (SNR=6.0 good); (5) irregular sample intervals. Sometimes this fails to capture the lesion enhancement event. The enhancement may be prolonged over 4–6 weeks as associated with the MR-defined lesions on the spin-density and the T_2-weighted MR scanning. The sensitive MRSI technique using reduced slice thickness visualizes the new MS lesion evolution after lipid detection (see Rovaris *et al.* [791]). After discussing several MS lesion characteristics, it is appropriate to realize the potentials of clinical MR metabolite screening and segmentation. These certainly throw light on the development of the MS disease process in the brain. Two distinct processes affect the myelin integrity or neuro-stability that are explainable based on ultrastructural findings. One, associated with the Gd enhancement, reflects the classic model of the T cell-mediated, macrophage-associated removal of the myelin from axons. The other process reflects the primary cell-mediated perivenous demyelination, independent of the blood-brain-barrier or inflammation changes (see Gutowski *et al.* [802], Trapp *et al.* [803], Gehrmann *et al.* [804], McManus *et al.* [805], Aquino *et al.* [806], Li *et al.* [807]). Moreover, lipids may be visible in the acute lesions but are absent in the Gd enhancement. Using the short TE, MRS studies demonstrate similar metabolite peaks' behavior in both these types.

Next, Sub-section 7.6.2 looks at the issues of segmentation and metabolite analysis in Alzheimer's Disease. Due to the ill-defined and diffuse pathology of plaques in AD, the major focus of this sub-section will be on the advantages of combining data from MRI and MRIS and/or MRSI in order to achieve better results.

7.6.2   Alzheimer's Disease Plaque Metabolite Characteristics

The MRSI examination is purely a non-invasive and sensitive neuro-imaging method. Initially, Point Resolved Spectroscopy (PRESS) proton MRSI study showed the reduced NAA in the supraventricular regions in the fronto-parietal and the hippocampal regions in the brain of AD, less than those in controls (see Constans *et al.* [808]). The segmented images showed the independent changes in the tissue composition and the hippocampal volume. Moreover, the superiority of MRSI was proven over MRI or MRS amounting up to 94% classification accuracy. Thus, tissue composition and metabolite analysis by segmentation and MRSI improves the diagnosis of AD. Figure 7.21 shows the slice orientation used for the H-1 MRSI study covering the frontal and the parietal cortex. The next section presents a discussion of MRSI.

7.7   Discussion

The automated program for spectroscopic imaging with the Magnetic Resonance Imaging post-processing method performs co-registered MRI segmentation. It provides significant information about AD plaque and MS lesions in the CSF suppressed White Matter around the ventricles. It offers quantitative tissue composition, completely free from operator dependent variability. Both our "Magnetic Resonance Image Analysis Package" and "Automated Proton Spectroscopic Image Processing" are routinely used for human studies. The segmentation algorithms in these software packages are robust and efficient, with less operator bias in the tissue composition analysis. The metabolite image processing algorithm performs quantification of the large arrays of the spectroscopic data. Furthermore, this fitting program for multi-slice processing performs improved curve fit by detecting and separating the broad, unresolved resonances without the local maxima on the target peaks. Several spectral fitting programs are available, such as SID, Peakfit, NMR-1, NMR-2 and others.

In the MS brain, several metabolites such as NAA, Creatine, Choline and Myo-inositol are prominent MR peaks. The lipids and amino acids MR spectral peaks are not well-defined but are MR-visible. The less MR-visible metabolites include lactate, alanine, acetate, glutamate, glutamine and taurine, which are indicative of protein regulation and energy deficiency. The overall abnormalities of these metabolites reflect the patho-biochemical state of the diseased locations in the MS brain. The MS lesions are indicative of neuronal loss, gliosis, and demyelination, as they are lipid rich. Our main emphasis has been on distinguishing the true lipid rich lesions in segmented images with GM/WM composition. These can be indicative of enhancing new lesions to distinguish progressive MS types.

Similarly, the H-1 multi-slice MRSI together with co-registered MRI segmentation could provide information on the metabolite and the tissue composition in Alzheimer's Disease. Sometimes, it is uncertain if the MR Spectroscopic Imaging findings are associated with the anatomical changes detected with the

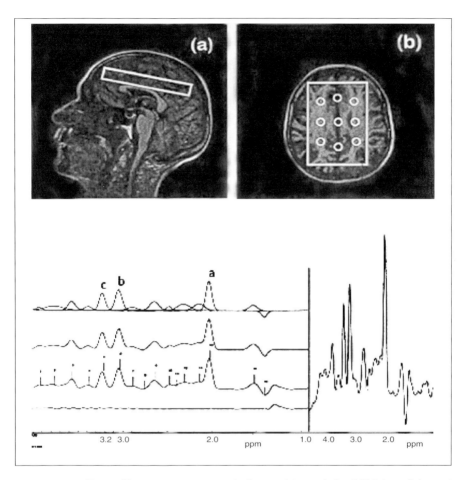

Figure 7.21: **Top**: Slice orientation and the position of the VOI box (a) used for H-1 MRSI studies covering the frontal and the parietal cortex in the brain (b) with Alzheimer's Disease. Bottom row: un-processed spectrum (right) and the post-processed spectrum (left) represent the NAA (a), Creatine (b) and Choline (c) (MRSI Data, Courtesy of MR Lab., University of California, San Francisco, CA.)

MR Imaging. Other differences seem to be due to the out-of-plane spatial extent of the chemical shift offset. This occurs whenever the slice section is used for the spatial localization. The chemical shift offset is determined by the tuning gradient strength, with the steeper gradients reducing the chemical shift offset. Thus, segmentation using differences in tissue type seems to be an important variable in the interpretation of MRSI studies. The obvious reason for this is the different metabolite composition of the Gray Matter and White Matter.

Some limitations in using these segmentation-MRSI methods still remain unresolved. These include magnetic field inhomogeneity across the brain, data acquisition from contiguous MRSI slices, using a short-echo time and tissue-water suppression methods. These limitations are trade-offs to achieving data with the maximum sensitivity. In this direction, several advancements have been reported emphasizing upgraded MR techniques, improved interpretations and new findings focused on robust automated segmentation and metabolic clinical imaging (see Bedell *et al.* [741], Pan *et al.* [809], Hirsch *et al.* [810], De Stefano *et al.* [811], Filippi *et al.* [812] Filippi *et al.* [813], Miller *et al.* [814], Filippi *et al.* [815], Erickson *et al.* [816], Zijdeenbos *et al.* [817], Filippi *et al.* [818], Michaelis *et al.* [819], Saunders *et al.* [794], Filippi *et al.* [820]). Other advanced, faster techniques which are only at experimental stages are not cited here.

7.8   Conclusion

Segmentation and MRSI are used as patho-chemical and anatomical research tools. These provide unique details of the brain's metabolism and function at different locations in a non-invasive manner. It is anticipated that improved segmentation analysis and the increased power of magnets will enhance the clinical acceptability of MRSI. The possibility of using MRSI and segmentation as a clinical modality depends upon easy data acquisition and processing and rapid display for routine MRSI examination by the radiologist. Data acquisition problems such as VOI selection, shimming, lipid and water suppression, co-registration, and magnetic field inhomogeneity can be minimized. Even simpler segmentation techniques are needed for automated, robust image processing and quantification data display. Success in MRSI essentially depends upon automated tissue composition analysis and spectral processing for clinical review. The combined MRSI and segmentation approach is being analyzed in Alzheimer's Disease and in serial longitudinal MS studies. State-of-the-art MRSI combined with segmentation to acquire data and perform processing in a clinical set-up seems far from perfect. Still, segmentation and metabolic MR screening techniques are improving in the interpretation of the pathology of diseases and the involvement of brain tissue in neurodegenerative diseases. In this chapter, the possibility of CSI and segmentation analysis has been highlighted as a future clinical tool in the analysis of Multiple Sclerosis lesions and Alzheimer's Disease plaques.

The prospects for segmentation and MRSI depend on improved fast switching gradients, 3-D phase encoding, Gibbs artifact removal, the use of short-echo times, automation in tissue segmentation incorporated with metabolite information from selected regions and faster data processing. Further information on Gray Matter, White Matter and CSF distribution and tissue composition enhances the power of metabolic imaging as a clinical tool. Fast and versatile spectral processing and statistical methods provide an opportunity for better image quality through automatic curve fitting and image reconstruction from signal deconvolution.

The future success of segmentation and MRS/MRSI depends on having higher spatial resolution, the ability to visualize regional heterogeneity as lesions, fluid accumulation, metabolite and tissue perfusion. Current reports suggest high hopes for MRSI and segmentation as a clinical modality in near future for the assessment of stroke, dementia, Alzheimer's Disease, Multiple Sclerosis, Parkinson's Disease, brain tumors, schizophrenia and other neurodegenerative diseases. Segmentation analysis further strengthens the possibility of assessing the temporal lobe, frontal lobe and basal ganglia in neuropsychiatric diseases by MRSI. It is anticipated that NAA will serve as a predictor of neuronal loss and possible neurotransmitters and amino acids may be valuable in solving neurochemical and pharmacological questions in research and clinical diagnosis.

7.8.1   Acknowledgements

Some of the data presented in this manuscript are part of an NIH research grant (1R01 NS 31499). I would like to acknowledge the copyright permissions from the editors and all the authors for reproducing their data. I would also like to acknowledge Professor P.A. Narayana, Radiology Department, University of Texas Medical School, Houston, Texas, for his research facilities and the Magnetic Resonance Spectroscopic Imaging data in this manuscript. I also wish to acknowledge Professor Michael W. Weiner, MR Spectroscopy, DVA Medical Center, University of California, San Francisco, CA, for the training program and for hosting me as a visiting scientist. Thanks also go to Professor Sameer Singh of the University of Exeter, UK and Dr. Jasjit Suri of Marconi Medical Systems, Inc., for their valuable suggestions on this chapter.

Chapter 8

Fast WM/GM Boundary Segmentation From MR Images Using The Relationship Between Parametric and Geometric Deformable Models[1]

Jasjit S. Suri

8.1 Introduction

The role of fast shape recovery has always been a critical component in 2-D and 3-D medical imagery since it assists largely in medical therapy such as image guided surgery applications. The applications of shape recovery have been increasing since scanning methods became faster, more accurate and less artifacted (see Chapter 4). Shape recovery of medical organs is more difficult compared to other computer vision and imaging fields. This is primarily due to the large shape variability, structure complexity, several kinds of artifacts and restrictive body scanning methods (the scanning ability is limited to acquiring images in three orthogonal and oblique directions only). The recovery of the White Matter (WM) and Gray Matter (GM) boundaries in the human brain slices is a challenge due to its highly convoluted structure (see Plate 3). In spite of the above complications, we have started to explore faster and more accurate software tools for shape recovery in 2-D and 3-D applications.

Brain segmentation in 2-D has lately been shown to be of tremendous interest and a number of techniques have been developed (see the classification tree as shown in Figure 8.1). The major success has been in deformation techniques. Deformation has played a critical role in shape representation and this chapter uses level sets as a tool to capture deforming shapes in medical imagery. In fact, the research on deformation started in the late 1980's when the paper called "snakes" (the first class of deformable models or classical deformable models) was published by Terzopoulous and co-workers (see Wikins *et al.* [209]). Since then, there has been an extensive burst of publications in the area of parametric deformable models and their improvements. For details on the majority of the parametric deformable model papers, see the recently published paper by Suri [139] and the references therein. A discussion of these references is out-

---

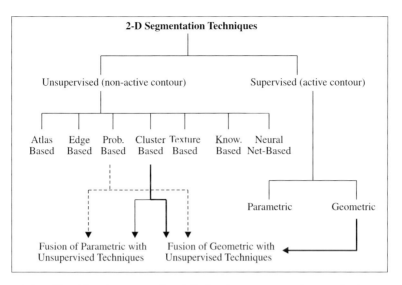

Figure 8.1: Classification tree for 2-D brain segmentation techniques. 2-D methods are primarily divided into two parts: unsupervised and supervised. They are also defined in terms of deformation models as: (**1**) non-active and (**2**) active contour methods. As seen in the figure, the unsupervised methods are futher classified into seven categories: (**1**) atlas-based, (**2**) edge-based, (**3**) probability-based, (**4**) cluster-based, (**5**) texture-based, (**6**) knowledge-based and (**7**) neural network-based. The supervised techniques are divided into two major classes: parametric and geometric. With the advancement in Computer Vision, Graphics and Image Processing techniques, we have started to see the fusion of unsupervised and supervised techniques. Also seen is the fusion of geometric and fuzzy clustering, the one used in this chapter. Complete details of segmentation techniques applied to Neuro imaging can be seen in Figure 4.7.

side the scope of this chapter. The second class of deformable models is level sets. These deformable models were introduced by Osher and Sethian [536] and formed the topic of Sethian's Ph.D. thesis [535]. The fundamental difference between these two classes is: parametric deformable methods are local methods based on an energy-minimizing spline guided by external and image forces which pulls the spline towards features such as lines and edges in the image. On the other hand, level set methods are based on active contour energy minimization which solves the computation of geodesics or minimal distance curves. Level set methods are governed by the curvature dependent speeds of moving curves or fronts. Those familiar in the field of parametric deformable models will appreciate the major advantages and superiority of level sets compared to classical deformable models. We will, however, briefly cover these in this chapter also.

The application of level sets in medical imaging was attempted by Sethian and his coworkers (see Malladi *et al.* [821]). Other authors who used level sets were: Kichenassamy *et al.* [545], Yezzi *et al.* [546] and Siddiqui *et al.* [547]. The work done above uses plain gradient-based techniques as the speed functions. These methods are very noise sensitive and are non-robust, especially in multi-spectral and multi-class brain volume scans. They fail to take advantage of the region-based statistics in the level set framework for curve propagation for WM/GM boundary estimation. Thus there is leaking or bleeding of the boundaries. Recently, Suri [614] tried to incorporate fuzzy statistics into the level set framework to prevent leaking of the boundaries.

This chapter presents a fast region-based level set system (so-called geometric snakes[2] based on regions) for the extraction of White Matter, Gray Matter and cerebrospinal fluid boundaries from two dimensional magnetic resonance images of the human brain. This method uses a new technique of introducing the fuzzy classifier into the level set framework besides keeping the traditional speed terms of curvature, shape and gradient.

The layout of this chapter is as follows: Section 8.2 presents the derivation of geometric snakes from parametric models. The numerical implementation of integrating the speed functions in the level set framework is discussed in Section 8.3. The methodology and the segmentation system are presented in Section 8.4. The results of synthetic and real data are presented in Section 8.5. The same section also discusses numerical stability issues related to this technique, the sensitivity of level set parameters, accuracy and speed issues. The superiority of geometric snakes when fused with fuzzy clustering in a level set framework is discussed in Section 8.6. Comparisons between region-based level sets and the previous techniques are discussed in Section 8.7. Finally, the chapter concludes in Section 8.8 with future directions.

8.2 Derivation of the Regional Geometric Active Contour Model from the Classical Parametric Deformable Model

Parametric Snake Model: in this section, we derive the level set equation by embedding the region statistics into the parametric classical energy model. This method is in the spirit of Xu *et al.*'s [613] attempt. We will discuss part of that derivation here. To start with, the standard dynamic classical energy model as given by Wikins *et al.* [209] was:

$$\gamma \frac{\partial \mathbf{X}}{\partial t} = \underbrace{\frac{\partial}{\partial s}(\alpha \frac{\partial \mathbf{X}}{\partial s}) - \frac{\partial^2}{\partial s^2}(\beta \frac{\partial^2 \mathbf{X}}{\partial s^2})}_{internal-energy} + \underbrace{F_{ext}(\mathbf{X})}_{external-energy} \quad , \qquad (8.1)$$

where $\mathbf{X}$ was the parametric contour[3] with parameter s and γ was the damping coefficient. As seen in Equation (8.1), the classical energy model constitutes

---

[2]Called the geometric active contour.

[3]For some details on classical energy models, readers can refer to Chapter 3; for complete implementation of these equations, see Wikins *et al.* [209].

an energy-minimizing spline guided by external and image forces that pulled the spline towards features such as lines and edges in the image. The energy-minimizing spline was called a "snake" because the spline softly and quietly moved while minimizing the energy term. The internal energy was composed of two terms: the first term was the first order derivative of the parametric curve which acted like a membrane and the second term was the second derivative of the parametric curve which acted as a thin plate (the so-called pressure force). These terms were controlled by the elastic constants α and β. The second part of the classical energy model constituted the external force given by $F_{ext}(\mathbf{X})$. This external energy term depended upon image forces which was a function of image gradient. Parametric snakes had the flexibility to dynamically control the movements, but there were inherent drawbacks when they were applied to highly convoluted structures, sharp bends and corners, or images with a large amount of noise. We therefore try to preserve the classical properties of the parametric contours but also bring the geometric properties which could capture the topology of the convoluted WM and GM. Next, we show the derivation of the geometric snake from the above model in the level set framework.

Derivation of the Geometric Snake: Since the second derivative term in Equation (8.1) did not significantly affect the performance of the active geometric snakes (see Caselles *et al.* [540]), we dropped that term and replaced it with a new pressure force term given as $F_p(\mathbf{X})$. This pressure force is an outward force which is a function of the unit normal, $\mathcal{N}$ of the deforming curve. Thus defining the pressure force as: $F_p(\mathbf{X}) = w_p(\mathbf{X})\mathcal{N}(\mathbf{X})$, where $w_p(\mathbf{X})$ is the weighting factor, the new parametric active contour could be written by replacing $\beta\frac{\partial^2 \mathbf{X}}{\partial s^2}$ by $w_p(\mathbf{X})\mathcal{N}(\mathbf{X})$:

$$\gamma\frac{\partial \mathbf{X}}{\partial t} = \frac{\partial}{\partial s}(\alpha\frac{\partial \mathbf{X}}{\partial s}) - w_p(\mathbf{X})\mathcal{N}(\mathbf{X}) + F_{ext}(\mathbf{X})\,. \tag{8.2}$$

If we adjust Equation (8.2) in terms of the curvature of the deformable curve by defining $\frac{\partial}{\partial s}(\frac{\partial \mathbf{X}}{\partial s})$ to be the curvature κ, and readjusting the terms by defining the constant $\epsilon = \frac{\alpha}{\gamma}$, $V_p = \frac{w_p(X)}{\gamma}\mathcal{N}(\mathbf{X})$ and $V_{ext} = \frac{F_{ext}}{\gamma}$, it can be rewritten as:

$$\frac{\partial \mathbf{X}}{\partial t} = (\epsilon\kappa + V_p + V_{ext}.\mathcal{N})\mathcal{N}\,. \tag{8.3}$$

The above equation is analogous to Sethian's [536] equation of curve evolution, given as: $\frac{\partial \phi}{\partial t} = V(\kappa)\mathcal{N}$, where $\mathcal{N} = -\frac{\nabla\phi}{|\nabla\phi|}$. Note, ϕ was the level set function and $V(\kappa)$ was the curvature dependent speed with which the front (or zero-level-curve) propagates. The expression $\frac{\partial \phi}{\partial t} = V(\kappa)\mathcal{N}$ described the time evolution of the level set function (ϕ) in such a way that the zero-level-curve of this evolving function was always identified with the propagating interface. We will interchangably use the term "level set function" with the term "flow field" or simply "field" during the course of this chapter. Comparing Equation (8.3) and $\frac{\partial \phi}{\partial t} = V(\kappa)\mathcal{N}$, and using the geometric property of the curve's normal $\mathcal{N}$

and considering only the normal components of internal and external forces,

$$\frac{\partial}{\partial s}\left(\alpha \frac{\partial \mathbf{X}}{\partial s}\right).\mathcal{N} = (\alpha \kappa), \qquad (8.4)$$

we obtain the level set function (ϕ) in the form of the partial differential equation (PDE):

$$\frac{\partial \phi}{\partial t} = (\epsilon \kappa + V_p)\,|\nabla \phi| - V_{ext}.\nabla \phi. \qquad (8.5)$$

Note, V_p can be considered as a regional force term and and can be mathematically expressed as a combination of the inside-outside regional area of the propagating curve. This can be defined as $\frac{w_R}{\gamma R}$, where R is the region indicator term that lies between 0 and 1, γ is the weighting constant and w_R is the term which controls the speed of the deformation process. An example of such a region indicator could come from a membership function of the fuzzy classifier (see Bezdek *et al.* [466]). Thus, we see that regional information is one of the factors which controls the speed of the geometric snake or propagating curve in the level set framework. A framework in which a snake propagates by capturing the topology of the WM/GM, navigated by the regional, curvature, edge and gradient forces is called a geometric snake. Also note that Equation (8.5) has three terms: $\epsilon \kappa$, V_p and V_{ext}. These three terms are the speed functions which control the propagation of the curve. These three speed functions are known as curvature, regional and gradient speed functions, as they contribute towards the three kinds of forces responsible for navigating the curve propagation. In the next section, we show the numerical implementation used for solving the partial differential equation (PDE) (Equation 8.5) to estimate the "flow field".

8.3 Numerical Implementation of the Three Speed Functions in the Level Set Framework for Geometric Snake Propagation

In this section, we mathematically present the speed control functions in terms of the level set function ϕ and integrate them to estimate ϕ over time. Let $I(x,y)$ represent the pixel intensity at image location (x,y), while $V_{reg}(x,y)$, $V_{grad}(x,y)$ and $V_{cur}(x,y)$ represent the regional, gradient and curvature speed terms at pixel location (x,y). Then, using the finite difference methods as discussed by Rouy *et al.* [822] and Sethian [823], the regional level set PDE Equation (8.5) in time can be given as:

$$\phi_{x,y}^{n+1} = \phi_{x,y}^{n} - \triangle t \left\{ V_{reg}(x,y) + V_{grad}(x,y) - V_{cur}(x,y) \right\}, \qquad (8.6)$$

where $\phi_{x,y}^{n}$ and $\phi_{x,y}^{n+1}$ were the level set functions at pixel location (x,y) at times n and $n+1$, $\triangle t$ was the time difference. The important aspect to note here is that the curve is moving in the level set field and the level set field is controlled by these three speed terms. In other words, these speeds are forces acting on the propagating contour. In the next three sub-sections, we discuss the speed terms mathematically in terms of the level set framework.

8.3.1 Regional Speed Term Expressed in Terms of the Level Set Function (ϕ)

The regional speed term at a pixel location (x, y) is mathematically given as: $V_{reg}(x, y) = max\,(V_p(x, y), 0)\, \nabla^+ + min\,(V_p(x, y), 0)\, \nabla^-$, where $V_p(x, y)$, ∇^+ and ∇^- were given as: $V_p(x, y) = \frac{w_R}{\gamma\, R_{ind}(x,y)}$, $R_{ind} = 1 - 2\, u(x, y)$, $\nabla^+ = [\nabla_x^+ + \nabla_y^+]^{\frac{1}{2}}$, and $\nabla^- = [\nabla_x^- + \nabla_y^-]^{\frac{1}{2}}$. ∇_x^+ and ∇_x^- were mathematically given as:

$$\begin{cases} \nabla_x^+ = [max\,(D^{-x}(x, y), 0))^2 + min\,(D^{+x}(x, y), 0))^2], \\ \nabla_y^- = [max\,(D^{-y}(x, y), 0))^2 + min\,(D^{+y}(x, y), 0))^2], \end{cases} \quad (8.7)$$

Note, $u(x, y)$ was the fuzzy membership function for a particular tissue class which had a value between 0 to 1 for a given input image I. R_{ind} was the region indicator function that falls in the range between -1 to +1. The fuzzy membership computation and pixel classification were done using fuzzy clustering to compute the fuzzy membership values for each pixel location (x, y). The number of classes taken was four corresponding to WM, GM, CSF and background. Note, ∇_x^+ and ∇_y^+ are the forward level set gradients in the x and y directions. Similarly, ∇_x^- and ∇_y^- are the backward level set gradients in the x and y directions. Also note, ∇_x^+, ∇_y^+, ∇_x^- and ∇_y^- are expressed in terms of $D^{-x}(x, y)$, $D^{+x}(x, y)$, $D^{-y}(x, y)$, $D^{+y}(x, y)$ which are the forward and backward difference operators defined in terms of the level set function ϕ given in Equation (8.9). We thus see that the regional speed term is expressed in terms of the "flow field" and the "flow field" is controlled by a regional force V_p, which in turn is controlled by a region indicator, which depends on the fuzzy membership function $u(x, y)$. Thus the pixel classifier is embedded in the level set framework to navigate the propagation of the geometric snake to capture the brain topology. The implementation details of this novel approach will be covered later in this chapter.

8.3.2 Gradient Speed Term Expressed in Terms of the Level Set Function (ϕ)

Here we compute the edge strength of the brain boundaries. The x and y components of the gradient speed terms were computed as: $V_{grad}(x, y) = V_{gradx}(x, y) + V_{grady}(x, y)$, where

$$\begin{cases} V_{gradx}(x, y) = max(p^n(x, y), 0)\, D^{-x}(x, y) + min(q^n(x, y), 0)\, D^{+x}(x, y), \\ V_{grady}(x, y) = max(q^n(x, y), 0)\, D^{-y}(x, y) + min(q^n(x, y), 0)\, D^{+y}(x, y), \end{cases} \quad (8.8)$$

$p^n(x, y)$ and $q^n(x, y)$ were defined as the x and y components of the gradient strength at a pixel location (x, y). These were given as: $p^n(x, y) =$

$\nabla_x(w_e \, \nabla(G_\sigma * I))$ and $q^n(x,y) = \nabla_y(w_e \, \nabla(G_\sigma * I))$. Note, w_e was the weight of the edge and was a fixed constant. Also note that G_σ is the Gaussian operator with a known standard deviation σ and I is the original gray scale image and $(G_\sigma * I)$ is the simple Gaussian smoothing. Here, ∇_x and ∇_y were the x and y components of the edge gradient image, which was estimated by computing the gradient of the smoothed image. Again, note that the edge speed term is dependent upon the forward and backward difference operators which were defined in terms of the level set function ϕ given in Equation (8.9).

$$\begin{cases} D^{-x}(x,y) = \frac{(\phi(x,y)-\phi(x-1,y))}{\triangle x} & \& \quad D^{+x}(x,y) = \frac{(\phi(x+1,y)-\phi(x,y))}{\triangle x} \\ D^{-y}(x,y) = \frac{(\phi(x,y)-\phi(x,y-1))}{\triangle y} & \& \quad D^{+y}(x,y) = \frac{(\phi(x,y+1)-\phi(x,y))}{\triangle y} \end{cases} \qquad (8.9)$$

where $\phi(x,y)$, $\phi(x-1,y)$, $\phi(x+1,y)$, $\phi(x,y-1)$, $\phi(x,y+1)$ were the level set functions at pixel locations (x,y), $(x-1,y)$, $(x+1,y)$, $(x,y-1)$, $(x,y+1)$, the four neighbours of (x,y). Note, $\triangle x$ and $\triangle y$ are the step sizes in the x and y directions.

8.3.3 Curvature Speed Term Expressed in Terms of the Level Set Function (ϕ)

This is mathematically expressed in terms of the signed distance transform of the contour as:

$$V_{cur}(x,y) = \epsilon \, \kappa^n(x,y)[\, (D^{0x}(x,y))^2 + ((\, D^{0y}(x,y))^2 \,]^{\frac{1}{2}}, \qquad (8.10)$$

where ϵ was a fixed constant. $\kappa^n(x,y)$ was the curvature at a pixel location (x,y) at n^{th} iteration, given as: $\kappa^n(x,y) = \frac{\phi_{xx}^2 \, \phi_y^2 - \phi_x^2 \, \phi_y^2 \, \phi_{xy}^2 + \phi_{yy}^2 \, \phi_x^2}{(\phi_x^2 + \phi_y^2)^{\frac{3}{2}}}$, and $D^{0x}(x,y)$ and $D^{0y}(x,y)$ were defined as: $D^{0x}(x,y) = \frac{(\phi(x+1,y)-\phi(x-1,y))}{2 \triangle x}$ and $D^{0y}(x,y) = \frac{(\phi(x,y+1)-\phi(x,y-1))}{2 \triangle y}$. Note that ϕ_x^2, ϕ_y^2 are the squares of the first order finite differences of the level set in the x and y directions. Similarly, ϕ_{xx}^2 and ϕ_{yy}^2 are the squares of the second order finite differences of the level set in the x and y directions. Also note that ϕ_{xy}^2 is the first order finite difference in x followed by y directions (details on finite difference can be seen in any book at undergraduate level). To numerically solve Equation (8.6), all we needed were the gradient speed values $[p(x,y), q(x,y)]$, curvature speed $\kappa(x,y)$ and the membership function $u(x,y)$ at pixel locations (x,y). These speeds are integrated to compute the new "flow field" (level set function, ϕ). The integrated speed term helps in the computation of the new "flow field" for the next iteration $n+1$, given the "flow field" of the previous iteration n. So far, we have discussed the "flow field" computation at every pixel location (x,y), but to speed up these computations, we compute the triplet speeds only in a "narrow band" using the "fast marching method", the so-called optimization, which is discussed next.

8.4   Fast Brain Segmentation System Based on Regional Level Sets

Having discussed the derivation of geometric snakes in Section 8.2 and its numerical implementation in Section 8.3, we can use this model to segment the brain's WM, GM and CSF boundaries. This section presents the system for a procedure to estimate these boundaries, given a gray scale MR brain scan. Due to large brain volumes (typically of the size of 256 cubed data), it is necessary to devise a method where one can optimize the segmentation process. We thus use the methodology as adapted by Sethian and his coworkers, so-called "narrow banding", since it is simple and effective.

The layout of this section is as follows: we first present the steps/procedure for a system and its components to estimate the WM/GM boundaries in Subsection 8.4.1. Since the system uses the triplets of speed control functions and the regional speed control is the crux of the system, we will then focus on the estimation of the membership function which gets integrated into the regional speed function. We will discuss the regional speed computation using the "Fuzzy C Mean" (FCM) in Sub-section 8.4.2. In Sub-section 8.4.3, we discuss how to solve the fundamental Eikonal equation. Given the raw contour, the Signed Distance Transform (SDT) computation is implemented using the "fast marching method" in Sub-section 8.4.4. Sub-section 8.4.4 presents the solution to the Eikonal equation when the speed is unity. A note on heap sorting is discussed in Sub-section 8.4.5. Finally, we conclude this section by discussing the segmentation engine in Sub-section 8.4.6, the so-called initialization and re-initialization loops.

8.4.1   Overall System and Its Components

The "WM/GM boundary estimation system" is presented using two diagrams: Figure 8.2 shows the overall system which calls the "segmentation engine" shown in Figure 8.3. The inputs to the overall system were: the user-defined closed contour and the input gray scale image. The input to the segmentation engine (see the center ellipse in Figure 8.2) included the level set constants, the optimization module, the so-called "narrow band" method, the speed terms and the signed distance transform of the raw input curve. The speed terms (regional and gradient) were computed first for the whole image just once, while the curvature speed terms were computed in the "narrow band". The segmentation engine was run over the initial field image (the so-called SDT image) which was computed for the whole image or for the "narrow band". The major components of the main system are:

1. *Fuzzy membership value computation/Pixel classification*:
   A number of techniques exists for classifying the pixels of the MR image. Some of the most efficient techniques are the Fuzzy C Mean (see Bezdek *et al.* [466]), k-NN, neural networks, (see Hall *et al.* [467]), and Bayesian pixel classification (see the patent by Sheehan, Haralick, Suri and Shao

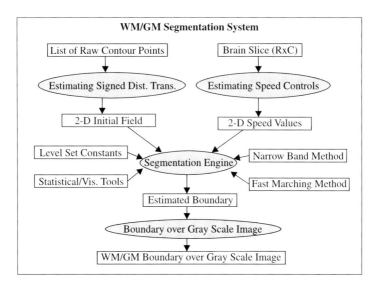

Figure 8.2: Overall system which calls the "segmentation engine". The user enters the raw contour and the initial field is estimated around that contour. A gray scale image is used to compute the gradient and regional speed functions. The segmentation engine receives the level set constants, gradient and regional speed values and the initial field to compute the final field in the narrow band using the "fast marching method" (four inputs to the central ellipse). The isocontour is extracted in the final field, which yields the WM/GM boundaries in the brain slice.

[235]). We used the FCM method for our system due to its simplicity and effectiveness.

2. *Integration of different speed components and solving the level set function (ϕ):*
   This includes the integration of regional, gradient and curvature-based speed terms, as discussed in Section 8.3.

3. *Optimization module (the "fast marching method" in the "narrow band"):*
   This involves the application of the curve evolution and the level set to estimate the new "flow field" distribution in the "narrow band" using the "fast marching method".

4. *Isocontour extraction:*
   The last stage of this system required the estimation of the WM/GM boundaries given the final level set function. This was accomplished using an isocontour algorithm at sub-pixel resolution (for details on these methods see, Berger [551], Sethian [552], Tababai *et al.* [553], Huertas *et al.* [554], and Gao *et al.* [555]).

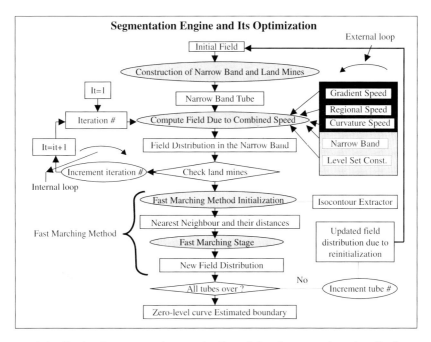

Figure 8.3: Brain "segmentation engine" and implementation details for running the region-based level set method in the narrow band using the "fast marching method". Given the initial field, we constructed the narrow tube of fixed thickness around the raw contour. The new field was computed using triplets of speed. The process exits if land mines are hit, or else the internal loop continues. The reinitialization process is activated and the next round of tubing starts, until all tubes are over.

8.4.2 Fuzzy Membership Computation/Pixel Classification

In this step, we classified each pixel. Usually, the classification algorithm expects one to know how many classes (roughly) the image would have. The number of classes in the image would be the same as the number of tissue types. A pixel could belong to more than one class and therefore we used the fuzzy membership function to associate with each pixel in the image. There are several algorithms used to compute membership functions and one of the most efficient ones is the Fuzzy C Mean (FCM) based on the clustering technique. Because of its ease of implementation for spectral data, it is preferred over other pixel classification techniques. We express the FCM algorithm mathematically below, but for complete details, readers are advised to see Bezdek *et al.* [466] and Hall *et al.* [467]. The FCM algorithm computed the measure of membership termed as the *fuzzy membership function*. Suppose the observed pixel intensities in a multi-spectral image at a pixel location j was given as:

$$\mathbf{y}_j = [y_{j1}\, y_{j2}\, ..., y_{jN}]^T, \qquad (8.11)$$

where j takes the pixel location and N is the total number of pixels in the data set (note, this should not be confused with the $\mathcal{N}$ used in the derivation in Section 8.2). In FCM, the algorithm iterates between computing the *fuzzy membership function* and the centroid of each class. This membership function is the pixel location for each class (tissue type) and the value of the membership function lies between the range of 0 and 1. This membership function actually represents the degree of similarity between the pixel vector at a pixel location and the centroid of the class (tissue type); for example, if the membership function has a value close to 1, then the pixel at the pixel location is close to the centroid of the pixel vector for that particular class. The algorithm can be presented in the following four steps. If $u_{jk}^{(p)}$ is the membership value at location j for class k at iteration p, then $\Sigma_{k=1}^{3} u_{jk} = 1$. As defined before, $\mathbf{y}_j$ is the observed pixel vector at location j and $\mathbf{v}_k^{(p)}$ is the centroid of class k at iteration p, thus, the FCM steps for computing the fuzzy membership values are:

1. Choose the number of classes (K) and the error threshold ϵ_{th} and set the initial guess for the centroids $\mathbf{v}_k^{(0)}$ where the iteration number $p=0$.

2. Compute the fuzzy membership function, given by the equation:

$$u_{jk}^{(p)} = \frac{||\mathbf{y}_j - \mathbf{v}_k^{(p)}||^{-2}}{\Sigma_{l=1}^{K}||\mathbf{y}_j - \mathbf{v}^{(p)}||^{-2}} \qquad (8.12)$$

where $j = 1, ..., M$ and $k = 1, ..., K$.

3. Compute the new centroids, using the equation:

$$\mathbf{v}^{(p+1)} = \frac{\Sigma_{j=1}^{N}(u_{jk}^{(p)})^2 \, \mathbf{y}_j}{\Sigma_{j=1}^{N}(u_{jk}^{(p)})^2}. \qquad (8.13)$$

4. Convergence was checked by computing the error between the previous and current centroids ($||\mathbf{v}^{(p+1)} - \mathbf{v}^{(p)}||$). If the algorithm had converged, an exit would be required; otherwise, one would increment p and go to step 2 for computing the fuzzy membership function again. The output of the FCM algorithm was K sets of fuzzy membership functions. We were interested in the membership value at each pixel for each class. Thus, if there were K classes, then we threw out K number of images and K number of matrices for the membership functions to be used in computing the final speed terms. Since the algorithm computed the region properties of the image, we considered this factor to be a region-based speed control term which was plugged into Equation (8.6).

8.4.3 Eikonal Equation and its Mathematical Solution

In this sub-section, we present the mathematical solution for solving the level set function with unity speed[4]. Such a method is needed to compute the signed distance transform when the raw contour crosses the background pixel grid. Let us consider a case of a "front" moving with a velocity $V = V(x, y)$, such that V is greater than zero. Using Sethian's level set equation, we can consider a monotonically advancing front represented in the form:

$$\phi_t = V(x, y) \, ||\nabla \phi||, \tag{8.14}$$

where ϕ_t is the rate of change of the level set and $\nabla \phi$ is the gradient of the ϕ. Let $T(x, y)$ be the time at which the front crosses the grid point (x, y). In this time, the surface $T(x, y)$ satisfies the equation:

$$||\nabla T|| \, . \, V = 1. \tag{8.15}$$

Details on the Eikonal equation can be seen in Osher and Sethian [536]. By approximation, the solution to the Eikonal equation would be given as:

$$max \, [\, max(D^{-x} T, 0), -min(D^{+x} T, 0) \,]^2 + \tag{8.16}$$
$$max \, [\, max(D^{-y} T, 0), -min(D^{+y} T, 0) \,]^2 = \frac{1}{V^2_{xy}},$$

where V^2_{xy} was the square of the speed at location (x, y) and $D^{-x} T$, $D^{+x} T$, $D^{-y} T$, $D^{+y} T$ are the backward and forward differences in time, given as:

$$
\begin{cases}
D^{+x} T = \frac{T(x,y+1)-T(x,y)}{2} \\
D^{-x} T = \frac{T(x,y)-T(x,y-1)}{2} \\
D^{+y} T = \frac{T(x+1,y)-T(x,y)}{2} \\
D^{-y} T = \frac{T(x,y)-T(x-1,y)}{2} \, .
\end{cases}
\tag{8.17}
$$

There are efficient schemes for solving the Eikonal Equation (8.15). For details, see Sethian [823], Cao *et al.* [542] and Chen *et al.* [543]. We implemented Equation (8.16) using Sethian's "fast marching" algorithm as referred to in patent [549], and discussed in the next sub-section.

8.4.4 Fast Marching Method for Solving the Eikonal Equation

The "fast marching method" (FMM) was used to solve the Eikonal equation, or a level set evolution with a given speed whose sign does not change. Its main usage was to compute the signed distance transform from a given curve (say, one with speed $= 1$). This signed distance function was the level set function that was used in the "narrow band" algorithm. FMM can also be used for a

---

[4]If one can perform the computation of curve evolution at unity speed, then the implementation can be done for any speed.

simple active contour model if the contour only moves either inward (pressure force in terms of parametric snakes) or outward (balloon force in terms of parametric snakes). The FMM algorithm consisted of three major steps: (1) initialization stage, (2) tagging stage and (3) marching stage (see Figure 8.3). We will briefly discuss these three stages.

1. *Initialization Stage*:
   Let us assume that the curve cuts the grid points exactly, which means that it passed through the intersection of the horizontal and vertical grid lines. If the curve did not pass through the grid points, then we found where the curve intersected the grid lines using the simple method recently developed by Adalsteinsson *et al.* [824] for curve-grid intersection (see Figure 8.4). We implemented a robust method, which was a modified version of Adalsteinsson *et al.* [824]. In this method, we checked four neighbors (E, W, N, S) of a given central pixel and found 16 combinations where the given contour could intersect the grid. Since the central pixel could be inside or outside, there were 16 positive combinations and 16 negative combinations. At the end of this process, we noted the distances of all the grid points which were closest to the given curve.

2. *Tagging Stage*:
   Here, we created three sets of grid points: *Accepted set*, *Trial set* and *Far set*. The *Accepted set* included those points which lay on the given curve. All these points obviously had a distance of zero. We tagged them as ACCEPTED. If the curve did not pass through the grid points, then those points were the points of the initialization stage and we also tagged them as ACCEPTED. The *Trial set* included all points that were nearest neighbors to a point in the *Accepted set*. We tagged them as TRIAL. We then computed their distance values by solving the Eikonal Equation (Equation 8.16). These points and their distances were put on the heap. The *Far set* was the grid points which were neither tagged as ACCEPTED nor TRIAL. We tagged them as FAR. They did not affect the distance computation of trial grid points. These grid points were not put onto the heap.

3. *Marching Stage*:

   (a) We first popped out a grid point (say P) from the top of the heap. It should have the smallest distance value among all the grid points in the heap. We tagged this point as ACCEPTED so that its value would not change anymore. We used the heap sort methodology for bubbling the least distance value on the heap.

   (b) We found the four nearest neighbors of the popped point P. This is what was done for these four points: if its tag was ACCEPTED, we did nothing; otherwise, we re-computed its distance by solving the Eikonal Equation (8.16). If it was FAR, it was relabeled as TRIAL and was put on the heap. If it was already labeled as TRIAL, its value was updated in the heap. This prevented the same point from appearing twice in the heap.

(c) We returned to step (a) until there were no more points in the heap, i.e. all points had been tagged as ACCEPTED.

Note that the above method was an exhaustive search like the greedy algorithm discussed by Suri *et al.* [550]. The superiority of this method is evidenced by the fact that we visited every grid point no more than four times. The grid or pixel location (x, y) was picked up by designing the back pointer method as used by Sethian *et al.* [549].

8.4.5   A Note on the Heap Sorting Algorithm

We used the heap sorting algorithm to select the smallest value (see Sedgewick *et al.* [825]). Briefly, a heap can be viewed as a tree or a corresponding ordered array. A binary heap has the property that the value at a given "child" position int(i) is always larger than or equal to the value at its "parent" position (int $(i/2)$). The minimum travel time in the heap is stored at the top of the heap. Arranging the tentative travel time array onto a heap effectively identified and selected the minimum travel time in the array. The minimum travel time on the heap identified a corresponding minimum travel time grid point. Values could be added or removed from the heap. Adding or removing a value to/from the heap included re-arranging the array so that it satisfied the heap condition ("heapifying the array"). Heapifying an array was achieved by recursively exchanging the positions of any parent-child pair violating the heap property until the heap property was satisfied across the heap. Adding or removing a value from a heap generally has a computation cost of order O(**log** n), where n is the number of heap elements.

8.4.6   Segmentation Engine: Running the Level Set Method in the Narrow Band

Having discussed the components of the brain segmentation system, we now present the steps for running the segmentation engine (see Figure 8.3). Below are the steps followed for computing the level set function ϕ in the "narrow band", given the speed functions (see Figure 8.3 and, for details on narrow banding, Malladi *et al.* [541]).

1. *Narrow Band and Land Mine Construction*:
   Here, we constructed a "narrow band" around the given curve where the absolute distance value was less than half the width of the "narrow band". These grid points are put onto the list. Now some points in the "narrow band" were tagged as land mines. They are the grid points whose absolute distance value was less than $\frac{W}{2}$ and greater than $(\frac{W}{2} - \triangle_l)$, where W was the band-width and $\triangle_l$ was the width of the land mine points. Note that the formation of the "narrow band" was equivalent to saying that the first external iteration or a new tube had been formed.

2. *Internal Iteration for computing the flow field (ϕ):*
   This step evolved the active contour inside the "narrow band" until the
   land mine sign changed. For all the iterations, the level set function
   was updated by solving the level set Equation (8.6). We then checked
   whether the land mine sign[5] of its ϕ had changed. If so, the system was
   re-initialized, otherwise the loop was continued (see Figure 8.3).

3. *Re-Initialization (ZLC[6] and SDT computation):*
   This step consisted of two parts: (i) Determination of the zero-level curve
   given the flow field ϕ. (ii) Given the zero-level curve, estimation of the
   signed distance transform was done. Part (i) is also called isocontour
   extraction since we estimated the front in the flow field which had a value
   of zero. We used the modified version of the Adalsteinsson *et al.* [824]
   algorithm for estimating the ZLC, however we needed the signs of the
   flow field to do so. In part (ii), we ran the "fast marching method"
   to estimate the signed distance transform (i.e., we re-ran Sub-sections
   8.4.4 and 8.4.3). The signed-distance-function was computed for all the
   points in the computational domain. At the end of step 3, the algorithm
   returned to step 1 and the next external iteration was started.

At the end of the process, a new zero-level curve was estimated which represented the final WM/GM boundary. Note, this technique used all the global
information integrated into the system. We will discuss in detail the major
advantages and superiority of this technique in Section 8.6.

8.5   MR Segmentation Results on Synthetic and Real Data

8.5.1   Input Data Set and Input Level Set Parameters

This sub-section presents the segmentation results obtained by running the
region-based level set technique in the "narrow band" using the "fast marching
method". We performed our experiments on several normal volunteers. MR
data was collected on five normal volunteers (in each of the three orthogonal
planes), thereby acquiring 15 brain volumes, each having around 256 slices.
Typical imaging parameters[7] were: $T_E = 12.1$ msec, BW (band width) = 15.6
kHz, $T_R = 500$ msec, FOV = 22.0 cm, PS = 0.812, flip angle = 90 degrees
and slice thickness = 5.0 mm using the Picker MR scanner. This data was
converted into an isotropic volume using internal Picker software and then the
MR brain slices were ready for processing. We ran our system over the sagittal,
coronal and transverse slices of the MR data set, but here only one complete

---

[5]If the sign of the ϕ was positive and changed to negative, then the sign changed occurred.
Similarly, if the sign of the ϕ was negative and changed to positive, then the sign change had
occurred.

[6]Zero-level curve.

[7]For definitions of these MR parameters, see Chapter 1.

cycle of results is shown over one sample MR brain scan.

Level Set Parameters: the following sets of parameters were chosen for all the experiments on real data. The factors which controlled the speed and error for the regional speed were: w_R=0.5 and ϵ_{th}=0.5. We took several combinations of the "narrow band" width (W) and land mine widths ($\triangle_l$). For W, we increased it from 10 to 25 in increments of 5. For ($\triangle_l$), we varied it from 2 to 10 in increments of 2. The level set constants α and γ and ϵ were fixed to 0.5, 1 and 1, respectively, for all of the experiments.

8.5.2   Results: Synthetic and Real

The inputs to the system (see Figures 8.2 and 8.3) were the gray scale image and the hand-drawn contour points. The speed model was first activated by computing three types of speed: curvature, gradient and region-based. The level set function was solved in the "narrow band" employing the "fast marching method" using these speed functions.

Results on Synthetic Data and its Validation:
Figure 8.5 shows the results of running the "fast marching" algorithm to compute the signed distance function in the "narrow band". Four kinds of synthetic shapes (from low convoluted shapes to high convoluted shapes) were taken into account to show the effect of signed distance transform on the convolution of shapes. The signed distance function performed well at the sharp curvature points. Also shown is the zero-level curve or the input contour. This serves as a measure of our validation of the "fast marching method" and 2-D field estimation, which is one of the most critical stages.

Results on Real MR Data and its Evaluation:
Figure 8.6 shows the results of pixel classification using the Fuzzy C Mean (FCM) algorithm. Also shown are the membership function results when the class number was 0, 1, 2 and 3. Figure 8.7 shows the results of running the "fast marching method" in the "narrow band" to compute the signed distance transform during the re-initialization stage of the segmentation process. Also shown are the associated zero-level curves (ZLCs). Figure 8.8 shows how the region evolved during the course of the external iterative process. Figure 8.9 shows how the raw contour grew during the level set function generation process. Currently, we make a visual inspection for the segmented boundary and overlay it over the gray scale boundary to see the difference. We also compare our results from the regional level set framework with the plain clustering-based technique. We are however working on a better technique where an experienced technologist can trace the WM/GM boundaries in the brain scans (slice-by-slice) and compare the error between the human traced boundaries and the boundaries estimated by the computer when the regional level set algorithm was run. We intend to use the polyline distance method as developed by Suri *et al.* [550], which has been well established and demonstrated over contours of the left

Curve Passing / Not Passing Through Grids Points

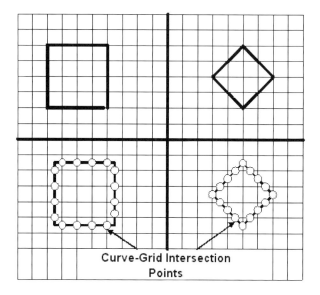

Figure 8.4: This figure shows the intersection of the curve with the background grid. Note that for implementation of level sets, one needs the points where the curve intersects the background grid. This is shown in circles.

ventricle of the heart and its segmentation.

8.5.3 Numerical Stability, Signed Distance Transformation Computation, Sensitivity of Parameters and Speed Issues

Numerical implementation requires very careful design and all variables should be of the float or double type. This is because the finite difference comparisons are done with respect to zero. Also, the re-initialization stage and isocontour extraction depend upon the sign[8] of the level set function which must be tracked well. During the signed distance transform computation, of all of the distances for the inside region were made positive and after computation of all the distances of the grid points, the distances were made negative.

There were two sets of parameters: one which controlled the accuracy of the results and the other which controlled the speed of the segmentation process.

---

[8]If it is positive or negative.

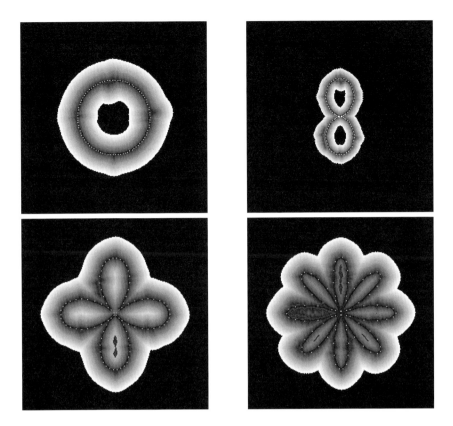

Figure 8.5: Results of running the "fast marching algorithm" in the "narrow band" on images of a synthetic circle, a flower with two petals, a flower with four petals and a flower with eight petal images. The synthetic shapes are sampled with white dots and the initial field (SDT) is estimated for the inner and outer regions (the so-called narrow band). The figure shows the field estimation to an accuracy of almost one hundred percent.

The accuracy parameter was the error threshold ϵ_{th} in fuzzy clustering. The smaller the ϵ_{th}, the better the accuracy of the classification and the crisper the output regions, however, it would take longer to converge. A good value for T_1-weighted MR brain images was between 0.5 to 0.7 with the number of classes kept to 4 (WM/GM/CSF/Background).

The brain segmentation system has two major loops, one for external tubing (called the "narrow band") and a second, internal loop for estimating the final field flow in the "narrow band" (see Figure 8.3). These two kinds of iterations were responsible for controlling the speed of the entire system. The outer loop speed was controlled by how fast the re-initialization of the signed distance transformation could be estimated given the zero-level curve. This was done by the "fast marching method" using Sethian's approach. The second kind of speed was controlled by how fast the "field flow" converged. This was con-

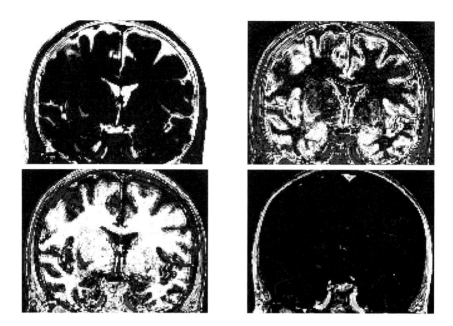

Figure 8.6: Results of the pixel classification algorithm with the number of classes equal to four on a sample MR brain scan. **Top Left**: class 0, **Top Right**: class 1, **Bottom Left**: class 2, **Bottom Right**: class 3.

trolled by the weighting factor w_R. Thus the parameters which controlled the speed were: (i) "narrow band width" (W) and land mine width ($\triangle_l$) and (ii) the regional term w_R. The larger the narrow band width, the longer it took to compute the "flow field". The range of w_R was kept between 0.1 to 0.5 and the best performance was obtained at 0.25, keeping the level set constants α, γ and ϵ fixed to 0.5, 1.0 and 1.0, respectively for all the experiments on the MR brain data set. We are continuing to explore in more depth the analysis of speed, sensitivity and stability issues as we get different types of pulse sequence parameters for human brain acquisitions and tissue characteristics.

8.6   Advantages of the Regional Level Set Technique

Overall, the following are the key advantages of this brain segmentation system. (**1**) The greatest advantage of this technique is its high capture range of "field flow". This increases the robustness of the initial contour placement. Regardless of where the contour was placed in the image, it would find the object to segment itself. (**2**) The key characteristic of this system is that it is based on region, so local noise or edges do not distract the growth process. (**3**) The technique is non-local and thus the local noise does not distract the final placement of the contour or the diffusion growth process. (**4**) The technique

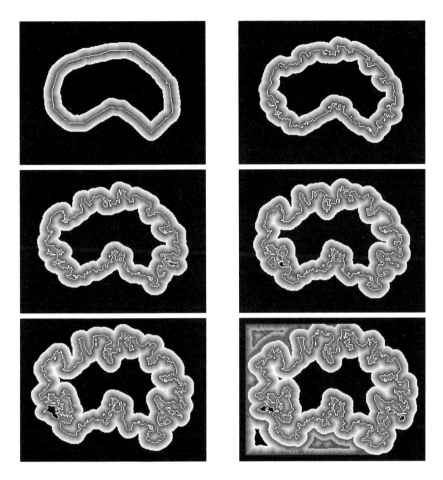

Figure 8.7: Results of the superimposition of the "zero-level curve" and its level set (field) function using the "fast marching method" in the narrow band. The figure show the six tubes in the order from left to right and top to bottom. The important aspect to note is that as we go along the deformation process, the system captures the White Matter topology. This topology characteristic is provided by the Fuzzy C Mean algorithm in the level set framework.

is not controlled by elasticity coefficients, unlike parametric contour methods. There is no need to fit the tangents to the curves and compute the normals at each vertex. In this system, the normals were embedded in the system using the divergence of the field flow. (**5**) The technique is very suitable for medical organ segmentation since it can handle all the cavities, concavities, convolutedness, splitting or merging. (**6**) The issue of finding the local minima, or global minima, does not arise, unlike the optimization techniques of parametric snakes. (**7**) This technique is less prone to normal computation error, which is very easily incorporated in the classical balloon force snakes for segmentation. (**8**) It is very easy to extend this model from semi-automatic to

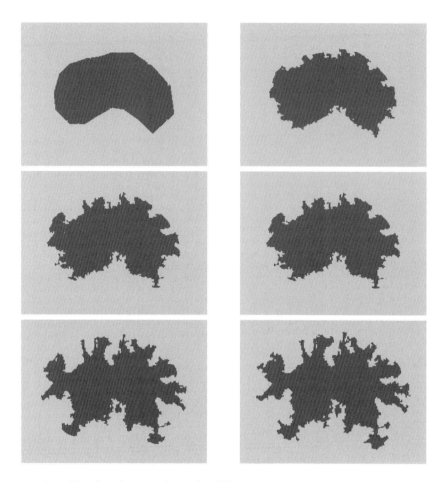

Figure 8.8: Results showing how the White Matter evolves using the regional level set method. The order is from left to right and top to bottom. Note, the power of the pixel classification process in the level set framework to capture the topology of the White Matter in the MR brain scan.

completely automatic because the region is determined on the basis of prior information. (**9**) This technique is based on the propagation of curves (just like the propagation of ripples in the tank or the propagation of flames in a fire) utilizing region statistics. (**10**) This method adjusts automatically to topological changes of the given shape. Diffusion propagation methods employ a very natural framework for handling topological changes (joining and breaking of the curves). (**11**) The technique can be applied to uni-modal, bi-modal and multi-modal imagery, which means it can have multiple gray level values. (**12**) It implements the "fast marching method" in the "narrow band" for solving the Eikonal equation for computing signed distances. (**13**) One can segment any part of the brain depending upon the membership function of the brain image. (**14**) It is easily extendable to 3-D surface estimation. (**15**) The methodology is

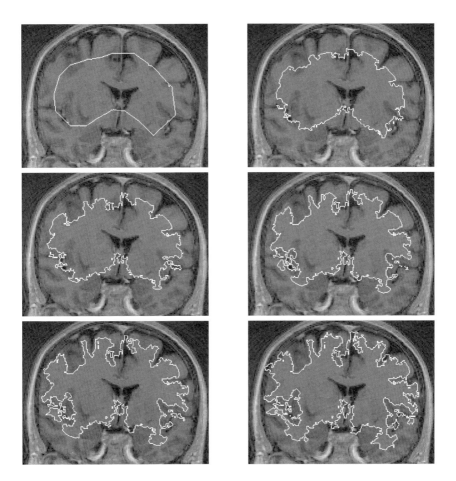

Figure 8.9: The above images show the growth of the zero-level curve to segment the White Matter in human brain MR images. The narrow band width was 25 pixels on either side of the zero-level curve, with the land mines as five pixels wide. Note, the deformation process has the ability to move in and out during the growth process.

very flexible and can easily incorporate other features for controlling the speed of the curve. This is done by adding an extra term to the region, gradient and curvature speed terms. (**16**) The system takes care of the corners easily, unlike parametric curves, which require special handling at the corners of the boundary. (**17**) The technique is extendable to multi-scale resolutions which means that at lower resolutions, one can compute region segmentations. These segmented results can then be used for the higher resolutions. (**18**) The technique is extendable to multi-phase, in which existing multiple level set functions automatically merge and split during the course of the segmentation process.

8.7 Discussions: Comparison with Previous Techniques

This section briefly presents a comparison between region-based level sets and the previous techniques for cortical segmentation. For comprehensive details on the comparison between different techniques, see the recent state-of-the-art paper by Suri *et al.* [826]. In the class of 2-D boundary-based techniques (as shown in Figure 8.1), current techniques are based on two approaches, parametric and geometric. These two techniques can be stand alone or fused with region-based techniques (so-called region-based parametric snakes or region-based geometric snakes). This chapter has described the region-based geometric snake because the propagation of the active contour is navigated by the regional forces computed using regional statistics such as fuzzy clustering. Earlier techniques such as stand alone parametric curves or regional-parametric snakes fail to estimate the deep convolutions of sulci and gyri (see Kapur *et al.* [594], [595]). The main reason for this is the instability of the elasticity constants of the parametric curves and the directionality of the normal computation of the propagating curves. Recently McInerney *et al.* [569] presented their work where the classical parametric snakes were made topologically adaptive, but they did not apply these to the cerebral cortex. In the case of region-based geometric snakes, Leventon *et al.* [588] very recently proposed a fusion of the shape model to the classical geometric level set snake. This work is similar to the work this chapter presents; the key difference is: we model the shape by statistical fuzzy clustering embedded in the level set snake, while Leventon *et al.* modeled the shape by adding an extra term to the curve evolution equation. A complete assessment of the pros and cons of this technique appears in Suri *et al.* [826].

8.8 Conclusions and Further Directions

Region-based level set snakes are a very powerful technique for segmenting White Matter/Gray Matter in MR slices of the human brain. We showed how one can apply the region-based level set technique for segmenting the brain using fast techniques. First, the chapter introduced the importance of 2-D brain segmentation in different fields of medicine. Then, we presented a significant amount of background information (based on Suri *et al.* [589]), along with the classification tree of the current state-of-the-art brain segmentation techniques based both on active (supervised) and non-active (unsupervised) contours. We then introduced the level set snake model and the incorporation of both regional forces and speed control methods. The core of the chapter explored fast brain segmentation system implementation, which solves the regional level set function in the "narrow band" using the "fast marching method". Then, we presented the results for the MR brain scan. Then, the chapter concluded with some critical advantages of current techniques compared to parametric snakes and non-active contour techniques. Finally, the chapter compared the suggested technique with other available techniques.

Note, the system used the fuzzy clustering method for computing the fuzzy membership values which were used in the regional speed computation. Recently, the authors have developed a mathematical morphology-based speed control function which acts as a regularizer for making the propagation more robust and leak free. It would also be worth exploring how either neural network or learning models would do in terms of the performance evaluation if clustering was to be replaced. A relationship between learning techniques and active contour models was attempted by Suri *et al.* [264]. The initial results on sagittal, coronal and transverse MR brain slices were very encouraging and need to be explored in three dimensions.

8.8.1 Acknowledgements

Special thanks go to John Patrick, Marconi Medical Systems, Inc., (MMS) for his encouragements during the course of this research. Thanks to IEEE Press for permitting me to reproduce this material from the *International Journal of Engineering in Medicine and Biology* (EMBS). Thanks are also due to Marconi Medical Systems, Inc. for the MR data sets and to Dr. Sameer Singh, Editor-In-Chief, *Pattern Analysis and Applications*, for his valuable suggestions.

Chapter 9

Medical Image Segmentation in Digitial Mammography

Sameer Singh, Keir Bovis

9.1 Introduction

Medical image segmentation is of primary importance in the development of Computer Assisted Detection (CAD) in mammographic systems. The identification of calcifications and masses requires highly sophisticated techniques that can isolate regions of interest from noisy backgrounds. The main objective of this chapter is to highlight the various issues related to digital mammography by providing a brief overview of the segmentation techniques used in this area. We first introduce the role of image segmentation in mammography in section 9.2. This section discusses a typical image analysis system for digital mammography and discusses the issues related to difficulties with segmentation. In order to understand the segmentation process, it is important to discuss some salient aspects of breast anatomy. This is detailed in Section 9.3. Various breast components are explained alongside the description of breast cancers. Image acquisition and storage formats are important as a predecessor to image analysis in mammography and these are discussed next in Section 9.4. This section also discusses different modes of mammography, image digitization and commonly used formats. Image segmentation cannot be isolated from some form of pre-processing that improves the visibility of objects of interest from their background. Section 9.5 discusses some of the enhancement techniques widely used in mammographic research. Often, the process of enhancement is difficult to verify, and therefore quantitative measures are sorely needed to select an optimal enhancement technique for a given data set. This issue is addressed in Section 9.6. A set of quantitative measures is shown based on the concept of target and background definitions. Sections 9.7 to 9.9 describe the various algorithms on the Segmentation of Breast Profile, Segmentation of Microcalcifications and Segmentation of Masses respectively. A breast profile must be segmented for studies dealing with bilateral subtraction or breast matching. Calcification detection is discussed with algorithms in the following section. A number of different successful algorithms for segmenting masses are discussed in Section 9.9. Global, edge-based and region-based segmentation techniques are explained. The segmentation process also needs to be evaluated for accuracy and it is important that the automatically segmented regions closely match the ground truth data marked by the radiologist. Quantitative measures of segmentation are discussed in Section 9.10. Once the regions have been automatically detected, features must be extracted from these to characterize them as either benign or malignant, fatty or dense, etc. The problem of feature extraction is discussed in Section 9.11 where a range of features are introduced including morphological features, texture features and others. We then discuss in Section 9.12 the four public domain databases: DDSM, LLNL-UCSF, Washington University database and MIAS. In Section 9.13 we describe in brief the process of classification and measuring performance of the classifiers using Receiver Operating Characteristic (ROC) analysis. The chapter concludes by describing possible future advances in this area.

9.2   Image Segmentation in Mammography

Image segmentation is a fundamental step towards the identification and analysis of regions of interest within an object. This section describes how and why we need to segment images. A large number of approaches towards image segmentation are available in the literature (e.g. see Haralick and Shapiro [244]; Rosenfeld [911]). We focus on those that are appropriate for digital mammogram segmentation. Segmentation is largely a qualitative process since in most cases we have nothing to measure the output against to determine the effectiveness of a segmentation procedure. We propose some basic techniques for identifying the quality of segmentation and illustrate how boundaries of regions of interest can be used for feature extraction.

In segmenting images it is important to differentiate between what we are interested in analyzing and other details that are not of interest. A simple example is to differentiate a dark point or a line from a white background. One of the fundamental assumptions in segmentation applications is that objects or regions of interest have different characteristics from the background that can be extracted using statistical procedures. These differences allow us to separate or segment regions of interest. Two important points of observation must be remembered in this context. First, it is not always the case that the background part of the image has uniform image intensity, and maybe sometimes we are more interested in the background than objects superimposed on it. Second, a computer should be used to iteratively reduce a starting set of possible objects or regions of interest from a segmented image to a final list that meets our specification. In other words, it is difficult to develop procedures that will automatically identify exactly what we need, but it is easier to develop methods that will start with a large set of regions of interest and prune them using statistical tests to a list that we are satisfied with.

A typical system based on digital mammography for the detection of masses is shown in Figure 9.1. X-ray images are acquired by compressing breasts within a plate. The X-rays are scanned by a digital scanner whose optical characteristics determine the quality of the digital image produced. Unfortunately, digital mammography, the process of acquiring digital images directly from the imaging equipment, is still being trialled in the US and Europe. This would eliminate some of the problems that we have with analogue to digital conversion. Enhancement can be performed in either the spatial or spectral domain. A variety of image enhancement algorithms are presented by Pratt [903]. If the quality of compression is poor or the scanning mechanism has low resolution, then the signal to noise ratio is poor in resultant images. Noise can be filtered from such images by taking their Fourier transforms and removing high-frequency components before taking an inverse to provide enhanced images. It is expected that the resultant images are of good quality for the detection of abnormalities using image processing tools. The next step is to find regions of interest that need further investigation to determine if they represent some form of abnormality. There are two common methods of isolating regions of interest (ROI) for mass detection. These include bilateral subtraction and single image decomposition. Bilateral subtraction techniques align left and right breasts taken with the same view using landmark information (for example the position of the nipple), and find differences between the two breasts by subtracting one image from the other. Asymmetries are widely thought to represent possible areas of abnormality and represent good starting points for analysis. The weakness of this approach lies in the fact we can get a large number of false positives as there are not enough accurate landmarks for aligning images and the two breasts can be differently imaged giving spurious gray level differences.

The single image decomposition approach assumes that uniform regions within an image require detailed investigation. Most masses when imaged show as regions with homogeneous gray level intensity. True masses usually have a convex contour, are at least as dense centrally as at the periphery, and can be seen in two projections (Mendez *et al.* [891]). These regions can be detected by pixel clustering. Using both methods (bilateral subtraction and single image decomposition), the aim is to have a set of regions that must ideally contain the abnormality if it exists. Yin *et al.* [931] compare the utility of single image processing method with bilateral subtraction. False positives are reduced using a range of criteria using tests on area, circularity and contrast. The results are shown to be better for bilateral subtraction; however this cannot be generalized to all circumstances.

Segmentation methods in themselves are not capable of judging the label of a region (normal or abnormal). Further shape or texture techniques must be applied to find this. However, regions of interest must be first detected to compute features from them – it would be highly uneconomical to do feature extraction for all parts of the image. From the computational point of view, a good image segmentation system should yield a small number of regions that have a higher probability of being the cases that we are looking for rather than, over segmentation, a lot of regions that have a low probability of being abnormal. In practice, shape and texture measures can be used to eliminate

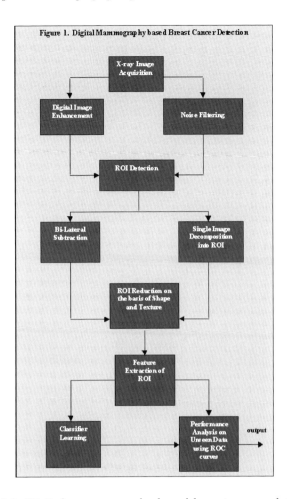

Figure 9.1: Digital mammography-based breast cancer detection.

those regions that appear unquestionably normal. For example, if regions are over a fixed size or have shapes that are hardly representative of true masses, then these can be eliminated from the analysis. For each region of interest, a set of features is extracted for its shape and texture. Haralick *et al.* [244] describe a set of 14 measures that can be used to characterize the texture of a region; Sonka *et al.* [917] describe a range of shape measures that can characterize the boundaries and area characteristics of regions. If known labels for a given set of regions within images exist, then their feature vectors can be used to train a classification system. Ideal candidates for these include linear methods, neural networks, nearest neighbor classifier and decision trees. The ability of the system is measured using ROC curves (see Metz [893]). In other studies other measures of performance have been used based on false and true positives, e.g. Petrick *et al.* [898] quote results as x false positives per image for an accuracy of $y\%$ true positives. A true positive is found when the centroid

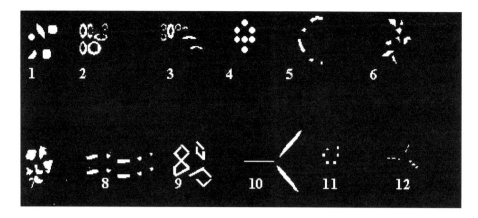

Figure 9.2: Various structures of calcifications: (1) calcified debris in ducts; (2) dense lucent centered calcifications; (3) precipitated calcifications in small cysts (milk of calcium); (4) concretions in small, cystically dilated lobules; (5) rim calcifications in the walls of a cyst; (6) early deposits in involuting fibrodenoma; (7) large deposits in involuting fibrodenoma; (8) vascular calcifications; (9) skin calcifications; (10) calcified rods in secretory disease; (11) pleomorphic deposits in intraductal cancer; (12) fine linear calcifications in comedocarcinoma (from Kopans [881] and © Lippencott, Williams and Wilkins. Reproduced with permission).

of the radiologist-marked region lies within the computer generated-boundary based on 50% or more overlap.

Image segmentation for digital mammography is based on the detection of objects within the breast that are of interest to radiologists for further analysis. Clinically, this interest can extend to several details within the breast, but most importantly, digital mammography research has focussed on the identification of calcifications and masses in mammograms. These two objects of interest are the most important indicators of whether further investigation is needed to identify the presence of breast cancer. Hence, image segmentation is used for the (a) identification of masses or calcifications including their shape and exact location using triangulation; (b) analysis of their granular or spatial structure to determine how suspicious these are; and (c) extraction of a feature vector that is unique to the region of interest and encodes information that can allow its automatic labeling on unseen cases. We briefly discuss these three aims in turn. First, image segmentation operates automatically to determine the exact shape, size and location of regions of interest that will include masses and calcifications. In clinical practice, two views of the same breast are taken. The Medio-Lateral Oblique (MLO) pair of X-rays takes a side view of the breasts and the Cranio-Caudal (CC) pair of X-rays takes the top view of the breasts. Through the identification of important landmarks within the breast and the position of the pectoralis muscle, it becomes possible to get very good positional coordinates of the region of interest if both views which are used as the

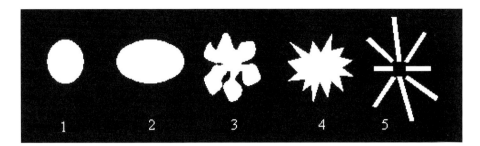

Figure 9.3: Variation on mass shape: (1) Round: A mass that is spheric, ball-shaped, circular or globular; (2) Oval: A mass that is elliptical or egg-shaped; (3) Lobular: A mass that has contours with undulations; (4) Irregular: The lesion's shape characterized by any previous shape; (5) Architectural Distortion: The normal architecture is distorted with no definite mass visible (from Kopans [881] and © Lippencott, Williams and Wilkins. Reproduced with permission).

object in one view will be available in another. As such, independent image segmentation in the two separate views can be used to triangulate objects (identifying their spatial location in 3D). Second, the granular or spatial structure of the regions of interest is extremely valuable in determining their significance. Masses in digital mammograms have a complex structure. Medical studies have pointed out that cancerous masses have a higher statistical probability of developing in certain regions. Kopans ([881] p. 14) points out that the majority of breast cancers develop in the 1 cm wide parenchyma zone that lies immediately beneath the subcutaneous fat or anterior to the retromammary fat. Masses appear as diffuse objects with variable structures that blend well with the surrounding tissue. The gray level of such regions is of little use in their identification as intensity levels in mammograms are affected by imaging conditions, image compression and the type of breast imaged. Their structure is better analyzed on the basis of texture and homogeneity. We briefly discuss these later on in this chapter. The spatial structure of segmented objects can be very useful in their taxonomic classification or other analysis as shown in the case of calcifications. The spatial density and structure of calcifications is useful in categorizing them as either punctuate, branching, linear, spherical, fine, coarse, cylindrical, smooth, jagged, regular in shape and size or heterogeneous (see Figure 9.2). Similarly masses can be categorized as round, oval, lobular, irregular, or an architectural distortion (see Figure 9.3). In order for proper categorization to take place, the image resolution must be very high and some form of relaxation labeling should be possible (Geman and Geman [457]; Hansen and Higgins [858]). Finally, all image segmented regions should be labeled on the basis of their unique signature or measurements on features that are unique to them. The quality of image segmentation has a direct bearing on what is extracted from them; segmented regions that include background pixels will have a negative effect on the quality of the measures extracted. On the other hand, very small segmented regions will not have enough pixels within the image to yield a meaningful measurement window. Hence, some optimal size of objects is necessary to have measures that we have some confidence in. Provided that a proper set of measurements is extracted over a number of cases, we should be able to learn the similarities between known suspicious cases to train an automated system to recognize these effectively. We will discuss this process later on.

Image segmentation is an effective method of focusing computational techniques on image areas that require investigation. If everything within an image were analyzed for signs of suspicious areas, it would be neither computationally sensible nor beneficial. When highlighting an area of interest, we benefit additionally by having information on its boundary that divides it from the background. Boundaries on their own can be of significant use in the diagnosis of suspicious regions. For example, boundaries of benign masses are well circumscribed and compact compared with malignant masses. As such, boundary information serves as an effective shape parameter that characterizes the nature of the object within.

Segmentation can be defined as either exact or approximate. Most of the methods discussed in the literature and in this chapter fall in the first category where a computer algorithm tries to find the best segmentation in an image. For this, a number of segmentation parameters are optimized. There is no guarantee that the best possible segmentation has been achieved; however the best possible approximation to the required result has been achieved under a given set of circumstances. In the last decade, it has become obvious that digital mammogram segmentation is a very difficult task indeed and computer-based systems could serve a better purpose in the clinical environment by highlight interesting regions to focus clinical attention on screening or diagnosis. As such, approximate segmentation would be concerned with the identification of areas that are worthy of manual inspection. The requirements in terms of quality expectations for such a system are much lower than that for an exact system. This allows us to build a different breed of systems that provide screening assistance rather than the replacement of manual mammographic screening.

In the next section we discuss the basics of breast anatomy. This is necessary to understand the significance of detail visible in breast X-rays. It is important to note that the level and quality of detail available in mammograms is dependent on the quality of the imaging device, the quality of the recording film, the age of the patient, and breast compression. Knowledge of breast anatomy is especially crucial for making decisions on detection with two views, model-based segmentation and diagnosis.

9.3   Anatomy of the Breast

In order to develop and implement segmentation techniques for digital mammograms, it is necessary to review the clinical aspects of mammography. The aim of this section, therefore, is to provide the reader with an understanding of the anatomy of the breast and structures that are contained within it to aid their

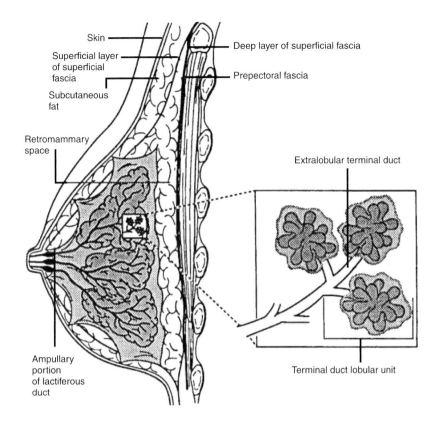

Figure 9.4: Anatomy of the breast (from Kopans [881] © Lippencott, Williams and Wilkins. Reproduced with permission).

basic understanding. Further details on breast anatomy and signs of breast cancer are available in Cardenosa [836], Egan [847] and Heywang-Köbrunner et al. [861].

Figure 9.4 shows the main components of the breast. The composition of the breast is extremely variable. Radiolucent adipose tissue forms a large portion of the breast. Other objects such as ducts, lobular elements and fibrous connective tissue are also be visible in varying degrees of radiographic density. These are described below:

Ducts   Ducts are typically seen as thin linear structures radiating back from the nipple that criss-cross other tissues. These ducts widen underneath the nipple as lactiferous sinuses and then empty (as between 5 and 9 nipple openings).

Lobules   The breast glandular tissue contains 15 to 20 lobules that enter into branching and interconnected ducts. Lobules contained within the breast consist of acini comprising of two different types of cell, epithelial and myoepithelial that surround a lumen. Lobules and the interlobular connective tissue appear as vague fluffy densities within mammograms whose architecture can be seen following the injection of contrast material.

Connective Tissue   There are two types of connective tissue in the breast:

(a) interlobular

(b) extralobular.

Interlobular connective tissue aids the visibility of the lobule. The majority of the radiographic density on a mammogram is attributed to the extralobular connective tissue.

Within this chapter we are primarily concerned with the identification of masses following the segmentation of mammographic images. Typically, several suspicious regions found within the breast are not necessarily malignant. Kopans [881] and Wolberg [930] identify the following benign objects and their associated characteristics:

Fibroadenoma   These are benign objects usually found in women under the age of 30 years. They are rounded in outline and easily movable. Though benign, they have a long-term risk factor for the subsequent development of breast cancer.

Fibrocystic Disease   This is an ambiguous term that includes most types of benign breast disease. Autopsies show that over half of all women have microscopic changes within their breast consistent with fibrosystic disease. Fibrocystic disease is not a precursor to malignancy and may be found as gross or micro cysts.

Atypical Hyperplasia of the Breast   This benign condition is characterized by marked proliferation and atypia of the epithelium (either ductal, or lobular). It is found in 3% of all benign breast biopsies. This condition is associated with 13% of subsequent breast cancer developments.

Phyllodes Tumor	This benign condition is a fibroepithelial tumor and approximately 10% of such cases metastasize from either histologically malignant or benign occurrences.
Periductal Mastitis	In its most acute form, this condition is the cause of most non-lactational breast inflammation. Aerobic or anaerobic bacteria may be involved or it may be sterile. Occurring chronically, it is the most frequent cause of nipple discharge in pre-menopausal women.
Papillomas	These masses are typically smaller that 1 cm and are often visible as intraductal growths. Patients frequently have nipple discharge and papillomas may occur solitarily or multiply. Patients with papillomas frequently develop cancer.

The diagnosis of malignant masses requires the radiologist to consider characteristics of each suspicious region. All malignant masses are different, some consisting of a single cell type that closely resembles normal breast cells while others consist of a great variety of different cell types with different appearances and different behavioral characteristics. Growth rates of tumors vary across patients. Typically the average breast cancer takes approximately nine years to reach a size of 1 cm. Breast cancer kills by spreading to other parts of the body (metastasis) and such spreading can occur at any time during the cancer's growth prior to it being detected. Typically by the time a mastectomy is performed, metastasis has already occurred, and exists as cancerous tissue that is too small to be detected by any clinical test. Certain cancers are more likely to metastasize than others, but at surgery malignancy cannot be classified as to its likelihood to spread.

Ductal Carcinoma *in situ* (DCIS) is a common manifestation of breast cancer. Malignant masses arise from the epithelial cells lining the ducts and lobules. Cancers that do not penetrate outside the confides of ducts of lobules where they arise rarely metastasize to the lymph nodes or to other distant sites in the body. Such non-infiltrating cancers are also termed *in situ* breast cancers. There are usually three conditions for metastases to occur:

1. Penetration of blood vessels or the lymphatic system.

2. The cancer cells must remain intact during transit.

3. The cells must lodge and proliferate at a distant site.

Typically breast cancer spreads from the breast to lymph nodes and from the breast to distant sites. A cancer that spreads to the lymph nodes is more likely to possess other bad characteristics. Wolberg [930] identifies two types of non-infiltrating breast cancer:

Lobular Carcinoma in situ	This type of cancer does not metastasize but gives a 20 to 30% risk of invasive carcinoma in the same or opposite breast. This type of cancer is typically treated by bilateral mastectomy.
Intraductal Carcinoma	Similarly this type of cancer does not metastasize and the risk of subsequent invasive cancer is confined to the same breast. This form of cancer is classified according to its morphology as cribiform, micropapillary or comedo. Often, the comedo form can travel extensively undetected through the breast. As such, there is a greater risk of developing invasive cancer after this has been removed. Radiotherapy or mastectomies are usually common additional forms of treatment.

Another common breast cancer is invasive breast cancer. These are types of cancers that penetrate outside the confines of ducts of lobules where they may arise, and frequently metastasize to lymph nodes or to other distant sites in the body. Increasing age is the main risk factor for developing this form of cancer. It may be associated with skin fixation, dimpling, or nipple retraction. Egan [847] identifies the following common types of invasive carcinoma; ductal, lobular, medullary, comedocarcinoma, papillary, scirrhous and tubular. On locating a mass within a suspicious region, the radiologist will review its key characteristics. Kopans [881] highlights the following features:

Location	Breast cancer can occur anywhere in the breast or wherever breast tissue is found. Statistically the most common location for breast cancer is in the upper outer quadrant of the breast.
Size	The size of a cancer is important for prognosis. The prognosis is much better for small tumors. Results from typical screenings indicate that more than 50% of invasive cancers detected are less than 1 cm in diameter.
Shape	Masses can be divided into the following shapes:

(a) round

(b) oval

(c) lobulated

(d) irregular

The probability of malignancy increases as the shape becomes more irregular.

Margins	Circumscribed masses that possess margins that form a sharp and abrupt interface with the surrounding tissue are almost always benign. Classic breast cancer has a spiculated margin. The majority of breast cancers have an irregular boundary as they invade the surrounding tissue thus producing an ill-defined boundary.

For a visual discussion of various forms and signs of breast cancer, refer to Kopans [881] and Gamagami [850]. We will now discuss how mammographic images are acquired and their formats.

9.4   Image Acquisition and Formats

In this section, a review of the main aspects of mammographic X-ray film acquisition is given. The aim of X-ray mammography is to produce detailed images of the internal structure of the breast, thereby permitting the early detection of breast cancer. As a high level of detail is needed for accurate screening and diagnosis, it is important to have radiographic images with high spatial resolution. Generating such images is a complicated process involving sophisticated hardware:

X-ray Device	This includes the X-ray tube and its cathode anode, focal spot, window, filtration, collimation of equipment, source-to-image distance, compression system and the automatic exposure control.
Detector	The detector detects the X-ray photons that pass through the breast on a phosphor screen and comprises the cassette, film and screen.
Interpretation System	A means to interpret the images generated from the mammographic system usually including a view box or computer display.

An X-ray tube is designed to take the electrical energy and convert it into X-ray photons. The electrical current is passed through the cathode filament causing some of the electrons to boil off. These electrons are accelerated towards an anode. On collision, a part of their energy is converted into X-ray photons and heat. The photons pass through the breast tissue and finally the detector forms the image. The requirements of the detector dictate the imaging parameters. For example, the screen and film combination requires sufficient exposure such that the processed image results in a picture optimized for viewing.

An important optimization parameter associated with an anode is its focal spot. The focal spot is the area where electrons from the cathode strike and determine the focus quality of the image. The design of the focal spot is a compromise between having a small spot that can produce a large number of photons and the need to protect the anode from excessive heat and perhaps melting. The composition of the anode determines the energy levels associated with each photon. Very low energy photons are completely absorbed by the breast thereby contributing to the dose but providing no advantage to the image output. To penetrate particularly dense breasts the energy of the beam must be increased. Filters can be used to adjust the energy level of the beam. In this discussion we are concerned with the interpretation of mammographic images. Such images have been seen to contain the following various characteristics (Haus [860]):

Contrast	The subject contrast is the difference in X-ray attenuation of various breast tissues determined by their thickness, density and composition. Contrast is also influenced by the amount of scatter reaching the film, which is influenced by the collimation of the beam, the thickness of the breast during breast compression, and any air gap in magnification. The tissue contrast is dependent on the film type and its method of processing.
Sharpness/Blur	Blurring in the mammographic image may be as a result of breast motion during the process. Reducing the exposure time and greater compression of the breast can reduce this. Other sources of blur include the size of the focal spot, the source-to-image distance, and the distance of the object from the detector. One goal for improving X-ray imaging is to minimize the blur.
Noise	This may be caused by the quality of the X-ray photons reaching the detector. Too few photons will lead to a noisy image with reduced definition of structures. If few photons reach the detector, the shadow of the object being imaged will be indistinct; the greater the number of photons, the clearer the image. The noise complicates the ability to detect anomalies.
Artefacts	There are many sources of artefacts that also compromise the image. These may be from the patient such as antiperspirant, ointments or powders. During handling, the film may be scratched or damaged and fingerprints may also cause positive artefacts. After developing, the presence of labels may further degrade the image quality.

To ensure that high-contrast resolution is achieved from low-contrast internal structures, high-contrast films have been developed. Films with a higher speed mean that a reduced radiation dosage is required to produce the proper film blackening for best viewing. The disadvantage of a reduced dose is that fewer photons reach the detector and these systems have increased noise. X-ray films consist of a backing material coated in gel on one side, containing a uniform spread of silver halide crystals. The crystals and the gel comprise the emulsion side of the film, and it is this side of the film that comes into direct contact with the phosphor layer of the screen. The contact between the screen and the film must be tight so that the light emitted from the screen by the X-ray's interaction with the phosphor cannot spread. The X-ray image is produced on the emulsion side of the film, and when exposed, the silver bromide of the crystals is converted to a silver ion by energy carried in the photons. These silver ions congregate forming structures containing silver atoms, and if enough atoms congregate then the silver halide grains becomes activated giving the foundation of an image. There are a variety of imaging methods in mammography:

Film-screen Mammography	In conventional radiography the film serves as image detector, display and storage medium. Film-screen mammography should be performed using a specially designed X-ray unit for mammography. The equipment should be capable of generating "clean beams" at a variety of focal spot sizes for high-resolution images and magnification. Accompanying the X-ray device must be apparatus for compressing the breast to a thickness preferably less than 5 cm. Compression reduces the object–film distance and thus reduces geometric unsharpness. The radiation dose is reduced.
Xero-mammography	Xero-mammography is performed using a general diagnostic machine with an overhead X-ray tube. Without the need for optimal breast compression, xero-mammography provides good visualization of the entire breast regardless of its thickness or density.
Digital Mammography	By capturing X-ray image information directly into a computer (not film), there are fewer constraints on the kinds of X-rays that can be used, since there is no film that has to be properly exposed. With specially designed X-ray tubes and filter systems, the X-ray energies can be tuned or customized for each woman's individual breast type, which is important since breasts vary dramatically in composition and size.

	Using the optimal X-ray energy for each woman's breasts will improve the overall quality of the resulting image while keeping the radiation dose to a minimum. In a digital mammography system, a phosphor screen that detects the X-ray photons leaving the breast replaces the film/screen cassette. The phosphor screen converts the X-ray photons into light that is transferred through a fibre optic reducer to the Charged Couple Device (CCD) detector. The CCD converts the incident light into a digitized analogue signal and this signal is displayed on a computer screen.
Ultrasound Imaging	Ultrasound imaging employs sound waves that are reflected from different tissue structures to create an image. For example, the most common cause of breast mass in premenopausal women is a cyst or cystic changes within the breast. The echogenic pattern of such fluid-filled spaces is very different to that produced by solid lesions such as tumors. Therefore, ultrasound complements screening mammography and palpation.
Magnetic Resonance Imaging (MRI)	MRI produces excellent three-dimensional images of the breast structure. It has a high sensitivity and identifies lesions of only 2–3 mm. However, MRI has a relatively low specificity in the detection of primary breast cancer and therefore more research is needed to improve this technique.
Scinti mammography	Scinti mammography is a nuclear imaging technique that can deliver breast imaging as sensitive as X-ray mammography and MRI in palpable tumors but with greater specificity. Scinti mammography requires the intravenous administration of a suitable radiotracer followed by the acquisition of an emission image using a gamma camera to identify the presence and site of a lesion. This non-invasive procedure provides functional and biological information complementing other anatomical imaging produced by mammography, ultrasonography or MRI.

Highnam *et al.* [863] and Highnam and Brady [864] propose a novel representation for mammographic image processing. By modeling the breast using a physics-based approach, they have developed a technique to calibrate the mammographic imaging process. This modeling process allows for a quantitative measure of "interesting" breast tissue, termed h_{int}, to be computed for each pixel within the image. This represents the thickness of interesting (non-fat) tissue between the pixel and X-ray source and can be observed as a surface providing anatomical breast information. From previous studies, the authors found that the intensity of a mammogram at any pixel $f(x, y)$ indicates the amount of attenuation (absorption and scattering) of X-rays in the column of breast tissue above the point (x, y) on the film. By estimating the scatter component, the representation differs from conventional approaches in that the technique aims to enhance mammograms by reducing image blurring. In addition the authors propose that the resultant enhanced column of breast tissue comprises the thickness of the interesting tissue, h_{int} and fat, h_{fat} (the reader is directed to the original paper for details regarding the estimation process). After removing the non-interesting h_{fat} layer, the resultant h_{int} representation is similar to intensity images in that the surface contains peaks and troughs. Highnam and Brady highlight an important difference in that it is a quantitative measure of anatomical tissue in columns of breast tissue. The h_{int} surface has many applications:

- *Mammographic enhancement.*
  The h_{int} representation provides images in which all the imaging conditions have been removed. In addition, as the images are based on the physics of the imaging process, they are less likely to introduce artefacts. The authors found that resultant representation is of radiographic structures that might not be otherwise visible. To this end, the h_{int} representation provides an enhancement.

- *Simulate the appearance of mammographic structures.*
  The h_{int} surface may be transformed prior to display in order to simulate change that might occur in the breast tissue or anatomical structure. In their studies, Highnam *et al.* [863] propose that the simulation of such structures might be useful in the development of a radiological training tool.

- *Image normalization.*
  By modeling the imaging characteristics within the h_{int} representation provides a more accurate method of normalizing images over varying radiographic conditions. Highnam *et al.* [863] argue that conventional means of normalization of mammograms simplify the complicated conditions associated with the acquisition process.

9.4.1 Digitization of X-Ray mammograms

Typically X-ray films are digitized using a scanning device with associated software. Prior to the digitization process, two decisions need to be made: what type of image is to be created, e.g. color, grayscale or binary, and the resolution. The image resolution is measured in dots per inch (dpi) or pixels per inch (ppi). This measurement dictates the number of dots per linear inch the scanner will record, and how much information each dot will record. The greater the dpi, the larger the resulting file. An alternative way of representing image resolution is in terms of the sampling rate, i.e. sampling rate of N

microns per pixel. For example the images in the DDSM database are scanned at a resolution of 42–50 microns per pixel. An image can be classified as follows:

1-bit Black and White	Images of this file type contain pixels that are coded either as black or white. Such images are termed binary images. Within digital mammography there is little reason to ever use this image type. The visual quality is poor and the internal structure of the breast is not apparent against its background.
8-bit Grayscale	This is the typical image type used in many existing studies. Each pixel within the image can be one of the 256 gray shades where 0 represents a black and 255 represent a white pixel. 8-bit grayscale works well for most non-color images, and gives a good, clear image.
12-bit Grayscale	Many studies conducted into digital mammography make use of 12-bit grayscale encoding. The larger range of grayscales allows more information to be extracted during the scanning process.
8-bit Color and 24-bit Color	8-bit and 24-bit color image types are not generally used to encode mammograms. The absence of color in the source makes this choice of image type unnecessary.

The choice of dpi to scan is dictated by practicalities. Inevitably though, if the original image does not have much detail, the resultant enlargement from a high dpi will gain little. Increasing the dpi also increases the resultant file size. Figure 9.5 shows the size of an uncompressed 1" × 1" image for different types.

9.4.2   Image Formats

A variety of different image file formats are available when saving the results of the scanning process to disk. Portable formats such as TIFF work over all platforms but suffer from the lack of built-in compression mechanisms. Other formats are applicable to particular operating systems, e.g. BMP (Microsoft Windows) and PICT (Apple Mac). Several image formats save the file in a compressed form, for example GIF, and the most common, JPEG. JPEG facilitates large compression levels to be applied to the image generating a file that is a fraction of the size of its TIFF equivalent. Subsequent processing of the JPEG file, e.g. enlargement or zoom-in, reveals its deficiencies as the JPEG image begins to "break down" much sooner than TIFF. With such limitations it is usual to save the scanned image in TIFF format and store it off-line on some form of archive media such as magnetic tape. These archived images contain a lot of information and may be used to create images of suitable types utilizing compression techniques for regular use. When scanning, it is advisable to use the color and contrast balance on the scanner and not to apply any additional color or contrast correction on the archived TIFF file. It is preferable to have images scanned with a consistent and known bias which is imposed by the particular scanning device. The majority of digital mammography research is current carried out using images stored in a Portable Gray Map (PGM) format, which is the lowest common denominator gray scale file format. A PGM file contains pixel grayscale values expressed as ASCII data values or in byte format.

9.4.2.1 PGM ASCII Data Value Representation

The image file contains the following information at the start of the file as an image header.

- A "magic number" for identifying the file type as an ASCII data representation. A PGM file's magic number is "P2".

- The image width w in pixels followed by the image height h in pixels.

- The maximum gray value expressed in ASCII decimal.

Following this, the image is expressed as $w \times h$ gray values. Each value is an ASCII decimal between zero and the specified maximum, separated by a white space starting at the top-left corner of the image gray map proceeding from left to right and top to bottom in direction. A value of zero indicates black, and the maximum value white. Characters from the symbol "#" to the next end-of-line are ignored (comments). The maximum line size is 70 characters.

9.4.2.2 PGM Byte Value Representation

The representation is the same as a PGM ASCII data value except that the magic number is "P5". This is followed by the image data expressed as $w \times h$ gray values although the gray values are stored as plain bytes instead of ASCII decimal. No white space is allowed in the gray section and only a single character of white space (typically a new line) is allowed after the maximum gray value. Images stored in this format of PGM are smaller and quicker to read and write. Note that this raw format can only be used for maximum gray values less than or equal to 255.

9.4.3 Image Quantization and Tree-Pyramids

As discussed in the previous section, scanning images at a high resolution results in large amounts of data. Subsequent processing of such large files may prove to be computationally time-consuming and lead to large amounts of output. One approach to reduce the amount of image information is to perform *image quantization*. This is the process of reducing the image data by removing some of the detail information by grouping data points into a single point. Quantization of spatial co-ordinates results in a reduction of the size of the image. This is accomplished by taking groups of pixels that are

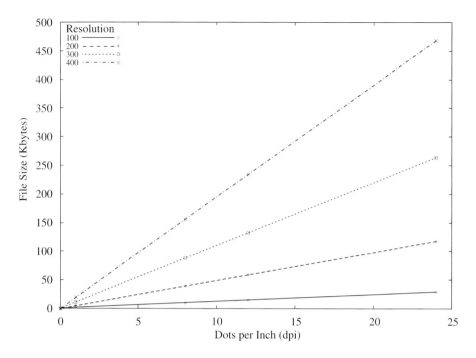

Figure 9.5: Comparison of dpi and image size at various resolutions.

spatially adjacent and mapping them to one pixel. Umbaugh [924] proposes three methods for calculating the mapped pixel value:

1. *Averaging:* We take all of the pixels in each group and find the average gray level.

2. *Median Method:* All pixels within the group are sorted in ascending order of intensity and we find the middle value.

3. *Sub-Sampling:* We simply eliminate some of the data, i.e. to reduce the image by a factor of two, and then take every other row and column and delete them. This technique may be used in conjunction with some form of smoothing filter to improve the resultant output.

In some applications it is desired to handle images at various scales (e.g. Zwiggelaar, [939]). To achieve this we need a data structure to represent an image at various scales. A common approach is the *tree-pyramid* (Sonka *et al.*, [917]), defined for an original image $f(i,j)$ of size 2^N with the algorithm below.

Tree Pyramid Definition Algorithm

1. A set of nodes $P = \{P = (k,i,j)$ such that level $k \in [0, N]; i, j \in [0, 2^k - 1]\}$.

2. A mapping F between subsequent nodes, P_{k-1}, P_k of the pyramid,

$$F(k, i, j) = (k - 1, i \text{ div } 2, j \text{ div } 2)$$

where div represents whole number division.

3. A function V that maps a node of the pyramid P to Z, where Z is the sub-set of the whole numbers corresponding to the brightness levels, for example $Z = \{0, 1, \ldots, 255\}$.

Every node of the pyramid has four child nodes except leaf nodes, which are nodes at level N that correspond to the original pixels in the image. Values of individual nodes of the pyramid are defined by the function V. Leaf nodes are of the same value as the gray-level in the original image at the finest resolution within the pyramid representation; the image size is 2^{N-1}. Values of the nodes in other levels are defined using one of the quantization techniques described above. The use of tree pyramids facilitates the retention of several image resolutions in memory simultaneously rather than just choosing one image scale.

9.5 Mammogram Enhancement Methods

There is a need to enhance digital mammograms before a reasonable segmentation can be achieved. This is to improve the poor signal to noise ratio found in most images. Image quality can suffer as a result of the X-ray imaging procedure itself, breast motion during its compression when imaged or its positioning in the plate. In addition, since the optical resolution of a film scanning device that converts data into digital form does not match with the true resolution of the X-ray image, subtle but important details are lost. One of the primary aims of image enhancement is to improve the contrast between region(s) of interest and the background. As such, the quality of enhancement has a direct bearing on the quality of segmentation. The enhancement process itself is dictated by the procedure adopted. Image enhancement can be accomplished using a range of spatial or spectral domain methods. Spatial domain methods are based on either histogram manipulation or the use of masks that are convolved with the original image to improve its quality. Spectral methods use appropriate transfer functions in the spectral domain that are convolved with the Fourier transform of the image before taking an inverse to yield an enhanced image. Some of the commonly used methods include lowpass, bandpass and highpass filters. Enhancement methods in the spatial domain are related to the redistribution of the pixel gray levels, e.g. histogram equalization and its variants.

Most mammograms have a poor signal to noise ratio. The Signal to Noise Ratio (SNR) of an image is defined as (Kitchen and Rosenfeld [878]): [SNR $= (h/\sigma^2)$] where h is the gray level difference between the object and the background and σ is the standard deviation of the noise. Mammograms are often blurred and unclear, and they are particularly difficult to segment unless properly enhanced. A range of standard techniques for enhancement are available

(Klette and Zamperoni [879]). In this section we initially review some of the pre-processing techniques commonly applied to mammograms to aid enhancement or provide a normalizing process typically necessary over a set of slides. Image pre-processing is important within digital mammography for a variety of important reasons: (i) to eliminate noise in the mammogram; (ii) to enhance the image, thereby improving the quality of segmentation; and (iii) to reduce the image size by image sub-sampling. Image enhancement typically has a variety of objectives such as the enhancement of edges within the image, the adjustment of image contrast, and the normalization of pixel values over sets of images. In several studies pre-processing techniques form an integral part of the methodology even though few report on the effectiveness of this step in a quantitative manner.

Noise found within an image is unwanted information that can result from the image acquisition process. Traditionally image processing applications make use of a variety of techniques to suppress accompanying noise by applying a range of spatial or frequency filtering techniques. Spatial filters work directly on pixels and attempt to remove noise by convolving spatial masks resulting in a smoother image (Gonzalez and Woods [852]). Conversely, frequency domain filters operate on the Fourier transformed representation of an image.

Histogram equalization is a popular technique for improving the appearance of a poor image. It is a technique where the histogram of the resultant image is manipulated to be as flat as possible. The theoretical basis for histogram equalization involves probability theory, where we treat the histogram as the probability distribution of the gray levels.

Histogram Equalization Algorithm

1. For a $N \times M$ image of L gray-levels, create an array H of length L initialized with 0 values.

2. Form the image histogram: Scan every pixel and increment the relevant member of H. If pixel p has intensity f_p, perform

$$H[f_p] = H[f_p] + 1$$

At the end of this, $H[f_p]$ contains the frequency of occurrence of pixel gray level f_p in the image.

3. Form the cumulative image histogram H_c as:

$$H_c[0] = H[0];$$
$$H_c[p] = H_c[p-1] + H[p], p = 1, 2, \ldots, L - 1.$$

4. Find a monotonic gray-level transformation $q = T(f_p)$ such that the desired output $G(q)$ is uniform over the whole range of gray values.

$$T[f_p] = round \left(\frac{L-1}{NM} H_c[f_p] \right)$$

5. Rescan the original image and for every pixel p write an output in the enhanced image with gray levels G_q, setting $G_q = T[f_p]$.

Yin *et al.* [931] have made use of the histogram equalization technique to normalize image pairs prior to their bilateral subtraction. Gupta and Undrill [856] report that histogram equalization aided the visualization of lesions and led to increased sensitivity in subsequent processing. In their study they make use of texture analysis for subsequent segmentation and found that in a textured image it allowed the smooth area of the lesion to be clearly distinguished.

Fuzzy image enhancement is another technique used to enhance the contrast of an image. Fuzzy image enhancement is mainly based on gray-level mapping into a fuzzy plane using a membership transformation function. Pal and Majumder [896] suggest that we can transform an image plane into its fuzzy plane using a fuzzy transformation function F. Each pixel in the original image $f(x, y)$ is mapped to its fuzzy plane value $P(x, y)$. The fuzzy plane is then manipulated using the arithmetic operator A with the purpose of contrast stretching. The modified fuzzy plane can be inverse transformed F^{-1} to produce a new image $f'(x, y)$ that is enhanced. The arithmetic operator A can be chosen either for contrast or smoothing. The process can be represented as:

$$F[f(x, y)] \rightarrow P(x, y)$$
$$A[P(x, y)] \rightarrow P'(x, y)$$
$$F^{-1}[P'(x, y)] \rightarrow f'(x, y)$$

Pal and Majumder [896] have outlined a general method of image enhancement which allows the user to set a reasonable choice of the operator A for their application. The transformation function A for transforming the original image into the fuzzy plane requires a membership function F and we present the one suggested by Zadeh [932]. The possibility distribution of the gray levels in the original image can be characterized using five parameters: $(\alpha, \beta_1, \gamma, \beta_2, max)$ as shown in Figure 9.6 where the intensity value γ represents the mean value of the distribution, α is the minimum, max is the maximum and β_1 and β_2 are the midpoints. The aim is to decrease the gray levels below β_1, and above β_2. Intensity levels between β_1 and γ, and β_2 and γ are stretched in opposite directions towards the mean γ.

The fuzzy transformation function for computing the fuzzy plane value P is defined as follows:

$$\alpha = min; \beta_1 = (\alpha + \gamma)/2; \beta_2 = (max + \gamma)/2; \gamma = mean$$

1. If $\alpha \leq u_i < \beta_1$ then $P = 2((u_i - \alpha)/(\gamma - \alpha))^2$

2. If $\beta_1 \leq u_i < \gamma$ then $P = 1 - 2((u_i - \gamma)/(\gamma - \alpha))^2$

3. If $\gamma \leq u_i < \beta_2$ then $P = 1 - 2((u_i - \gamma)/(max - \gamma))^2$

4. If $\beta_2 \leq u_i \leq max$ then $P = 2((u_i - \gamma)/(max - \gamma))^2$

Membership

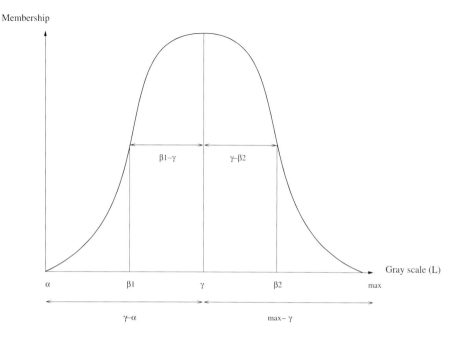

Figure 9.6: Possibility distribution function for calculating membership values.

where $u_i = f(x, y)$ is the ith pixel intensity.

$P(x, y)$ is given by equations (1–4) above depending on the pixel's gray level. The operator A used is a square operator, and the inverse operation is given by: $F^{-1}[P'(x, y)] = P'(x, y).f(x, y)$.

In their study, Singh and Al-Mansoori [916] attempted to improve performance of subsequent mammogram processing by evaluating the use of the histogram equalization and fuzzy enhancement techniques. In the study, 30 mammograms at 512×512 complete with hand-drawn ROIs were taken from the University of South Florida DDSM public database (Heath and Bowyer [862]). The authors found that the best results were obtained with the fuzzy enhancement technique based on a set of quantitative measures which will be discussed later.

Wei *et al.* [926] describe an *adaptive background correction* technique to remove the low-frequency background thus facilitating the comparison of masses from different slides on a common background. The technique was originally reported by Chan *et al.* [839]. The authors in this latter study noted that certain textural features for a particular ROI derived from a Spatial Gray Level Dependency (SGLD) matrix, may be affected by the X-ray density and density of overlapping tissues. Their technique is described below (see Figure 9.7).

Adaptive Background Correction Algorithm

1. Calculate the running average of the gray-level values along the perimeter within a series of 32×16 pixel box filters for an ROI of 256×256 pixels. The box filter is applied at the four ROI edges top, bottom, left and right $(g_i^0, g_i^{180}, g_i^{90}, g_i^{270} \; \forall i = 0, ..., N_b)$ respectively, where N_b = number of box filters in edge direction, here $N_b = 8$.

2. For each pixel (i, j) in the ROI, the gray level $G(i, j)$ of a given pixel $f(i, j)$ is calculated as:

$$G(i,j) = [\sum_{k=1}^{4} g_k^\theta / d_d^\theta]/[\sum_{k=1}^{4} 1/ d_k^\theta]$$

where g_k^θ is the gray value from the lowpass filtered perimeter found at the intersection of a boundary box and a constructed normal from pixel (i, j) and $\theta \in (0°, 90°, 180°, 270°)$. d_k^θ is the distance from pixel (i, j) to the perimeter along the constructed normal where $\theta \in (0°, 90°, 180°, 270°)$.

3. This background image is then subtracted from the original image giving a new image with a flattened ROI background leaving the high frequencies of the ROI unchanged.

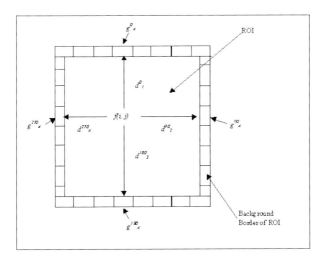

Figure 9.7: Adaptive background correction technique.

Ng and Bischof [895] have used Gaussian filters to remove high-frequency noise. The Gaussian filter G is defined as:

$$G(x, y) = (2\pi\sigma^2)^{-1} \exp[-(x^2 + y^2)/2\sigma^2]$$

where the standard deviation σ dictates the amount of smoothing. In this study, it was found that a compromise is necessary between adequate noise removal whilst retaining the fine spicules that delineate a spiculated mass. Following experimentation, a value of $\sigma = 1.5$ was used to generate the Gaussian filter subsequently convolved with the original image. The resultant smoothed image is then used in the segmentation process. Li *et al.* [885] and Qian *et al.* [905] make use of a Tree Structured Filter (TSF) for image noise or artefact suppression. TSF is a three-stage filter based on a median filter. In the first stage, the filter is applied generating an image that is compared with the original. In the second and third stages, details such as parenchymal tissue structures and mammographic directional features are preserved.

Rangayyan *et al.* [908] used an *Adaptive Neighbourhood Contrast Enhancement (ANCE)* method and evaluated it to determine the improvement in breast cancer diagnosis sensitivity. Their algorithm is shown below.

Adaptive Neighbourhood Contrast Enhancement (ANCE) Algorithm

1. Nearly homogeneous regions are identified by region growing.

2. The visual contrast of the region is computed by comparing the intensity of the region with its surrounding pixels.

3. Modifying intensity selectively increases the region contrast provided that the region contrast is low and the pixels in the region background have a standard deviation with respect to a mean of less than 0.1.

4. This process is applied to each pixel in the image in order to enhance the contrast of all objects and features in the image.

The algorithm is applied to two image sets (i) 21 difficult cases (malignant $n = 7$, benign $n = 7$) digitized at a resolution of 4096×2048 pixels. (ii) 222 interval cancer films digitized at a resolution of 2048×1536 pixels. Using ROC analysis, the area under the ROC curve (the value of Az) is computed for the two image sets. For the difficult cases, the values obtained are $Az = 0.67$ (original slide); $Az = 0.62$ (digitized slide) and $Az = 0.67$ (ANCE enhanced image). For interval cases the values obtained for Az were: $Az = 0.39$ (original slide); $Az = 0.46$ (digitized slide) and $Az = 0.54$ (ANCE enhanced slide).

Petrick *et al.* [899] have described a Density Weighted Contrast Enhancement (DWCE) segmentation for detecting masses. The study aims to perform a high-quality contrast enhancement followed by an edge detection algorithm to identify regions of interest. The enhancement process and segmentation are performed in two stages – first, globally on the whole image, and then on regions of interest. Normalized images are passed through a band pass filter to obtain a contrast image and then through a low pass filter to obtain a density image. A product is taken between this and multiplication factors (determined experimentally) to obtain an enhanced image. The output is passed through a non-linear band pass filter to obtain the final enhanced image. A Laplacian-Gaussian edge detection is then used to find edges in the enhanced image that enclose regions of interest. The method is very successful but needs an efficient postprocessing stage to reduce false positives. The criteria used includes the number of edge pixels, total object area, object contrast, circularity, rectangularity, perimeter to area ratio, and five normalized radial length features including NRL mean, standard deviation, entropy, area ratio and zero crossing count. The DWCE algorithm is shown below.

Density Weighted Contrast Enhancement (DWCE) Algorithm

1. A breast profile map is created.

2. Scale all pixels in the original image breast map to lie between 0 and 1. This prevents outliers from skewing the data.

3. The normalized image is split into a density image by applying a low-pass filter and a contrast image by applying a high-pass filter.

4. Each pixel in the density image is used to define a multiplication factor that modifies the corresponding pixel in the contrast image.

5. The output of the DWCE filter is a non-linear re-scaled version of the weighted contrast image.

9.6 Quantifying Mammogram Enhancement

One important question is: "How do we measure the quality of enhancement in digital mammograms using a given method?" The quality of image enhancement can be measured in the context of how well the contrast between the region of interest (target) and the background has improved relative to the original image. Fortunately in mammography, target regions in ground truth data are specified by a radiologist (details of size and location of calcifications and masses are available). In a number of studies, such improvement can be evaluated subjectively. However, it would be beneficial if we could have a more quantitative measure of the quality of enhancement. We can consider the problem shown in Figure 9.8.

In Figure 9.8, we have an original image (a) that is enhanced to produce image (b). For our example, we do not need to know the details of the enhancement process. We are primarily concerned with finding whether this enhancement has improved our ability to differentiate target T from the background B. The background B here is shown as the region outside the target

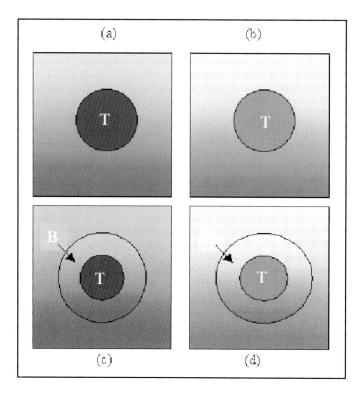

Figure 9.8: Target T and background B (original image (a) is enhanced as (b), analysis images are (c) and (d)).

as a concentric circle. The following measures can be used for analyzing the improvement in image quality as a result of the enhancement process (Bovis and Singh, [833]).

1. Target to background contrast ratio using entropy

$$TBC_\epsilon = \left(\frac{(\mu_T^E/\mu_B^E) - (\mu_T^o/\mu_B^o)}{\epsilon_T^E \: / \: \epsilon_T^o} \right)$$

2. Target to background contrast ratio using standard deviation

$$TBC_\sigma = \left(\frac{(\mu_T^E/\mu_B^E) - (\mu_T^o/\mu_B^o)}{\sigma_T^E/\sigma_T^o} \right)$$

where μ is the mean of a region, σ its standard deviation and ϵ the entropy. The indices E and O refer to the enhanced and original images and T and B refer to target and background. It is expected that as a result of enhancement, both measures should give a value greater than zero. When considering a number of images, such measurements can be scaled between zero and one to get a reasonable idea of how well the different images in that set have been enhanced. For regions of uniform intensity, both of the above measures are not directly usable as the value of σ will tend to be zero. Hence the above schemes can use an additive constant c to the σ term to avoid division by zero problems.

Another approach to measuring the quality of enhancement is based on its ability to increase the contrast between object and background. Good quality enhancement should lead to sharper differences between objects and the surrounding area. Gradient information can be obtained from the image using any of the edge detection operators. Two useful methods include Sobel and Prewitt operators. These operators can be used to find the gradient image in both horizontal and vertical directions which is combined to give the overall gradient. The position of the edges themselves is given by the zero-crossing of the Laplacian operator. If we apply the Laplacian operator on the gradient image within the region labeled B in Figure 9.8 including the area covered by target T, then this edge position provides a better estimate of the object boundary. Once a good boundary separating the target and background has been established, gradient histograms showing the probability of different gradients can be calculated for both background and target. In particular, it is desired that the probability of large target gradients should be reduced after enhancement. This is shown in Figure 9.9.

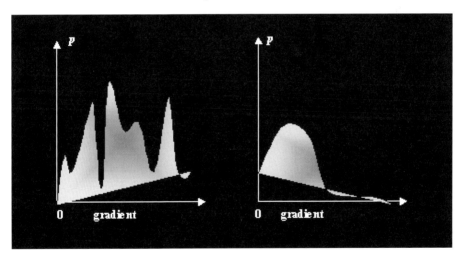

Figure 9.9: The probability of large gradients in target gradient histograms is reduced.

In addition to minimizing the gradient changes within the target, the enhancement process should ideally maximize the gradient differences between the object and the target. Since the edge position is known, it is possible to find the gradients at this position for every point on the boundary before and after enhancement. If the boundary consists of N pixels, then the following measure should be used to quantify enhancement.

$$G_{TB} = \frac{1}{N}\left(\sum_{i=1}^{N}|g_i^E| - \sum_{i=1}^{N}|g_i^O|\right)$$

Here g_i is the gradient of pixel i on the boundary separating the object and the background. Ideally, the value of G_{TB} should be positive. The higher the value, the better the quality of enhancement. In mammography, a better estimate of the effectiveness of the enhancement process is possible if we consider a tube-shaped boundary which is more than one pixel thick. Gradient changes for all pixels within this tubular structure can be computed before and after enhancement.

In Figure 9.10 we plot the overlap between target and background gray-levels. In mammography, this is representative of the overlap found between masses and their backgrounds. A good enhancement technique should ideally reduce the overlap shown as the highlighted region. In particular, we expect that the enhancement technique should help reduce the spread of the target distribution and shift its mean gray-level to a higher value thus separating the two distributions and reducing their overlap.

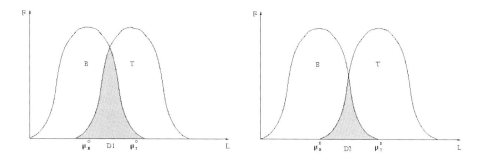

Figure 9.10: Distribution overlap between background and target before and after enhancement.

The best decision boundary for the original image between the two classes, assuming both classes have a multivariate normal distribution with equal co-variances is given by (Weszka *et al.* [927]):

$$D_1 = \frac{\mu_B^O \sigma_T^O + \mu_T^O \sigma_B^O}{\sigma_B^O + \sigma_T^O}$$

Similarly, the best decision boundary for the original image after enhancement is given by:

$$D_2 = \frac{\mu_B^E \sigma_T^E + \mu_T^E \sigma_B^E}{\sigma_B^E + \sigma_T^E}$$

Another approximation to D_1 and D_2 can found using the cutting score (Hair *et al.* [857]). If the groups are assumed to be representative of the population, a weighted average of the group centroids will provide an optimal cutting score given as:

$$D_1 = \frac{N_B^O \mu_T^O + N_T^O \mu_B^O}{N_B^O + N_T^O}$$

and

$$D_2 = \frac{N_B^E \mu_T^E + N_T^E \mu_B^E}{N_B^E + N_T^E}$$

where N_B^O and N_T^O are the number of samples in the background and target prior to enhancement, and N_B^E and N_T^E the respective sample numbers after the enhancement. Again this approximation assumes that the two distributions are normal and that the group dispersion structures are known.

A final approximation to an optimal decision boundary may be found using Bayes' theorem. Assume that the probability that a pixel belongs to the target T, given that it has gray level x, is denoted by $P(T|x)$. Similarly, the probability that a pixel belongs to the background B, given that it has gray level x is denoted by $P(B|x)$. We can compute the optimal decision boundary if we assume the densities are continuous and overlapping as: $P(T|x) = P(B|x)$. Substituting Bayes' theorem and cancelling $p(x)$ gives $P(T)P(x|T) = P(B)P(x|B)$ at the optimal decision boundary. If we assume that the gray-level x in the target and background areas is normally distributed, this equation can be represented as:

$$P(T)\frac{1}{\sigma_B\sqrt{2\pi}}e^{-\frac{1}{2}(x-\mu_T/\sigma_T)^2} = P(B)\frac{1}{\sigma_B\sqrt{2\pi}}e^{-\frac{1}{2}(x-\mu_B/\sigma_B)^2}$$

Solving these equations, we calculate the decision boundary x. The distance between the decision boundaries and the means of the targets and background, before and after segmentation, is a good measure of the quality of enhancement. This measure, termed as *Distribution Separation Measure (DSM)*, is given by:

$$DSM = \left(|(D2 - \mu_B^E)| + |(D2 - \mu_T^E)|\right) - \left(|(D1 - \mu_B^0)| + |(D1 - \mu_T^O)|\right)$$

Ideally the measurement should be greater than zero; the higher the positive figure, the better the quality of the enhancement. For comparing any two enhancement techniques, we should choose the technique that gives a higher value on the *DSM* measure. Once the images have been enhanced, they need to be segmented for isolating regions of interest. These regions may represent single or a cluster of microcalcifications or masses. In the next three sections we discuss the algorithms that are useful for segmenting breast profile, microcalcifications and masses.

9.7 Segmentation of Breast Profile

The segmentation of the foreground breast object from the background is a fundamental step in mammogram analysis. The aim is to generate a breast profile (map) as shown in Figure 9.11.

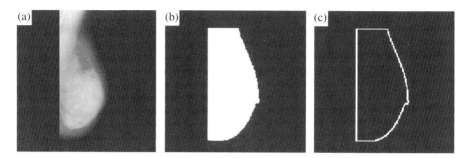

Figure 9.11: Segmented breast profiles (a) original image, (b) binarized image, (c) edge generated profile.

Several studies have attempted to segment the breast from its background by applying a simple thresholding criterion. Lau and Bischof [883] segmented the breast profile from which control points are found for alignment of left and right breast image pairs. They defined the generation of a binary map $m(x, y)$ of the breast area with the algorithm below.

Breast Profile Segmentation Algorithm

1. Define a binary map of the original image $f(x, y)$ as

$$m(x, y) = \left\{ \begin{array}{lll} 1; & if & f(x, y) \geq T \\ 0; & if & f(x, y) < T \end{array} \right\}$$

   where the threshold T was found to be the trough between the two major peaks in the gray-scale histogram.

2. The resultant image has a noisy boundary and it is smoothed using an averaging filter $a_2(x, y)$ defined as:

$$a_2(x, y) = \left\{ \begin{array}{lll} (2n + 1)^{-2}; & if & |x| \leq n, |y| \leq n \\ 0; & & otherwise \end{array} \right\}$$

   where n is the total number of pixels.

3. The averaging filter is convolved with the binary breast map giving a smoothed image $m_s(x, y)$ as:

$$m_s(x,y) = \left\{ \begin{array}{lll} 1; & if & a_2(x,y) * m(x,y) \geq \frac{1}{2} \\ 0; & if & a_2(x,y) * m(x,y) < \frac{1}{2} \end{array} \right\}$$

where $a * b$ denotes convolution of a and b.

In their study, Mendez *et al.* [892] found the location of the nipple within their digital mammograms using an edge-generated profile with an edge-tracking algorithm. The identification of edge profile points $f(x_i, y_i)$ was based on the condition that nine previous pixels in the tracking direction satisfy the following condition:

$$f(x_1, y_1) < f(x_2, y_2) < ... < f(x_7, y_7) \leq f(x_8, y_8) \leq f(x_9, y_9) \leq f(x, y)$$

Chandrasekhar [842] investigated fixed and adaptive thresholding techniques, for breast profile segmentation and concluded that they were not fully effective in their application due to underlying image noise. In his study, he proposes that the noise element of the mammogram should be modeled using a polynomial of order n. The algorithm is given below.

Breast Profile Segmentation Algorithm

1. Orientate the image such that the nipple faces right and threshold at a suitable intensity such that the resultant image contains the entire background and a small portion of the breast adjoining it.

2. Fit a polynomial $P_n(x, y)$ in the direction of x and y to the thresholded image and apply to every pixel $f(x, y)$ giving a model image $I_m(x, y)$.

3. Subtract the modeled image from the original image giving a difference image $I_d(x, y)$.

4. Threshold the difference image with a suitable value k, such that the breast is segmented from the background giving a binary image $I_b(x, y)$.

5. Apply a labeling algorithm to label connected pixels as belonging to labeled regions.

6. Take the largest labeled region and remove remaining island regions giving an image of two disjoint regions: a background and a foreground breast profile.

Goodsitt *et al.* [855] observe that all borders can be characterized by symmetric or asymmetric polynomials. Within their study, border irregularities are removed by run-length averaging. The y-axis of profile was found by least square fitting a line between midpoints of line segments. The intersection of this line with the border is the origin and the x-axis of the border is perpendicular to the y-axis. The border was then rotated and translated to find the best fit (root mean square error minimization) of the polynomial. The authors subsequently attempted to classify the border shape, polynomial coefficients were passed to a K-means clustering classifier in an attempt to develop an external filter for equalizing the X-ray exposure during the mammographic acquisition process.

9.8   Segmentation of Microcalcifications

Calcifications are small structures of calcium that appear brighter than the surrounding tissue in mammograms and are seen in one or both projections of the breast (Kallergi *et al.* [872]) (see Figure 9.2). On digital mammograms, the smallest microcalcifications are of size 0.1 to 0.2 mm. Calcifications appear as isolated or a part of a group. Their clusters are important for detection. Commonly defined groups are of size five or more calcifications with a 1 cm^3 volume, each less than 0.5 mm in size and less than 5 mm apart (nearest neighbor distance). These are difficult to detect as the noise level on high density parts of the image is higher.

Karssemeijer [873] describes an automated calcification detection procedure consisting of two steps – thresholding and postprocessing based on shape, gray-level, size or cluster size. The approach used to segment microcalifications is based on Random Field Models described in greater detail in Besag [829]. Another approach to the segmentation and detection of microcalcifications is based on the top hat and watershed algorithms as described by Betal *et al.* [830]. One of the key features of this study is the use of both views (lateral-oblique and cranio-caudal) for detection based on the previous work suggesting this approach (Spiesberger [918]). The authors report that using both views, the area under the ROC curve increased to a value of 0.79 (the area was 0.73 using only the CC view and 0.63 using only LO view). Microcalcifications appear as bright spots on the mammogram. The top hat algorithm is used when the background signal intensity is highly variable. Image intensities can be thought of as three-dimensional topographic surfaces. We can imagine a top hat being placed on each part. The features with high contrast are detected as they poke out of the top of the hat. The hat dimensions can be controlled to detect features with varying diameter and relative contrast. A circular disc is used as a local neighborhood. First, morphological opening is applied (erosion followed by dilation). During erosion, the pixel value at the center of the kernel is replaced by the minimum value of neighboring pixels reducing regions of high signal intensity. At the time of dilation, pixel values at the center of the kernel are replaced by the maximum of the neighborhood restoring regions of high intensity which were not completely eroded earlier. The second part of the top hat algorithm involves the subtraction of the opened image from the original image – the predominant features now left are microcalifications.

A triple ring filter approach to detecting microcalcifications is shown by Ibrahim *et al.* [867] on the MIAS database. The approach involves the determination of breast region, segmentation of skinline area, contrast correction, density gradient calculation, triple ring filter analysis, variable ring filter analysis, feature analysis and classification of cluster areas. The gradient density of the images is first calculated using a Sobel filter. A triple ring filter is used to analyze the calculated gradient. The filter has three subfilters of size 3 pixels, 5 pixels and 7 pixels (see Figure 9.12).

The triple ring filter is convolved with the contrast enhanced image. For each point, a directional feature D and magnitude feature I are computed and if they are above certain thresholds, the pixel is considered as a part of the microcalcification. The directional feature D is calculated as follows. First, pixels are numbered according to the number of pixels with the kth address on the subfilter written as ν_k and the difference of its direction from the basic vector pattern is $\theta_k (0 \leq \theta_k \leq \pi)$. For a subfilter of n pixels, we calculate:

$$D = \frac{1}{n} \sum_{k=1}^{n} (1 + \alpha \sin \theta_k) \cos \theta_k.$$

```
          3   3   3
      3   2   2   2   3
  3   2   1   1   1   2   3
  3   2   1   .   1   2   3
  3   2   1   1   1   2   3
      3   2   2   2   3
          3   3   3
```

Figure 9.12: Triple ring filter: filters 1, 2 and 3.

For the first filter A, $n = 8$, for the second filter B, $n = 12$ and for the third filter C, $n = 16$. The value of D lies between -1 and $+1$. It is equal to $+1$ when the candidate pattern is close to the basic pattern and -1 when it is not. α is the directional feature coefficient – by setting it to a different value for each subfilter, irregularly-shaped microcalcifications can be found. The magnitude feature I is determined as:

$$I = \frac{1}{n} \sum_{k=1}^{n} |v_k| (1 + \alpha \sin \theta_k) \cos \theta_k$$

The detection of microcalcifications is now based on a look-up table of conditions that specify for what values of D and I a calcification is present.

Once microcalcifications have been detected, further information on them can be collated for their classification. Chan *et al.* [841] develop a signal extraction approach that can determine the size, contrast, signal to noise ratio and shape of microcalcifications in mammograms based on their coordinates. A

range of morphological features and texture features based on SGLD matrices
are proposed which we will discuss in the feature extraction section later.

Wavelet Analysis has also been frequently used for the detection of microcalcifications. Microcalcifications can be considered as high-frequency components of the image spectrum and their detection can be accomplished by
decomposing a mammogram into different frequency sub-bands and then suppressing the low-frequency sub-band. It is proposed by several researchers that
conventional image processing techniques are not well suited to the analysis
of mammographic images (e.g. Wang and Karayiannis [925]). Large variation
in feature size and shape reduces the effectiveness of classical neighborhood
techniques such as unsharp masking. At the same time, fixed neighborhood or
global techniques may adapt to local features within a neighborhood but do not
adapt the size of the neighborhood. Wavelets are considered as an attractive
option for microcalcification detection as they require fewer parameters to be
tuned related to local image statistics, thereby resulting in a smaller number
of false positives.

Non-stationary signals can be analyzed using Short Term Fourier Transform
(STFT). Wavelet Transform (WT) allows the use of short windows at high
frequencies and long windows at low frequencies for attaining better signal
resolution (Rao and Bopardikar [906]). A signal can be decomposed into a
set of basis functions called wavelets that are obtained from a single parent
wavelet by dilations and contractions (scalings), as well as translations and
shifts. In practice, continuous or discrete transforms can be used. A signal
$f(t)$ is represented as a weighted sum of basis functions:

$$f(t) = \sum_i c_i \psi_i(t),$$

where $\psi_i(t)$ are basis functions and c_i the coefficients or weights. The functions are fixed so that all of the information is contained in weights. Impulse
functions will yield information only on the time behavior of the signal and
sinusoid functions will yield information only on the frequency domain. Fortunately, wavelets allow both of these aspects to be represented. The product of
the time resolution (Δt) and frequency resolution ($\Delta \omega$) is lower bounded. Basis
functions can be designed to act as cascaded octave bandpass filters which repeatedly split the bandwidth in half. A wavelet representation can be obtained
by scaling and translating the basis functions $\psi(t)$ to get different versions.
Since ψ has finite support, it should be translated along the time axis to cover
the entire signal. This transform is accomplished by considering all integral
shifts of ψ, that is $\psi(2^a t - b)$, and hence

$$f(t) = \sum_a \sum_b c_{ab} \psi_{ab}(t),$$

where $\psi_{ab}(t) = 2^{a/2} \psi(2^a t - b)$. The coefficients c_{ab} are computed via a wavelet
transform.

Wang and Karayiannis [925] have used the standard wavelet methodology
for the detection of microcalcifications. The procedure involves decomposing

the original mammogram into a set of orthogonal subbands of different resolution and frequency component. This is based on wavelet analysis filtering and downsampling of rows and columns of the image. The microcalcifications which correspond to the highest frequencies are carried to other subbands. The detection of calcifications is accomplished by setting the wavelet coefficients in the upper left subband to zero in order to suppress the image background before reconstructing the image. The reconstructed image contains high-frequency components including microcalcifications.

9.9 Segmentation of Masses

Li *et al.* [885] state: "Mass detection poses a more difficult problem in terms of sensitivity of detection and FP detection rate compared with microcalcification cluster detection because: (a) masses are of varying size, shape and density; (b) masses often exhibit poor image contrast; (c) masses may be highly connected to surrounding parenchymal tissue (this is particularly true for spiculated lesions), and (d) background tissues surrounding the mass are non-uniform and have similar characteristics". Segmentation taxonomy can be represented with four classes of techniques: threshold techniques, boundary-based techniques, region-based techniques and hybrid methods (Adams and Bischof [439]). A simpler classification can be *global*, *edge-based* or *region-based*. In global methods, the aim is to analyze images as a whole and investigate the probability distributions of pixel gray-levels for finding the appropriate threshold. Edge-based methods utilize information about gradient changes within an image to locate edges that separate objects from their background. Region-based methods are aimed at differentiating regions on the basis of some statistical characteristic. Starting with a very small region that meets some gray-level homogeneity criteria, we can expand this region with its surrounding pixels as long as the expanded region meets our fixed criteria. Following this process over the complete image, we can generate a set of regions that are of interest. A reverse procedure can be adopted by splitting an image into regions till some criteria of uniformity within the regions derived is satisfied. This approach is discussed later on. The number of approaches proposed in the literature on image segmentation is enormous. It is beyond the scope of this chapter to review every single image segmentation method. However, we will discuss some of the commonly used methods and their relative merits in the context of mammography.

First, it is important to identify the components of an X-ray mammogram. An example of a right breast digital mammogram taken as the Medio-lateral view is shown in Figure 9.13.

The digitized image contains the actual breast, tags on whether it is left or right and its view, plus noise outside the breast region. In our example image, the gray-level varies between 0 and 255 and the original image resolution is 1024×1024 pixels. The first step is to remove labels. Several studies have used their own methods for removing labels from the mammograms (e.g. Masek *et*

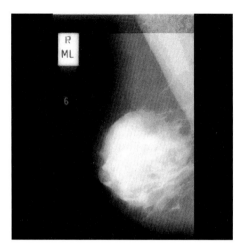

Figure 9.13: Digital mammogram from the MiniMias database [919].

al. [888]). The easiest method is to crop the image manually to remove areas that are not useful for the analysis. The main drawback of this approach is the amount of work required can slow down the overall analysis. If we had a template for what the background looks like, and subtracted it from the image, we could possibly get the object of interest. Unfortunately, the position of the labels is varied, and the noise is variable over backgrounds in different mammograms, and therefore background subtraction does not help. One of the standard automated techniques for finding labels is to write a program that detects rectangular objects with bimodal histograms (for background and text), and removes this from the mammogram. Another technique based on detecting the envelope or profile of the breast as one extreme and the pectoralis muscle at the end can be used to determine the work area for image processing techniques. Once the labels have been removed, isolated pixels (with no neighbors in a 4 or 8 pixel neighborhood) can be removed. A range of noise filters are available that can be applied to reduce noise. The elimination of the high-frequency component of the Fourier image of the mammogram can also reduce the noise in images. Salt and pepper noise can be eliminated using masks that take out isolated pixels. When dealing with a set of mammograms for the same patient (left and right breast), it helps the segmentation process if images are scaled between the full range of gray-levels available. This allows a direct comparison between the data for two different breasts for the same patient and facilitates a better image subtraction between the pairs if needed (bi-lateral subtraction). Often, we are dealing with a set of mammograms rather than an individual case. In order to treat them on an equal footing, the following procedures should be completed as the initial pre-processing step: (a) noise management and tag removal; (b) scaling of the mammograms so that their pixel gray-levels are comparable; scaling will have no effect on the shape of their gray-level distributions; (c) ensure that data is sampled with the same resolution and the process of analogue to digital conversion is as uniform as possible for different samples; and (d) ensure that any enhancement procedures applied are not biased in favour of specific cases. The last observation is hard to achieve in practice as quite often the enhancement process may need to be optimized on a case-specific basis. It is not computationally feasible to optimize enhancement on a case-by-case basis. However, the process selected should maximize the average improvement over a set of images. The improvement itself can be quantified using measures suggested in the previous section. Once the above pre-processing steps are finished, image segmentation procedures can be used. The following sections discuss global, edge-based and region-based methods of image segmentation used in digital mammography for detecting masses.

9.9.1 Global Methods

Global methods of segmentation involve utilizing information on the gray level distributions from the image for its segmentation. **Thresholding methods** are based on finding an optimal value of threshold T as a gray level. All pixels with a gray level greater than T are identified as objects and those below form the background. Ideally, we would like to have an automated method of finding T. If image objects have sharp boundaries, then the gray level of the boundary pixels can serve as the threshold. Boundary pixels can be identified using gradient methods and the use of zero crossings of the Laplacian operator. If there is only one object imposed on the background, and the object/background intensities are considerably different but uniform within them, then the resultant histogram will be bimodal. Often when dealing with more than one object or variable object and background gray level intensities, the histogram will be multimodal. It is not very easy to label a histogram as multimodal rather than bimodal. For bimodal histograms, two peaks separated by a minimum gray level distance D can be detected, and the minimum gray level found in the valley between them is chosen as the threshold T. The distance D can be computed as the difference in mean gray levels of the object and the background. The catch is that we do not know D before the segmentation process itself. So D is either set manually or computed on other training data for which correct segmentation is already available. It is important to have a good peak-to-valley ratio in histograms to get a good threshold. A better histogram can be obtained if we remove the contribution made by pixels that have high gradient values, i.e. those pixels that lie on the edge between the object and the background. Another approach can be used to plot the histogram of pixels that have the highest image gradient. This histogram will be unimodal. The gray level corresponding to the peak gives the threshold T, or the average of N values surrounding the peak can be used as a reliable estimate of T. One of the advantages of the above methods of thresholding is their ability to work in real time. The other methods described later may require slightly longer to compute. Figure 9.14 shows an example of using multiple thresholds for a multimodal histogram to divide it into several regions of interest. The threshold is chosen as the minimum value between peaks of the histogram provided that the peaks are at least 25 gray levels apart.

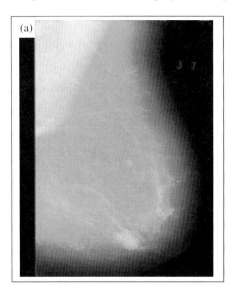 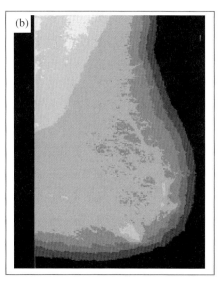

Figure 9.14: Original mammogram (a) and multimodal histogram thresholded mammogram (b).

Optimal thresholding can be used as another alternative (see example in Figure 9.15).

Optimal Threshold Algorithm

1. For an image $f(x, y)$ of size $M \times N$ (M rows and N columns), assume that pixels $f(0,0)$, $f(0, N)$, $f(M, 0)$ and $f(M, N)$ belong to the background and the rest of the image is the object. Compute the mean gray level for the background and the object (target), called μ_B and μ_T respectively. At time step $t = 0$, these can be represented as the initial approximations μ_B^0 and μ_T^0 respectively.

2. Compute at step $t + 1$, the segmentation threshold Z as

$$Z^{t+1} = (\mu_B^t + \mu_T^t)/2.$$

3. Find the background pixels and object pixels using this revised threshold and calculate the object and background means for the next step.

4. Repeat steps (2) and (3) until $Z^{t+1} = Z^t$.

Adaptive thresholding is another method that can work well with digital mammograms. The basic idea is to divide the image into a number of parts of

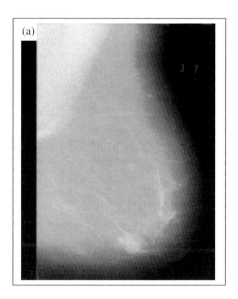 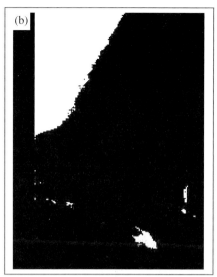

Figure 9.15: Original mammogram (a) and optimal thresholded mammogram (b).

equal size, e.g. we can divide it into 4×4 or 3×3 windows. For each window, a thresholding procedure based on histograms or optimal thresholding can be applied. As such, a better estimate of thresholds in local regions is possible that yields good results. If for each window w, a threshold T_w is detected, then we can label pixels with gray levels greater than T_w as objects and others as background. The following algorithm can be used for detecting multiple objects using adaptive thresholds.

Adaptive Threshold Algorithm

1. For an image $f(x, y)$ of size $M \times N$ (M rows and N columns), divide it into equal sized windows so that we have a total of W $m \times n$ sized windows.

2. For each window, determine the optimal threshold and find regions that correspond to object and background.

3. For each of the total of R regions found in w windows, $R = 2w$, find which regions are similar across windows with a t-test. Using this statistical test, find whether the pixels of a pair of recognized regions are statistically different or similar.

4. Two or more regions that are not statistically different are treated as a single object (geographically if similar disjoint regions are found, it shows the presence of the same region in more than one location).

5. If after the t-test, we identify r statistically different regions, where $r \leq R$, then allocate r different gray levels to these regions for segmentation labeling.

The adaptive threshold algorithm is able to detect multiple regions of interest that are statistically different. For optimal results, the size of the windows used must be larger than the largest object to be detected for a meaningful threshold detection (see Figure 9.16 as an example).

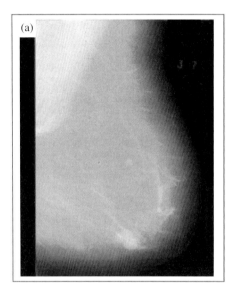 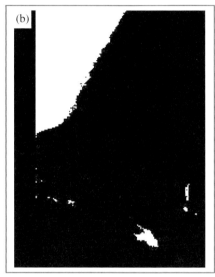

Figure 9.16: Original mammogram (a) and adaptive thresholded mammogram (b).

Hierarchical data structures have been used frequently in image processing (see previously mentioned algorithm for tree pyramid definition). One example is the popular pyramid data structure for image analysis. **Thresholding** in hierarchical data structures can give good segmentation results. If an image I is a square matrix of elements, then a pyramid can be derived as a set of images $\{I_L, I_{L-1}, \ldots, I_0\}$. The image I_{j-1} is derived from I_j by reducing the resolution by half using pixel averaging. So I_0 has the lowest resolution and I_L is the original image with the highest resolution. The image having one degree smaller resolution in the pyramid contains four times less data which allows it to be processed four times faster. Two separate approaches can be adopted for image segmentation using an image pyramid constructed using a given mammogram. The first approach can be termed for convenience the *Iterative Pyramid Segmentation* approach and the second is called *Hierarchical Thresholding using Significant Pixel*. The following algorithms define their operational characteristics.

Iterative Pyramid Segmentation Algorithm

1. For a pyramid structure $\{I_L, I_{L-1}, \ldots, I_0\}$, start with the image having the lowest resolution $I_j = I_0$. The region R to be segmented is initially the full image.

2. Find a threshold T_j using any histogram-based method in region R. Identify the boundary pixels using this threshold and their 8-connected neighbors.

3. Identify the pixels in the image in the next level I_{j+1} that correspond to the boundary pixels and neighbors identified in step (2) for image I_j. These constitute region R for the next step.

4. Re-segment the region R identified in step (3) by using the same thresholding method as used in step (2).

5. Repeat the cycle of steps (2) to (4), until we find the final threshold T_L for the original image. This threshold will be used for segmenting the original image.

Hierarchical Thresholding using Significant Pixel Algorithm

1. For a pyramid structure $\{I_L, I_{L-1}, \ldots, I_0\}]$, in each level of the pyramid, find significant pixel positions and their neighbors in a 3×3 window where the center of the window is the significant pixel. Significant pixels represent those pixels whose gray level is significantly different from their neighbors. These can be found by convolving a mask that responds well to such differences, e.g. the center of the mask is a high positive value compared with its neighbors. Large image gradients can be detected easily using this procedure.

2. For each significant pixel p found in level j, find a threshold T_{pj} defined as:

$$T_{pj} = \frac{c + \frac{1}{8}\sum_i n_i}{2}$$

where c is the gray level of the significant pixel p, and n_i are the gray levels of its neighbors in the window.

3. For each significant pixel detected in level j and its window of neighbors, find the area in the original image that corresponds to this surrounding and segment it with threshold T_{pj}. This will give the segmented image.

9.9.2   Edge-Based Methods

Edge-based methods of image segmentation are an important class of techniques that can be effectively used for separating regions of interest from their backgrounds in mammograms. The fundamental assumption when using such methods is that the separation between two regions (object and background or two objects) is feasible using gradient information. The gradient of an image represents the rate of change with which pixel gray levels change in a given direction. Gradient detection is performed using masks that are convolved with the image to give a gradient image. The image gradient magnitude in the horizontal and vertical directions can be combined to give an overall magnitude of gradient and its direction. The magnitude of the gradient represents the strength of the edge. Provided that all edges of strength greater than some threshold can be detected, further processing can yield regions of interest. Laplacian operators can be used to find the exact position of the edge. One of the simplest methods using edge information in mammography is to simply remove from the original image those pixels that have a gradient magnitude greater than a threshold. If a low threshold is set, a large number of pixels can be removed. On the basis of our assumption that masses are relatively homeogeneous in their gray level, and therefore contain a small number of edges, we will be ultimately left with regions of interest. This is however a gross technique of using edge information for identifying regions of interest. Another simple method can be based on edge image thresholding to find strong edges and edge linking to determine closed regions.

More sophisticated techniques based on edge manipulation first identify borders and then determine the regions that lie within them. As such, border detection in itself becomes the primary task. It is not always easy to construct regions on the basis of borders detected. Often, the quality of prior analysis has considerable impact on finding optimal regions. Fortunately, methods exist that are able to find regions even when the boundaries are not closed. Hong *et al.* [865] describe a good method for finding regions using partially connected boundaries. An algorithm for this is given below (Sonka *et al.* [917]):

Region Formation from Partial Borders Algorithm

1. For each border pixel x, search for an opposite edge pixel y that lies within a distance M. M is chosen using *a priori* information on the maximum region sizes. If this edge pixel is found, mark it as a potential region member. If no edge pixel is found, move on to the next border pixel. For pixels x and y to be opposite, the following condition must be satisfied:

$$\frac{\pi}{2} < |(\phi(x) - \phi(y)) \bmod (2\pi)| < \frac{3\pi}{2},$$

where $\phi(x)$, and $\phi(y)$ represents the direction of the edge at x and y respectively.

2. Compute the total number of markers for each pixel (this represents how often the pixel was on a connecting line between opposite edge pixels). Let $b(x)$ be the number of markers for pixel x.

3. We can determine a score $B(x)$ as follows:

$$B(x) = 0.0 \text{ for } b(x) = 0$$
$$B(x) = 0.1 \text{ for } b(x) = 1$$
$$B(x) = 0.2 \text{ for } b(x) = 2$$
$$B(x) = 0.5 \text{ for } b(x) = 3$$
$$B(x) = 1.0 \text{ for } b(x) > 3$$

4. The confidence C that the pixel x is a member of the region is given by summing $B(x)$ in a 3×3 neighborhood.

5. If $C \geq 1$, then pixel x is in the region, otherwise it is a part of the background.

6. Segmentation can be achieved by recording all pixels within the region.

The above method works well for both bright regions on dark backgrounds, and for dark regions on white backgrounds. The above algorithm is applied once we have an array of data representing border pixels. The process of detecting borders themselves is a complicated task. Sonka *et al.* [917] detail a range of methods for tracing borders in edge images. A number of these methods use graph theory to maintain a record of linked pixels called nodes. In order to find optimal borders, appropriate cost functions must be evaluated. These include strength of the edges forming the border and border curvature. In particular, the role of border curvature for mass detection in mammography cannot be underestimated. If the curvature of the regions is known beforehand, then techniques such as the Hough transform can be used (Illingworth and Kittler [868]). The Hough transform is a very powerful technique that can effectively isolate lines or curves of predefined nature. As such, it can be applied to either the original image or the edge image. In digital mammograms, the removal of labels for example can be effectively performed using the Hough transform that will detect straight lines. However, since we do not know the exact form of regional borders in advance for a given mammogram, it is difficult to use the Hough transform for detecting masses as a whole. However, if we were to develop a system that detected small curves and lines, a partially broken border of regions of interest could be effectively constructed. Partially connected border segments can be linked to form closed boundaries in such cases.

9.9.3   Region-Based Segmentation

This is the most popular range of methods of image segmentation in digital mammography. One of the key attractions of region-based segmentation is that the amount of prior information needed or parameter setting for region identification is minimal. Region-based segmentation involves the analysis of regional properties within an image. Some popular techniques for such segmentation include region merging, region splitting, a combination of these, the watershed method, and clustering of various types. The principle of homogeneity in segmented regions is critical to all of these methods. Homogeneity refers to uniformity in either gray level or gradient information within the pixels. Our confidence in the segmentation process is based directly on how well homogeneous regions in the original image are clustered in the segmented image. It should be stressed that various segmentation methods based on regional processing do not yield exactly the same result. This is because as regions are formed as a result of expansion or reduction of a set of pixels, the order in which processing takes place has a direct and often irreversible impact on the final regions obtained. We briefly discuss some of the important region-based segmentation techniques.

Region merging is based on the concept of grouping pixels that satisfy merging criteria. This criteria is based on whether the region formed after the combination of two or more pixels will be homogeneous. As the region grows, the homogeneity of the resultant regions must be maintained. Simple criteria to check this include average gray level, gray level variance, histogram properties and texture properties. As long as these properties remain stable before and after new pixels are added to a growing region, the process can continue. The implementation of this class of methods varies depending on what properties are chosen for monitoring the region growing process and what limits have been set as acceptable for measuring the stability of these properties. The definition of a region starts as a single pixel and becomes an aggregate pixel region with time. The start pixel for initiating the process is user-specified and depending on this, different segmentation results can be finally achieved. There are two methods of finding regions. First, we can start with the N brightest pixels in an image and grow regions based on their neighborhood. Second, we can start with a 2×2 or 4×4 pixel window labeled as a region. Adjacent windows or pixels can be merged if the merged region satisfies the homogeneity criteria.

Sonka *et al.* [917] describe how we can use state space search methods based on super-grid data structures for region merging. This method is also referred to as region merging via boundary melting. The basic principle is to merge two regions if their common boundary consists of weak edges. The boundary is determined on the basis of the strength of the crack edges along their common border (four crack edges are attached to each pixel as its four neighbors – the direction of the crack edge is that of increasing brightness and its magnitude is the absolute difference between the brightness of the relevant pair of pixels). A weak edge is defined as an edge whose gradient magnitude is less than a predefined threshold. The weakness of the boundary as a whole is computed as a ratio of the number of weak edges and the total length of the boundary. By recursively removing common boundaries with most weak edges, we can merge adjacent regions effectively.

Region splitting follows an opposite approach to image segmentation by splitting the image into smaller homogeneous regions. The same criteria for homogeneity apply as in region-merging algorithms. Region splitting will not necessarily lead to the same results as region merging. A more frequently used approach involves a combination of region splitting and merging to obtain the computational advantages of both. **Split and merge** approaches are based on pyramid data structure representation of image data and a homogeneity criterion. If any region in the pyramid data structure is not homogeneous, then it is split into four child-regions. At the same time, if any four child-regions of any parent are found to be homogeneous, then they can be merged together into a single region. Once no more splits and merges are possible, then identify any possibilities of merging regions R_i and R_j into a homogeneous region even if these regions are in two different pyramid levels. Merge these plus any other regions that are too small with their adjacent region. Split and merge methods have been successfully used for mammogram segmentation (e.g. Bovis and Singh [834]). A simple algorithm defining the procedure is illustrated by Jain *et al.* [871] as follows (see example in Figure 9.17).

Split and Merge Region Segmentation Algorithm

1. Start with the entire image as a single region.

2. Pick a region R. If $H(R)$ is false, then split the region into four sub-regions. Here $H(R)$ is the homogeneity test for the region.

3. Consider any n more neighboring sub-regions, $R_1, R_2, \ldots, R_n$, in the image. If $H(R_1 \cup R_2 \cup \ldots \cup R_n)$ is true, merge the n regions into a single region.

4. Repeat these steps until no further splits or merges take place.

A Fast Adaptive Segmentation (FAS) algorithm that merges regions that are homogeneous has been proposed by Chang and Li [844]. The image is divided into many small, equal sized, primitive regions that are assumed to be homogeneous. Traditionally, a threshold test is used. If the difference between features in adjacent regions is less than a given threshold, then homogeneity is assumed. The adaptive element of the algorithm is captured in its adaptive homogeneity test. The test is based on the feature distributions of the two regions. From the feature histogram of a region, the adaptive range (t_1, t_2) is computed within which the central λ portion of the region feature values lie $(0 \leq \lambda \leq 1)$. For two regions to be considered homogeneous, it is required that each region's mean falls within the other region's adaptive range. For $\lambda = 0.8$, regions R_1 and R_2 are considered homogeneous if the mean of a given feature within R_1 falls within the central 80% range of the same feature in R_2. For regions that are too small, a Mann–Whitney test is used to determine if two region means are significantly different from each other or not.

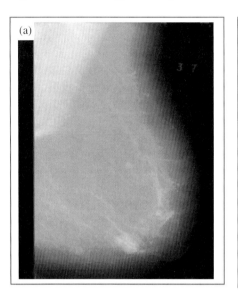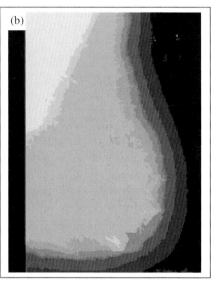

Figure 9.17: Original mammogram (a) and split and merge thresholded mammogram (b).

The research on **watershed algorithms** for image segmentation dates back to over a hundred years ago. The seminal papers by Cayley [837] and Maxwell [889] describe how smooth surfaces could be decomposed into hills and dales by studying the critical points and slope lines of the surfaces. Earlier work on watersheds involved processing digital elevation models and were based on local neighborhood operations on square grids (Collins [845]; Marks *et al.* [887]; Puecker and Douglas [904]). Improved gradient-following methods were later introduced to overcome problems with intensity plateau and square pixel grids (Blom [832]; Griffin *et al.* [853]). Another approach has used immersion algorithms to identify watershed regions by flooding the image with water starting at intensity minima. Watershed segmentation is essentially based on the topographic surface interpretation of images where gradient image gray-levels represent altitudes such that region edges correspond to high watersheds and low-gradient region interiors correspond to catchment basins. Catchment basins represent areas of the image with low gradient gray-levels and their identification becomes the prime goal of a watershed segmentation algorithm. There are two basic approaches to identifying catchment basins. We can move either downstream or upstream. In the downstream approach, we first identify the paths from each pixel to a local minimum by following the gradient altitude information. All pixels whose paths downstream lead to the same altitude minimum are labeled as belonging to the same catchment basin.

One of the weaknesses of this approach is that we have few rules to specify unique and valid paths. A different approach for segmentation by moving upstream has been given by Vincent and Soille [923]. This approach allows the catchment basin to fill from the bottom. The implementation of this approach is based on sorting pixels in increasing order of their gray level values followed by a flooding step which requires a breadth-first scanning of pixels in order of their gray levels.

Betal *et al.* [830] explain the watershed algorithm in detail for detecting microcalcifications. The first step is to locate all local minima within the image and these are given a unique label. All pixels that have gray scale value one higher than the minimum value are identified and pixels adjacent to a catchment basin are labeled as belonging to the catchment basin associated to that local minima. Those pixels not included are put in a queue and given an appropriate label at such time as their neighbors have been assigned a particular catchment basin. This flooding procedure is repeated for successively large gray scale values up to the maximum signal intensity of the image. Divide lines are constructed at points where floods tend to merge – these constitute the watersheds. In cases where a local minima identifies each object of interest uniquely, the watershed lines represent the object boundary. In order to avoid over-segmentation of the image, because of too many minima, the following enhancements can be made to the standard watershed algorithm.

Rather than applying flooding on the original image, it can be applied on the difference image obtained by the difference of dilation and erosion of the image that represents the largest change at the boundaries of microcalcifications. Furthermore, only those catchment basins that correspond to objects of interest (microcalcifications) are flooded. For each microcalcification, a unique internal marker with an external marker is needed. Internal markers are given by the top hat algorithm. An external marker is obtained by applying the watershed algorithm to the inverted image constrained by the internal markers. The flooding proceeds as normal but this time catchment basins forming at minima that do not correspond to markers are flooded by overflow from neighboring catchment basins.

Belhomme *et al.* [828] propose a revised version of watershed segmentation for detecting regions of interest in mammograms. The standard watershed algorithm is based on the following two steps: (a) image simplification conducted from a set of markers extracted by procedures which take into account some knowledge about the objects, the image class and also the image processing operators being used; and (b) building the watershed lines of the simplified image which is thus split into regions designated as "catchment basins". Serra [477] has shown that the first step is of great significance because watershed transformation leads to a strong over-segmentation when applied on the raw image. It is therefore useful to detect object and background markers (seeds) using techniques based on image class properties (Vincent and Soille [923]). Once the interesting seeds are found, images can be simplified by modifying homotopy by imposing some minima on the location of the markers and removing unwanted regional minima. Belhomme *et al.* consider the traditional watershed algorithm as a region growing operator with only one topographical criterion (the value of points in the gradient image). The revised version of the watershed algorithm is suggested to take into account several pieces of image information such as contrast, topographical attributes and statistical parameters calculated on regions. The revised algorithm is based on the use of FIFO stacks and its details are beyond the scope of this chapter. However, the advantages claimed include: (a) the potential image does not have to be transformed in order to change its homotopy since the flooding stage starts directly from markers and not from region minima; (b) the revised algorithm is fast and linear with respect to the points processed; and (c) the algorithm makes it possible to integrate additional local and global information by modifying point properties during the flooding stage. In order to consider local and global information during the flooding stage, point priorities are computed iteratively by combining local criteria (gradient modulus, gray or color levels) with global information about regions (area, mean gray or color level, standard deviation, and range statistics).

Multiscale analysis of intensity minima in watershed algorithms provides a mechanism for imposing a scale-based hierarchy on the watersheds associated with these minima (Gauch [851]). This provides a valuable insight into the multiscale properties of edges in the image without following these curves through the scale space. Once an image has been decomposed into visually sensible atomic regions and a meaningful hierarchy has been imposed on these regions, the process of segmenting an image is greatly simplified. Users can point to the regions or objects of interest and use the hierarchy to combine atomic regions into meaningful image regions associated with objects of interest. Gauch [851] highlights three main advantages of using the multiscale approach over standard methods. First, multiscale analysis is fast and easy with a one-to-one relationship between intensity extrema and watershed regions in the image. Second, visually sensible measurements of importance to individual curve segments make up the boundaries of watershed regions. Finally, interactive segmentation tools can be constricted that use gradient watershed region hierarchies to quickly and easily identify image regions associated with objects of interest.

Clustering methods are one of the best known techniques for identifying regions (see Jain and Dubes [869] for a review). Clustering methods can be applied directly on image pixels to separate regions that are homogeneous. Clustering can be applied using either statistical or connectionist approaches. Statistical approaches include simple and fuzzy clustering techniques. Connectionist approaches include unsupervised neural networks such as Kohonen's Self Organising Map (SOM). Here we shall focus on the statistical approaches. A brief criticism of some classical statistical clustering methodologies is given below (Pauwels and Frederix [848]):

- *K-means clustering:* This is one of the classic clustering methods. Unfortunately, the number of clusters to be found needs to be specified in advance and may not be known. The method is also unable to handle unbalanced clusters, i.e. one cluster that has significantly more points than another cluster. Elongated clusters are another problem – it can erroneously split a large cluster into artificial sub-clusters. Also, since the algorithm produces a voronoi tessellation of data space, the resulting clusters are convex by construction.

- *Hierarchical clustering:* Starting with as many clusters as data points, clusters are successively merged if they are sufficiently close to each other. The result is a partially ordered tree in which the number of clusters decreases monotonically, rather than a single cluster. The method suffers from the "chaining effect" – nearby, but distinct clusters are often lumped together whenever there is a chain of data points bridging the gap.

- *Parametric density estimation:* This approach hinges on the assumption that the underlying data density is a mixture of g Gaussian densities. The aim is to find g means and covariances of these Gaussians and partition data among them. Some of the key limitations of clustering algorithms based on this include the need for specifying the number of clusters in advance and the performance is poor for irregular clusters (e.g. the EM algorithm).

- *Non-parametric density estimation:* In these algorithms, we do not assume that Gaussian distributions exist. Density is determined by data convolution with a density kernel of limited support. Clusters are then identified by locating local density maxima. There are usually no *a priori* restrictions on the shape of the resulting density and there is no need to specify the number of clusters (see Roberts [910] for a discussion of parametric and non-parametric methods).

The first two types of clustering methods are widely available in standard software packages. We present the generic methodology for data density based clustering methods. Pauwels and Frederix [848] develop a robust and versatile non-parametric clustering algorithm that is able to handle unbalanced and highly irregular clusters and introduce two new cluster validity measures. Their clustering algorithm is described below:

Non-parametric Clustering Algorithm

1. The process starts with the construction of data densities obtained by convolving the data set by a density kernel. Given an n-dimensional data set $\{x_i \in R^n, i = 1...N\}$, a density $f(x)$ is obtained by convolving the data set by a density kernel $K_\sigma(x)$ where σ is the spread parameter.

$$f(x) = \frac{1}{N} \sum_{i=1}^{N} K_\sigma(x - x_i)$$

2. Take K_σ to be a rotation invariant Gaussian density with σ^2 variance.

$$K_\sigma(x) = \left(\frac{1}{2\pi\sigma^2}\right)^{n/2} \cdot e^{-||x||^2/2\sigma^2}$$

3. After convolution, identify clusters using gradient descent (hill climbing). To pinpoint the local minima of density f, the k-nearest neighbors of every point are determined where each point is linked to the point of highest density among these neighbors (possibly itself). Thus, data is carved into compact and dense clumps.

4. σ is picked as a small value initially. Find candidate clusters by locating the local minima of the density f. This will result in overestimation of the number of clusters. Using data density, a hierarchical family of derived clustering is used to systematically merge clusters. The order of merging is based on comparing density values at neighboring maxima with respect to the data density at a saddle-point in between, which is defined as the point of maximal density among the boundary points (points having neighbors in both clusters).

5. Judge the cluster validity using newly introduced Isolation and Connectivity cluster validity measures.

6. Isolation measure calculation: This is measured using the k-nearest neighbor norm (NN-norm). For a given K, $V_K(x)$ is defined for a data point (x) as the fraction of k-nearest neighbors of x that have the same cluster label as (x). Ideally, $V_K(x) = 1$. The isolation measure is defined as:

$$N^{(K)} = \frac{1}{N}\sum V_K(x).$$

Connectivity measure calculation: This measure relates to the fact that for any two points in the same cluster, there is always a path connecting both along which data density remains high. Two random points (a and b) are chosen in the same cluster and connected using a straight line. A test point t is picked halfway along this line and we find its local density maximum. The location of t is changed but it must remain halfway. If for point t_i, the maximum intensity is $f(t_i)$, then the connectivity measure is defined as:

$$C^K = \frac{1}{K}\sum_{i=1}^{K} f(t_i)$$

for k randomly chosen pairs (a_i, b_i).

7. Typically, the isolation measure will decrease and the connectivity measure will increase as the number of clusters increase. Compute z-scores to

make indices comparable. If $Z(x) = \frac{x-\bar{x}}{\sigma}$, then compute $Z_p = Z(N_p) + Z(C_p)$ for the pth clustering. Plot this index to choose the number of clusters that give maximum Z_p.

In the above algorithm, isolation and connectivity measures have been used for cluster validity. There are several other measures that can be used, such as the fuzzy compactness-separation ratio (Zahid *et al.* [933]).

A large number of medical imaging studies use Fuzzy C-Means (FCM) clustering and its variants due to several attractive properties. Pham and Prince [469] describe the standard FCM and an improved Adaptive Fuzzy C-Means Clustering (AFCM) approach, comparing these on segmenting MR images of the brain. The standard FCM algorithm for scalar data sets seeks the membership functions μ_k and centroid ν_k such that the following objective function J_{FCM} is minimized:

$$J_{FCM} = \sum_{i,j} \sum_{k=1}^{c} \mu_k(i,j)^q ||y(i,j) - \nu_k||^2$$

where $\mu_k(i,j)$ is the membership value at pixel location (i,j) for class k such that

$$\sum_{k=1}^{c} \mu(i,j) = 1.$$

$y(i,j)$ is the observed image intensity at location (i,j) and ν_k is the centroid of class k. The total number of classes c is assumed to be known. Parameter q is a weighting coefficient exponent on each fuzzy membership and determines the amount of fuzziness. The aim of the algorithm is to minimize function J_{FCM}. High membership values are assigned to pixels that are close to the centroid and low to those far away from the centroid. An example segmentation of our chosen mammogram is shown in Figure 9.18 using standard the FCM technique.

The updated algorithm AFCM preserves the advantages of FCM while being applicable to images with intensity homogeneities. The algorithm tries to minimize the following objective function with respect to μ, ν and m.

$$\begin{aligned}
J_{AFCM} = &\sum_{i,j} \sum_{k=1}^{c} \mu_k(i,j)^2 ||y(i,j) - m(i,j)\nu_k||^2 \\
&+ \lambda_1 \sum_{i,j} \left((D_i * m(i,j))^2 + (D_j * m(i,j))^2 \right) \\
&+ \lambda_2 \sum_{i,j} (D_{ii} * m(i,j))^2 + 2(D_{ij} * *m(i,j))^2 + (D_{jj} * m(i,j)^2)
\end{aligned}$$

where D_i and D_j are standard forward finite difference operators (similar to derivatives in the continuous domain) along the rows and columns and

$D_{ii} = D_i * D_i, D_{jj} = D_j * D_j, D_{ij} = D_i * D_j$ are second order finite differences. The symbol * represents a one-dimensional convolution and ** represents a two-dimensional convolution operation. The coefficients λ_1 and λ_2 are regularization terms. The first term penalizes a large amount of variation and the second term penalizes multiplier fields that have discontinuities. These two terms are set on the basis of image inhomogeneity. The multiplier field $m(i,j)$ is a slowly varying function.

Frigui and Krishnapuram [849] provide a summary of the relative abilities of various clustering methods. The K-means and fuzzy c-means methods have been criticized for their sensitivity to initialization. Other clustering programs mentioned with references include the k-Medoids algorithm, Robust C-Prototypes (RCP) algorithm, Robust Fuzzy C-Means (RFCM) algorithm, Fuzzy C Least Median of Squares (FCLMS) algorithm, Fuzzy Trimmed C Prototypes (FTCP) algorithm, and Cooperative Robust Estimation algorithm (CRE). Frigui and Krishnapuram also detail their own Robust Competitive Agglomeration (RCA) algorithm which is supposed to improve upon existing clustering methods. Their procedure starts with a large number of clusters and reduces them by competitive agglomeration. Noise immunity is achieved using robust statistics. RCA can be used to find clusters of any shape as it fits an unknown number of parametric models simultaneously. The results produced on image segmentation tasks are very encouraging. This study also provides different distance measures for detecting clusters of different shapes (ellipses or circles).

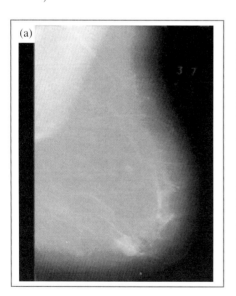 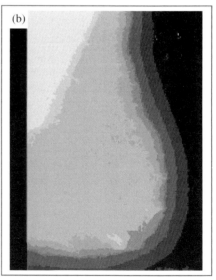

Figure 9.18: Original mammogram (a) and FCM thresholded mammogram (b).

Li *et al.* [885] have used **wavelet analysis** as a method of image segmentation and feature extraction. The analysis is used to classify masses as suspicious or normal based on a multi-orientation or Directional Wavelet Transform (DWT) decomposition. This methodology provides texture domain and morphological domain data alongside gray scale data, allowing features to be extracted from all domains. This study demonstrates the FROC results using a fuzzy decision tree. In the gray level domain, the features used include the intensity variation in the extracted region, the mean intensity difference between the extracted region and its surrounding area, and the mean gradient of region boundary. In the morphological domain, features include region area, circularity in shape, and normalized deviation of radial length. In the directional feature domain, a tracing algorithm is designed to extract the spicules – features include the number of spiculations and mean length of normalized spiculations.

A **model-based approach** to segmentation is described by Polakowski *et al.* [902]. The overall system consists of five modules. The focus of attention (FOA) module segments suspicious regions in the mammogram. The indexing module separates the regions into size-dependent categories and reduces the number of false positives. The prediction module develops models for each tissue type in each category. The feature extraction module obtains features from suspicious ROIs and finally the matching module classifies the regions. In a model-based system, information on what constitutes a reasonable mass needs to be incorporated. The use of a Difference of Gaussian (DoG) filter has been suggested as one method of modeling the presence of masses. The DoG filter is constructed by subtracting two Gaussians of different standard deviations and taking the Fourier transform. This results in a transfer function that can be convolved with the original image for its segmentation. The resulting filter has a bandpass characteristic which is tuned to leave out masses in the image. Breast tissue is segmented using a simple threshold. Artifacts from the wrap-around error by Fourier transform convolution are removed by a horizontal gradient fill algorithm. Once the DoG filter is implemented, the mass and interior structure of the breast become more visible in the resultant image.

Region-growing approaches have been used by a range of studies. Region growth starts from a given pixel of interest (called the seed) and tests the similarity between the seed and surrounding pixels. A region is grown around the seed iteratively testing the homogeneity between pixels at the periphery of the growing region and its inside. Region-growing algorithms can also use homogeneity criteria between the spatial and histogram neighborhoods (Revol and Jourlin [909]). Adams and Bischof [439] illustrate the operation of a seeded region-growing algorithm that has similarities with the watershed algorithm. Theoretically speaking, segmentation in the watershed algorithm is equivalent to flooding the topography from the seed points. The seeded region algorithm (SRG) is described below (see the example segmentation in Figure 9.19).

Seeded Region Growing (SRG) Algorithm

1. Start with a number of seeds grouped into n sets $A_1 \ldots A_n$. Some of these sets may consist of single points.

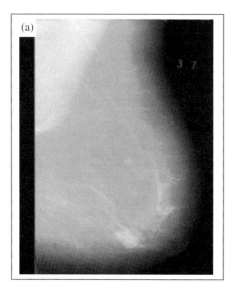
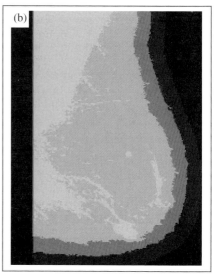

Figure 9.19: Original mammogram (a) and seeded region-growing thresholded mammogram (b).

2. Each step of the process involves the addition of one pixel to one of the above sets.

3. Consider the state of sets A after m steps. Let T be the set of all as yet unallocated pixels which border at least one of the regions:

$$T = \left\{ x \notin \bigcup_{i=1}^{n} A_i \middle| N(x) \cap \bigcup_{i=1}^{n} A_i \neq \emptyset \right\},$$

where $N(x)$ is the set of immediate neighbors of pixel (x). A rectangular grid with 8 connectivity is used.

4. If for $x \in T$ we have that $N(x)$ meets just one of the A_i, then we define $i(x) \in \{1, 2, ..., n\}$ to be that index such that $N(x) \cap A_{i(x)} \neq \emptyset$ and define $\delta(x)$ to be a measure of how different x is from the region it adjoins.

$$\delta(x) = |(g(x) - \operatorname*{mean}_{g \in A_{i(x)}} |g(x)|)|$$

where $g(x)$ is the gray value of the input image (x). If $N(i)$ meets two or more of the A_i, we take $i(x)$ to be that value of i such that $N(x)$ meets A_i and $\delta(x)$ is minimized.

5. We then take an $x \in T$ such that $\delta(x) = \min\{\delta(x)\}$ and append it to A_i.

6. The process is repeated until all pixels have been allocated.

One of the criticisms of the above algorithm is that it is dependent on the order of pixel processing. Hence raster order processing and anti-raster processing do not, in general, lead to the same tessellation. This problem is resolved in a revised version proposed by Mehnert and Jackway [890] whose seeded region-growing algorithm is pixel order independent.

Kupinski and Giger [882] present two more algorithms based on region analysis. The first algorithm is based on the calculation of the Radial Gradient Index (RGI) and uses an index calculation to determine which region of interest represents a true abnormality. The second algorithm is based on probability-based segmentation. These two algorithms are defined below:

Algorithm for Automated Seeded Lesion Segmentation using RGI
Definitions: The study is performed on normalized images (gray level range 0 to 1). ξ is the partition (region) containing the lesion. Lesions tend to be compact meaning that shapes are convex.

1. Start the segmentation process using seed point (μ_x, μ_y).

2. Multiply the original image by a constraint function that suppresses distant pixels. Choose an isotropic Gaussian function centered on the seed point with fixed variance σ_c^2. The resulting function $h(x, y)$ is defined as: $h(x, y) = f(x, y)N(x, y : \mu_x, \mu_y, \sigma_c^2)$, where $N(x, y : \mu_x, \mu_y, \sigma_c^2)$ is a circular normal distribution. Partitions are now defined on $f(x, y)$ for which $h(x, y)$ exceeds a certain threshold.

3. For each region (partition), an RGI function is calculated and the region with the maximum RGI value is selected. The function is computed on the original image even though the partitions are generated on the processed image $h(x, y)$. To compute RGI, the following steps are undertaken:

   (a) All pixels on the margin are first computed. Let the margin be M_i for partition i.

   (b) The RGI function is now given by:

$$RGI = \left(\sum_{(x,y)\in M_i} ||\hat{G}(x,y)|| \right)^{-1} \cdot \sum_{(x,y)\in M_i} \hat{G}(x,y) \cdot \frac{\hat{r}(x,y)}{||\hat{r}(x,y)||}$$

where the gradient vector of $f(x, y)$ is $\hat{G}(x, y)$ at position (x, y) and

$$\frac{\hat{r}(x,y)}{||\hat{r}(x,y)||}$$

is the normalized radial vector at (x, y).

(c) The RGI for a circular region is equal to 1. Select the region that has the highest RGI index.

In the above algorithm, RGI is the measure of the average proportion of gradients that are radially directed outwards. When it is equal to 1, it means that all gradients around the margin are pointing directly outwards along the radius vector and a value of -1 indicates that all gradients are pointing inwards. Kupinski and Giger [882] also present the probabilistic segmentation algorithm that is shown below. This algorithm uses probability distributions of regions that have been detected using seeded region growing.

Algorithm for Automated Seeded Lesion Segmentation using Probabilistic Method

1. Start the segmentation process using seed point (μ_x, μ_y).

2. The probability of pixel gray levels in region i is modeled as:

$$p(f(x,y)|i,\sigma_l^2) = \left\{ \begin{array}{ll} N(f(x,y) : f(\mu_x,\mu_y), \sigma_l^2) & : (x,y) \in i \\ z(f(x,y)) & : (x,y) \notin i \end{array} \right\}$$

where $N(f(x,y) : f(\mu_x,\mu_y), \sigma_l^2)$ is a normal distribution centered at the seed point gray level $f(\mu_x,\mu_y)$ with a variance of σ_l^2, and $z(f(x,y))$ is a function.

3. The uniformity of lesions is accounted for by a small variance Gaussian function centered around the seed pixel value. The probability of an ROI is:

$$p(ROI|i,\sigma_l^2) = \prod_{(x,y) \in ROI} p(f(x,y))|i,\sigma_l^2).$$

4. The region which has maximum p(ROI) is chosen.

Kupinski and Giger compare the above two algorithms with the standard region-growing technique in mammography and conclude that the regions grown by these algorithms are superior to those by region growing on the basis of how well the grown regions overlap with the hand-sketched boundaries drawn by radiologists.

One of the principal tasks of any Computer Aided Detection (CAD) system should be to automatically detect suspicious areas or ROIs and a variety of techniques have been used to meet this goal. These can be categorized as follows:

- ROI detection techniques using single views

- ROI detection techniques using multiple views.

9.9.4 ROI Detection Techniques Using a Single Breast

For single-view detection techniques, Parr *et al.* [897] and Zwiggelaar *et al.* ([938, 941, 942]) and Zwiggelaar [939], investigated the classification of linear structures within digital mammograms, especially those associated with spiculated lesions. The authors have extracted linear structure information including line strength, orientation and scale from mammograms using multi-scale line detection techniques. An algorithm for the extraction of linear information is given below:

Detect Linear Structures Algorithm

1. Define a line operator within an $n \times m$ window centered at target pixel t_i.

2. For each pixel p_i within the image, a linear neighborhood is tested with the line operator window centered at t_i:

   - Calculate the mean gray level of pixels lying on an orientated local line.

   - Subtract the average intensity of all pixels in the locally-orientated neighborhood.

3. Compute the line strength in q orientations.

4. Take the line orientation as the direction producing the maximum line strength.

5. The process is repeated over a set of scaled images obtained by sub-sampling and represented in a tree pyramid. For each pixel, the optimum scale can be found by determining where the maximum line strength is obtained.

6. Associate the scale-orientated signature with each pixel and thus build a probability image.

The line operator generates a high response for thin lines and a low response for thick lines. Zwiggelaar *et al.* [942] describe various approaches to represent patterns of linear structures. After application of the line operator, non-maximal suppression was applied to the line-strength image. The resultant image is thinned such that only the pixels lying within the center lines of linear structures were preserved resulting in a skeleton image.

The authors have carried out further research focused on detecting the central mass associated with spiculated lesions. Zwiggelaar *et al.* ([940, 942]) use scale-orientated signatures at each pixel. These scale-orientated signatures are constructed using a Recursive Median Filter (RMF), a class of filters known as sieves, that remove image peaks or troughs of less than a chosen size. Through their application with increasing sizes to an image and then finding the difference between previous sieves, it is possible to isolate features of a specific size. An outline algorithm for their application for the detection of masses is given below:

Detect Central Mass Algorithm

1. Define a 1-D RMF whose output is the median gray-level within the local neighborhood.

2. For a chosen angle θ, cover the image with lines such that every image pixel belongs to only one line.

3. For each pixel at orientation θ, perform 1-D RMF to obtain a scaled signature at this orientation.

4. Repeat the process at different orientations θ, resulting in a scale-orientated signature for each pixel.

5. Associate the scale-orientated signature with each pixel and thus build a probability image.

Many studies directed towards abnormality detection use a probability image (Astley *et al.* [827], Kegelmeyer *et al.* [876], Karssemeijer [874]) as a traditional method of classifying a pixel as being normal or abnormal. The algorithm for the formation of a probability image is given below:

Algorithm Probability Image

1. Assume an n-dimensional normally distributed feature vector x_i for each pixel i.

2. Assume for each class w_j (normal or abnormal) the mean m_{wj} and covariance C_{wj}. These have been estimated from a training set of images where an expert has annotated each pixel with the appropriate class.

3. The probability density of obtaining a feature vector x_i for a pixel of class w_j is given by

$$p(x_i|w_j) = \frac{1}{(2\pi)^{n/2}|C_{wj}|^{1/2}} \exp\left(\frac{-\delta_{ij}}{2}\right)$$

where δ_{ij}, is the Mahalanobis distance to the class mean given by

$$\delta_{ij} = (x_i - m_{ij})^T C_{wj}^{-1}(x_i - m_{wj}).$$

4. Applying Bayes' theorem, a probability image for class w_j (e.g. normal or abnormal) is obtained by calculating the following for each pixel:

$$p(w_j|x_i) = \frac{p(x_i|w_j)p(w_j)}{\sum_n p(x_i|w_n)p(w_n)}.$$

5. Detection can be performed by thresholding the resultant image, the results of which can be summarized using ROC analysis.

---

te Brake *et al.* [921] propose three methods of detecting suspicious areas: (i) detection of radiating patterns of linear spicules; (ii) detection of bright regions, and (iii) a combination of (i) and (ii). Kegelmeyer *et al.* [876] present the Analysis of Local Orientated Edge Feature (ALOE) method that is sensitive to stellate lesions. Probability-based methods assign a measure of suspiciousness to each pixel within the input image on the basis of spicules, masses or both. It is on the basis of suspiciousness that features are then subsequently extracted from each pixel. Ng and Bischof [895] propose two methods to detect masses: (i) a segmentation approach by detecting image regions that are brighter than adjacent areas and then constraining the results based on shape; and (ii) use of templates similar to the one shown in Figure 9.20 to detect the central mass, the matching process controlled with a cross-correlation function.

```
                -1 -1 -1
             -1 -1 0  -1 -1
          -1 -1 0  1  0  -1 -1
       -1 -1 0  1  1  1  0  -1 -1
    -1  0  1  1  1  1  1  0  -1
       -1 -1 0  1  1  1  0  -1 -1
          -1 -1 0  1  0  -1 -1
             -1 -1 0  -1 -1
                -1 -1 -1
```

Figure 9.20: Central mass template for a central region with diameter of 5 pixels.

In their experiments the authors used a variety of templates varying in diameter from 12 to 56 pixels. Kegelmeyer *et al.* [876] used a Binary Decision Tree (BDT) classifier to label each pixel of a mammogram with its probability of being abnormal. For every pixel in the image, a 5-D feature vector was extracted and BDT was used to determine the probability of a pixel being suspicious. These probabilities are then assembled into a probability image. The probability image is then thresholded and suspicious regions are colored red and superimposed onto the original image as an aid to direct the attention of the radiologist reading the film.

Kobatake *et al.* [880] propose the use of an *Iris filter* in the enhancement of low contrast images. The Iris filter is applied to the gradient image obtained using the generation of gradients in two orthogonal directions (authors adopt a Prewitt 3×3 operator) using the algorithm below (see Figure 9.21).

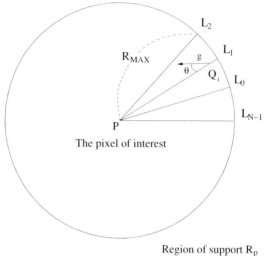

Figure 9.21: Central mass template for a central region diameter of 5 pixels (from Kobatake *et al.* [880]; © 1999, IEEE).

Iris Filter Algorithm

1. A region of support R_p is defined around the pixel of interest P at $f(x, y)$ as a combination of N radiating lines of maximum length R_{max}.

2. For each pixel Q_i on line PL_i, the convergence index of the gradient vector g at Q_i towards P is defined as:

$$F(Q_i) = \left\{ \begin{array}{ll} \cos\theta, & |g| \neq 0 \\ 0, & |g| = 0 \end{array} \right\}.$$

3. Subsequently the average convergence degree of gradient vectors on line PQ_i given as C_i is defined:

$$C_i = \frac{\int_P^{Q_i} f(Q)dQ}{\overline{PQ_i}}.$$

4. The maximum convergence degree, C_{io}, is calculated for each radiating line PL_i and is defined as $C_{io} = \max C_I$ such that $Q_i \in [P, R_i]$.

5. The output of the Iris filter at the pixel of interest $P(x, y)$ is defined as

$$C(x, y) = \frac{1}{N} \sum_{i=0}^{N-1} C_{io}.$$

On application to every pixel within the gradient image, the authors use the output from the Iris filter as means of detecting masses on the assumption that the output is typically large near the center of rounded convex regions such as tumor masses. Polakowski *et al.* [902] devised a focus of attention model as a mechanism for selecting likely target ROIs. The breast mass is convolved with the difference of Gaussian convolution kernel to filter masses of a particular size and generate a binary image. The difference of Gaussian filter is constructed by subtracting two Gaussians of different standard deviations and taking the Fourier transform. Within their study the authors found that values of $\sigma_1 = 20$ and $\sigma_2 = 50$ were capable of matching masses approximately 1 cm in diameter. In their study, Li *et al.* [885] and Qian *et al.* [905] employed a novel mass detection method using the computation of features in three domains (gray level, morphology and directional texture). The wavelet model used can be described as a multi-channel frequency decomposition filter containing frequency and directional information. The Directional Wavelet Transform (DWT) generates two output images from an input image:

- Directional texture image following directional feature analysis.

- A smoothed version of the original image in which the directional texture information is absent and subsequently analyzed by a segmentation module resulting in two classes of pixels.

- Details of fatty or parenchyma tissue, and suspicious masses.

Petrick *et al.* [899, 900] proposed the previously discussed Density Weighted Contrast Enhancement method (DWCE) which when applied to the original image gives a re-scaled weighted-contrast image and in addition provides significant background reduction. A Laplacian-Gaussian edge detector is applied to the resultant image to identify suspicious closed regions that are then subjected to ROI segmentation.

9.9.5   ROI Detection Techniques Using Breast Symmetry

Many studies have used the clinical observation of asymmetry between left and right breast images for detecting suspicious areas (see Figure 9.22). When mammographic images of breast pairs are inspected, clinicians typically make comparisons as if they were symmetric. Kopans [881] makes two important mammographic observations in this context:

1. Though one breast may be larger than the other, internal structures are quite symmetric over broad areas.

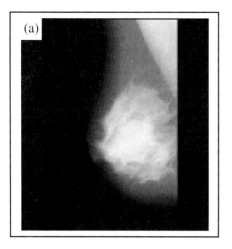 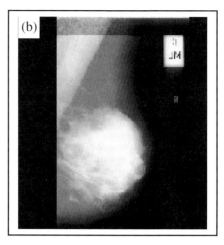

Figure 9.22: (a) Right and matching (b) left breast (from MiniMias Database [919]).

2. Overlapping tissue structures that form summation shadows and normal tissue variations on the mammogram highlights unimportant asymmetries.

In order to distinguish focal asymmetric densities from asymmetric breast tissue, the clinician should determine the following characteristics (Kopans [881]):

Size   Focal asymmetric densities should be considered suspicious if they are usually smaller than asymmetric breast tissue.

Density   Typically, the asymmetric density is concentrated towards the center of the mass tapering towards the periphery.

Projections   Asymmetry will be present in two mammographic projections.

Boundaries   Asymmetry contains definable margins that fade into the surrounding tissue.

Within a CAD scheme, the simplest method of seeking asymmetries within breast pairs is to register one image against the other. This is achieved using either a rigid alignment employing translation and rotation operators around one or more pre-defined control points, or by employing a non-point based deformable alignment. Finally a simply subtraction of the images in a bilateral manner results in asymmetries. The resulting images contain suspicious areas that are then subsequently segmented using techniques described in later sections.

One of the earliest studies on bilateral subtraction is by Winsberg *et al.* [928]. A more recent study by Mendez *et al.* [892] outlines the procedure for finding true asymmetries as a result of bilateral subtraction. Aligned images are subtracted and thresholded. The experiments demonstrate that there is no relationship between optimal thresholds (determined visually) and the absolute gray level distributions of different cases. Thresholding determines the regions selected for analysis and its optimization is essential. The method used selects a high threshold and finds the object and background pixels using this. A region-growing algorithm is used to find regions that have object pixels in them before applying an area and shape eccentricity tests. The process continues iteratively, each time lowering the threshold by a small constant until at least one region satisfies area and eccentricity requirements. Any false positives appearing at the end can be reduced using a texture test (Mendez *et al.* [891]).

9.9.6   Detection of Spicules

Masses are commonly described as spiculated or circumscribed. Spiculated masses have been traditionally considered more likely to be malignant and their detection is an important goal of computerized analysis. Spiculated masses have a central tumor mass that is surrounded by a radiating structure of sharp, dense and fine lines called "spicules" emanating from the central mass. Ng and Bischof [895] give a detailed account of how spicules and their associated central mass can be detected in mammograms. Their study also describes the **edge-**, **field-** and **spine-oriented** approaches for finding these. Three main approaches presented for spicule and central mass detection adopt different criteria for determining which pixels lie on the spine of the spicule. Once these pixels have been identified, the Hough transform can be used to find the center of the mass. If points lying on different spicules have been identified, then the lines passing through them intersect at the center of the mass. In particular, the spine-oriented approach has been recommended as the most successful and we will describe this in greater detail. Spicule detection is assisted by pre-processing the mammograms by stretching their contrast to full 256 levels and using a Gaussian filter to remove the high frequency component in digitized mammograms. The **edge-oriented** method assumes that if a line is drawn passing through an edge point of a spicule and in a direction normal to the edge gradient, it should pass through the center of the radial structure. First, all edges in the mammogram whose gradients exceed a threshold T are extracted using a Canny edge detector based on zero-crossings of the second directional derivative in the direction of the principal gradient. Edge pixels (x_k, y_k) with orientation θ_k normal to the edge gradient are then used with the Hough transform to find the radial center. The **field-oriented** method does not attempt to find spicules directly. It is based on the assumption that spicules produce a brightness pattern for which the brightness gradient field follows concentric circles, i.e. the vector field normal to the gradient field has a radial structure. These patterns do not appear within the central mass itself. Unfortunately, neither of these methods produce a peak at the center of the stellate tumor but instead produce an annular response. The **spine-oriented** method has been shown to produce the best results by Ng and Bischof. The method is complicated and detailed compared with the edge- and field-oriented approaches. We provide brief details on the spine-oriented method with an algorithm. One of the preliminary assumptions is that spicules are distinctly visible and show a unique microstructure.

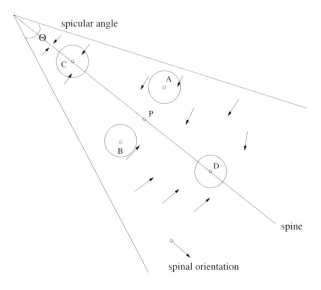

Figure 9.23: Ideal microstructure of a spicule where the gradient field on both sides is indicated by arrows. Around spinal pixel P, gradient is coherent in areas A and B and incoherent in areas C and D (from Ng and Bischof [895]; © Academic Press).

In Figure 9.23, the central line of a spicule is called the *spine*, and its orientation *spinal orientation* points towards the center of the tumor. Pixels lying on the spine are called *spinal pixels* and other pixels within the spicule are called *spicular pixels* and have *spicular orientation* defined by the gradient at that pixel. Spicular orientation is usually in the direction between the direction normal to the spine and the spine itself. The areas where the gradient is coherent (A and B), and areas where gradient is incoherent (C and D) are better shown in Figure 9.24 to illustrate how spinal pixels can be detected. In coherent areas, the gradient vectors point in the same direction and in incoherent areas they point in different directions.

The detection of spinal pixels is based on the *gradient coherence rule*. This rule uses a *gradient coherence measurement* χ. If at a point (x, y) in the image, the gradient is given by $g(x, y) = [g_x(x, y), g_y(x, y)]$ with magnitude $|g(x, y)|$, then using a Gaussian weighting function G, we can compute the following convolutions: $J(x, y) = G * g$; $J_x(x, y) = G * g_x$; and $J_y = G * g_y$. *Gradient coherence measurement* χ is defined as:

$$\chi(x,y) = \frac{(J_x^2(x,y) + J_y^2(x,y))^{1/2}}{J(x,y)}.$$

The coherence ranges from 0 in the absence of any dominant orientation in the neighborhood of (x,y), to 1 for a highly oriented pattern. The angle ω of $J(x,y)$ with the horizontal axis is given by

$$\arctan\left(\frac{J_y(x,y)}{J_x(x,y)}\right).$$

If P is a spinal pixel and A and B are as shown in Figure 9.24, then the spinal orientation s pointing towards the radial center can be estimated as:

$$s = \frac{\mathbf{a}}{|\mathbf{a}|} + \frac{\mathbf{b}}{|\mathbf{b}|}$$

where $\mathbf{a} = \mathbf{J}(A)$ and $\mathbf{b} = \mathbf{J}(B)$. The gradient coherence rule states that if P is a spinal pixel then it is possible to find two areas A and B in its neighborhood where the gradient is coherent and two other areas C and D where it is incoherent. The process of determining whether a pixel is spinal or not is shown in Figure 9.24. First the area centered at P is divided into four quadrants $Q_1 \ldots Q_4$, and four pixels A, B, C, D are chosen equidistant at a fixed distance from P. If both measures $\chi(A)\chi(B)$ and $\chi(C)\chi(D)$ are less than threshold T, then P is rejected as the spinal pixel ($T = 0.8$ in Ng and Bischof's study). The position of the potential spine can be determined by comparing $\chi(A)\chi(B)$ with $\chi(C)\chi(D)$. Further tests are conducted to confirm if a pixel is spinal. Ng and Bischof use the position of vectors $\mathbf{a}$ and $\mathbf{b}$ to reject any pixel as spinal if the gradients at A and B either or both move away from the spine or if both gradients are parallel. Another set of conditions rejects pixels as spinal if the spinal orientation is neither fully horizontal nor vertical within 10 degrees and $\mathbf{a}$ and $\mathbf{b}$ lie in certain quadrants. In Figure 9.24(c), a better estimate of spinal orientation s is illustrated. Here two new positions A$'$ and B$'$ are determined on a line normal to s and at the same distance as PA and PB. The new estimate of spinal orientation is given by:

$$s = \frac{\mathbf{a}'}{|\mathbf{a}'|} + \frac{\mathbf{b}'}{|\mathbf{b}'|}$$

where $\mathbf{a}' = \mathbf{J}(A')$ and $\mathbf{b}' = \mathbf{J}(B')$. If the estimates s and s' differ by more than a preset angle threshold ($15°$ in Ng and Bischof's study), then pixel P is rejected as a spinal pixel.

Spinal pixels are characterized by the following attributes: (i) location given by the pixel position; (ii) orientation given by estimate s; and (iii) spicular angle ϕ defined as

$$\phi = \pi - \arcsin\left(\frac{|a \times b|}{|a||b|}\right).$$

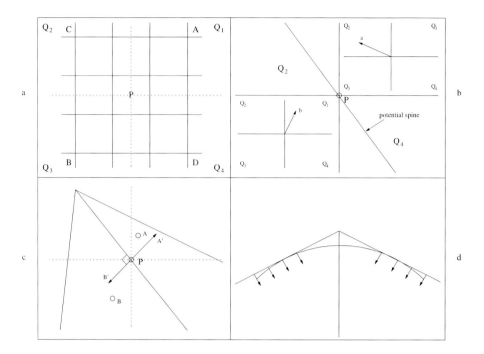

Figure 9.24: Detection of the spinal pixel P: (a) Measurement of the gradient field at pixel positions A, B, C and D in the four quadrants Q_1–Q_4 in the neighborhood of spinal pixel P. (b) Vectors **a** and **b** denote the average gradient fields at pixel positions A and B; (c) A$'$ and B$'$ gradients provide improved estimates of spinal orientation s. These two points lie on a line normal to the initial estimate of s; (d) Pixels on the boundary of large objects could pass spinal consistency tests but will be rejected if spicular angle ϕ is too large (from Ng and Bischof [895]; © Academic Press).

Very obtuse spicular angles indicate that the spinal pixel is responding to the boundary of a central mass or of some large object as shown in Figure 9.24(d). If the spicular angle is greater than say 130°, then P is rejected as a spinal pixel. Once all spinal pixels have been detected, the detection of the central mass using the Hough transform is relatively straightforward. Given a spinal position P and spinal orientation vector s, the radial center will lie on the line P + γs where $\gamma > 0$. It is assumed that the central mass is brighter than the background. Hence, the brightness along the line from P to the central mass in the direction of spinal orientation s should first increase, reach a local maximum at the mass center, and then decrease. The endpoint of the radial line is set as a point where brightness drops by a fixed amount.

Often in image segmentation, we might be interested in finding circular objects within the breast. A number of methods will respond best for a bright circular disc area superimposed on a dark background. The presence of spicules can weaken the response of such methods. In cases where we are primarily interested in finding a circular mass or the mass area first before spicules, it is a good idea to remove all spicules from the image. Spicule removal is achieved using a simple image filter or mask that removes all spinal pixels. The spinal pixel intensity is replaced by the median gray level of their neighboring pixels provided that the new gray level is darker than the old one. The detection of circular masses becomes an easier task once all spicules have been removed. The mask shown in Figure 9.25 can be used to respond positively to circular masses of a given size.

$$
\begin{array}{ccccccccc}
 & & & -1 & -1 & -1 & & & \\
 & & -1 & -1 & 0 & -1 & -1 & & \\
 & -1 & -1 & 0 & 1 & 0 & -1 & -1 & \\
-1 & -1 & 0 & 1 & 1 & 1 & 0 & -1 & -1 \\
-1 & 0 & 1 & 1 & 1 & 1 & 1 & 0 & -1 \\
-1 & -1 & 0 & 1 & 1 & 1 & 0 & -1 & -1 \\
 & -1 & -1 & 0 & 1 & 0 & -1 & -1 & \\
 & & -1 & -1 & 0 & -1 & -1 & & \\
 & & & -1 & -1 & -1 & & &
\end{array}
$$

Figure 9.25: A mask for detecting a central mass of diameter 5 pixels.

Masks of varying diameter can be used to detect masses of different sizes. A cross-correlation function can be used to find the response of applying the mask on a given area in the mammogram. If T is the template (mask), D is the mask size, and $f(x, y)$ represents the gray level at position (x, y) in the mammogram, then the cross-correlation function R at position (x, y) is given by:

$$
R = \frac{\sum_{i=1}^{D} \sum_{j=1}^{D} T(i,j).f(x+i, y+j)}{\left(\sum_{i=1}^{D} \sum_{j=1}^{D} T^2(i,j). \sum_{i=1}^{D} \sum_{j=1}^{D} f^2(x+i, y+j) \right)^{1/2}}
$$

By observing local maxima of R, the position of the central mass can be found.

9.9.7 Breast Alignment for Segmentation

9.9.7.1 Studies Involving Rigid Breast Alignments

Yin *et al.* [931] have investigated the performance of bilateral breast image subtraction with single-image processing. For the bilateral subtraction technique left and right image pairs were aligned, histogram equalized, thresholded, subtracted and run-length images are extracted. The resultant images were then binarized to which morphologic operators were applied. For the comparative single-view study, the gray-level thresholding was used to identify initial masses. Each image is divided into 100×100 pixel blocks and each sub-image is subjected to local contrast analysis and local thresholding. Using Free-response Receiver Operating Characteristic (FROC) analysis to evaluate the performance of each technique, the authors found that the bilateral subtraction technique was superior to the single view method. Mendez *et al.* [892] also proposed a computerized method to automatically detect malignant masses on digital mammograms based on bilateral subtraction. The breast border is first extracted using a tracing algorithm, then smoothed, and finally thresholded. The nipple was detected to align images using the maximum spatial height of the breast border if the nipple was in profile, otherwise its location is computed using the second derivative of the profile of gray levels across radial segments orientated towards the center. Alignment involved the translation of one image and the rotation around the nipple to maximize the correlation between the pixels of the two images. Image pairs are then normalized and subtracted giving images containing suspicious areas. In contrast to complete bilateral subtraction, Lau and Bischof [883] proposed an asymmetry measure as a method for detecting breast tumors. The asymmetry measures used are a compromise between absolute bilateral subtraction and asymmetry detection. Their method employs elements of a rigid rotation and image warping using three control points. A breast profile is initially extracted by adaptive threshold based on the analysis of the histogram of the breast image. The resultant profile is then smoothed using an averaging filter and the process of approximating plane curves using B-splines identifies control points. Initial translation and rotation of the image pairs around control points achieve alignment, then finally scaling along a baseline accounts for differences in breast shape. An asymmetry measure is then calculated based on the features extracted from each of the aligned images.

9.9.7.2   Studies Involving Deformable Breast Alignments

Wirth *et al.* [929] proposed a novel deformable method to align left and right breast images. The stages involved in the alignment include:

1. Image registration by establishing a frame of reference matching the corresponding mammograms using uniformity criteria.

2. Generation of a difference measure between the two mammograms and using that measure to generate an image that accentuates suspicious entities.

3. Use of a fusion technique where information contained in separate mammograms combined in a coherent manner by image subtraction.

The authors use a multi-quadratic function with a locality parameter to provide a 2-D deformation of a breast. The nipple was used as a control point found using Chandrasekhar's method (Chandrasekhar and Attikiouzel

[843]). The study was applied to selected images in the MIAS database (Suckling *et al.* [919]). Unfortunately, the authors do not report any quantitative results even though their qualitative results show that deformable alignment using Radial Basis Functions (RBF) results in fewer suspicious regions to subsequently segment. Karssemeijer *et al.* [875] employ a non-rigid mapping of breast pairs based on thin-plate splines. Seven equally spaced control points are selected along the edge of the breast border and pectoral boundary. Alignment is achieved by nonlinearly deforming the regions between these points in a manner that requires minimal warping energy. A simple contrast correction method is necessitated as a result of exposure differences when matching breast pairs. Following the subtraction process, the resultant images are smoothed with a large Gaussian kernel to account for anatomical variations and inaccuracies in their alignment.

9.10   Measures of Segmentation and Abnormality Detection

Segmentation evaluation and segmentation comparison are two distinctly different processes. The purpose of evaluation (intra-technique) is to quantitatively recognize how an algorithm treats various images in order to set appropriate parameters in a given domain. The purpose of segmentation comparison (inter-technique) is to rank different algorithms on the basis of their performance so that they can be selected in a given domain and their strong features can be retained in the development of new algorithms. A generic approach to the evaluation and comparison of different segmentation algorithms based on the use of synthetic images has been demonstrated by Zhang [937]. The images are designed to contain disks of varying size and shape. The complexity of the task is set according to the number of disks, their size and orientation and addition of Gaussian noise. The segmentation algorithms can be evaluated by: (i) evaluating their ability and consistency in treating images with different contents and/or acquired under different conditions, (ii) evaluating on a given set of images how the algorithm behaves with different parameter settings. Zhang proposes the use of the measure RUMA (Relative Ultimate Measurement Accuracy) which is defined as: $RUMA_f = (|R_f - S_f|).100\%$, where R_f denotes the feature value obtained from a reference image (ground truth) and S_f denotes the feature value from the segmented image. The smaller the value of this index, the better the quality of segmentation. The features to be selected depend on the problem domain (taken as *eccentricity* in Zhang's study). Other studies for reference on evaluation of segmentation algorithms include Pal and Pal [433], Sahoo [915], Zhang and Gerbrands [934, 935] and Zhang [936]. The criticism of these studies lies in the fact that no intra-evaluation of particular algorithms has been reported.

Kallergi *et al.* [872] have described in detail how the performance of detection algorithms can be evaluated in mammography. For the evaluation of automated techniques we need to have the ground truth and the guidelines for matching the computer-detected output to ground truth. The segmented region must be compared with the ground truth to see whether appropriate segmentation has been achieved and the degree of success in pinpointing the location of the abnormality. The definition of ground truth data is important. It usually includes information on the coordinates of the object centroid or the coordinates of the circle or ellipse encompassing the object. The size of the object is determined by finding its largest dimension, or recording major and minor axes of the ellipse surrounding it, or through the outline of its margins. In the case of calcifications, their inner distances are useful. The most common method of finding how well the object of interest has been segmented is to find some degree of overlap between the segmented region and the ground truth. Kallergi *et al.* suggested six possible approaches on how this could be accomplished. A detected area is defined as a true positive:

1. If the common area between the segmented and ground truth regions divided by the sum of the two is greater than a certain percentage, e.g. 30%. In this manner, an area detected by the computer that is too large is ignored.

2. If there is a certain percentage overlap of say 50% or more between segmented and ground truth regions. The overlap can be calculated on the basis of surrounding circles or ellipses. Additionally, the detected area can not be greater than twice the area of the true mass.

3. If it overlaps the centroid of the area of the mass defined by the radiologist. The weakness lies in the fact that there is no lower or upper limit on the size of the segmented region.

4. If the pixel with the maximum probability of suspiciousness is inside the truth file area.

5. In this case the true and false positives are defined at the pixel level as truth-and-test area and test-not-truth area respectively. We can separate those pixels that overlap with the truth region from those outside. The pixels of the true lesion W are specified and the TP% rate is now given as $(TP/W) \times 100$ and the FP% rate is $(FP/W) \times 100$. This approach requires an accurate definition of the margins.

6. If, for microcalcifications, its spatial location is within a distance of about 0.35 mm (0.5 mm is also used) from the location of a microcalcification in the truth file. The truth file consists of coordinates of the centers of the individual calcifications.

For microcalcification clusters, the definitions of true positive and false positive can be revised. A hit or true positive identification indicates the detection of at least N_{min} calcifications from the true center or a percentage in the area occupied by the true cluster. A false positive identification indicates the presence of N_{min} or more signals in a specific area that do not correspond to true calcifications. A microcalification cluster is defined as a true positive:

1. If a specified minimum number of signals is found inside the area containing the true cluster. Regions of interest often vary between 5×5 mm^2 and 15×15 mm^2. The area of the region of interest is used as a definition of the maximum area of the cluster. The number of minimum signals range from 1 to 5 and false positive clusters are those found outside the area of the true cluster. There is no requirement for the detected signals to correspond to true calcifications which can in turn lead to overestimated performance and misleading results.

2. If three or more signals are identified within a certain area and correspond to actual calcifications. This is an improved version of the above, but requires correlation between calcifications in true and segmented areas.

3. If the centroid of the cluster lies within the convex hull of the true calcifications marked by the radiologist or is within a certain distance (e.g. 5 mm) and a minimum number of its member signals are scored as true positives.

4. If the nearest neighbor distances are less than 5 mm and there are more than three or five signals linked in this way that correspond to true calcifications.

5. If the cluster contains at least three true calcifications within 1 cm^3.

It is obvious that if different definitions of what constitutes a true and false positive are used in different studies, their results can not be meaningfully compared. Hence, the same evaluation criteria must be followed for direct comparison. These criteria are discussed by Kallergi *et al.* in greater detail.

Chalana and Kim [838] describe a methodology for evaluating boundary detection algorithms on medical images. The authors identify the following reasons why medical image segmentation is hard to evaluate:

1. Lack of a definitive gold standard due to observer bias, inter, and intraobserver variability.

2. Difficulty in defining a metric for segmentation due to the complex multidimesionality of the segmentation data.

3. Lack of standard statistical protocols attributable to the lack of a gold standard and the absence of a segmentation metric.

4. Tedious and time-consuming data collection.

The authors propose a metric to measure the distance between a computer-generated boundary and a hand-outlined boundary. The metric is based on finding the Hausdorff distance between two curves that represent the two boundaries. Artificial correspondence between the two curves is determined in the absence of landmarks. In addition they describe a procedure for averaging multiple expert observers' outlines to generate a gold standard boundary, and finally propose statistical methods for validating the computer-generated boundaries against the boundaries identified by experts. Within the study, the authors use the methodology to evaluate image segmentation algorithms in ultrasound images. The authors conclude that the objective and quantitative evaluation and comparison of various medical image segmentation algorithms are important steps to their acceptance and clinical use.

The measurement of segmentation performance is a nontrivial task. The quality of segmentation depends on the complexity of the object and its background. In mammography, it is suggested that measures reported on the success of segmentation algorithms should relate performance to the size of masses detected. Polakowski *et al.* [902] have indexed the size of masses as: small (diameter < 0.5 cm); medium (diameter ≥ 0.5 cm and < 2 cm); large (diameter ≥ 2 cm and < 4 cm); and extra large (diameter ≥ 4 cm). Data can also be ground truthed on the basis of levels of subtlety. Mendez *et al.* [892] have used five levels: (i) obvious mass that is easy to detect by untrained observer; (ii) relatively obvious mass detectable by untrained observer; (iii) subtle mass detectable by observers with little mammographic experience; (iv) very subtle mass requiring more mammographic experience; and (v) extremely subtle mass detectable only by an expert mammographer. At the same time, it is very important that any segmentation program can be ranked against its competitors. Hoover *et al.* [866] describe the measures needed for comparing the machine-segmented image with the ground truth image to classify regions in one of the following five categories: (1) correct detection; (2) oversegmentation; (3) undersegmentation; (4) missed; and (5) noise. The accuracy of segmentation is quantified by computing the average and standard deviation of the differences between the angles made by all pairs of adjacent regions that are instances of correct detection in machine-segmented and ground truth images.

9.11   Feature Extraction From Segmented Regions

After mammogram enhancement where needed, and the segmentation of images, the next stage in a Computer Aided Detection (CAD) system is feature extraction. Features are extracted to characterize the region. Feature vectors from masses are assumed to be considered different from normal tissue, and based on a collection of their examples from several subjects, a system can be trained to differentiate between them. The main aim is that features should be sensitive and accurate for reducing false alarms. Typically a set or vector of features is extracted for a given segmented region. Features can be broadly classified as of type:

1. Morphological features relating to the morphology of the region.

2. Texture features characterizing the underlying texture of the region.

3. Clinical features extracted manually on the basis of clinical observations.

4. Gray scale distribution features relating to the gray-scale histogram of the image.

5. Other features including asymmetry measures, linear patterns and edge strengths.

6. Shape features.

A suitably designed classifier to discriminate between regions that are masses, non-masses, malignant and benign, uses the feature vectors. This section describes types of features that have been extracted in various mammographic studies from segmented regions together with an indication of their performance.

9.11.1 Morphological Features

Several studies have used morphological features that relate to the general morphology of a region. Yin *et al.* [931] extracted an area feature (the number of pixels that comprise the region) and a border feature (the distance in pixels from the region and the breast border). These were used to eliminate false positives resulting from the bilateral subtraction of breast pairs. The remaining regions were then subjected to a further area test and circularity test. The measure of the circularity of the region is calculated by forming a circle centered at the centroid of the region with the same area as the region. Circularity is then defined as the ratio of the area of the region within the circle to the total area of the region. In their study this feature was used to discard elongated suspicious regions. Petrick *et al.* [899] and Sahiner *et al.* [912] use a similar shape measure. The circularity measurement is defined as:

$$circularity = \frac{area(F_{OBJ} \cap F_{EQ})}{area(F_{OBJ})}$$

where bounding circle F_{EQ} has a center $F_{EQ}(x,y)$ bounded by a circle with an area equivalent to the region's area with a radius

$$r_{EQ} = \sqrt{\frac{area(F_{OBJ})}{\pi}}$$

as shown in Figure 9.26. The circularity measure gives a value between 0 and 1; the higher the number, the more circular the region. In addition the authors define a contrast test defined as the ratio of the average gray scale value for a selected portion inside the region to that outside the region. The test is used to eliminate those regions with low local contrasts. The definition of circularity by Ibrahim *et al.* [867] is as follows:

$$circularity = \frac{4\pi}{(contour\_length)^2}.$$

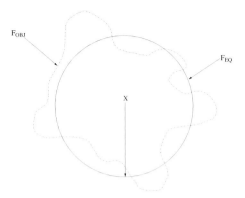

Figure 9.26: Calculation of Circularity Measure (from Petrick *et al.* [899]; ©
1996 IEEE).

Qian *et al.* [905] define an additional circularity measure as $Cl = p^2/S$
where p is the number of pixels making up the perimeter of the region and S
is area.

Morphological features have been widely used in a range of mammographic
studies. As an example, Polakowski *et al.* [902] have successfully used area,
contrast and circularity tests for finding medium-sized masses (more than 0.5
cm but less than 2 cm in diameter). The contrast test is conducted by finding
mass contrast defined as the ratio of the difference in the average gray scale in
ROI obtained finally and the average value of the gray scale outside the final
ROI but within the original pixel region, to the sum of the above averages.
The area test eliminates all regions greater than 1000 pixels, the circularity test
eliminates masses with circularity less than 0.58 and the contrast test eliminates
regions with contrast greater than 0.2. Similarly for microcalcifications, area
and circularity tests can be used. As an example, Ibrahim *et al.* [867] use an
area test to eliminate spots of size greater than 50 pixels. Using their circularity
measure, all regions of circularity greater than 0.5 are retained.

Petrick *et al.* [899] extract a rectangularity measure by constructing the
minimum bounding box F_{BB} to contain the object as shown in Figure 9.27.
The rectangularity of the region F_{OBJ} is then defined as the ratio of its area
to that of the box:

$$rectangularity = \frac{area(F_{OBJ})}{area(F_{BB})}.$$

The authors define five Normalized Radial Length (NRL) features based on
a radial length vector, r_k. The calculation is based on the Euclidean distance
from the centroid of F_{OBJ} at point X, as shown in Figure 9.28, to each of the
edge pixels where the maximum number of edge pixels is N_E. The results are
then normalized for a maximum radial length. Also the histogram of the radial
length was calculated giving a probability vector P_j. From these two vectors,
the features extracted include NRL mean (μ_{NRL}), standard deviation (σ_{NRL}),

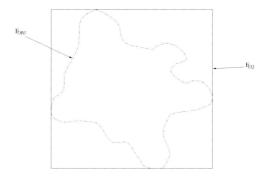

Figure 9.27: Calculation of Rectangularity Measure.

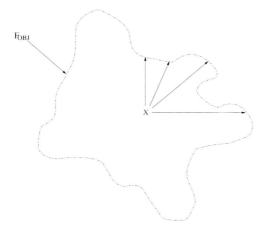

Figure 9.28: Calculation of Normalized Radial Length Features.

entropy (E_{NRL}), area ratio (AR_{NRL}) and zero-crossing count (ZCC_{NRL}).

The NRL vector is given by $\mathbf{r} = \{r_k : 0 \le k \le N_E - 1\}$, where N_E is the number of edge pixels in the object. The histogram of the radial length is calculated yielding the probability vector given by $\mathbf{p} = \{p_j : 0 \le j \le N_H - 1\}$, where N_H is the number of bins used in the histogram.

The calculation of these NRL features is given by (Petrick *et al.*, [898]) as follows:

$$\mu_{NRL} = \frac{1}{N_E} \sum_{k=0}^{N_E - 1} r_k$$

$$\sigma_{NRL} = \sqrt{\frac{1}{N} \sum_{k=0}^{N_E - 1} (r_k - \mu_{NRL})^2}$$

$$E_{NRL} = - \sum_{j=0}^{N_H - 1} p_j \log(p_j)$$

$$AR_{NRL} = \left\{ \frac{1}{N_E \mu_{NRL}} \sum_{k=0}^{N_E - 1} (r_k - \mu_{NRL}) : r_k > \mu_{NRL} \right\}$$

$$ZCC_{NRL} \equiv \text{number of zero crossings of } \{r_k - \mu_{NRL}\}_{k=0}^{N_E - 1}$$

In their study, Rangayyan *et al.* [907] extract a variety of morphological features. These include:

1. *Compactness (C)*
   A measure of contour complexity versus the enclosed area, defined as $C = p^2/a$ where p and a are the object perimeter length and region area in pixels respectively. The authors noted that a malignant spiculated border could be expected to have a higher C value than a smooth and round benign mass.

2. *Fourier Descriptors (FD)*
   In order to calculate the *FD*s, the (x, y) co-ordinates of the perimeter pixels are represented as complex values given by the equation $Z_i = x_i + jy_i; i = 0, 1, ..., N - 1$. The *FD*s are now defined as:

   $$A(n) = \frac{1}{N} \sum_{i=0}^{N-1} Z_i \exp[-j2\pi ni/N], n = 0, 1, \ldots, N - 1$$

   for $n = 0, 1, \ldots, N - 1$. Using only the magnitude of the *FD*s, normalized *FD*s (*NFD*s) may be obtained as:

   $$NFD(k) = \left\{ \begin{array}{ll} 0; & k = 0 \\ A(k)/A(1); & k = 1, 2, ..., N/2 \\ A(k + N)/A(1); & k = -1, -2, ..., -N/2 + 1 \end{array} \right\}.$$

   The final *FD* based shape factor is given by:

   $$FF = 1 - \frac{\sum\limits_{k=-N/2+1}^{N/2} \|NFD(k)\| \, / \, \|k\|}{\sum\limits_{k=-N/2}^{N/2} \|NFD(k)\|}.$$

   The authors found that the *FF* feature was insensitive to noise and invariant to translation, rotation, starting point and contour size. Its value becomes larger as the object shape becomes more complex and rough but remains in the range $(0, 1)$.

Ng and Bischof [895] developed a tumor differentiation technique to discriminate between spiculated and circumscribed lesions. A spicularity measure was defined as the number of spicules connected to a lesion. These spicules were detected during the segmentation process. Two conditions must be met in order for a spicule to be considered connected: (i) it should not be located inside any of the central mass, and (ii) the spinal direction line should cross the boundary of the mass. Using these two criteria, the authors were able to correctly classify 90% of the regions within their data set as spiculated or circumscribed.

Chan *et al.* [841] propose a set of morphological features that may be selected from mammographic microcalcifications. The authors have developed an automated signal extraction process to determine the size, contrast, Signal-to-Noise Ratio (SNR) and shape of the microcalcification from a mammogram based on the co-ordinates of each individual microcalcification. A detailed list of the feature descriptors is given below:

1. *Size of Microcalcification (SA)*
   This is estimated as the number of pixels in the signal region.

2. *Mean Density (MD)*
   The mean density is the average of the pixel values above the background level within the signal region.

3. *Eccentricity (EC)*
   The eccentricity is the effective ellipse that can be derived from the major and minor axes given as $\varepsilon = \sqrt{a^2 - b^2}/a$ where the lengths of the major axis, $2a$ and minor axis, $2b$ are given by:

$$2a = \sqrt{2[M_{xx} + M_{yy} + \sqrt{(M_{xx} - M_{yy})^2 + 4M_{xy}^2}]}$$

and

$$2b = \sqrt{2[M_{xx} + M_{yy} + \sqrt{(M_{xx} - M_{yy})^2 + 4M_{xy}^2}]}.$$

The axes are derived from the second moments calculated as:

$$M_{xx} = \sum_i g_i(x_i - M_x)^2/M_0$$

$$M_{yy} = \sum_i g_i(y_i - M_y)^2/M_0$$

$$M_{xy} = \sum_i g_i(x_i - M_x)(y_i - M_y)/M_0$$

where g_i is the pixel value above the background, and (x_i, y_i) are the coordinates of the ith pixel. The moments M_o, M_x and M_y are defined as follows:

$$M_0 = \sum_i g_i$$

$$M_x = \sum_i g_i x_i / M_0$$

$$M_y = \sum_i g_i y_i / M_0$$

4. *Moment Ratio (MR)*
   This is defined as the ratio of M_{xx} to M_{yy} with the larger second moment in the denominator.

5. *Axis Ratio (AR)*
   The axis ratio is the ratio of the major axis to the minor axis of the effective ellipse.

9.11.2   Texture Features

Texture features provide a measure of the underlying texture within a given region. A variety of methods are used to extract texture characteristics. Some of the commonly-used approaches include the use of spatial frequencies, edge frequencies, run lengths, pixel's joint probability distribution and special masks such as Law's masks. It has been demonstrated in different studies that different feature extraction methods can yield different results based on the application domain. Here we define the above approaches of feature extraction.

9.11.2.1   Features Based on Spatial Frequency – Autocorrelation Texture Description

The textural character of an image depends on the spatial size of texture primitives. Large primitives give rise to coarse texture (e.g. rock surface) and small primitives give fine texture (e.g. silk surface). An autocorrelation function can be evaluated that measures this coarseness. This function evaluates the linear spatial relationships between primitives. If the primitives are large, the function decreases slowly with increasing distance whereas it decreases rapidly if the texture consists of small primitives. However, if the primitives are periodic, then the autocorrelation increases and decreases periodically with distance. The set of autocorrelation coefficients shown below are used as texture features:

$$C_{ff}(p,q) = \frac{MN}{(M-p)(N-q)} \frac{\sum\limits_{i=1}^{M-p} \sum\limits_{j=1}^{N-q} f(i,j)f(i+p,j+q)}{\sum\limits_{i=1}^{M} \sum\limits_{j=1}^{N} f^2(i,j)},$$

where p, q is the positional difference in the i, j direction, and M, N are image dimensions.

9.11.2.2 Features Based on Edge Frequency

A number of edge detectors can be used to yield an edge image from an original image. We can compute an edge-dependent texture description function E as follows:

$$E = |f(i,j) - f(i+d,j)| + |f(i,j) - f(i-d,j)|$$
$$+ |f(i,j) - f(i,j+d)| + f(i,j) - f(i,j-d)|$$

This function is inversely related to the autocorrelation function. Texture features can be evaluated by choosing specified distances d.

9.11.2.3 Features Based on SGLD Matrices

Statistical methods use second order statistics to model the relationships between pixels within the region by constructing Spatial Gray Level Dependency (SGLD) matrices. A SGLD matrix is the joint probability occurrence of gray levels i and j for two pixels with a defined spatial relationship in an image. The spatial relationship is defined in terms of distance d and angle θ_k. If the texture is coarse and distance d is small compared with the size of the texture elements, the pairs of points at distance d should have similar gray levels. Conversely, for a fine texture, if distance d is comparable to the texture size, then the gray levels of points separated by distance d should often be quite different, so that the values in the SGLD matrix should be spread out relatively uniformly. Hence, a good way to analyze texture coarseness would be, for various values of distance d, some measure of scatter of the SGLD matrix around the main diagonal. Similarly, if the texture has some direction, i.e. is coarser in one direction than another, then the degree of spread of the values about the main diagonal in the SGLD matrix should vary with the direction d. Thus texture directionality can be analyzed by comparing spread measures of SGLD matrices constructed at various distances d.

Conners and Harlow [846] examined the effects of distortion caused by variations in the image acquisition process, including exposure time, development time and scanner settings in radiographic images. The authors observed that equal probability quantization normalizes the image contrast and provides a near optimal way to reduce the number of gray levels in the image whilst retaining an accurate representation. In addition the technique makes the SGLD matrices invariant to the distortions described. Haralick *et al.* [859] describe an algorithm to iteratively quantize the remaining unquantized gray levels into the remaining number of levels. This is summarized below.

SGLD Quantization Algorithm

1. Let x be a non-negative random variable with a cumulative probability distribution function F_x.

2. Let G_x, the K-level equal probability quantization function for x, be defined as $G_x = k$ if and only if $g_{k-1} \leq x < g_k$, where g_{k-1} and g_k are the end points of the kth quantization level and $k = 1, \ldots, K$.

3. Iterate to find the quantization levels g_k as follows:

   - Let $g_0 = 0$.
   - Assume g_{k-1} is defined.
   - Then g_k is the smallest number such that $\forall g$

$$\left| \frac{1 - F_x(g_{k-1})}{K - (k-1)} - (F_x(g_k) - F_x(g_{k-1})) \right| \leq \left| \frac{1 - F_x(g_{k-1})}{K - (k-1)} - (F_x(g) - F_x(g_{k-1})) \right|.$$

From SGLD matrices, a variety of features may be extracted. The original investigation into SGLD features was pioneered by Haralick *et al.* [859]. From each SGLD matrix, fourteen statistical measures are extracted using the nomenclature given in Table 9.1.

$p(i,j) = p(i,j)/R$

(i,j)th entry in a normalized SGLD matrix, $p(i,j,d,\theta)$ where i, j are the gray scale values of pixels at distance d pixels apart, and angle θ is the angle of the line joining the centers of these pixels in the creation of the SGLD matrix.

$p_x(i) = \sum_{j=1}^{N_g} p(i,j)$

ith entry in the marginal-probability matrix obtained by summing the rows of $p(i,j)$.

N_g

Number of gray levels in the image.

$$p_y(j) = \sum_{i=1}^{N_g} p(i,j)$$

jth entry in the marginal-probability matrix obtained by summing the columns of $p(i,j)$.

$$p_{x+y}(k) = \sum_{i=1}^{N_g} \sum_{j=1}^{N_g} p(i,j); k = 2, 3, ..., 2N_g$$

The result of adding the ith and jth entries calculated above from the marginal-probability matrix.

$$p_{x-y}(k) = \sum_{i=1}^{N_g} \sum_{j=1}^{N_g} p(i,j); k = 0, 1, 2, ..., 2N_g - 1$$

The result of subtracting the ith and jth entries calculated above from the marginal-probability matrix.

Table 9.1: Statistical measures nomenclature

The 14 texture features given by Haralick *et al.* [859] are shown in Table 9.2.

Angular Second Moment (ASM)

$$f_1 = \sum_{i=1} \sum_{j=1} (p(i,j))^2$$

Contrast

$$f_2 = \sum_{n=0}^{N_g-1} n^2 \left(\sum_{i=1}^{N_g} \sum_{j=1}^{N_g} p(i,j) \right)$$

Correlation

$$f_3 = \frac{\sum_i \sum_j (i,j) p(i,j) - \mu_x \mu_y}{\sigma_x \sigma_y}$$

where $\mu_x = \sum\limits_{i=0}^{n-1} i p_x(i)$

$\sigma_x^2 = \sum\limits_{i=0}^{n-1} (i - \mu_x)^2 p_x(i)$

$\mu_y = \sum\limits_{j=0}^{n-1} j p_y(j)$

$\sigma_y^2 = \sum\limits_{j=0}^{n-1} (j - \mu_y)^2 p_y(j)$

Sum of Squares: Variance

$$f_4 = - \sum_i \sum_j (i - \nu)^2 p(i,j)$$

Inverse Different Moment

$$f_5 = - \sum_i \sum_j \frac{1}{1+(i-j)^2} p(i,j)$$

Sum Average

$$f_6 = \sum_{i=2}^{2N_g} i p_{x+y}(i)$$

Sum Variance

$$f_7 = \sum_{i=2}^{2N_g} (i - f_6)^2 p_{x+y}(i)$$

Sum Entropy

$$f_8 = - \sum_{i=2}^{2N_g} p_{x+y}(i) \log(p_{x+y}(i))$$

Entropy

$$f_9 = - \sum_i \sum_j p(i,j) \log(p(i,j))$$

Difference Variance

f_{10} = variance of p_{x-y}

Difference Entropy

$$f_{11} = -\sum_{i=0}^{N_g-1} p_{x-y}(i)\log(p_{x-y}(i))$$

Information Measure of Correlation I

$$f_{12} = \frac{HXY-HXY1}{\max(HX,HY)}$$

where $HXY = -\sum_i\sum_j p(i,j)\log(p(i,j))$

and $HXY1 = -\sum_i\sum_j p(i,j)\log(p_x(i)p_y(j))$

and $HXY2 = -\sum_i\sum_j p_x(i)p_y(j)\log(p_x(i)p_y(j))$

and HX and HY are entropies of p_x, p_y.

Information Measure of Correlation II

$$f_{13} = (1-\exp[-2.0(HXY2-HXY)])^{\frac{1}{2}}$$

where $HXY = -\sum_i\sum_j p(i,j)\log(p(i,j))$

and $HXY1 = -\sum_i\sum_j p(i,j)\log(p_x(i)p_y(j))$

and $HXY2 = -\sum_i\sum_j p_x(i)p_y(j)\log(p_x(i)p_y(j))$

and HX and HY are entropies of p_x, p_y.

Maximal Correlation Coefficient

f_{14} = (second largest eigenvalue of Q)$^{\frac{1}{2}}$

where $Q(i,j) = \sum_k \frac{p(i,k)p(j,k)}{p_x(i)p_y(k)}$

Table 9.2

The *angular second moment* is a measure of the homogeneity of the image. In a homogenous image there are very few dominant gray tone changes and the SGLD matrix will have only a few entries of a large magnitude. Conversely in a less homogenous image there will be many entries in the SGLD matrix of smaller magnitude and hence the ASM will be smaller in magnitude. The *contrast* feature is the difference moment of the SGLD matrix and is a measure of the amount of local variation in the image. A low value of contrast results from uniform images whereas images with large variation produce a high value. *Correlation* is a measure of gray level linear-dependency within the image. It measures the degree to which the rows and columns of the SGLD matrix resemble each other. High values are obtained when the matrix elements are uniformly equal and low values are obtained for a matrix with large differences in element values. The *entropy* of the image is a measure of the randomness of gray pixel values. When the SGLD matrix is equal, the entropy is the highest. Low values for entropy are obtained when matrix elements are very different from each other (large variability). Hence higher values for entropy indicate greater randomness in the image. For a complete description of these features, please refer to Haralick and Shapiro [244].

Several researchers have applied techniques proposed by Haralick *et al.* [859] to find a discriminatory set of features for subsequent feature analysis. Chan *et al.* [839] evaluated eight of the fourteen features: correlation, entropy, energy, inertia, inverse difference moment, sum average, sum entropy and difference entropy. After running discriminant analysis, six features were selected as most discriminant: correlation ($45°$), correlation ($135°$), difference entropy ($45°$), difference entropy ($135°$), entropy ($135°$) and inertia ($90°$). The performance of the technique was evaluated using ROC analysis resulting in the maximum value of $Az = 0.83$ for training and $Az = 0.82$ for testing. These results were achieved by constructing the SGLD matrices at a distance of 20 pixels. Sahiner *et al.* [914] extracted the SGLD texture features from ROI identified using the Rubber Band Straightening (RBST) algorithm. Matrices were constructed at distances ($d = 1, 2, 3, 4, 6, 8, 12$ and 16) and in four directions ($\theta = 0°, 45°, 90°$ and $135°$) and the following features were extracted: correlation, energy, difference entropy, inverse difference moment, entropy, sum average, sum entropy and inertia. Classification results obtained from an RBST image for these texture features were evaluated using ROC analysis and gave a maximum $Az = 0.95$ in training and $Az = 0.90$ in testing. Wei *et al.* [926] extracted two types of global and local texture features from the whole ROI image and partitions of the ROI respectively. For the global texture features, the authors calculated 13 statistical texture features from SGLD matrices constructed for the original image and sub-images resulting from an application of a wavelet transform. The extraction of the local texture features involved the segmentation of the ROI into a mass and a periphery background. From the segmented suspicious mass and periphery, SGLD matrices were constructed and 13 texture features were extracted. Their data set comprised ROI that had been subjected to the previously described DWCE algorithm. Using linear discriminant analysis and following ROC analysis, the global texture features gave $Az = 0.93$, the local texture features gave $Az = 0.96$ and combined global and local texture features gave $Az = 0.97$. The authors concluded that the study demonstrated the effectiveness of multi-resolution feature analysis in the reduction of false positives for mass detection. In a similar study, Petrick *et al.* [898] extracted 13 texture features at various distances and angles from SGLD matrices constructed from the ROI within multi-resolution images obtained from a wavelet transform giving 364 global multi-distance texture features for each ROI. Local texture features were also extracted from the segmented ROI. Classification of the feature sets was performed using linear discriminant analysis. The results from the best test data set gave a global True Positive (TP) detection of 82 out of 84 and local TP detection of 81 out of 84. The global texture features gave a higher false-positive rate of 32.6 false positives per image, the local texture features performed better with 12.4 false positives per image. Using all data sets and extracting the most salient features from both local and global texture feature sets, stepwise feature selection after Free Receiver Operating Characteristic (FROC) analysis gave 3.77 false positives per image at a 90% TP fraction threshold.

9.11.2.4 Features Based on GLDS Vectors

The use of Gray Level Difference Statistics (GLDS) features (Weszka *et al.* [927]) have been investigated by Sahiner *et al.* [913] for differentiating between masses and normal breast tissue. GLDS features extracted from the GLDS vector of an image provide a measure of the image coarseness. An algorithm to compute the GLDS vector is given below.

GLDS Vector Formation Algorithm

1. Assume a displacement vector for a pixel pair displacement in the horizontal and vertical direction given as $d = (d_1, d_2)$ respectively.

2. For a given ROI $H(i, j)$, compute a difference image H_d as $H_d(i, j) = |H(i, j) - H(i + d_1, j + d_2)|$.

3. Assign the kth entry in the GLDS vector p_d as the probability of occurrence of the pixel value k in the difference image $H_d(i, j)$ where a maximum pixel value is given as K.

If the image texture is coarse and the length of the displacement vector d is small compared with the texture element size, then the pixel values separated by d will have similar pixel values. This implies that all the elements of the GLDS vector will be concentrated around zero, i.e. $p_d(k)$ will be large for small values of k and small for large values of k. If the length of the vector d is comparable to the texture element size, then the elements of the GLDS vector will be distributed more evenly. Sahiner *et al.* [913] give the following four features that may be extracted from the GLDS vector $p_d(k)$.

1. Contrast

$$CON = \sum_{k=0}^{K-1} k^2 p_d(k).$$

2. Angular Second Moment

$$ASM = \sum_{k=0}^{K-1} p_d(k)^2.$$

3. Entropy

$$G\_ENT = \sum_{k=0}^{K-1} p_d(k) \log p_d(k).$$

4. Mean

$$MEAN = \frac{1}{K} \sum_{k=0}^{K-1} p_d(k).$$

9.11.2.5   Features Based on SRDM

Kim and Park [877] detail a comparative evaluation of various texture-based features including features extracted using their previously developed Surrounding Region-Dependence Method (SRDM). The SRDM is based on a second-order histogram in two surrounding regions whose window sizes are determined based on the lesion size to be detected. Details on the construction of these types of matrices can be found in Kim and Park [877]. The authors found that analysis of the matrix provided an insight into the underlying texture of the image. If the texture is smooth, it is very possible that a pixel and its surrounding pixels will have a similar gray-level. This means that the distribution of the elements will be concentrated in or near the upper left corner of the matrix. If the image has a fine texture then it is possible that the difference between a pixel and its surrounding area will be large, therefore the distribution of the pixels within the matrix will be spread out along the diagonal. From these characteristics of the distribution in the region-dependence matrix, the authors propose the following four features:

1. *Horizontal-Weighted Sum (HWS)*

$$HWS = \frac{1}{N} \sum_{i=0}^{m} \sum_{j=0}^{n} j^2 r(i,j)$$

2. *Vertical-Weighted Sum (VWS)*

$$VWS = \frac{1}{N} \sum_{i=0}^{m} \sum_{j=0}^{n} i^2 r(i,j)$$

3. *Diagonal-Weighted Sum (DWS)*

$$DWS = \frac{1}{N} \sum_{i=0}^{m+n} k^2 \left(\sum_{\substack{i=0 \\ i+j=k}}^{m} \sum_{j=0}^{n} r(i,j) \right)$$

4. *Grid-Weighted Sum (GWS)*

$$GWS = \frac{1}{N} \sum_{i=0}^{m} \sum_{j=0}^{n} ijr(i,j)$$

where m and n are the total number of pixels within the region and $r(i,j)$ is the reciprocal of the element from the region-dependence matrix given as

$$r(i,j) = \left\{ \begin{array}{ll} \frac{1}{\alpha(i,j)}, & if\, \alpha(i,j) > 0 \\ 0, & otherwise \end{array} \right\}.$$

N is the total number of elements in the surrounding region dependence matrix, given by:

$$N = \sum_{i=0}^{m} \sum_{j=0}^{n} \alpha(i,j),$$

where $\alpha(i,j)$ is the element of the matrix.

In addition to the above features, fractal geometry has been used in many studies as a feature to discriminate between masses and non-masses. Fractal models typically relate a metric property such as line length or surface area to an elementary length or area used as a basis for determining the metric property. Mandelbrot [886] illustrates the concept using the example task of measuring a coastline with a 1 km ruler laid end to end. The same procedure can be repeated with a shorter ruler and it can be seen that using a shorter ruler will result in an increased total measured length. The relationship between the ruler length and the coast length can be considered as a measure of the coastline's geometric properties, e.g. roughness. The functional relationship between the measured length L and the ruler size r can be expressed as: $L = cr^{1-D}$ where c is a scaling constant and D is the fractal dimension using this concept. Byng *et al.* [835] investigated the relationship between mammographic texture and carcinoma risk. The fractal dimension measure was used to quantify the underlying texture of the image and the authors concluded that the fractal dimension was related to the risk of developing breast carcinoma. Taylor *et al.* [920] used the fractal dimension measure to determine whether a breast was fatty or dense. Using ROC analysis, the authors found that the fractal dimension measure was more discriminatory than Laws' $R5R5$ texture energy and standard deviation based measure. Pohlman *et al.* [901] used the fractal dimension as a feature to discriminate between benign and malignant lesions segmented using a region growing technique. Using ROC analysis, the authors found that the fractal measure performed better than the morphological feature of compactness and shape roughness giving a high value of $Az = 0.812$ after ROC analysis.

9.11.2.6   Features based on special masks

Laws [884] observed that certain gradient operators such as Laplacian and Sobel operators accentuated the underlying microstructure of texture within an image. This was the basis for a feature extraction scheme based on a series of pixel impulse response arrays obtained from combinations of 1-D vectors shown in Figure 9.29. Each 1-D array is associated with an underlying microstructure and labeled accordingly using an acronym. The arrays are convolved with other arrays in a combinatorial manner to generate a total of 25 masks, typically labeled as $L5L5$ for the mask resulting from the convolution of the two L5 arrays.

$$
\begin{aligned}
\text{Level} \quad L5 &= \begin{bmatrix} 1 & 4 & 6 & 4 & 1 \end{bmatrix} \\
\text{Edge} \quad E5 &= \begin{bmatrix} -1 & -2 & 0 & 2 & 1 \end{bmatrix} \\
\text{Spot} \quad S5 &= \begin{bmatrix} -1 & 0 & 2 & 0 & -1 \end{bmatrix} \\
\text{Wave} \quad W5 &= \begin{bmatrix} -1 & 2 & 0 & -2 & 1 \end{bmatrix} \\
\text{Ripple} \quad R5 &= \begin{bmatrix} 1 & -4 & 6 & -4 & 1 \end{bmatrix}
\end{aligned}
$$

Figure 9.29: Five 1-D arrays identified by Laws [884].

These masks are subsequently convolved with a texture field to accentuate its microstructure giving an image from which the energy of the microstructure arrays is measured together with other statistics. The energy measure for a neighborhood centered at $F(j, k), S(j, k)$, is based on the neighborhood standard deviation computed from the mean image amplitude, (Pratt [903]):

$$
S(j, k) = \frac{1}{W^2} \left[\sum_{m=-W}^{W} \sum_{n=-W}^{W} [F(j + m, k + n) - M(j + m, k + n)]^2 \right]^{\frac{1}{2}}
$$

where $W \times W$ is the pixel neighborhood and the mean image amplitude $M(j, k)$ is defined as:

$$
M(j, k) = \frac{1}{W^2} \sum_{m=-w}^{w} \sum_{n=-w}^{w} F(j + m, k + n)
$$

In its application to mammography, Laws' texture measures were used by Kegelmeyer *et al.* [876]. In their study, the authors found that the masks *L5E5*, *E5S5*, *L5S5* and *R5R5* were shown to be superior to other masks. Gupta *et al.* [856] drew on previous work by Miller and Astley [894] that the *R5R5* mask combination gave the best results. In their study they found that this mask produced a true lesion outline for 70% of the abnormalities. Polakowski *et al.* [902] applied Laws masks to a segmented image following false positive reduction using morphological analysis. A derivative-based neural network feature saliency algorithm was used to select the features that have the largest effect on determining the neural network classifier's decision boundary. The authors found the *W5R5* mask combination had the highest ranking; their results were supported by observations made by Kegelmeyer *et al.* [876] in their identification of the most important masks. Polakowski *et al.* [902] obtained results giving 100% classification accuracy for true positive lesions with a false positive rate of 1.8 per image.

9.11.3 Other Features

9.11.3.1 Edge Strengths

Kegelmeyer *et al.* [876] investigated the use of Analysis of Local Orientated Edges (ALOE) features. These features were designed specifically for the detection of spiculated lesions. The clinical basis for ALOE features is the presence of architectural distortion within the breast associated with such a lesion. A spiculated lesion changes the underlying image gradient radial pattern causing localized gradients to emanate from the structure, as shown in Figure 9.30.

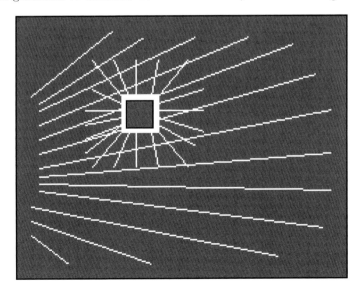

Figure 9.30: Radial patterns present within a breast containing a lesion (from Kegelmeyer *et al.* [876]; © RSNA).

Figure 9.30 shows the two texture properties exhibited in a breast with a spiculated lesion: uniform edge direction (long lines) and localized mixed edge detection (short lines). ALOE features aim to detect areas where the edge direction is mixed in order to identify lesions. The technique is implemented by centring a 4 cm × 4 cm moving window around each pixel and computing the edge orientations using a Sobel operator in that window. From these orientations, a histogram is constructed and the flatness of the histogram is computed by determining the standard deviation of the bin height. The standard deviation is the ALOE feature for that pixel. Typically flat histograms are associated with spiculated lesions whereas a peaked histogram is associated with normal tissue. The authors reported that whilst this feature is sensitive to spiculated lesions, it generates a large number of false positives and therefore it should be used in conjunction with other features. In another study te Brake *et al.* [921] extended the ALOE features to include the use of relative orientations. The authors reported a sensitivity of 60% with a specificity of 3 false positives per image. Rangayyan *et al.* [907] extracted an actuance measure A, as a measure of the edge strength. As part of the segmentation process the authors used polygons to approximate the boundary of the region. The authors noted that since malignant tumors have fuzzy (ill-defined) boundaries, it is expected that the actuance measure would be low for malignant masses and high for benign masses. Their algorithm is summarized below.

9.11.3.2 Actuance Measure

For every point on the perimeter, a normal of 160 pixels is drawn comprising of 80 pixels inside the region, $f(i)$ and 80 pixels outside $b(i)$ for $i = 1, 2, ..., n_j$ where n_j is the number of pixels inside and outside the ROI as shown in Figure 9.31. Calculate the sum of the differences $d(j)$ along the normal to each boundary point $j = 0, 1, ..., N - 1$, where N is the number of boundary points of the region as

$$d(j) = \frac{\sum\limits_{i=1}^{n_j} f(i) - b(i)}{2i}.$$

The normalized value of $d(j)$ is then computed over all boundary pixels to obtain the actuance measure A as

$$A = \frac{1}{d_{\max}} \sqrt{\frac{1}{N} \sum_{j=0}^{N-1} \frac{d^2(j)}{n_j}}$$

where $d_{\max}$ is a normalization factor dependent on the maximum gray-level range.

9.11.3.3 Asymmetry Measures

Lau and Bischof [883] investigated the use of an asymmetry feature for use with a breast pair approach to mass classification. The authors proposed that

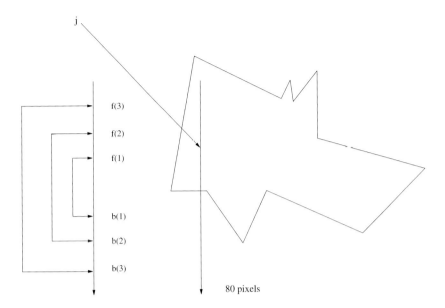

Figure 9.31: Calculation of Actuance Measure A (from Rangayyan *et al.* [907]; © 1997 IEEE).

strong structural asymmetries between corresponding regions in the left and right breast are taken as evidence for the possible presence of a tumor in that region. The asymmetry measure for a point (x, y) is given as:

$$A(x, y) = [B(x, y) + R(x, y) + Q(x, y)] * W(x, y),$$

where:

Brightness $B(x, y)$:
On the basis of clinical asymmetry observations, large gray-level differences between aligned breast corresponding regions can indicate the presence of a tumor. Differences in image acquisition conditions are accounted for by normalizing breast pairs $N_L(x, y)$ and $N_R(x, y)$ for left and right breast pairs, and inaccuracies in alignment are resolved using an averaging filter $a_2(x, y)$. The brightness is defined as:

$$B(x, y) = |(N_L(x, y) - N_R(x, y)) * a_2(x, y)|$$

where * denotes convolution.

Roughness $R(x, y)$:
Roughness is a measure of texture. It is based on the variance measure extracted from the local normalized variance window. Given a variance window V and a large normalization window W with variance σ_v^2 and σ_w^2, the normalized local variance at $f(x, y)$, is given as: $v(x, y) = \sigma_v^2/\sigma_w^2$. Roughness

is the difference between the two regions in the left and right breast pairs: $R(x,y) = |v_L(x,y) - v_R(x,y)|$.

Brightness-to-Roughness $Q(x,y)$:
Given a digitized mammogram $M(x,y)$, the authors hypothesized that the brightness to roughness ratio may also help discriminate between region types. In this measure, the authors provide a more specific definition of roughness within a window W of size $n \times n$ pixels using the running sum of absolute gray-level differences in horizontal, h, and vertical, v, directions. Hence:

$$p_j = \frac{1}{n^2} \sum_{(x,y) \in W} (h_j(x,y) + v_j(x,y))$$

where

$$h_j = \left\{ \begin{array}{ll} 1; & |M(x+1,y) - M(x,y)| = j \\ 0; & otherwise \end{array} \right\}$$

and

$$v_j = \left\{ \begin{array}{ll} 1; & |M(x,y+1) - M(x,y)| = j \\ 0; & otherwise \end{array} \right\}.$$

Now roughness is defined as

$$\sigma_W = \sum_{j=0}^{255} j^2 p_j$$

and the brightness-to-roughness ratio for window W centered at (x,y) is defined as

$$q(x,y) = \frac{\mu_W^2}{(1+\sigma_W)}$$

where μ_W is defined as the average gray-level within the window W.

Finally the brightness-to-roughness difference is calculated as: $Q(x,y) = |q_L(x,y) - q_R(x,y)|$.

9.11.3.4   Directionality

Directionally strong responses are typically associated with blood vessels or glandular tissue, whereas tumors rarely appear as highly orientated patterns. A directionality measure D is computed from a Fourier transform of the brightness profile within a window W. The vertical directionality D within a window W, is given as $D = P_v/P_w$ where P_v is the total power for a given direction and P_W is the total power in W. The authors observed that for non-orientated patterns, the value of D is $1/2$ whereas for highly orientated vertical patterns it approaches 1 and for highly orientated horizontal patterns it is close to 0. The directionality measure is incorporated into a weighting factor $W(x, y)$ defined as: $W(x, y) = \max[0, 1 - D_p(x, y)]$ where

$$D_p(x, y) = D_L^p(x, y) + D_R^p(x, y),$$

where D_L^p and D_R^p are the directionality measures for the left and right breast both raised to the pth power.

On evaluating the performance of the asymmetry measure, the authors final result showed 12 out of 13 suspicious areas were detected with an average of 4.9 false positives per image.

9.11.3.5 Grayscale Histogram Frequency and Distribution

Statistical features based on the gray-scales of pixels making up a segmented region have been used extensively by many researchers in the field of digital mammography. Li *et al.* [885] extracted three features: the intensity variation within the extracted region, the mean intensity difference between the extracted region and the surrounding area, and the mean gradient of the boundary. Taylor *et al.* [920] used statistical measures of standard deviation and skewness in their investigation into the classification of breast tissue as fatty or dense. From a 128×128 pixel ROI, five sub-sampled images were extracted and the two statistical features calculated from each. The authors found that the skewness feature outperformed Laws $R5R5$ texture energy and fractal dimension in discrimination. In the classification of suspicious ROI as a result of bilateral subtraction, Mendez *et al.* [892] extracted the following features based on the absolute values of the gray scales contained within: maximum grayscale, minimum grayscale, average grayscale, gray levels at 5% of cumulative frequency distribution, and gray levels at 95% of cumulative frequency distribution. In their results, the authors found that following the classification using linear discriminant analysis, the features *95% of CFD*, *maximum*, and *minimum* contributed to the formation of the resultant discriminant function. Qian *et al.* [905] identified three features based on pixel intensity.

Intensity Variation (IV)
The intensity variation, IV, is a measure of the smoothness of the pixel intensity in the extracted region and is defined as:

$$IV = \sqrt{\frac{1}{N_a} \sum_{(i,j) \in A} [I(i,j) - m_a]^2}$$

where N_a is the total number of pixels within the region A and m_a is the mean intensity value of the region A given as:

$$m_a = \frac{1}{N_a} \sum_{(i,j) \in A} I(i,j).$$

Mean Intensity Difference (MID)
This feature measures the intensity difference between the extracted region and its surrounding area.

$$MID = \frac{1}{N_a} \sum_{(i,j)\in A} I(i,j) - \frac{1}{N_a} \sum_{(i,j)\in A_s} I(i,j)$$

where N_a is the total number of pixels in the region A, N_s is the total number of pixels in region A_s surrounding region A.

Mean Gradient of Region Boundary (MG)
This feature measures the edge contrast of the extracted region and is defined as:

$$MG = \frac{1}{N_b} \sum_{k=1}^{N_b} g_k,$$

where N_b is the total number of pixels on the boundary of the extracted region and g_k is the edge gradient value of the kth boundary pixel calculated with a Sobel operator.

In their study to discriminate masses from non-masses, the authors used ROC analysis to evaluate the performance of the features in conjunction with wavelet-based segmentation. For the intensity difference IV, the value of $Az = 0.75$ is obtained, for the mean intensity difference MID, the value of $Az = 0.85$ is obtained, and for the mean gradient of region boundary MG, the value of $Az = 0.72$ is obtained.

Finally, we discuss in the next section brief details of some popular international databases used by researchers. International databases are important as various studies can compare their results on the same set of images. We present brief details on four important databases which can be retrieved through the Internet.

9.12   Public Domain Databases in Mammography

9.12.1   The Digital Database for Screening Mammography (DDSM)

The DDSM database (Heath *et al.* [862]) is publicly available from the University of South Florida. The database provides high-resolution digitized film screen mammograms with associated ground truth specified by an expert radiologist. The primary motivation for its development was to produce a mammography database to facilitate comparative analysis of computer-aided detection and diagnosis methods. Mammograms are scanned at a sampling rate of 42-50 microns per pixel and scanned at either 12 or 16 bits per pixel. Images are compressed using a truly lossless JPEG compression algorithm. The patient age and breast density indicators are provided for all cases. Each abnormality is specified by a chain-coded boundary and includes a subtlety rating, and a description coded using the BI-RADS nomenclature. Each abnormality is assigned one of the following categories:

- *Benign* – findings made after additional workup performed (biopsy, ultrasound, etc.).

- *Benign without call back* – findings obtained without any additional workup.

- *Malignant* – proven by pathology.

Cases of the same type, scanned on the same scanner, are grouped into volumes as processed. The completed database comprises 2620 cases in 43 volumes which total over 230 GB of compressed data.

9.12.2   LLNL/UCSF Database

The Lawrence Livermore National Laboratories (LLNL), along with University of California at San Fransisco (UCSF) Radiology Dept. have developed a 12 volume CD Library of digitized mammograms featuring microcalcifications. For each digitized film image, there exist two associated "truth" images (full-size binary images) that show the extent of all calcification clusters, and the contour and area of a few individual calcifications in each cluster.

Along with the "truth" images, a file with case history, radiologist's comments, and other information is provided. The library contains 198 films from 50 patients (4 views per patient, but only 2 views from one mastectomy case), selected to span a range of cases of interest. The films are digitized to 35 microns. Each pixel is sampled at 12 bits of grayscale. As a result, each digitized mammogram results in an image that is about 50 megabytes in size, nearly 6 gigabytes for the entire library.

9.12.3   Washington University Digital Mammography Database

This database contains digitally acquired images of pathologically proven breast pathology. Each case consists of a single scout image of a breast lesion obtained during the course of stereotactic core needle biopsy. Cases are organized according to lesion histopathology. Patient demographic data will be added to the database in the near future. Images have been acquired on a LORAD CCD-based, stereotactic core biopsy table. Each image is 512×512 pixels in size with 12 bits of gray scale data per pixel. Raw image data can be downloaded via FTP to any Unix-based system.

9.12.4   The Mammographic Image Analysis Society (MIAS) Database

The Mammographic Image Analysis Society (MIAS) (Suckling *et al.* [919]) is an organization of UK research groups interested in the understanding of mammograms. Films are taken from the UK National Breast Screening Programme. The mammograms are all medio-lateral oblique view, the UK screening view. All mammograms were digitized with a scanning microdensitometer (Joyce-Loebl, SCANDIG3) to 50-micron × 50-micron resolution. The gray-scale response of the instrument is linear in the optical density range of 0–3.2 OD. The data is in byte-stream format without any of the standard image format headers. The database has been handled and written to Exa-Byte tape in UNIX "tar" format using SUN Microsystems Workstations. The data is compressed using the UNIX "compress" command. All of the data is from examinations done as part of mass screening. There are four image sizes: small (1600 × 4320 pixels); medium (2048 × 4320 pixels); large (2600 × 4320 pixels) and extra large (5200 × 4000 pixels). The data has been reviewed by a consultant radiologist and abnormalities have been identified and marked. The ground truth data consists of the location of the abnormality and the radius of a circle which encloses it. No other information is included. This is partly to protect patient confidentiality and partly due to the large effort required in collecting this data. The age of subjects varies between 50 and 65 years which is the call-up range for the UK Screening Programme. The MIAS data set contains a variety of different anomalies contained with a variety of breast tissue types. Left and right breast tissue types, anomalies and frequencies are shown in Table 9.3. The table shows the number of individual images. The whole data set comprises 322 breast image pairs from 161 patients.

9.13   Classification and Measures of Performance

9.13.1   Classification Techniques

As previously discussed, for each suspicious area segmented, we extract measurements or properties called *features* to classify the objects. Automating the classification of objects based on extracted vector of features can be a difficult task. There are techniques such as clustering for unsupervised learning (Bishop [831]) or class discovery that attempt to divide data sets into naturally occurring groups without a pre-determined class structure. Typically in mammography we know the class structure, for example malignant or normal tissue for the two-class mass detection schemes. Using supervised learning techniques we are able to train a classifier based on a *training set* (a feature set with known classes). Subsequently we use a *test set* (a feature set with known classes used) to test the classifier following the training process. The choice of classifier used is determined by the complexity of the problem, commonly

	Breast Type			Totals	
	Fatty	Fatty-Glandular	Dense		
Calcification	B: 2 M: 4	B: 5 M: 4	B: 5 M: 5	B: 12 M: 13	25
Circumscribed Mass	B: 7 M: 2	B: 6 M: 2	B: 3 M: 0	B: 16 M: 4	20
Spiculated Mass	B: 2 M: 4	B: 4 M: 3	B: 6 M: 2	B: 12 M: 9	21
Miscellaneous (ill-defined mass)	B: 4 M: 4	B: 3 M: 2	B: 1 M: 1	B: 8 M: 7	15
Architectural Distortion	B: 4 M: 2	B: 2 M: 4	B: 4 M: 4	B: 10 M: 10	20
Asymmetry	B: 2 M: 3	B: 3 M: 2	B: 3 M: 4	B: 8 M: 9	17
Normal	66	64	74	204	
Abnormal	40	40	38	118	
Totals	106	104	112	322	

Table 9.3: MIAS Data set composition (B = Benign, M = Malignant). [Nomenclature: B: 2 is two benign cases, M: 9 is nine malignant cases.]

dictated by the feature set. Jain *et al.* [870] provide a comprehensive review of statistical pattern recognition classifiers including statistical classifiers, syntactic approaches, neural networks, evolutionary methods, and decision trees. It is beyond the scope of this chapter to discuss different classification techniques. The main criteria in the choice of the classifier are data distribution and overlap between different classes. Linear approaches are tested first, followed by non-linear analysis. As a result of the classification process, we get a confusion matrix and final result of classification quoted as the recognition rate. Further analysis involves the use of ROC curves described below.

9.13.2 The Receiver Operating Characteristic Curve

Receiver Operating Characteristic (ROC) analysis is a statistical technique that provides information about the overlap within a two-class classification. The analysis allows for a plot of the sensitivity or True Positive Fraction (TPF) against the specificity or False Positive Fraction (FPF) at differing thresholds so that inaccuracies, which arise from assuming findings are absolutely normal or abnormal, are avoided (Goddard *et al.* [854]; Metz [893]). Within mammographic studies that are using ROC analysis, the following nomenclature is typically used:

- *True Positive* (TP): lesions that are classified cancer and prove to be cancer

- *False Positive* (FP): lesions that are classified cancer and prove to be benign

- *False Negative* (FN): lesions that are classified benign and prove to be cancer

- *True Negative* (TN): lesions that are classified benign and prove to be benign.

On the basis of this terminology, we can evaluate the performance of a CAD technique by calculating True Positive Fraction and False Positive Fraction and using ROC analysis. These fractions are defined as:

$$TPF = \frac{TP}{TP + FN}, FPF = \frac{FP}{FP + TN}$$

To understand the mechanism by which ROC analysis works, take the following example of two distributions belonging to categories normal, w_1 and abnormal, w_2, together with a suitable threshold (Theodoridis and Koutroumbas [922]).

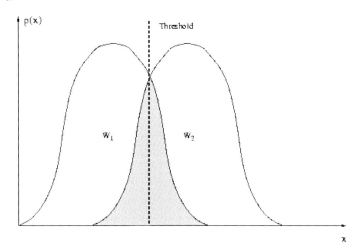

Figure 9.32: ROC Analysis and the two-class problems.

For any member of one of the two distributions, we assign it to class w_1 for values of x on the left of the threshold and w_2 for values on the right. This threshold or decision boundary is associated with a certain error, a (FPF), of reaching a wrong decision for class w_1 and an error b (FNF), of reaching a wrong decision for class w_2 (see Figure 9.32). It is seen that by moving the threshold over all possible positions, different values of a and b will be obtained. If the two distributions have complete overlap, then for any position of the threshold we get $a = 1 - b$ shown in Figure 9.33 by the dotted line in the graph. As the two distributions move apart, the curve departs from the straight line as shown by the solid line. The smaller the overlap of the classes, i.e. the smaller the confusion in the classification, the larger the area between the curve and the straight line. A quantitative measure of the accuracy of the classification technique may be obtained by finding the area under the constructed ROC curve termed Az. Values that may be obtained for this metric vary between 0 for poor classification performance, and 1 for high classification performance. Free response operating characteristic (FROC) curves plot sensitivity as a function of the number of false positives detected per image.

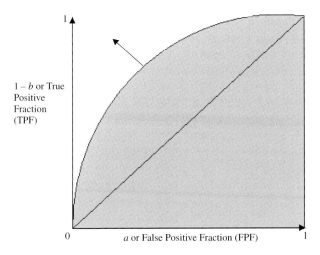

Figure 9.33: The ROC Curve. The arrow indicates the direction of movement as classification performance increases. The shaded area represents Az.

9.14 Conclusions

In this chapter we have highlighted some of the important issues in mammogram image segmentation. Our approach to the discussion is based on modular components needed to process mammograms from the acquisition stage to their final classification. The quality of segmentation, the central theme of this chapter, has a strong impact on the quality of final results produced. It is not possible to present all possible approaches in the literature for mammogram segmentation but we have put together a reasonable collection of image segmentation algorithms that have been widely used in mammography. These approaches have been specifically developed for mammography in most cases or demonstrated to work successfully in this domain, as it is well known that not all image analysis techniques work well in this difficult area. It is through empirical analysis that one can judge which techniques perform better on a given data. In addition to segmentation algorithms, we have also highlighted the various feature extraction approaches suited to mammography. A number of these are used to reduce the number of false positives before the final stage of classification. We have not detailed classification methods as a range of standard techniques is used for this purpose. One of the main changes required to a standard approach will be to use a *loss matrix* penalizing false positives and true negatives as per our requirement. This matrix can be used for optimizing the parameters of the classifier during the training process.

Another important area for investigation is *multiple classifier combination.* Recent research in this field has highlighted the benefits of classifier combination resulting in solutions that cannot be effectively solved by a single classifier, or that can more effectively be performed by a modular classification approach. One classic approach to classifier combination is the ensemble approach. Here a collection of different classifiers gives a solution to the same problem. The aim is to increase the overall classification performance by combination of classifier outputs fused using a suitable combination strategy. An alternative modular approach is built on the basis that the problem cannot be solved by a single classifier but must be broken into sub-tasks. By developing specialized classifiers capable of providing solutions to particular tasks, and combining them in a hierarchical framework, the aim is to develop a solution strategy based using the efficiency of modular problem decomposition.

It is important that further research focuses on *standard databases* in order for researchers to test their work on a uniform benchmark. Studies need to report results on full databases rather than a selective portion as is most often the case. This consistency is also necessary in the manner in which images are used for analysis; for example, some form of standard image correction process is needed for ensuring that minor variations created during acquisition can be eliminated.

It is becoming increasingly important to *correlate image analysis techniques* with our deeper understanding of anatomical structures. For example, linear structures can be removed from the mammogram to aid the quality of segmentation. Similarly, a three-dimensional surface can be generated from the two-dimensional view for better detection of masses. Image analysis techniques in the future based on hierarchical representation of images will allow suspicious areas to be highlighted in a lower resolution image before a detailed analysis of the granular structure of the mass or microcalcification is performed in the higher resolution. This will allow less storage space and faster computational processing.

9.15   Acknowledgements

We would like to acknowledge the help and support offered by Mona Sharma in creating segmented images and Jonathan Fieldsend for reading the final draft. Mona and Jonathan are members of PANN Research, Department of Computer Science, University of Exeter.

Chapter 10

Cell Image Segmentation for Diagnostic Pathology

Dorin Comaniciu, Peter Meer

10.1 Introduction

The colors associated with a digitized specimen representing peripheral blood smear are typically characterized by only a few, non-Gaussian clusters, whose shapes have to be discerned solely from the image being processed. Nonparametric methods such as mode-based analysis [952], are particularly suitable for the segmentation of this type of data since they do not constrain the cluster shapes. This chapter reviews an efficient cell segmentation algorithm that detects clusters in the $L^*u^*v^*$ color space and delineates their borders by employing the gradient ascent mean shift procedure [950], [951]. The color space is randomly tessellated with search windows that are moved till convergence to the nearest mode of the underlying probability distribution. After the pruning of the mode candidates, the colors are classified using the basins of attraction. The segmented image is derived by mapping the color vectors in the image domain and enforcing spatial constraints.

The segmenter is the core module of the Image Guided Decision Support (IGDS) system [956], [955] which is discussed next. The IGDS architecture supports decision-making in clinical pathology and provides components for remote microscope control and multi-user visualization. The primary and long term goal of IGDS-related research is to reduce the number of false negatives during routine specimen screening by medical technologists. The Decision-Support component of the system searches remote databases, retrieves and displays cases which exhibit visual features consistent to the case in question, and suggests the most likely diagnosis according to majority logic. Based on the Micro-Controller component, the primary user can command a robotic microscope from a distance, obtain high-quality images for the diagnosis, and authorize other users to visualize the same images. The system has a natural man-machine interface that contains engines for speech recognition and voice feedback.

Section 10.2 concentrates on the segmentation algorithm. In Section 10.3

we underline the idea of diagnosis support through the presentation of relevant cases and show how the IGDS system was developed based on the robust handling of the image features.

10.2   Segmentation

We explain first the advantages of nonparametric methods for the analysis of feature spaces. An iterative, gradient ascent procedure for mode seeking is presented next. The section concludes with a description of the cell segmentation algorithm and segmentation examples.

10.2.1   Feature Space Analysis

Feature space analysis is a widely used tool for solving image understanding problems. An image feature is defined as a local, meaningful, and detectable part of the image [983, p.68]. Given the input image, feature vectors representing color, texture, or parameters of curves or surfaces, are extracted from local neighborhoods and mapped into the space spanned by their components. Significant features in the image then correspond to high density regions in this space.

The feature space provides an intrinsic tolerance to noise but a reduced sensitivity to features represented by only a few points. The space the features originate is often used to compensate for allocation errors. For example, the image domain is used during the task of color segmentation to compensate for errors resulting from the analysis of the color space. The feature space can be regarded as a sample drawn from an unknown probability distribution. Analyzing this distribution based on a parametric model (e.g., Gaussian mixture) will introduce severe constraints since the shape of the delineated clusters is predefined. By contrast, nonparametric cluster analysis uses the *modes* of the underlying probability density to define the cluster centers and the *basin of attraction* to define the boundaries separating the clusters.

The nonparametric methods, however, require *multidimensional range searching* [980, p.373], that is, the search for the data points falling into a given neighborhood. Since the optimization of this task is difficult [980, p.385] the nonparametric analysis of large data sets is computationally expensive, with a complexity proportional to the square of the number of data points. Therefore, a practical algorithm for cluster delineation should involve the tessellation of the feature space and selective processing of data points. Following this idea, we have developed a general technique for the analysis of multi-modal data based on the *mean shift* property, first described in [961], and more recently discussed in [948].

10.2.2   Mean Shift Procedure

Let $\{\mathbf{x}_i\}_{i=1\ldots n}$ be a set of n points in the d-dimensional Euclidean space R^d, i.e., the feature space. Define the hypersphere $S_h(\mathbf{x})$ of radius h centered on

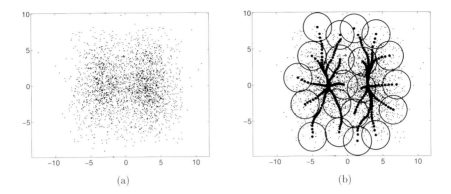

Figure 10.1: 2-D mode seeking through mean shift iterations. (a) Input data. (b) Trajectories of 20 mean shift procedures.

$\mathbf{x}$ and containing $n_\mathbf{x}$ data points. It can be shown [952] that the sample mean shift is

$$M_h(\mathbf{x}) = \frac{1}{n_\mathbf{x}} \sum_{\mathbf{x}_i \in S_h(\mathbf{x})} \mathbf{x}_i - \mathbf{x} \sim \frac{\hat{\nabla} f(\mathbf{x})}{\hat{f}(\mathbf{x})}, \tag{10.1}$$

where $\hat{f}(\mathbf{x})$ is the local density estimate and $\hat{\nabla} f(\mathbf{x})$ is the local density gradient estimate. Note $\sim$ means proportional. The expression (10.1) indicates that a local estimate of the normalized gradient can be obtained by computing the sample mean shift and that the mean shift vector always points towards the direction of the maximum increase in the density. Moreover, the procedure defined by recursively moving the hypersphere by the mean shift vector defines a path leading to a local density maximum, i.e., to a mode of the density. For a more detailed discussion, as well as proof of convergence of the mean shift procedure, see [952].

As an example, Figure 10.1b presents the trajectories of 20 mean shift procedures started from random locations and applied in parallel on the data shown in Figure 10.1a. The entire process results in two convergence points that correspond to the two modes of the underlying density. In addition, by associating the points with the modes, the structure of the data (number of clusters and their shapes) is revealed. The analysis needs only one parameter, the radius h of the searching sphere and no other *a priori* knowledge. It is simple and straightforward to implement, being based on the iterative shifting of a fixed size window to the average of the data points within. However, a practical method must handle artifacts such as poor convergence over the low density regions or plateaus without a clear local maximum.

10.2.3   Cell Segmentation

This section briefly describes the cell segmentation based on the mean shift procedure (see [950], [951] for details). Figure 10.2 shows a summary of the

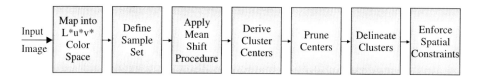

Figure 10.2: The processing flow of the segmentation algorithm.

algorithm. The RGB input vectors are first transformed into $L^*u^*v^*$ vectors to obtain a perceptually uniform color space [984, Section 3.3.9].

Then, a set of m points called the *sample set* is randomly selected from the data. Distance and density constraints are imposed on the points retained in the sample set, fixing the sample set cardinality. The distance between any two neighbors should be larger than h, the radius of a searching sphere $S_h(\mathbf{x})$, and the sample points should not lie in sparsely populated regions. Whenever the number of points inside the sphere is below a threshold T_1, a region is regarded as sparse.

The mean shift procedure is applied to each point in the sample set, and the resulting convergence points define m *cluster center candidates*. Since a local plateau in the color space can prematurely stop the mean shift iterations, each cluster center candidate is perturbed by a random vector of small norm and the mean shift procedure is allowed to converge again.

The candidates are then pruned to obtain $p \leq m$ cluster centers. The mean of any subset of cluster center candidates which are less than h close to each other defines a *cluster center*. In addition, the presence of a valley between each pair of cluster centers is tested [952] and if no valley is found, the tested center of lower density is removed.

Cluster delineation has two stages. First, each sample point is allocated to a cluster center based on the trajectory of its initial window. Then, each data point is classified according to the majority of its k-nearest sample points. Finally, small connected components containing less than T_2 pixels are removed, and region growing is performed to allocate the unclassified pixels.

10.2.4   Segmentation Examples

Three parameters control the segmentation: the searching sphere radius h, the threshold T_1 which enforces the density constraint, and the threshold T_2 which determines the minimum connected component size. The results presented here were obtained with $h = 4$, $T_1 = 50$, and $T_2 = 1000$.

A typical leukocyte image is shown in Figure 10.3a. The segmented image is presented in pseudogray-levels in Figure 10.3b. Pseudocolors are used to display the cluster delineation in Plate 12e, where the clusters are shifted for better visualization. Plates 12a–d present, respectively, the corresponding $n = 6005$ color vectors, sample set with $m = 73$, cluster center candidates, and $p = 4$ cluster centers.

The resulting decomposition is meaningful in both the spatial domain and

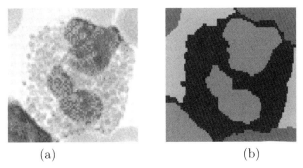

(a)   (b)

Figure 10.3: (a) Original image. (b) Segmented image.

the color space, the cytoplasm texture, for example, being classified as one cluster.

The segmentation quality can also be evaluated from Figure 10.4 which shows the original, contour, and segmented images of a stained specimen of Mantle Cell Lymphoma (upper) and two stained specimens of Chronic Lymphocytic Leukemia (lower) [947]. Additional results are presented in Figure 10.5 where the nucleus of each cell was delineated using the algorithm from above and no further post-processing was necessary. The data set contains images of different color, sharpness, contrast, noise level and size (for convenience, they are displayed at the same size).

The algorithm running time is linear with the number of pixels in the image. It takes fractions of a second to segment a 256×256 pixel image on a standard PC/workstation.

10.3   Decision Support System for Pathology

This section reviews a prototype system for clinical pathology that assists the user in the diagnostic process. The IGDS system [956], [955] segments and analyzes the elemental structures of the input image, searches remote databases and retrieves relevant images based on their content.

After a short description of the problem domain, we present an overview of the system and the currently used database of ground truth cases. The analysis of the visual attributes of the query is explained next. The optimization of the overall dissimilarity measure is then presented, together with the retrieval performance assessment by cross-validation. Finally, comparisons to the human experts performance on the same database are given.

For more information about the IGSD system, including demonstration videos, the reader is referred to

        http://www.caip.rutgers.edu/∼comanici/jretrieval.html

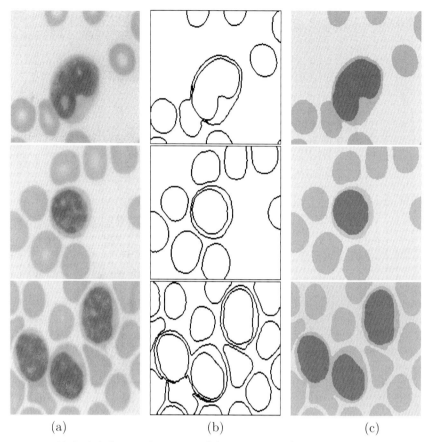

(a)   (b)   (c)

Figure 10.4: (a) Original images. (b) Contours. (c) Segmented images.

10.3.1   Problem Domain

The subjective, visual analysis of malignant lymphomas and chronic lympho-cytic leukemia gives rise in practice to a significant number of false negatives (malignant cells classified as benign). If suspicious cells are detected, subse-quent morphological evaluation of specimens by even experienced pathologists is often inconclusive. In these cases differential diagnosis can only be made after expensive supporting tests such as immunophenotyping by flow cytometry.

Mantle Cell Lymphoma (MCL) [944], [946] is of particular interest among the indolent lymphomas since it is often misdiagnosed as Chronic Lymphocytic Leukemia (CLL) or Follicular Center Cell Lymphoma (FCC) [947]. In addi-tion, the survival of patients with MCL is much shorter than that of patients with other low-grade lymphomas, and standard therapy for CLL and FCC is ineffective with MCL. Timely and accurate diagnosis of MCL has therefore significant therapeutic and prognostic implications.

The literature in diagnostic hematopathology ascribes much of the difficulty in rendering consistent diagnoses to subjective impressions of observers and

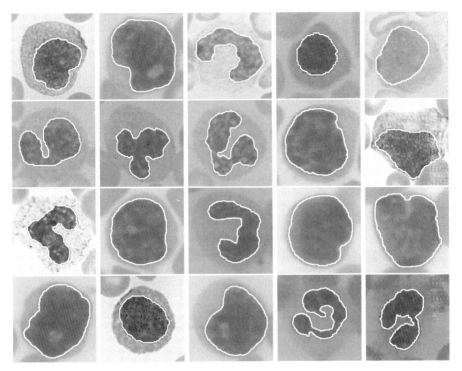

Figure 10.5: Nucleus segmentation for various cell categories. The nucleus border is marked with a white contour.

shows that when morphologic cell classification is based upon computer aided analysis, the level of objectivity and reproducibility improves [945]. However, only recently has the potential of diagnosis support through the presentation of relevant cases (as opposed to automatic diagnosis) been recognized [982].

The technologies that capture, describe, and index the content of multi-media objects rely on methods from image analysis, pattern recognition, and database theory. A new family of information retrieval systems emerged in recent years, exploiting the richness of visual information and covering a large spectrum of applications [958], [960], [968], [972], [973]. These systems differ according to their degree of generality (general purpose versus domain specific), level of feature abstraction (primitive features versus logical features), overall dissimilarity measure used in retrieval ranking, database indexing procedure, level of user intervention (with or without relevance feedback), and evaluation methodology.

The problem domain of the IGDS system, discriminating among lympho-proliferative disorders, contrasts with that of general retrieval systems engines. It is well defined and allows the quantitative evaluation of the system's performance and comparison with the human expert results. The reason for this comparison however is only to assess the usefulness of the system. In a real analysis scenario, a lot of context information that is difficult to quantize is taken into account for the diagnosis and no technique can ever replace the pathologist and light microscopy. Our system is designed as a tool to help the physician during analysis, by presenting cases consistent to the case in question, and not as an automatic cell classifier.

10.3.2 System Overview

The IGDS system has a platform-independent implementation in Java and consists mainly of two software components that are described below.

10.3.2.1 Micro-Controller Component

The Micro-Controller allows one primary user and multiple secondary users to connect to the image server located at the microscope site. The primary user can control the remote microscope (AX70 Olympus equipped with motorized stage), receive and visualize diagnostic-quality images of tissue samples. The transfered images can simultaneously be observed and analyzed by the secondary users. Thus, the IGDS system provides support for consultation, when a fellow pathologist is logged in as secondary user, or teaching, when a group of students is connected to the image server.

A display capture of the Micro-Controller is shown in Figure 10.6. Image 1 is obtained during the initialization and represents the low resolution panoramic view of the specimen at the robotic stage. Image 2 is the current view using a lens of 100× and corresponds to the small rectangular region marked on the panoramic image. The primary user can adjust the light path or focus of the

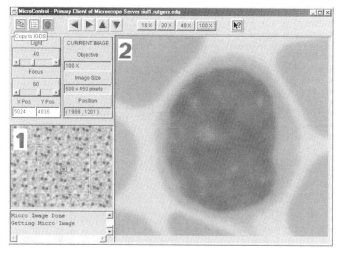

Figure 10.6: The Micro-Controller component. 1 – Panoramic image. 2 – Current view of the selected region in the panoramic image using the 100× lens.

microscope, change the objective lens, move the specimen on the robotic stage, or copy the current image to the Decision-Support part for further analysis. These actions are possible by mouse input or by speech.

A distinct feature of the IGDS system is its bi-modal human-computer interaction [981]. A fusion agent capable of multi-modal inputs interprets the commands, calls the appropriate method, and gives voice feedback. Currently the system employs a speech recognizer engine with finite-state grammar. The use of a small, task-specific vocabulary results in very high recognition rate. The recognition is speaker-independent. Examples of voice commands for the Micro-Controller are: Set Light ##, Set Focus ##, Change #, Transfer, Move Right (Left, Up, Down), Update the System.

10.3.2.2 Decision-Support Component

This component allows the user to load a (remote) query image and select a rectangular region which contains the cells of interest. The elemental structures from the selected region (e.g., leucocyte nuclei and cytoplasm areas) are then delineated through the segmentation described in Section 2. By choosing a cell nucleus, the user first initiates the analysis of the nucleus attributes (shape, texture, area, and color), then the search in a remote database of digitized specimens. As a response, the system retrieves and displays the images from the database that are the closest to the query.

A display capture of the Decision-Support component is shown in Figure 10.7, containing the query image with the region of interest, the selected nucleus during texture analysis, the normalized shape of the nucleus, eight retrieved images, and the control panel. The user can modify the color resolution and spatial resolution of the segmentation, which are defined as the inverses of the segmentation parameters h and T_2, respectively (see Section 10.2.4). Access to the resolution parameters is only for experiments and maintenance, in normal operations of the system they are set by default. While the segmentation produces reliable results for almost all the images in the database, the system provides a user-handled contour correction tool based on cubic splines. It is also possible to select different query attributes, browse the retrievals, select a different scale for visualization, and display specific clinical data and video clips.

As in the Micro-Controller case, the commands can be initiated using speech recognition or graphical input. Typical voice commands for the Decision-Support are: Open Image ##, Save Image ##, Segment the Image, Search the Database, Show 2 (4, 8) Retrievals, Show First (Next, Previous) Retrievals, Show Video, Clinical Data #. Examples of voice feedback are: Image ## Opened, Segmentation Completed, Analyzing Texture, Database Search Completed, Suggested Class: CLL (FCC, MCL, Normal).

The Decision-Support component has the client-server architecture shown in Figure 10.8. The client part is intended to be used in small hospitals and laboratories to access through the Internet the database at the image server site.

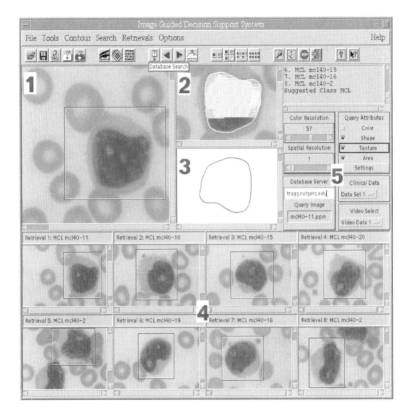

Figure 10.7: The Decision-Support component. 1 – Query image. 2 – Delineated nucleus. 3 – Normalized shape of the nucleus. 4 – Retrieved images. 5 – Control panel.

The I/O module loads the query image from a local or remote microscope and saves the retrieved information. It also includes the Speech Recognizer and TTS (Text to Speech) engines. The Client Processor contains the query formation stages, performing region of interest selection, color segmentation and feature extraction. Based on the retrieval data, the Client Presenter communicates the suggested classification to the user, and allows the browsing of cases of interest including their associated clinical data and video clips.

The server consists of two parts: the Retrieval and Indexing modules. The retrieval process is multi-threaded, simultaneous access to the database being authorized. During feature matching, the query data and logical information in the database are compared to derive a ranking of the retrievals. For indexing the server uses the same client processing stages plus an optimization stage.

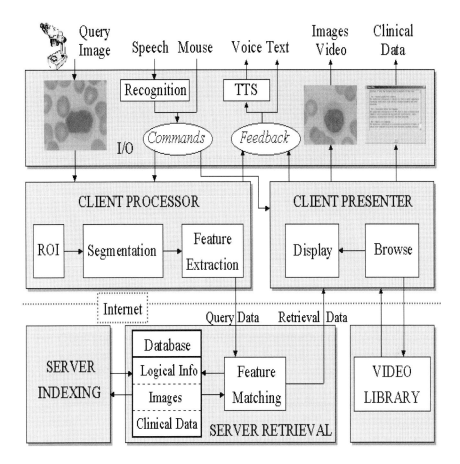

Figure 10.8: The Decision-Support Architecture. The client part includes the I/O module, the Client Processor, and the Client Presenter. The server part contains the Retrieval and Indexing modules.

10.3.3 Current Database

The IGDS system is currently using a database containing 98 CLL, 38 FCC, 66 MCL, and 59 Normal cells, a total of 261 images. The ground truth of the recorded cases was obtained off line through immunophenotyping and used to maximize the probability of correct classification.

Immunophenotyping is the characterization of white blood cells by determining the cell surface antigens they bear. The cells are isolated and incubated with fluorescently-tagged antibodies directed against specific cell-surface antigens. Then, they pass through the flow cytometer past a laser beam. When the cells meet the laser beam, they emit fluorescent signals in proportion to the amount of the specific cell surface antigen they have and a computer calculates the percentage of cells expressing each antigen.

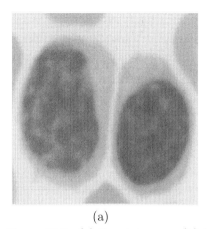
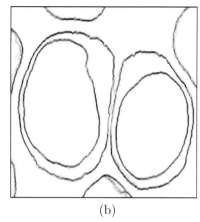

(a)   (b)

Figure 10.9: (a) Input image. (b) Contours showing the stability of the segmentation. The input image has been segmented 25 times and the resulting contours were superimposed. The regions between two cells are the least stable.

10.3.4   Analysis of Visual Attributes

The query data is determined by four visual attributes of the delineated cell nucleus: shape, texture, area, and color. Medical literature frequently employs the first three of the above attributes to morphologically describe the appearance of malignant cells [944]. The Fourier coefficients describing the nuclear shape are made invariant to changes in location, orientation, and scale (i.e., similarity invariant), by following the approach of Kuhl and Giardina [965]. The texture analysis is based on a Multiresolution Simultaneous Autoregressive (MRSAR) Model [969].

10.3.4.1   Similarity Invariant Shape Descriptors

The number of Fourier harmonics that reliably represent a nuclear shape is dependent on the uncertainty introduced by the prior processing stages (e.g., region of interest delineation, segmentation). Since the segmentation process is global, any change in the region of interest selected by the user may have effect on the nucleus delineation. In addition, due to its probabilistic nature the segmentation produces slightly different results when repeatedly applied to the same image. For example, a procedure composed of 25 segmentations of the image from Figure 10.9a, followed by the superposition of the derived contours, yields the result shown in Figure 10.9b. The darker a pixel in the contour image, the more stable is the contour passing through that pixel. To estimate the influence of this uncertainty on the Fourier coefficients, experiments with several images were conducted and the normalized variance (variance over the squared mean) of each coefficient was computed. For a given image, a user delineated 25 times the region of interest (a leukocyte). The region was then segmented and the first 64 Fourier coefficients were determined for the nucleus. Since the normalized variances of the coefficients were typically rapidly increasing for the coefficients with index larger than 40, we concluded that the segmentation is sufficiently stable for the use of only the first 40 coefficients (10 harmonics). Consequently, we compare a query contour with a reference contour in the database by computing the Euclidean distance between the corresponding 40-dimensional vectors of Fourier invariants

$$D_1 = \sqrt{(\mathbf{f}_{query} - \mathbf{f}_{reference})^T (\mathbf{f}_{query} - \mathbf{f}_{reference})} \,. \qquad (10.2)$$

10.3.4.2   Texture, Area, and Color Metrics

The nuclear texture is a representation of the chromatin density, being relatively unstructured. It is characterized by random patterns, and shows no presence of periodicity or directionality. We therefore describe the gray level texture data with the Multiresolution Simultaneous AutoRegressive (MRSAR) model [969]. This is a second-order noncausal model that contains five parameters at each resolution level. For a given resolution, the center pixel value in a neighborhood is expressed as a linear combination of the neighboring pixel values and an additive white Gaussian noise term. Four model parameters (the weights associated with selected pixel values) are estimated through least squares. The model parameters and the estimation error define a five-dimensional feature vector for the given neighborhood. The multiresolution feature vector is obtained by varying the neighborhood size and concatenating the obtained features.

In [976] it was shown that the MRSAR features computed with 5×5, 7×7, and 9×9 neighborhoods provide the best overall retrieval performance for the entire Brodatz database. The same neighborhoods were used here to form fifteen-dimensional multiresolution feature vectors whose mean and covariance were computed for each database entry.

Thus, the texture dissimilarity has to be measured on the basis of the distance between two multivariate distributions with known mean vectors and covariance matrices. We use the Mahalanobis distance between the MRSAR feature vectors to express this dissimilarity

$$D_2 = \sqrt{(\mathbf{t}_{query} - \mathbf{t}_{reference})^T \, \Sigma^{-1}_{reference} \, (\mathbf{t}_{query} - \mathbf{t}_{reference})} \,, \qquad (10.3)$$

where $\Sigma^{-1}_{reference}$ represents the inverse of the covariance matrix of $\mathbf{t}_{reference}$. For each entry in the database $\Sigma^{-1}_{reference}$ is obtained and stored off-line for each indexed nucleus.

Note that for the current database, the use of $\Sigma_{reference}$ for Mahalanobis computation resulted in better classification than that obtained with Σ_{query}. By using the Mahalanobis distance, the assumption we make is that the covariance of the query Σ_{query} and the covariances of the references from the database $\Sigma_{reference}$ are similar.

However, our own research [954] showed that the retrieval performance can be improved by using the Bhattacharyya distance [962, p. 99] as a dissimilarity measure. This distance takes into account not only the separation induced by different mean vectors, but also the separation due to the difference in covariance matrices. In addition, we showed that efficient computation of the Bhattacharyya distance is possible when most of the energy in the feature space is restricted to a low dimensional subspace. The improved representation will be implemented into the IGDS system.

The digitized specimens in the database have all the same magnification, therefore, the nuclear area is computed as the number of pixels inside the delineated nucleus. The dissimilarity between two nuclei in terms of their areas is expressed as:

$$D_3 = \sqrt{(a_{query} - a_{reference})^2} \ . \tag{10.4}$$

The nuclear color is expressed as a 3-D vector in the $L^*u^*v^*$ space and is determined during the segmentation as the center of the associated color cluster. However, since the colors of the nuclei in the database cannot discriminate among the digitized specimens, the current implementation of the system uses the color attribute only for nucleus separation from the background.

10.3.5 Overall Dissimilarity Metric

Recall that the cases in the reference database fall into one of the four categories: CLL, FCC, MCL, or normal (benign). The suggested classification of the query image is based on the voting kNN rule [962, p. 305] among the classes of the closest k matches. That is:

$$k_i = max\{k_1, \ldots, k_4\} \ \rightarrow \ X \in \omega_i \tag{10.5}$$

where k_i is the number of neighbors from the class ω_i $(i = 1, \ldots, 4)$ among the kNN's, and $k_1 + \cdots + k_4 = k$. In addition to the four original cell classes, the kNN rule may also produce a NO DECISION class, in the case when the value of i verifying (10.5) is not unique.

We measure the system performance through the *confusion matrix* $\mathbf{R}$ defined as having as element $r_{j,i}$ the empirical probability of classification in class j when the query image belonged to class i, $P(j|i)$. The criterion that should be maximized is the sum of conditional probabilities of correct decision:

$$J = \sum_{j=1}^{4} P(j|j) \ . \tag{10.6}$$

The dissimilarity between two cell nuclei is expressed as a linear combination of the distances corresponding to each query attribute. Thus, for three attributes (e.g., shape, texture, and area) we have the overall distance:

$$D = \sum_{i=1}^{3} w_i D_i \ , \tag{10.7}$$

where w_i represents the relevance of the i-th attribute and $\sum_{i=1}^{3} w_i = 1$.

The best weights w_i were derived off-line by employing the downhill simplex method [978, p. 408] with the objective function J (10.6). A simplex in N

dimensions consists of $N + 1$ totally connected vertices. The optimization is based on a series of steps which reflect, expand, and contract the simplex such that it converges to a maximum of the objective function. As an advantage, the downhill simplex requires only function evaluations and no computation of derivatives.

Table 10.1: Best weights and the value of optimization criterion corresponding to the global maximum.

Shape	Texture	Area	J
0.1140	0.5771	0.3089	3.4207

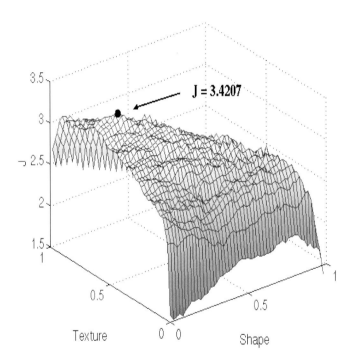

Figure 10.10: Plot of the objective surface (resolution is 0.02 on each dimension). The downhill simplex converged in this case to the global maximum.

Table 10.1 presents the best set of weights, obtained by running the optimization with seven retrievals over the entire database. It corresponds to the highest obtained value ($J = 3.4207$) of the objective function (10.6). Figure 10.10 shows the objective surface as a function of the two independent weights.

10.3.6 Performance Evaluation and Comparisons

At present, the IGDS system is being evaluated in real retrieval scenarios at the Department of Pathology, University of Medicine and Dentistry of New Jersey, Robert Wood Johnson Medical School. Since the sequential searching and ranking of the logical database take about 50 ms on a Pentium II at 266 MHz, the extension of the current database to thousands of images is possible with no noticeable increase in the delay at the end user. The retrieval delay depends mostly on the bandwidth available for the client-server communication.

To obtain a more realistic estimation of the retrieval performance, we performed the ten-fold cross-validated classification [959, p. 238] of the entire database. The data set was randomized and split into 10 approximately equal test sets, each containing about 9 CLL, 3 FCC, 6 MCL, and 5 Normal cases. For the q-th test set its complement was used to obtain the best weights through the downhill simplex method described above. The confusion matrix $\mathbf{R}_q$ of the resulting classifier was then computed over the q-th test set for seven retrievals. The elements of the cross-validated confusion matrix were defined as

$$P_{cv}(j|i) = \frac{1}{10} \sum_{q=1}^{10} P_q(j|i) \,, \tag{10.8}$$

for $i = 1 \ldots 4$, and $j = 1 \ldots 5$. According to the data in Table 10.2, the system performance is satisfactory, especially when related to the current difficulties in differentiating among lymphoproliferative disorders based solely on morphological criteria [946].

Table 10.2: Ten-fold cross-validated confusion matrix (7 retrievals): IGDS system.

	CLL	FCC	MCL	NRML	NO DEC
CLL	**.8389**	.0200	.0711	**.0700**	.0000
FCC	.0250	**.9000**	.0000	**.0500**	.0250
MCL	.1357	.0143	**.8333**	.0000	.0167
NRML	.1333	.1200	.0000	**.7300**	.0167

The confusion matrices representing the results of three human experts classifying the digitized specimens from the same database are presented in Table 10.3. The human experts were shown one digitized specimen at a time on a high resolution screen with no other distractor displayed.

Table 10.3: Confusion matrix: Human experts.

	CLL	FCC	MCL	NRML	NO DEC
CLL	**.5647**	.0352	.2117	**.1764**	.0117
FCC	.0285	**.9428**	.0000	**.0285**	.0000
MCL	.1538	.0769	**.5538**	**.1692**	.0461
NRML	.1228	.0000	.1053	**.7543**	.0175

	CLL	FCC	MCL	NRML	NO DEC
CLL	**.4000**	.0588	.1647	**.3765**	.0000
FCC	.0000	**1.000**	.0000	**.0000**	.0000
MCL	.0769	.0923	**.5538**	**.1692**	.0923
NRML	.0000	.0877	.1053	**.7719**	.0351

	CLL	FCC	MCL	NRML	NO DEC
CLL	**.4941**	.0235	.2118	**.2000**	.0471
FCC	.0000	**.8857**	.0857	**.0286**	.0000
MCL	.4308	.0154	**.3077**	**.0308**	.2154
NRML	.2000	.0364	.1455	**.3455**	.2727

By comparing Tables 10.2 and 10.3 we observe that the human performance is slightly better for FCC and Normal cases, but it is worse for the CLL and MCL cases, both in terms of probabilities of correct decision (the marked diagonals) and probabilities of false negatives (the NRML[1] column). The correlation between the human and machine results is also noteworthy. The classification of the FCC cells proved to be the easiest task while the CLL and MCL cells resulted in similar levels of difficulty.

We note here that in a real classification scenario, the human expert uses a lot of context information including both patient data and additional data inferred from the digitized specimens. We therefore stress the Decision Support function of the IGDS system. The system is not intended to provide automatic identification of the disorder, but to assist the pathologist to improve his/her own analysis. The pathologist combines the objective classification suggested by the system with the context information to obtain a robust diagnostic decision.

10.4   Conclusion

This chapter discussed an effective algorithm for cell segmentation and showed its integration in a real-time system that supports decision making in clinical

---

[1]Normal.

pathology. The nonparametric nature of the segmentation and its robustness to noise allowed the use of a fixed resolution for the processing of hundreds of digital specimens captured under different conditions.

The segmentation has been indirectly evaluated through the IGDS system which demonstrated satisfactory overall performance. As a broader conclusion, however, this research proved that the segmentation, although a very difficult task in its general form, can become a successful processing step when the goal of the vision application is well defined.

Acknowledgment

We thank Professor David J. Foran of the Department of Pathology, University of Medicine and Dentistry of New Jersey, Robert Wood Johnson Medical School, for help and advice with the development of the IGDS system. Dorin Comaniciu and Peter Meer were supported by the NSF under the grant IRI-9530546 and IRI-9618854.

Chapter 11

A Note on Future Research in Segmentation Techniques Applied to Neurology, Cardiology, Mammography and Pathology

Jasjit S. Suri, Sameer Singh, S. K. Setarehdan, Rakesh Sharma, Keir Bovis, Dorin Comaniciu, Laura Reden

11.1 Future Research in Medical Image Segmentation

In previous chapters, we saw the application of segmentation in different areas of the body, such as the brain, heart, breast and cells. We covered many different kinds of models of CVGIP[1] and PR[2], but with the pace at which research in segmentation is progressing, this book would be incomplete if it did not also envision the future of segmentation techniques for the above mentioned areas. Therefore, we present in this chapter the future aspects of the segmentation techniques covered in this book.

The layout of this chapter is as follows: Sub-section 11.1.1 discusses the future of MR image generation and physical principles. Sub-section 11.1.2 presents a discussion of future research and development in the area of cardiac imaging. This applies to MR, CT, X-ray and PET/SPECT. Sub-section 11.1.3 discusses future topics of research in the area of neurological segmentation. Sub-section 11.1.4 discusses the future in digital mammography. The chapter concludes with the future of pathology and cytology imaging in Sub-section 11.1.5.

11.1.1 The Future of MR Image Generation and Physical Principles

In Chapter 1, we discussed the principles of image generation of X-ray, CT, MR and PET. New developments in image generation through software improvements involve applying these physical principles in two directions: obtaining

---

[1]Computer Vision, Graphics and Image Processing.
[2]Pattern Recognition.

better image generation in less time and minimizing image acquisition errors. Included in these developments are: to increase the speed of the acquisition, reduce the T_E, increase the spatial and contrast resolution, reduce aliasing, increase tissue ROI[3] coverage, achieve contiguous tissue slices, achieve better CNR[4], increase SNR[5], obtain better tissue or lipid/water suppression, along with the use of flow correction, cardiac gating, spatial presaturation, gradient moment nulling, stronger and faster gradients with rise time, low flip angle imaging, acquiring multiple overlapping thin slices, even or odd echo numbers in image generation and metabolite characterization.

On the other hand, hardware issues are being surmounted by improvements in areas such as using better gradients to provide a homogeneous magnetic field, RF[6] receiver coils for desired imaging protocols, minimizing eddy currents and artifacts. Limited magnet power is still an active research problem that needs to be solved in order to obtain better image quality. Moreover, both intrinsic and extrinsic physical parameters play a part in determining the image generation and its quality.

With the advancements in MR technology[7] for the clinical MR scanner setup, pulse sequences play an important role and will continue to do so in the future developments in the fields of non-invasive diagnostic, research and therapeutic modalities, which are currently in development. These fields of application including interventional, ultrasound-thermography-MR, gated MR, ultra-fast MR image-guided surgery, and functional MR imaging, continue to demand better and better algorithms. For example, co-registered interventional MR tomography during surgery needs problem-solving skills in the generation of an imaging strategy. The status of clinical MR spectroscopy and an integrated MRI/MRSI approach is still embryonic. It is hoped that better and more reliable ultra-fast MR spectroscopic imaging will soon become available and MRSI metabolite images with spectral information will be used clinically. The following techniques are some of the major advancements in the direction of ultra-fast generation: dynamic contrast-enhanced breast MRI using two- and three-dimensional variable flip angle fast low-angle shot T_1-weighted measurement; dynamic breathing MRI; hepatic lesion fat-suppressed T_2-weighted MR imaging; coronary MR angiography fast-FLAIR MTC pulse sequence; Single Shot Fast Spin-Echo (SSFSE); Fast Spin-Echo Diffusion Coefficient Mapping MRI; adiabatic multiple Spin-Echo pulse sequence; half-Fourier Turbo Spin-Echo MRI (HASTE); 3-D Time of Flight MR Angiography (Ultra-fast MP-RAGE); Coherent and Incoherent Steady-State Spin-Echo (COSESS and INSESS) sequences; phase-modulated binomial RF pulses for spectrally-selective imaging; Dual Echo Steady-State Free Precession (SSFP). These are among the new techniques currently in development. We hope to obtain better and better MR imaging methods with growing insights into applicable image

---

[3]Region of interest.
[4]Contrast to noise ratio.
[5]Signal to noise ratio.
[6]Radio frequency.
[7]Techniques becoming faster and more robust.

generation through the quick availability of a supercomputer setup and the possible integration of other imaging and diagnostic-surgical procedures. Another possibility is the use of these methods for drug monitoring and therapies. Although this is still a long way off, it is already being reported as an MRI success in those fields.

11.1.2 The Future of Cardiac Imaging

With the advancement of digital imaging in the areas of MR, CT, X-ray, Ultrasound, PET and SPECT, it has become very important to understand computer vision and image processing algorithms in order to obtain the full benefit in diagnostic and clinical cardiovascular research. Temporal and spatial resolution help the CVPR algorithms in post-processing and quantification. To cite an example, we saw in Chapter 3 by Suri how important it is to have the models developed, trained and applied to extract diagnostic information and heart motion information, whether it is in MR, CT, X-ray, PET or SPECT. In the future, we will continue to see more model-based algorithms coming into use. These models will be trained, taught to learn the shape of the cardiac anatomy, and are likely to mimic cardiac motion on the basis of neighborhood correspondence. Furthermore, validation algorithms will be needed to evaluate the reliability of the models and to establish the generality of the cardiac behavior. We will see links between CVPR algorithms, digital cardiac imaging and cardiac electrification.

The Future of Cardiac Ultrasound Imaging: as discussed in Chapter 2, there has been remarkable progress made in ultrasonic imaging and echocardiography, such as in Doppler and duplex techniques and color-coded Doppler imaging, particularly during the past 15 years. There are still many opportunities for further improvements. The future promises an important role for digital signal and image processing techniques in both pulse-echo ultrasonic imaging systems and echocardiography. For pulse-echo systems, this can be in the field of electronic beam formation and steering, image resolution improvements, speckle noise reduction, scan conversion, image enhancement, display methods, portable and handheld systems, picture archiving and communication systems. For experimental applications and in particular echocardiography, progress can be expected in myocardial tissue characterization, automatic edge detection, boundary extraction and region segmentation, with complete 3-D and 4-D reconstruction of the objects and heart chambers, which will lead to fully automatic cardiac functional assessment.

One of the major weak points in ultrasound cardiac imaging is the speckle noise that is inherent in pulse-echo imaging, which causes many anatomical features to break up and meaningless fine detail to appear where there should be a uniform gray scale level. As a long-term goal, speckle reduction makes ultrasound images easier to interpret with the possible outcome of improved diagnostic accuracy, shorter reading times, decreased observer variability and greater similarity in results using different systems. To achieve this, there are a number of suggested signal processing-based speckle reduction techniques under investigation including spatial, temporal, frequency and angle compounding, non-linear filtering and adaptive processing [985]. Among the improvements in instrument performance that can be anticipated naturally in a few years time, it is likely that some of the most significant progress will result from the incorporation of hardware and software developments to take advantage of one or more of these methods.

The development of new methods for beam formation and steering can improve the temporal and spatial resolution of ultrasound images. In traditional ultrasound scanning, a single pulse in an ultrasound signal is transmitted along a narrow beam in some particular direction and another pulse is not transmitted until all the echoes have been received. In principle, however, it is possible to transmit a rather broad ultrasound beam and simultaneously receive separate echoes corresponding to different lines at slightly different angles within the broad transmitted beam. This spatial multiplexing process, called Explososcan [13], allows the image frame rate to be increased (perhaps by a factor of 4), which will maintain a corresponding increase in temporal resolution that is necessary for 3-D and 4-D imaging.

A pragmatic and relatively easily realized approach to spatial resolution improvement could be in system optimization [987], [986]. In this approach, a two-dimensional real-time scan would be produced in the usual way; however, a Region of Interest containing the structures to be displayed with enhanced resolution would then be localized within the scan area by using a higher number of scan lines in that region.

With the higher quality images which can be expected in the future and the above mentioned improvements in pulse-echo systems, further progress in experimental applications, such as the processing of echocardiographical images, can be expected in the near future.

11.1.3   The Future of Neurological Segmentation

As shown in Chapter 4 by Suri *et al.*, Chapter 5 by Sharma *et al.*, Chapter 6 by Gopal, Chapter 7 by Sharma and Chapter 8 by Suri *et al.*, neurological segmentation is still a very active area of research. The main theme of segmentation is to obtain a distinct clear classification of tissue features which may be color-coded. Several approaches have been in common use including manual tracing, intensity-based threshold application of single-image segmentation and multi-spectral methods. Recently, emphasis was diverted to automated feature space-based or non-feature space-based classification by unsupervised methods using non-parametric statistical methods. Several new approaches are available in the latest state-of-the-art techniques in MR image segmentation, each one having its own advantages and limitations. For the sake of a multi-directional approach, these are significant in many ways and are discussed here as a guideline for future research and to show the advantages of these methods.

Artificial neural networks for two- and three-dimensional applications can be used to measure the brain's distinctive structures. A new LEGION segmentation method for medical images was proposed in Chapter 5. A 3-D multi-spectral discriminant analysis method was used with automated training class selection to provide better qualitative tissue classification. Segmentation classifies brain tissue into White Matter, Gray Matter and CSF brain components with cortex surfaces obtained by several methods, such as local parametric modeling and Bayesian segmentation, surface generation and local quadric coordinate fitting, surface editing using a combined method for several macaque brains, automated and surface generation. However, segmentation still faces many challenges. The segmentation method for classifying false MS lesions using dual echo MR images was discussed in Chapter 5. This method applied the following techniques: **1**) improved lesion-tissue contrast on MR images; (**2**) using a fast spin-echo sequence involving both CSF signal attenuation and magnetization transfer contrast; and (**3**) flow information from MR images. Using the dual approach of tissue segmentation, it is possible to reduce false lesion classification by 87%. However, segmentation suffers from several *in-vivo* tissue artifacts. Segmentation by fuzzy algorithm for learning vector quantification uses updating of all prototypes of a competitive network by an unsupervised learning process. It performs feature extraction on brain tissue to yield well-defined boundaries. The experiments evaluated a variety of Fuzzy Algorithms for Learning Vector Quantization (FALVQ) in terms of their ability to differentiate abnormal tissues from normal tissue.

Cortical surface-based analysis for segmentation and surface reconstruction is used routinely for functional brain imaging. This highlights active areas in the brain. A pyramidal approach for automatic segmentation of multiple sclerosis lesion in brain MRI was proposed for the quantitative assessment of a lesion load. The systematic pyramidal decomposition in the frequency domain provided a robust and flexible low-level tool for MR image analysis. The best MR correlations were evaluated using surface-based thresholding segmentation techniques to obtain $\frac{T_1}{T_2}$ ratio[8] and magnetization transfer ratio lesion parameters. The split and merge segmentation technique for magnetic resonance images was analyzed for performance evaluation and extension into three dimensions. Hybrid artificial neural network segmentation and classification of dynamic contrast-enhanced MR imaging (DEMRI) for osteosarcoma was reported as a non-invasive visualization technique for necrotic and viable tumors without inter-operator and intra-operator errors.

Another area of development in segmentation is the identification and extraction of brain pathological information. A comparison of pre-contrast vs. post-contrast loads and of manual vs. semi-automated threshold techniques for lesion segmentation demonstrated a T_1 hypointense lesion load in secondary progressive Multiple Sclerosis. An algorithm for the automated unsupervised connectivity-based thresholding segmentation of mid-sagittal brain MR images was evaluated for developing a robust method. A semi-automatic windows-based image processing method using a graphical interface has enabled a combination of different segmentation methods to be used. Automatic tumor segmentation using multi-spectral analysis by knowledge-based segmentation pro-

---

[8]See Chapter 1 for this definition.

vided the separation of the intracranial region extraction along cluster centers for each class. A fully robust automatic brain MRI scan using anisotropic filters and the "snake contour" technique with *a priori* knowledge-based method was evaluated for multi-stage refining of the brain outline. The stochastic relaxation-intensity corrected method uses image enhancement using homomorphic filtering to correct for magnet or coil inhomogeneities. It can perform morphological post-processing by the thresholding method.

Tissue morphology is a challenge which is still to be overcome in segmentation analysis. It is contributed by the evaluation of ventricular CSF, sulcus CSF tissues vs. CSF segmentation on the lowest axial sections, in the regions of the frontal, temporal and occipital lobes. These regions appear on MRI as contiguously positioned between the superior aspect of the temporal lobes and the inferior aspect of the temporal lobes. These remain visible in the apical section and contain 50% or more tissue with clear sulci and gyrate features. These represent supra-ventricular and superior brain volume. These desired regions on MRI images need be corrected, especially in diffused neurodegenerative disease processes like Alzheimer's Disease. Another common artifact due to RF inhomogeneity could be corrected in images by the use of a threshold application and inhomogeneity subtraction in the segmented images to obtain a combination of T_2-PD-weighted training sets. Further improvements in "discriminant analysis" are needed for specific pixel intensities classifying CSF or non-CSF regions in the ventricle and sulcus regions.

Spatial resolution enhancement in MRSI is still a major problem. "Spatial response function" data generation methods still need further improvement to perform better in the spatial resolution of Gray Matter and White Matter tissues for the use of H-1 MR Spectroscopic Imaging and segmentation. This has excellent potential in localized neurodegeneration like demyelination in MS. In this direction, the VOI location for each metabolite was computed, usually by the use of metabolite-specific chemical shift offsets. This method still suffers from the discrepancy that it allows the assignment of the VOI area with high metabolite signal intensities in the center and zero outside the VOI. It needs further improvement to be able to perform a homogeneous assignment. Another artifact of these composite MR images is that of tissue atrophy affecting each MR image column. Presumably, the representation of tissue types in each VOI region corresponding to each MR image column is not correct and it needs to be atrophy corrected for the correct image representation of GM, WM, CSF and Normal Appearing White Matter (NAWM) at each pixel. Significantly, the percentage variation in ventricular size measured by segmentation analysis (the involvement of posterior mesial Gray Matter metabolite variations such as the NAA/Cho ratio) remains positively significant as a predictive power of MR imaging. The use of MR spectroscopic imaging for treatment, detection and quantification of the neurodegenerative diseases using Gadolinium-contrast-enhanced lesions on MRI may further improve the characterization of the disease state in Multiple Sclerosis (MS) in the near future.

A recent trend is using flow dephasing gradient flow-suppression to minimize signal from flow spins. This further removes false classification due to static enhancing structures and flow artifacts for the rapid and robust quantification of lesion enhancements. The local intensity of MS lesion visualization by the threshold application was based on a "seed growing" algorithm. This is accepted as a computer assisted segmentation technique and is currently used at the MR Laboratory, University of Texas Medical School, Houston for MS lesions in Quadruple Contrast images. A unique feature of this is that it allows the operator to select an intensity threshold in addition to an ROI by putting a "seed" in the desired area by pointing the cursor to the appropriate position. Other pixels with similar intensities are determined by using the connectivity algorithm which provides a clear visual of yellow colored lesions seen in a darker background of White Matter.

Future work will include improving the pre-processing segmentation steps of image scaling, image enhancements and RF homogeneity corrections. A graphical user interface will serve as a guide to the pathological staging by automated segmentation algorithms. This will empower speedy segmentation of large data sets. Another approach would be to perform data compression and assess its effect on the segmentation of images of serially-scanned MS patients on a drug trial.

11.1.3.1   The Future of Brain Segmentation in Relation to fMRI

As seen in Chapter 4 by Suri *et al.*, the role of computer vision, graphics and image processing (CVGIP) is very significant in both 2-D and 3-D WM/GM/CSF segmentation techniques. Fast growing applications of the fusion of functional and anatomical information will be one of the challenging tasks. Much of the research is likely to provide a break-though for studying neurological disorders.

Blood Oxygenation Level Dependent functional Magnetic Resonance Imaging (BOLD-fMRI) mainly determines activation in the oxygen rich area in the brain during its functional activities. Its main advantage was utilized in language perception. Phonological processes map[9] the sound information. This can provide the mechanism for verbal information to be temporarily stored in the working memory area in the brain. For this activity to occur, the left lateralization and distributed encoding in the anterior and posterior perisylvian language areas need to be well defined. The trend for using the fMRI segmentation application was to investigate the conditions under which the lateral frontal areas can be activated during speech-discrimination tasks. The segmentation processing may distinguish phonological sub-processes by brain encoding. Subjects perform "same/different" judgements based on the sound of pairs of words. A speech stimulus[10] to an initial consonant may require *overt segmentation* to distinguish it from the rest of the word. So, segmentation allows "different" pairs with varying phonetic voicings of the initial consonant such as dip-tip.[11] Speech stimuli require segmentation since "different" pairs vary in initial consonant voicing and contain different vowels and final con-

---

[9]Activity to recognize and perceive voice message.
[10]Stimulus is singular and stimuli is plural.
[11]It is MRI defined consonants.

sonants. Speech conditions could also be compared to a tonal-discrimination control condition. Segmentation of the fMRI data indicated that speech shows superior temporal activation areas. This was compared to tone discrimination with consistent evidence of frontal activity. In phonological processing, frontal areas may not be involved much. Frontal activation is the net outcome of segmentation processes in speech perception. Other applications of segmentation of fMRI may be useful in the assessment of optic centers of visualization in the near future. Cortical surface-based analysis and surface reconstruction can be used routinely for fMRI segmentation (see Chapter 4 for details).

11.1.3.2   The Future of Spectroscopic Imaging

Several neuro-degenerative brain diseases are still widely reported today as frontline health hazards. As of yet, the mechanism of neuro-degeneration remains unsolved. The main reasons for this include poor assessment of neuronal loss, shrinkage of neuron cell bodies, glial loss and brain volume measurements. Moreover, these may not be specific indicators of neuronal integrity. This highlights the need for future clinical metabolic imaging with the capability to measure and monitor these changes in different regions of the brain. Recent developments in clinical metabolic imaging also suggest the need for further improvement in automatic segmentation, image processing and spectra processing algorithms to obtain the full advantage in diagnostics and therapeutic monitoring. Today, major improvements are focused in two directions independently, as described in Sub-section 7.6. One direction is the identification and classification of the MRI-defined anatomical and tissue composition changes in diseased areas. The other direction is in *in-vivo* metabolic variation and regional imaging. Currently, MR spectroscopic imaging measures the regional distribution of cerebral metabolites at a much coarser spatial resolution. Most metabolite imaging studies of the brain appear to explore the possibility of the metabolic turnover of amino acids in the near future. N-Acetyl Aspartate (NAA), Choline (Cho) and Creatine (Cr) will continue to be used as predictive markers of metabolism in neurons and glial cells in the future.

For MR Spectroscopic Imaging (MRSI) and Single Voxel Spectroscopy (SVS), internal metabolite reference and calibrations of the metabolite absolute concentration are major unsolved problems. Identification of important neuro-chemically active lesion metabolites such as lipids, lactate, myo-Inositol, alanine and acetate is still under investigation for active lesion detection. Today, these metabolites are identified and used as research tools. Other physical artifacts seen are bleed-through, insufficient brain registration, Partial Volume Averaging (PVA) effects, false classification of the tissue disease burden and its quantitation. Segmentation Spectroscopic Imaging algorithms suffer from a variety of issues, including operator-bias, its semi-automatic nature, magnetic field and Radio-Frequency inhomogeneity, CSF contamination, lesion volumetry and assessment of functional motor pathways. Most of the recent segmentation approaches are focused on image analysis for diagnostic accuracy rather than on solving the *in-vivo* physiological and physical artifacts in data acquisition. Several of them have been identified but many others are still poorly understood or poorly implemented.

Despite these technical difficulties, cost-effect benefits and technical advancements continue to strengthen the need for an integrated routine MRI-MRSI as a future clinical assessment modality. The future success of the H-1 clinical metabolic imaging-segmentation approach depends on the expectation and realization of faster, well-equipped, user-friendly systems with improved quality of clinical trials for newer therapeutic agents. Let us now focus on the limited successes in technical improvements relevant to diagnostic use.

Successfully improved spatial resolution techniques may exhibit a strong possibility of solving the issue of brain regional patho-chemical characterization and metabolite regional variations. This unique example was considered in Sub-section 7.3 in a serial follow-up study on brain tissue and MS lesion volumetry. Other potentials of this approach are identified for normal appearing morphological features, metabolite differences in Normal Appearing White Matter (NAWM) or Normal Appearing Gray Matter (NAGM). The advantage of contrast enhanced MS lesions was described in order to better understand the rationale behind the biochemical mechanism during sub-physiological changes during the progression of the MS disease. This advantage could be extrapolated as an *in-vivo* metabolite fingerprinting of the diffused neurodegeneration in Alzheimer's Disease. This was highlighted with an example of Alzheimer's Disease metabolite regional changes in Normal Appearing White Matter (NAWM) in Sub-section 7.5.

Some specific benefits of metabolite characterization and regional distribution by lesion Single Voxel Spectral analysis and/or Chemical Shift Imaging combined with segmentation appear to be future assets for brain imaging. In the future, segmentation algorithms and metabolic imaging will be able to answer unresolved questions. Basal *in-vivo* metabolite absolute concentrations in normal vs. definitive disease have not yet been established. Exciting examples of this are: glutamate which occurs at 4 Tesla using a short-echo time as a TCA marker, N-Acetyl Aspartate flux, as a marker for functional motor pathway and dementia. All these are key future trends in clinical segmentation-metabolic imaging.

The present trend in research on clinical segmentation-localized proton MR spectroscopy (H-1 MRS) indicates several possibilities for neuro-anatomical assessment. As an example, Alzheimer's Disease is characterized by cortical tissue loss, reduced hippocampus volumes, and regional metabolites by related signal hyper-intensities. H-1 MRS in Multiple Sclerosis exhibits enhanced lesions based on the metabolite distribution in the brain. Present day studies demonstrate the future of non-invasive MRI and MR Spectroscopic Imaging integrated approaches to assess significant regional metabolite variations possibly free from physiological artifacts. This was highlighted by the reports from others authors in Sub-section 7.7. H-1 MRSI predicts these metabolite levels better in White Matter for signal hyper-intensities relative to contra-lateral Normal Appearing White Matter (NAWM) regions. This offers the comparison of different metabolite levels in diseased areas with a normal control group.

It further demonstrates White Matter Signal Hyper Intensities (WMSH). The future possibilities of using clinical MRSI and segmentation are anticipated to define neurodegenerative diseases and other diseases of the brain. Furthermore, this research will improve the quality of spectroscopic imaging pulse sequences, automation in MR spectroscopic imaging and spectral analysis methods. Another advantage of this technique is to predict the comparison in left versus right hemisphere metabolites and MR signal intensities. This information is needed urgently as effective therapies are introduced in clinical trials. Regional metabolic characterization in the MS brain is an unavoidable issue and needs to be addressed. The effect of drug treatment on contrast enhanced lesions over several months was highlighted in Sub-section 7.6. The use of clinical segmentation-metabolic imaging further suggests the ability to classify chronic or acute Relapsing Remitting MS or Primary Progressive MS (RRMS, PPMS) with the normal appearing tissue image characteristics described in Sub-section 7.6.

Several of these issues, such as quantification in tissue composition and metabolite screening by Magnetic Resonance Spectroscopic Imaging, were covered in Chapter 5 and Chapter 7. Furthermore, our main goal in the future will be in the direction of improved and definitive answers for MS serial studies, neuro-chemical characterization of Alzheimer's Disease, Myocardial Ischemia, and MS lesions. Other goals of our clinical segmentation include: that MRSI will be an active research study focused on absolute concentration measurement of metabolites, improvements in Chemical Shift Imaging, critical evaluation of lesions bearing single voxel spectral analysis, validation of seeing contrast enhanced MS lesions, and single voxel metabolite abnormalities in neuro-degenerative diseases. In the future, we are likely to see drug trials, MS lesion identification and Myocardial Therapy using high field 4.2 T Magnetic Resonance Imaging.

Success in high spatial resolution and the detection of many more proton resonances will help in MRSI. We hope to see proton MRSI implemented in animal studies primarily and later in routine human clinical studies. It seems that the future diagnostic tool will be complementary to the standard MRI examination for diffused and focal brain diseases with the possible assessment of psychiatric and functional disorders.

Possible major clinical applications of clinical segmentation such as clinical metabolic imaging are expected in the precise assessment of three major groups of neurodegenerative diseases. First among these with a high chance of clinical success seem to be focal diseases such as stroke, epilepsy, Multiple Sclerosis, Alzheimer's Disease, dementia due to HIV and others. Second among them with a moderate chance of success appear to be the group of disorders such as Parkinson's Disease and movement disorders, coma and brain injury. The third group with some probability of success appear to be the psychiatric disorders of the temporal and frontal lobes or basal ganglia mainly seen in schizophrenia, anxiety and mood disorders.

Despite these challenging tasks, MR spectroscopic imaging still suffers from several drawbacks. The main drawbacks are its high cost, long acquisition times, expensive software and lengthy image post-processing modules, uncertain tissue pathology rich regions, poor baseline metabolite screening data and nonspecific internal calibration techniques.

11.1.4   The Future in Digital Mammography

Current research is addressing a range of issues related to mammography including the use of computers for training radiologists, assisting them in their daily work and as the final frontier, automating the screening and diagnostic process. The area of medical image segmentation remains central to the detection of micro-calcifications and masses. The area of image analysis is very mature. Several techniques for identifying image objects have been detailed over the last few decades. However, at the same time, as more research occurs, the inadequacy of applying standard techniques to specialised problems becomes increasingly evident. In this vein, we continue to explore methods that are better suited to digital mammography. These methods are designed to either improve the quality of image segmentation, or generate novel image representation methods that improve our chances of detecting malignancies.

The analysis of digital mammograms is based on a series of steps – a chain of processes before a system can be trained to screen unseen cases. The three components, image analysis, classification and performance analysis, demand their own improvements. The overall chain works effectively only if all of these components are based on state-of-the-art research. The methodologies, therefore, need to be exhaustively tested and compared with other available techniques and their parameters adjusted to the requirements of different images.

In the area of image analysis, significant improvements are needed in image acquisition and standardization. The process of acquiring x-ray mammograms is not straightforward. The image quality depends on a range of factors related to the equipment, methods and subject. Image blurring and loss of detail are common problems. Once the images have been taken on analog media, their conversion to digital format and possible compression have a considerable impact on the level of detail. Compression is needed in the future for techniques to become available that generate a level of standardization across the images. In simple terms this process is implemented as some form of gray level normalization in various studies. However, proper standardization is impossible without a deeper understanding of the optical nature of the image. In the area of image processing including enhancement and segmentation, better quality tools are needed for objective evaluation, rather than choosing methods based on intuition or visual inspection. In this book, we have presented a formalism for comparing image enhancement methods objectively based on the concept of defining targets and their borders. Further work in this area is necessary.

In addition, it is becoming increasingly important to correlate image analysis techniques with our deeper understanding of anatomical structures. For example, linear structures can be removed from the mammogram to aid the quality of segmentation. Similarly, 3-D information can be generated from 2-D views for better detection of masses. Image analysis techniques in the future based on the hierarchical representation of images will be useful, allowing suspicious areas to be highlighted in a lower resolution image before a detailed analysis of the granular structure of the mass or microcalcification is performed in the higher resolution. This will require less storage space and allow faster computational processing.

In the area of classification, sophisticated classifiers are needed. Non-linear classification techniques are necessary to generate better recognition performances. One of the main changes required for a standard approach will be to use a loss matrix penalizing false positives and true negatives as per user requirement. This matrix can be used for optimizing the parameters of the classifier during the training process. Another important area for investigation is the multiple classifier combination. Recent research in this field has highlighted the benefits of classifier combination resulting in solutions that cannot be effectively solved by a single classifier, or that can be performed more effectively by a modular classification approach. One classic approach to classifier combination is the ensemble approach. Here, a collection of different classifiers gives a solution to the same problem. The aim is to increase the overall classification performance by classifier output fusion using a suitable combination strategy. An alternative modular approach is built on the basis that the problem cannot be solved by a single classifier but must be broken into sub-tasks. By developing specialized classifiers capable of providing solutions to particular tasks and combining them in a hierarchical framework, the aim is to develop a solution using the efficiency of modular problem decomposition.

Performance analysis of various image analysis and classification tools is extremely important. The performance of individual components within the chain or the chain itself can be evaluated. One of the most important areas of research that remains an unknown territory is on evaluating segmentation algorithms in medical imaging. Previous work in this area within the image processing community has focused on determining segmentation accuracy on synthetic objects of various shapes and sizes. In the case of mammography, ground truth does not accurately define the boundary of the mass to be found, and hence the degree of overlap between the ground truth and the actual segmented area does not accurately quantify the quality of the segmentation. Benchmark data at a greater degree of detail and accuracy for ground truth images is needed for better quality segmentation evaluation. In order for the techniques to be comparable, therefore, some standard benchmarks from real applications need to be developed. It is also important that experimental results across studies can be compared. Therefore, it is necessary that more research focuses on available standard databases, in order for researchers to test their work on a uniform benchmark. Studies need to report results on full databases rather than on a selective portion, as is so often the case. In the area of image analysis, the conceptual importance of the relative utility of various algorithms can not be ignored. Without some form of comparative measurement on standard data and standard evaluation measures, the broader area of medical imaging can not benefit. At the same time, it is also important to understand what qualifies as a benchmark – publishing the benchmark data and making it available on the Internet is not sufficient. In the future, digital mammography promises to bring a significant improvement over conventional film-screen mammography in the early detection of breast cancer. Digital mammography assists in the early detection of breast cancer by incorporating modern electronics and computers into x-ray mammography methods. Instead of using x-ray film, an image is acquired electronically and can be stored directly into a computer. This will still involve mammography through x-ray, as it is the least expensive and the best method of screening subjects for breast cancer. This transition from analog to digital is slowly taking over all areas of medical imaging. This change will make computer-based techniques even more popular in mammography. The segmentation techniques presented in this book will remain equally relevant in the face of such a change. It is quite difficult to know how well computers can actually perform in a clinical setting, as a range of studies has shown results on selective data using selective evaluation measurements. However, the general trend has been an improvement in the quality of computer aided detection techniques for screening mammograms. Computers also have a key role to play as second screeners or for aiding the radiologist in a variety of ways. A system that can automatically separate normal mammograms from suspicious ones will be extremely valuable. Initial clinical trials in the U.S. by the Food and Drug Administration (FDA) found that a trial digital system should help doctors store, manipulate and transmit images. However, until more research is carried out, the FDA concluded that data still need to be collected to demonstrate "that the digital images are more helpful in finding cancer" than standard analog/film images. Undoubtedly, digital technology will allow doctors to store and transfer images electronically, making it easier for them to retrieve and send to specialists for evaluation. In addition, digital images may also be manipulated to correct for under- or over-exposure, saving women from the need for another mammogram.

The primary role for breast imaging is in the detection of breast cancer through breast screening, thus allowing for the early detection of malignancy and preventing early death. Though many of the structures found may be benign so long as early stage clinical cancers are detected, mammography will prove to be beneficial. As a diagnostic technique, mammography suffers from an inability to differentiate between solid breast lesions and other types of lesions. On the basis of such observations, it is unlikely that mammography will be of use in both areas. However, it will continue to be used as an inexpensive and effective means of screening women for the early detection of breast cancer.

11.1.5 The Future of Pathology Image Segmentation

The purpose of the segmentation of digitized specimens representing blood samples consists in the detection of the cells of interest and their partition into elemental regions which are believed to be significant to the diagnosis. These regions satisfy a homogeneity criterion and their further automatic analysis should provide objective clues to the diagnosis decision. However, while the cell segmentation task can be formulated as a general paradigm, its implementation is application specific. Issues such as the features to be analyzed, the homogeneity of the elemental structures, the scale and stability of the segmentation, the fusion of local and global information, the parameter selection and evaluation of the segmentation quality should always be defined according to the final goal of the entire processing sequence.

Applying a segmentation model to a scenario that is different from the original design can, therefore, lead to unsatisfactory results. For example, the segmenter presented in Chapter 10 yields very good results in delineating the nucleus and cytoplasm regions of various types of cells. By employing a robust clustering analysis of the color vectors associated with the input image, the regions of interest are recovered, most often based only on some preset parameters. Nevertheless, the piecewise constant structure which we assumed is in many other pathology applications is violated. Indeed, a slowly changing illumination may generate an elongated cluster whose delineation is difficult, due to its increased probability of merging with other clusters. A similar problem appears in the case of cluttered images, when high density regions in the color space are not necessarily meaningful in the image. When these artifacts are present, they can be eliminated by taking into account the spatial information carried by the pixel coordinates, as suggested in [953].

Although the automatic parameter selection for segmentation has been addressed by many scientists, it is still an open research problem. The difficulty consists in translating the top-down constraints, which are usually vague and imprecise, in mathematical expressions employed in the optimization of certain criteria. The analytical methods that include high level constraints are limited to simple frameworks, while the numerical methods based on different segmentation instances require extensive simulations and are not suitable for real-time processing. With the advance of computational technology, however, we expect that the complexity of the latter will prevail, allowing the integration of more advanced statistical procedures [949], [959] in the online analysis of the input data.

Bibliography

[1] Geiser, E. A. and Oliver, L. H., Cardiac Imaging and Image Processing, Chapter 1: Echocardiography: Physics and instrumentation, pp. 3-23, McGraw-Hill, 1986.

[2] Dunn, F., Ultrasound, IEEE Trans. on Education, Vol. 34, No. 3, pp. 266-268, 1991.

[3] McDicken, W. N., Diagnostic Ultrasonics (3rd ed.), Churchill Livingstone, Inc., NY, ISBN: 0-4430-4132-6, 1991.

[4] Carr, J., Surface Reconstruction in 3-D Medical Imaging, Ph.D. Thesis, University of Canterbury, New Zealand, 1996.

[5] Edler, I. and Hertz, C. H., Use of ultrasonic reflectoscope for continuous recording of movements of heart walls, Kurgl Fysiogr. Sallad i Lund Forhandl, Vol. 24, No. 5, 1954.

[6] Feigenbaum, H., Echocardiography (3rd ed.), Chapter 1. Instrumentation, pp. 1-50, ISBN: 0812107586, Lea and Febiger, 1980.

[7] Skorton, D. J., Collins, S. M. and Kerber, R. E., Cardiac Imaging and Image Processing, Chapter 9: Digital image processing and analysis in echocardiography, pp. 171-205, McGraw-Hill, 1986.

[8] Wells, P. N. T., Technical introduction to echocardiography, British Medical Bulletin, Vol. 45, No. 4, pp. 829-837, 1989.

[9] Wells, P. N. T., Advances in ultrasound techniques and instrumentation, Churchill Livingston, Inc., New York, N.Y., 1993.

[10] Fish, P., Physics and Instrumentation of Diagnostic Medical Ultrasound, ISBN: 0-4719-2651-5, John Wiley and Sons, Ltd., Chichester, England, 1990.

[11] Geiser, E. A., Echocardiography: Physics and instrumentation. In Marcus, M. L., Schelbert, H. R., Skorton, D. J. and Wolf G. L. (eds), Cardiac Imaging, pp. 348-364, W. B. Saunders, 1991.

[12] Gregg, E. C. and Palogallo, G. L., Acoustic impedance of tissue, Invest. Radiol., Vol. 4, No. 6, pp. 363-375, 1969.

[13] Harris, R. A. and Wells, P. N. T., Ultimate Limits in Ultrasound Image Resolution, In Wells, P. N. T., Advances in Ultrasound Techniques and Instrumentation, Chapter 9, pp. 109-123. Churchill Livingstone, Inc., New York, NY, 1993.

[14] Kremkau, F. W., Diagnostic Ultrasound, (4th ed.), ISBN: 0-7216-4308-6, W. B. Saunders Company, Philadelphia, PA, USA, 1993.

[15] Rohling, R. N., 3-D Ultrasound Imaging: Optimal volumetric reconstruction. First year report, Cambridge University, Engineering Department, 1996.

[16] Hood, Jr., W. P. and Rackley, C. E., Ventriculography, In Grossman, William (Ed.), Cardiac Catheterization and Angiography, ISBN: 0-8121-0504-4, Lea and Febiger, Philadelphia, PA, pp. 111-121, 1974.

[17] Zissermann, D., Strand, E. M., Smith, L. R., Wixson, S. E., Hood, Jr., W. P., Mantle, J. A., Rogers, W. J., Russell, R. O. Jr. and Rackley, C. E., Cardiac catheterization and angiographic analysis computer applications, Progress in Cardiovascular Diseases, Vol. 25, No. 5, pp. 409-434, 1983.

[18] Conti, C. R. and Ross, R. S., The risks of cardiac catheterization, American Heart Jour., Vol. 78, No. 3, pp. 289-291, 1969.

[19] Shung, K. K., Smith, M. B. and Tsui, B. M. W., Principles of medical imaging, Academic Press, San Diego, Calif.: ISBN: 0-1264-0970-6, 1992.

[20] Rickerd, C. L., Cardiac Catheter, US Patent #: 5,322,509, June 21, 1994.

[21] Stephen, B. G., Goldman, M. R. and Leonard, M. Z., Cardiac Catheter and method of using same, US Patent #: 4,033,331, July 5, 1977.

[22] MacCallum, J. B., On the muscular architecture and growth of the ventricles of the heart, Johns Hopkins Hospital Rep., Vol. 9, pp. 307-335, 1900.

[23] Mall, F. P., On the muscular architecture of the ventricules of the human heart, Am. J. of Anat., Vol. 11, pp. 211-266, 1911.

[24] Moodie, D. S. and Yiannikas, J., Digital subtraction angiography of the heart and lungs, Grune and Stratton, Orlando, Florida, ISBN: 0-8089-1775-7, 1986.

[25] Mancini, G. B. J., Clinical applications of cardiac digital angiography, Raven Press, NY, ISBN: 0-8816-7361-7, 1988.

[26] Moore, R. J., Imaging Principles of Cardiac Angiography, Aspen Publishers, Rockville, Maryland, ISBN 0-8342-0120-8, pp. 1-258, 1990.

[27] Trenholm, B. G., Winter, D. A. and Dinn, D. F., Digital Computer Analysis of Left Ventricular Volume from Videoangiograms, Biomedical Sciences Instrumentation, Vol. 7, pp. 1-3, 1970.

[28] Suri, J. S., Contouring of Motion Objects In Fuzzy Low Contrast Multiple Image Frames: An Application in Cardiological X-ray Imaging, Ph.D. Thesis, University of Washington, Seattle, 1997.

[29] Stark, D. D. and William, Jr., G. B., Magnetic Resonance Imaging (2nd ed.) Mosby, ISBN: 0-8016-4930-7, 1992.

[30] Lauterbur, P. C., Image formation by induced local interactions: Example employing nuclear magnetic resonance, Nature, Vol. 242, pp. 190-191, 1973.

[31] Bedell, B. J., Narayana, P. A. and Wolinsky, J. S., A dual approach for minimizing false lesion classification on magnetic resonance images, Magnetic Resonance in Medicine, Vol. 37, No. 1, pp. 94-112, 1997.

[32] Bedell, B. J. and Narayana, P. A., Volumetric analysis of white matter, gray matter and CSF using fractional volume analysis, Magnetic Resonance in Medicine, Vol. 39, No. 6, pp. 961-969, 1998.

[33] Wild, J. M. and Marshall, I., Normalization of metabolite images in 1-H NMR spectroscopic imaging, Magnetic Resonance Imaging, Vol. 15, No. 9, pp. 1057-1066, 1997.

[34] Sharma, R., Studies on NMR Relaxation Times of Biological Tissues and MR-Biochemical Correlation in Medicine, Ph.D. Thesis, Indian Institute of Technology, Delhi, India, pp. 28-35, 1995.

[35] Brookes, J. A., Redpath, T. W., Gilbert, F. J., Murray, A. D. and Staff, R. T., Accuracy of T1 measurement in dynamic contrast enhanced breast MRI using two- and three-dimensional variable flip angle fast low-angle shot, Journal of Magnetic Resonance Imaging, Vol. 9, No. 2, pp. 163-171, 1999.

[36] Suga, K., Tsukuda, T., Awaya, H., Takano, K., Koike, S., Matsunaga, N., Sugi, K. and Esato, K., Impaired respiratory mechanics in pulmonary emphysema: evaluation with dynamic breathing MRI, Journal of Magnetic Resonance Imaging, Vol. 10, No. 4, pp. 510-520, 1999.

[37] Outwater, E. K., Ultrafast MRI imaging of the pelvis (Review), European Journal of Radiology, Vol. 29, No. 3, pp. 233-244, 1999.

[38] Kanematsu, M., Hoshi, H., Itoh, K., Murakami, T., Hori, M., Kondo, H., Yokoyama, R. and Nakamura, H., Focal hepatic lesion: comparison of four fat suppressed T2-weighted MR imaging pulse sequences, Radiology, Vol. 211, No. 2, pp. 363-371, 1999.

[39] Duerinckx, A. J., Coronary MR angiography, Radiology Clinics North America, Vol. 37, No. 2, pp. 273-318, 1999.

[40] Filippi, M., Lesion load measurements in multiple sclerosis: the effect of incorporating magnetization transfer contrast in fast-FLAIR sequence, Magnetic Resonance Imaging, Vol. 17, No. 3, pp. 459-461, 1999.

[41] Kadoya, M., Gabata, T., Matsui O., Kawamori, Y., Takashima, T., Matsuura, Y., Kurata, Y. and Kawahara, K., Usefulness of T2-weighted images using Single Shot Fast Spin Echo (SSFSE) pulse sequence for the evaluation of pancreatobiliary diseases: comparison with MRCP using SSFSE, Nippon Rinsho, Vol. 56, No. 11, pp. 2836-2841, 1998.

[42] Brockstedt, S., Thomsen, C., Wirestam, R., Holtas, S. and Stahlberg, F., Quantitative Diffusion Coefficient Maps using Fast Spin-Echo MRI, Magnetic Resonance Imaging, Vol. 16, No. 8, pp. 877-886, 1998.

[43] Zweckstetter, M. and Holak, T. A., An adiabatic multiple spin-echo pulse sequence: removal of systematic errors due to pulse imperfections and off-resonance effects, Journal of Magnetic Resonance, Vol. 133, No. 1, pp. 134-47, 1998.

[44] Coates, G. G., Borello, J. A., Mc Farland, E. G., Mirowitz, S. A., and Brown, J. J., Hepatic T2-weighted MRI: a prospective comparison, including breath-hold, Half-Fourier Turbo Spin Echo MRI (HASTE),

Journal of Magnetic Resonance Imaging, Vol. 8, No. 3, pp. 642-649, 1998.

[45] Yamashita, Y., Mitsuzaki, K., Tang, Y., Namimoto, T. and Takahashi, M., Gadolinium-enhanced breath-hold three-dimensional time-of-flight MR Angiography of abdominal and pelvic vessels: the value of Ultra-fast MP-RAGE sequences, Journal of Magnetic Resonance Imaging, Vol. 7, No. 4, pp. 623-628, 1997.

[46] Werthner, H., Krieg, R., Ladebeck, R. and Saemann-Ischenko, G., COSESS and INSESS: coherent and incoherent spin-echo in the steady state, Magnetic Resonance in Medicine, Vol. 36, No. 2, pp. 294-305, 1996.

[47] Thomasson, D., Purdy, D. and Finn, J. P., Phase-modulated binominal RF pulses for fast spectrally-selective musculoskeletal imaging, Magnetic Resonance in Medicine, Vol. 35, No. 4, pp. 563-568, 1996.

[48] Hardy, P. A., Recht, M. P., Piraino, D. and Thomasson, D., Optimization of a dual echo in the steady state (DESS) free-precession sequence for imaging cartilage, Journal of Magnetic Resonance Imaging, Vol. 6, No. 2, pp. 329-335, 1996.

[49] Zha, L. and Lowe, I. J., Optimized Ultra-Fast Imaging Sequence (OUFIS), Magnetic Resonance in Medicine, Vol. 33, No. 3, pp. 377-395, 1995.

[50] Foo, T. K., Sawyer, A. M., Faulkner, W. H. and Mills, D. G., Inversion in the steady state contrast optimization and reduced imaging time with fast three-dimensional inversion-recovery-prepared GRE pulse sequences, Radiology, Vol. 191, No. 1, pp. 85-90, 1994.

[51] Tien, R. D., Felsberg, G. J., Friedman, H., Brown, M. and MacFall, J., MR imaging of high-grade cerebral gliomas: value of diffusion-weighted echoplanar pulse sequences, American Journal of Roentgenology (AJNR), Vol. 162, No. 3, pp. 671-677, 1994.

[52] Tkach, J. A., Ruggieri, P. M., Ross, J. S., Modic, M. T., Dillinger, J. J. and Masaryk, T. J., Pulse sequence strategies for vascular contrast in time-of-flight carotid MR angiography, Journal of Magnetic Resonance Imaging, Vol. 3, No. 6, pp. 811-820, 1993.

[53] Urhahn, R., Drobnitzky, M., Klose, K. C. and Gunther, R. W., Incremental flip angle snapshot FLASH MRI of hepatic lesions: improvement of signal-to-noise and contrast, Journal of Computer Assisted Tomography, Vol. 16, No. 2, pp. 219-225, 1992.

[54] Gyngell, M. L., The application of steady-state free precession in rapid 2DFT NMR imaging: FAST and CE-FAST sequences, Magnetic Resonance Imaging, Vol. 6, No. 4, pp. 415-419, 1988.

[55] Seeram, E., Computed Tomography; Physical Principles, Clinical Applications and Quality Control, W. B. Saunders, ISBN: 0-7216-6710-4, 1994.

[56] Peters, T. M. and Williams, J., The Fourier Transform in Biomedical Engineering, Birkhauser, Boston, ISBN: 0-8176-3941-1, 1998.

[57] Glaspy, J. A., Hawkins, R., Hoh, C. K. and Phelps, M. E., Use of positron emission tomography in oncology. Oncology (Huntingt), Vol. 7, No. 7, pp. 41-46, Jul. 1993.

[58] Bergmann, S. R., Cardiac positron emission tomography, Semin. Nucl. Med., Vol. 28, No. 4, pp. 320-40, Oct. 1998.

[59] Watson, J. D., Images of the working brain: Understanding human brain function with positron emission tomography, J Neurosci Methods, Vol. 74, No. 2, pp. 245-56, Jun 27, 1997.

[60] Schiller, N. B., Two-dimensional echocardiographic determination of left ventricular volume, systolic function and mass. Summary and discussion of the 1989 recommendations of the American Society of Echocardiography. Circulation, Vol. 84 ([suppl I]), pp. 280-287, 1991.

[61] Berne, R. M. and Levy, M. N., Principles of Physiology, Chapter 17, pp. 214-227, Wolfe Publishing, 1990.

[62] Force, T. L., Folland, E. D., Aebischer, N., Sharma, S. and Parisi, A. F., Echocardiographic Assessment of Ventricular Function, In Marcus, M. L., Schelbert, H. R., Skorton, D. J. and Wolf, G. L. (eds), Cardiac Imaging, pp. 374-401, W. B. Saunders, 1991.

[63] Gibson, D. G., Assessment of left ventricular structure and function by cross sectional echocardiography. British Med. Bulletin, Vol. 45 No. 4, pp. 1061-1075, 1989.

[64] Salcedo, E., Atlas of Echocardiography (2nd ed.), Chapter 11, The Left Ventricle, pp. 197-215, W. B. Saunders, 1985.

[65] Xiao, H., How to do echocardiography, part 2: Assessment of LV function by echocardiography. British J. of Cardiology, Vol. 2 (Supp. 2), pp. 48-51, 1995.

[66] Stamm, R. B., Carabello, B. A., Mayers, D. L. and Martin, R. P., Two-dimensional echocardiographic measurement of left ventricular ejection fraction: prospective analysis of what constitutes an adequate determination, American Heart J., Vol. 104, No. 1, pp. 136-144, 1982.

[67] Konstam, M., Dracup, K., Baker, D., *et al.*., Heart Failure: Evaluation and Care of Patients With Left-Ventricular Systolic Dysfunction, Rockville, MD: Agency for Health Care Policy and Research, Public Health Service, U.S. Department of Health and Human Services, Clinical Practice Guideline No. 11, AHCPR Publication No. 94-0612, June 1994.

[68] Moynihan, P. F., Parisi, A. F. and Feldman, C. L., Quantitative detection of regional left ventricular contraction abnormalities by two-dimensional echocardiography, I. Analysis of methods, Circulation, Vol. 63, No. 4, pp. 752-760, 1981.

[69] Garrison, J. B., Weiss, J. L., Maughan, W. L., Tuck, O. M., Guier, W. H. and Fortuin, N. J., Quantifying regional wall motion and thickening in two-dimensional echocardiography with a computer-aided contouring system, In Proc. of Computers in Cardiology, IEEE Press, pp. 25-35. 1977.

[70] Skorton, D. J., Collins, S. M. and Kerber, R. E., Cardiac Imaging and Image Processing, Chapter 9: Digital image processing and analysis in echocardiography, pp. 171-205, McGraw-Hill, 1986.

[71] Adam, D., Hareuveni, O. and Sideman, S., Semiautomated border tracking of cine echocardiographic ventricular images, IEEE Trans. on Med. Imag., Vol. 6, No. 3, pp. 266-271, 1987.

[72] Bijnens, B., Van Hamme, M., Vandekerckhove, J., Herregods, M. C., Nuyts, J., Suetens, P. and Van de Werf, F., Segmentation of echocardiographic images using classification in the radiofrequency feature space, In Proc. of Computers in Cardiology, IEEE Press, pp. 733-736, 1995.

[73] Brennecke, R., Hahne, H., Wessel, A. and Heintzen, P. H., Computerized enhancement techniques for echocardiographic sector scans, In Proc. of Computers in Cardiology, IEEE Press, pp. 7-11, 1981.

[74] Canny, J., A computational approach to edge detection, IEEE Trans. on Pattern Analysis and Machine Intelligence, Vol. 8, No. 6, pp. 679-698, 1986.

[75] Chu, C. H., Delp, E. J. and Buda, A. J., Detecting left ventricular endocardial and epicardial boundaries by digital two-dimensional echocardiography, IEEE Trans. on Med. Imag., Vol. 7, No. 2, pp. 81-90, 1988.

[76] Chalana, V., Linker, D. T., Haynor, D. R. and Kim, Y., A Multiple Active Contour Model for Cardiac Boundary Detection on Echocardiographic Sequences, IEEE Trans. on Med. Imag., Vol. 15, No. 3, pp. 290-298, 1996.

[77] Coppini, G., Poli, R. and Valli, G., Recovery of the 3-d shape of the left ventricle from echocardiographic images, IEEE Trans. on Med. Imag., Vol. 14, No. 2, pp. 301-317, 1995.

[78] Collins, S. M., Skorton, D. J., Geiser, E. A., Nichols, J. A., Conetta, D. A., Pandian, N. G. and Kerber, R. E., Computer assisted edge detection in two-dimensional echocardiography: Comparison with anatomic data, American Journal of Cardiology, Vol. 53, No. 9, pp. 1380-1387, May 1984.

[79] Chou, W. S., Wu, C. M., Chen, Y. C. and Hsieh, K. S., Detecting myocardial boundaries of left ventricle from a single 2DE image, Pattern Recognition, Vol. 23, No. 7, pp. 799-806, 1990.

[80] Detmer, P. R., Bashein, G. and Martin, R. W., Matched filter identification of left-ventricular endocardial borders in transesophageal echocardiograms, IEEE Trans. on Med. Imag., Vol. 9, No. 4, pp. 396-404, 1990.

[81] Dias, J. and Leitao, J., Wall position and thickness estimation from two dimensional echocardiograms. In Proceedings of the Nuclear Science Symposium and Medical Imaging Conference Vols. 1-3, Ch 394, pp. 1246-1250, 1993.

[82] Dias, J. and Leitao, J., Wall position and thickness estimation from sequences of echocardiographic images, IEEE Trans. on Med. Imag., Vol. 15, No. 1, pp. 25-38, 1996.

[83] Eltoft, D. A., Aylward, P. E., Collins, S. M., Skorton, D. J., Noel, M. P., Knosp, B. N., Berbaum, K. S., Taylor, A. L. and Kerber, R. E., Real-time image in two-dimensional echocardiography, In Proc. of Computers in Cardiology, IEEE Press, pp. 481-484, 1984.

[84] Ezekiel, A., Garcia, E. V., Areeda, J. S. and Corday, S. R., Automatic and intelligent left ventricular contour detection from two-dimensional echocardiograms, In Proc. of Computers in Cardiology, IEEE Press, pp. 261-264, 1985.

[85] Friedland, N. and Adam, D., Automatic ventricular cavity boundary detection from sequential ultrasound images using simulated annealing, IEEE Trans. on Med. Imag., Vol. 8, No. 4, pp. 344-353, 1989.

[86] Feng, J., Lin, W. C. and Chen, C., Epicardial boundary detection using fuzzy reasoning, IEEE Trans. on Med. Imag., Vol. 10, No. 2, pp. 187-199, 1991.

[87] Garcia, E., Ezekiel, A., Levy, R., Zwehl, W., Ong, K., Corday, E., Areeda, J., Meerbaum, S. and Corday, S., Automated computer enhancement and analysis of left ventricular two-dimensional echocardiograms, In Proc. of Computers in Cardiology, IEEE Press, pp. 399-402, 1982.

[88] Garcia, E., Gueret, P., Bennet, M., Corday, E., Zwehl, W., Meerbaum, S., Corday, S. R., Swan, H. I. C. and Berman, D., Real-time computerization of two-dimensional echocardiography, American Heart Journal, Vol. 102, pp. 783-792, 1981.

[89] Han, C. Y., Lin, K. N., Wee, W. G., Mintz, R. M. and Porembka, D. T., Knowledge-based image analysis for automated boundary extraction of transesophageal echocardiographic left-ventricular images, IEEE Trans. on Med. Imag., Vol. 10, No. 4, pp. 602-610, 1991.

[90] Hunter, I., Soraghan, J., Christie, J. and Durrani, T., A novel artificial neural network based system for automatic extraction of left ventricular edge features, In Proc. of Computers in Cardiology, IEEE Press, pp. 201-204, 1993.

[91] Klinger, J. W., Vaughan, C. L., Fraker, T. D. and Andrews, L. T., Segmentation of echocardiographic images using mathematical morphology, IEEE Trans. on Biomed. Eng., Vol. 35, No. 11, pp. 925-934, 1988.

[92] Karras, T., Wilson, D. C., Geiser, E. A. and Conetta, D. A., Automatic identification of papillary muscle in left ventricular short-axis echocardiographic images, IEEE Trans. on Biomed. Eng., Vol. 43, No. 5, pp. 460-470, 1996.

[93] Linker, D. T., Pearlman, A. S., Lewelien, T. K., Huntsman, L. H. and Moritz, W. E., Automated endocardial definition of 2-D echocardiograms: A comparison of four standard edge detectors and improved thresholding techniques, In Proc. of Computers in Cardiology, IEEE Press, pp. 395-398, 1982.

[94] Lindower, P. D., Rath, L., Preslar, J., Burns, T. L., Rezai, K. and Vandenberg, B. F., Quantification of left ventricular function with an automated border detection system and comparison with radionuclide ventriculography, American Journal of Cardiology, Vol. 73, pp. 195-199, 1994.

[95] Maes, L., Bijnens, B., Suetens, P. and Van de Werf, F., Automated contour detection of the left ventricle in short axis view in 2d echocardiograms, Machine Vision and Applications, Vol. 6, No. 1, pp. 1-9, 1993.

[96] Perez, J. E., Klein, S. C., Prater, D. M., Fraser, C. E., Cardona, H., Waggoner, A. D., Holland, M. R., Miller, J. G. and Sobel, B. E., Automated, on-line quantification of left ventricular dimensions and function by echocardiography with backscatter imaging and lateral gain compensation, American Journal of Cardiology, Vol. 70, No. 13, pp. 1200-1205, 1992.

[97] Parker, D. L., Pryor, T. A. and Ridges, J. D., Enhancement of two-dimensional echocardiographic images by lateral filtering, Comput. Biomed. Res., pp. 12-265, 1979.

[98] Ruiz, E. E. S. and Fairhurst, M. C., Dynamic Boundary Location for 2-D Echocardiographic Images in a Semi-Automated Environment, In Proc. Int. Conf. Img. Proc. and its Appl., Edinburgh, pp. 134-138, 1995.

[99] Skorton, D. J. and Collins, S. M., Echocardiography: A Review of Cardiovascular Ultrasound, Chapter 1. Digital computer image analysis in echocardiography, McGraw-Hill, pp. 1-15, 1984.

[100] Skorton, D. J. and Collins, S. M., Garcia, E., Geiser, E. A., Hillard, W., Kroppes, W., Linker, D. and Schwartz, G., Digital signal and image processing in echocardiography, American Heart Journal, Vol. 110, pp. 1266-1283, 1985.

[101] Suri, J. S., Haralick, R. M. and Sheehan, F. H., Accurate Left Ventricular Apex Position and Boundary Estimation From Noisy Ventriculograms, In Proc. of Computers in Cardiology, IEEE Press, pp. 257-260, 1996.

[102] Skorton, D. J., McNary, C. A., Child, J. S., Newton, F. C. and Shah, P. M., Digital image processing of two-dimensional echocardiograms: identification of endocardium. American Journal of Cardiology, Vol. 48, pp. 479-486, 1981.

[103] Tamura, S. and Nakano, S., Three-dimensional reconstruction of echocardiograms on orthogonal sections, Pattern Recognition, Vol. 18, pp. 115-124, 1985.

[104] Vitale, D. F., Lauria, G., Pelaggi, N., Gerundo, G., Bordini, C., Leosco, D., Rengo, C. and Rengo, F., Optimal number of averaged frames for noise reduction of ultrasound images, In Proc. of Computers in Cardiology, IEEE Press, pp. 639 -641, 1993.

[105] Vandenberg, B. F., Rath, L. S., Stuhlmuller, P., Melton, H. E. and Skorton, D. J., Estimation of left ventricular cavity area with an on-line semiautomated echocardiographic edge detection system, Circulation, Vol. 86, pp. 159-166, 1992.

[106] Wilson, D. C., Geiser, E. A. and Li, J. H., The use of matched filters for extraction of left ventricular features in 2-dimensional short-axis echocardiographic images, In Wilson, D. (ed.), Proc. of Mathematical Methods in Medical Imaging, Vol. 1768, SPIE - The International Society for Optical Engineering, San Diego, ISBN 0-8194-0941-3, pp. 37-49, 1992.

[107] Setarehdan, S. K. and Soraghan, J. J., Automatic left ventricular feature extraction and visualisation from echocardiographic images, In Proc. of Computers In Cardiology, IEEE Press, pp. 9-12, 1996,

[108] Setarehdan, S. K. and Soraghan, J. J., Fully Automatic Echocardiographical Feature Extraction Applied to Left Ventricular Wall Motion and Volume Changes Visualization, 18th IEEE Int. Conf. Of Engineering in Medicine and Biology (EMBS), pp. Vol. 2, 877-878, 1996.

[109] Setarehdan, S. K. and Soraghan, J. J., Cardiac Left Ventricular Volume Changes Assessment by Long Axis Echocardiographical Image Processing, International Conference of Image Processing and its Applications, July 14-17, 1997.

[110] Setarehdan, S. K. and Soraghan, J. J., Cardiac Left Ventricular Volume Changes Assessment by Long Axis Echocardiographical Image Processing, IEE Proceedings – Vision, Image and Signal Processing (Special Section from IPA97), Vol. 145, No. 3, pp. 203-212, 1998.

[111] Setarehdan, S. K. and Soraghan, J. J., Fuzzy Multiresolution Signal Processing, Proc. of the 3rd World Multiconference on Systemics, Cybernetics and Informatics (SCI) and 5th International Conference on Information Systems Analysis and Synthesis (ISAS), 1999.

[112] Setarehdan, S. K. and Soraghan, J. J., Automatic Cardiac LV Boundary Detection and Tracking Using Hybrid Fuzzy Temporal and Fuzzy Multiscale Edge Detection, IEEE Trans. on Biomed. Eng., Vol. 46, No. 11, pp. 1364-1378, 1999.

[113] Xiao, H., How to do echocardiography. Part 2: Assessment of LV function by echocardiography, British Journal of Cardiology, Vol. 2 (Supp. 2), pp. 48-51, 1995.

[114] Zhang, L. and Geiser, E. A., An effective algorithm for extracting serial endocardial borders from 2-dimensional echocardiograms, IEEE Trans. on Biomed. Eng., Vol. 31, No. 6, pp. 441-447, 1984.

[115] Zwehl, W., Levy, R. and Garcia, E., Haenchen, R. V., Child, W., Corday, S. R., Meerbaum, S. and Corday, E., Validation of computerized edge detection algorithm for qualitative 2-D echocardiography, Circulation, Vol. 68, No. 5, pp. 1127-1135, 1983.

[116] Bellman, R. E. and Zadeh, L., Decision-making in a fuzzy environment, Manage. Sci., Vol. 17, No. 4, pp. B141-B164, 1970.

[117]   Dubois, D. and Prade, H., Fuzzy sets and systems: Theory and applications, ISBN: 0-1222-2750-6, Academic Press, Inc., 1980.

[118]   Golub, G. H. and van Loan, C. F., Matrix Computations, (2nd ed.), ISBN: 0-8018-3739-1, Johns Hopkins Press, Baltimore, Maryland, 1989.

[119]   Sonka, M., Hlavac, V. and Boyle, R., Image Processing, Analysis and Machine Vision, ISBN: 0-5349-5393-X, Chapman and Hall Computing, 1993.

[120]   Wang, L. and Mendel, J., Generating fuzzy rules by learning from examples, IEEE Trans. on Systems, Man and Cybernetics, Vol. 22, No. 6, pp. 1414-1427, 1992.

[121]   Zimmerman, H. J., Methods and applications of fuzzy mathematical programming, In: Yager, R.R. and Zadeh, L.A., An introduction to fuzzy logic applications in intelligent systems, pp. 97-120, Kluwer Academic Publishers, 1992.

[122]   Bergholm, F., Edge focusing, IEEE Trans. on Pattern Analysis and Machine Intelligence, Vol. 9, No. 6, pp. 726-741, 1987.

[123]   Lu, Y. and Jain, R. C., Reasoning about edges in scale space. IEEE Trans. on Pattern Analysis and Machine Intelligence, Vol. 14, No. 4, pp. 450-467, 1992.

[124]   Mallat, S., A Theory for Multiresolution Signal Decomposition: The Wavelet Representation, IEEE Trans. on Pattern Analysis and Machine Intelligence, Vol. 11, No. 7, pp. 674-693, 1989.

[125]   Mallat, S. and Hwang, W. L., Singularity detection and processing with wavelets, IEEE Trans. on Information Theory, Vol. 38, No. 2, pp. 617-643, 1992.

[126]   Mallat, S. and Zhong, S., Characterization of signals from multiscale edges, IEEE Trans. on Pattern Analysis and Machine Intelligence, Vol. 14, No. 7, pp. 710-732, 1992.

[127]   Rosenfeld, A. and Thurston, M., Edge and curve detection for visual scene analysis, IEEE Trans. on Computers, Vol. 20, No. 5, pp. 562-569, 1971.

[128]   Xu, Y., Weaver, J. B., Healy, Jr., D. M. and Jian, L., Wavelet transform domain filters: A spatially selective noise filtration technique, IEEE Trans. on Med. Imag., Vol. 3, No. 6, pp. 747-757, 1994.

[129]   Setarehdan, S. K. and Soraghan, J. J., Automatic Left Ventricular Centre Point Extraction in Echocardiographic Images, Signal Processing Vol. 61, No. 3, pp. 275-288, 1997.

[130]   Gustavsson, T., Pascher, R. and Caidahl, K., Model Based Dynamic 3-D Reconstruction and Display of the Left Ventricle from 2-D Cross-Sectional Echocardiograms, Computerized Medical Imaging and Graphics, Vol. 17, Nos. 4/5, pp. 273-278, 1993.

[131]   Taratorin, A. M. and Sideman, S., Constrained Detection of Left Ventricular Boundaries from Cine CT Images of Human Hearts, IEEE Trans. on Med. Imag., Vol. 12, No. 3, pp. 521-533, 1993.

[132] Thomas, J. D., *et al.*, Improved Accuracy of Echocardiographic Endocardial Borders by Spatiotemporal Filtered Fourier Reconstruction: Description of the Method and Optimization of Filter Cutoffs, Circulation, Vol. 77, No. 2, pp. 415-428, 1988.

[133] Bartels, R. H., Beatty, J. C. and Barsky, B. A., A simple approximation technique-uniform cubic B-Splines, An introduction to splines for use in computer graphics and geometric modeling, Morgan Kaufmann, pp. 19-46, 1987.

[134] Marr, D. and Hildreth, E., Theory of edge detection, Proceedings of the Royal Society of London, Vol. B207, No. 1, pp. 187-217, 1980.

[135] Stytz, M. R., Frieder, G. and Frieder, O., Three-Dimensional Medical Imaging: Algorithms and Computer Systems, ACM Computer Surveys, Vol. 23, No. 4, pp. 421-499, Dec. 1991.

[136] Research report by the American Heart Association, Dallas, TX, pp. 1-29, 1998.

[137] Report by Associated Press, London, England, Herald Newspaper, 1997.

[138] Robb, G. P. and Steinberg, I., Visualization of the chambers of the heart, the pulmonary circulation and great vessels in man, American Journal of Roentgenol., Vol. 41, pp. 1-17, 1939.

[139] Suri, J. S., Computer Vision, Pattern Recognition, and Image Processing in Left Ventricle Segmentation: Last 50 Years, Journal of Pattern Analysis and Applications, Vol. 3, No. 3, pp. 209-242, 2000.

[140] Zerhouni, E. A., Parish, D. M. and Rogers, W. J., Human heart: Tagging with MRI imaging, a method of non-invasive assessment of myocardial motion, Vol. 16, No. 9, pp. 59-63, 1988.

[141] Axel, L. and Dougherty, L., Heart wall motion: Improved method of spatial modulation of magnetization of MR imaging, Radiology, Vol. 172, No. 2, pp. 349-350, Aug. 1989.

[142] Axel, L., System and method for magnetic resonance imaging of 3-D heart wall motion with spatial modulation of magnetization, US Patent #: 511820, May 12, 1992.

[143] Creswell, L. L., Wyers, S. G., Pirolo, J. S., Perman, W. H., Vannier, M. W. and Pasque, M. K., Mathematical Modeling of the Heart Using Magnetic Resonance Imaging, IEEE Tran. on Med. Img., Vol. 11, No. 4, pp. 581-589, Dec. 1992.

[144] Barth, K., Braeckle, G., Lenz, G., Weikl, A. and Reinhardt, E. R., Principles for the study of heart dynamics with Magnetic Resonance Imaging, Computer Assisted Radiology, pp. 38-43, 1985.

[145] Richey, J. B., Wake, R. H., Walters, R., Hunt, W. and Cool, S. L., Cardiac imaging with CT scanners, US Patent #: 4547892, Oct. 15, 1985.

[146] Huang, H. K. and Mazziotta, J. C., Heart Imaging from computerized tomography, J. of Computerized Tomography, Vol. 2, No. 1, pp. 37-44, 1978.

[147] Seppi, E., Harell, G. and Charles, M., Method and system for cardiac computed tomography, US Patent #: 4,182,311, January 8, 1980.

[148] Ritman, E. L., Kinsey, J. H., Robb, R. A., Gilbert, B. K., Harris, L. D. and Wood, E. H., 3-D Imaging of Heart, Lungs and Circulation, Science Journal, Vol. 210, pp. 273-280, 1980.

[149] Von Behren, P. L., Method and apparatus for cardiac nuclear imaging, US Patent #: 4,458,688, July 10, 1984.

[150] Strauss, H. W., McKusick, K. A. and Bingham, J. B., Cardiac Nuclear Imaging: Principle, Instrumentation and Pitfalls, American Jour. of Cardiology, Vol. 46, No. 7, pp. 1109-1115, Dec. 18, 1980.

[151] Leitl, G. P., Buchanan, J. W. and Wagner, Jr., H. N., Monitoring Cardiac function with nuclear techniques, Am. Jour. of Cardiology, Vol. 46, No. 7, pp. 1125-1132, Dec. 1980.

[152] Heather, C., 3-D Echo assist study of dynamic structures, Diagnostic Imaging, Vol. 19, No. 7, pp. 77-80, July 1997.

[153] Herlin, I. L. and Ayache, N., Feature extraction and analysis methods for sequences of Ultrasound images, Image Vision Computation, Vol. 10, No. 10, pp. 673-682, 1992.

[154] Herlin, I. L., Nguyen, C. and Graffigne, C., A deformable region model using stochastic processes applied to echocardiographic images, Proc. of CVPR, Urbana, IL, IEEE Computer Society, pp. 534-539, 1992.

[155] Yin, F. C. P., Strumpf, R. K., Chen, P. H. and Zeger, S. L., Quantification of the mechanical properties of non-contracting canine myocardium, J. of Biomech, Vol. 20, No. 6, pp. 577-589, 1987.

[156] Meier, G. D., Ziskin, M. C., Santamore, W. P. and Bove, A. A., Kinematics of the beating heart, IEEE Trans. on Biomedical Engineering, Vol. 27, No. 6, pp. 319-329, June 1980.

[157] Plonsey, A., Mathematical modeling of activity of the heart, J. Electrocardio, Vol. 20, No. 3, pp. 219-226, 1987.

[158] Netter, F. H. and Colacino, S., consulting editor, Atlas of human anatomy, Ciba-Geigy Corp., Summit, N.J., ISBN: 0-9141-6818-5, 1989.

[159] Wolferth, C. C. and Margolies, A., The excursion of the apex and base of the LV compared with that of the left border, In Movements of Roentgen-Opaque Deposits in Heart Valve Areas, pp. 197-201, 1947.

[160] Higgins, W. E. and Ritman, E. L., 3-D image enhancement technique for volumetric cardiac images, Proceedings of SPIE - The International Society for Optical Engineering, Biomedical Image Processing, Vol. 1245, pp. 159-170, 1990.

[161] Wilson, D. L. and Bertram, C., Morphological enhancement of coronary angiograms, In Proc. of Computers in Cardiology, IEEE Press, pp. 313-316, 1991.

[162] Nagao, M. and Matsyyama, T., Edge Preserving Smoothing, Computer Graphics and Image Processing, Vol. 9, No. 4, pp. 394-407, 1979.

[163] Vonesh, M. J., Kequing, C. and Radvany, M., Digital Subtraction for noise reduction in Intravascular Ultrasound Data, In Proc. of Computers in Cardiology, IEEE Press, pp. 329-327, 1991.

[164] Lamberti, C. and Sgallari, F., Edge Detection and Velocity Field for the Analysis of Heart Motion, in Digital Signal Processing, V. Cappellini and A. G. Constantinides (eds), Elsevier Science Publishers, B.V., pp. 603-608, 1991.

[165] Weszka, J. S. and Rosenfeld, A., Threshold Evaluation Techniques, IEEE Trans. on System, Man And Cybernetics, Vol. SMC-8, No.8, pp. 622-629, Aug. 1978.

[166] Tanaka, N., Method of judging the presence or absence of a limited irradiation field, method of selecting a correct irradiation field and method of judging correctness or incorrectness of an irradiation field, U.S. Patent #: 4,952,805, Aug. 28, 1990.

[167] De Jong, L. P. and Slager, C. J., Detection of the Left Ventricle outline in angiographs using TV Signal processing technique, IEEE Trans. on Biomedical Engineering, Vol. 22, No. 3, pp. 230-237, May 1975.

[168] Reiber, J. H. C., Contour Detector and Data Acquisition System for the left ventricular outline, US Patent #: 4,101,961, July 18, 1978.

[169] Han, C. Y., Porembka, D. T. and Lin, Kwun-Nan, Method for automatic contour extraction of a cardiac image, US Patent #: 5,457,754, Oct. 10, 1995.

[170] Hideya, T. and Shimura, K., Method of recognizing layout and subdivision patterns of radiation images, U.S. Patent #: 4,962,539, Oct. 9, 1990.

[171] Nakajima, N., Method of adjusting image processing conditions, U.S. Patent #: 5,028,782, July 2, 1991.

[172] Muhammed, I. S., Digital image processing method employing histogram peak detection, U.S. Patent # 4,731,863, March 15, 1988.

[173] Jang, B. K., Method for automatic foreground and background detection in digital radiographic images, U.S. Patent #: 5,268,967, Dec. 7, 1993.

[174] Capozzi, J. R. and Schaetzing, R., Method and apparatus for automatic tonescale generation in digital radiographic images, U.S. Patent #: 5,164,993, Nov. 17, 1992.

[175] Wollschleger, H., Tenspiel, R. W., Solzbach, U., Zeiher, A. M. and Just, H., Reliable Automatic Frame-By-Frame Contour Detection of Digitized LV Cine-Angiograms, In Proc. of Computers in Cardiology, IEEE Press, pp. 353-356, 1988.

[176] Revankar, S., Sher, D. and Rosenthal, S., Collaborative processing to extract myocardium from a sequence of 2-D echocardiograms, Proceedings of SPIE - The International Society for Optical Engineering, Vol. 1459, pp. 268-273, 1991.

[177] Revankar, S., Sher, D. and Rosenthal, S., An interactive thresholding scheme to extract myocardium from a sequence of 2-D echocardiograms, In Proc. of the IEEE 17th Annual North East Bioengineering Conference, pp. 197-201, April 1991.

[178] Sher, D. B., Revankar, S. and Rosenthal, S. M., Computer methods in quantification of cardiac wall parameters from 2-D echocardiograms: A Survey, Int. Journal of Cardiac Imaging, Vol. 8, No. 1, pp. 11-26, 1992.

[179] Chow, C. K. and Kaneko, T., Border Detection based on Local Characteristics, Computers in Biomedicine Research, Vol. 5, pp. 388-410, Aug. 1972.

[180] Otsu, N., A Threshold Selection Method from Gray Scale Histograms, System, Man and Cybernetics, Vol. 9, No. 1, pp. 62-66, Jan. 1979.

[181] McAdams, H. P., Histogram Directed Processing of Digital Chest Images, Investigative Radiology, Vol. 21, No. 3, pp. 253-259, 1986.

[182] Fu, K. S. and Mui, J. K., A Survey on Image Segmentation, Jour. of Pattern Recognition, Vol. 13, No. 1, pp. 3-16, 1981.

[183] Haralick, R. M. and Shapiro, L. G., A Survey: Image Segmentation Techniques, Jour. of Computer Vision, Graphics and Image Processing, Vol. 29, No. 1, pp. 100-132, 1985.

[184] Haralick, R. M., Digital Step Edges from Zero Crossing of Second Directional Derivatives, Pattern Analysis and Machine Intelligence Vol. 6, No. 1, pp. 58-68, Jan. 1984.

[185] Haralick, R. M., Cubic Facet Model Edge Detector and Ridge Valley Detector, in Pattern Recognition in Practice II, Gelsema, E. S., and Kanal, L. N., (ed.), Implementation Details, Elsevier Science Publishers B.V., (North Holland) pp. 81-90, 1986.

[186] Davis, L. S., A survey of edge detection techniques, Computer Graphics and Image Processing, Vol. 4, No. 3, pp. 248-270, Sept. 1975.

[187] Lee, J. S., Haralick, R. M. and Shapiro, L.G., Morphologic Edge Detection, IEEE Jour. of Robotics and Automation, Vol. RA-3, No. 2, pp. 142-156, April 1987.

[188] Sezan, M. I., Tekalp, A. M. and Schaetzing, R., Automatic Anatomically Selective Image Enhancement in Digital Chest Radiography, IEEE Trans. on Med. Imag., Vol. 8, No. 2, pp. 154-162, 1989.

[189] Setarehdan, S. K. and Soraghan, J. J., Fully Automatic Left Ventricular Myocardial Boundary Detection in Echocardiographic Images, In Proc. of IEEE Engineering in Medicine and Biology, The Netherlands, ISBN: 90-9010005-9 (CD-ROM) SOE 9609001, pp. 877-878, 1996.

[190] Setarehdan, S. K., Eschocardiographical cardiac function assessment and wall motion visualisation using fuzzy logic and the wavelet transformation, Ph.D. Thesis, University of Strathclyde, Glasgow, 1998.

[191] Zadeh, L. A., Fuzzy Sets, Information and Control, Vol. 8, No. 3, pp. 338-353, 1965.

[192] Tu, H.-K. and Goldgof, D. B., Spatio-Temporal Edge Detection, Proc. of the 5th Florida Artificial Intelligence Research Symposium, Fort Lauderdale, FL, pp. 243-246, 1992.

[193] Turin, G. L., An introduction to digital matched filters, Proc. IEEE, Vol. 64, No. 7, pp. 1092-1112, July 1976.

[194] Grattoni, P. and Bonamini, R., Contour detection of the left ventricle cavity from angiographic images, IEEE Trans. on Med. Imag., Vol. 4, pp. 72-78, June 1985.

[195] Grattoni, P., Pollastri, F. and Dimino, G., Detection of moving contours from left-ventricle cineangiograms, In Time-Varying Image Processing and Moving Object Recognition 2, V. Cappellini, Elsevier Science Publishers, 1990, pp. 197-204.

[196] Beucher, S., Segmentation Tools in Mathematical Morphology, Image Algebra and Morphological Image Processing, Proceedings of SPIE - The International Society for Optical Engineering, Vol. 1350, pp. 70-84, 1990.

[197] Beucher, S., Segmentation Tools in Mathematical Morphology, Proceedings of SPIE - The International Society for Optical Engineering, Vol. 1769, Image Algebra and Morphological Image Processing, pp. 70-84, 1992.

[198] Vincent, L. and Soille, P., Watersheds in Digital Spaces: An efficient algorithm based on immersion simulations, IEEE Trans. on Pattern Analysis and Machine Intelligence, Vol. 13, No. 6, pp. 583-598, June 1991.

[199] Lantuejoul, C. and Maisonneuve, F., Pattern Recognition, Vol. 17, No. 2, pp. 177-187, 1984.

[200] Wang, T. C. and Karayiannis, N. B., Detection of microcalcification in digital mammograms using wavelets, IEEE Tran. on Med. Imag., Vol. 17, No. 4, pp. 498-509, 1998.

[201] Lee, C. K., Automated Boundary Tracing Using Temporal Information, Ph.D. Thesis, Department of Electrical Engineering, University of Washington, Seattle, 1994.

[202] Sheehan, F. H., Lee, C. K. and Haralick, R. M., Method for determining the contour of an in vivo organ using multiple image frames of the organ, US Patent #: 5,570,430, Oct. 29, 1996.

[203] Santago, P. and Gage, H. D., Quantification of MR brain images by mixture density and partial volume modeling, IEEE Trans. on Medical Imaging, Vol. 12, pp. 566-574, 1993.

[204] Shattuck, D. W. and Leahy, R. M., BrainSuite: An Automated Cortical Surface Identification Tool, Medical Image Computing and Computer-Assisted Intervention (MICCAI), pp. 50-61, 2000.

[205] Wilson, A., Statistical Models for Shapes and Deformations, Ph.D. Thesis, Institute of Statistical and Decision Sciences, Duke University, Durham, NC, 1994.

[206] van Bree, R. E., Pope, D. L. and Parker, D. L., Improving Left Ventricular Border Recognition Using Probability Surfaces, In Proc. of Computers in Cardiology, IEEE Press, pp. 121-124, 1989.

[207] Pope, D. L., Parker, D. L., Gustafson, D. E. and Clayton, P. D., Dynamic Search Algorithms in Left Ventricular Border Recognition and Analysis of Coronary Arteries, In Proc. of Computers in Cardiology, IEEE Press, pp. 71-75, 1984.

[208] Pope, D. L., Parker, D. L., Clayton, P. D. and Gustafson, D. E., Ventricular Border Recognition Using Dynamic Search Algorithms, Radiation Physics, Vol. 155, No. 2, pp. 513-518, 1985.

[209] Wikins, K. and Terzopoulos, D., Snakes: Active Contour Models, International Jour. of Computer Vision, Vol. 1, No. 4, pp. 321-331, 1988.

[210] Singh, A., Kurowski, L. and Chiu, M. Y., Cardiac MR Image Segmentation Using Deformable Models, Proceedings of SPIE - The International Society for Optical Engineering, Vol. 1905, No. 8, pp. 8-28, 1993.

[211] Richens, D., Rougon, N., Bloch, I. and Mousseaux, E., Segmentation by deformable contour of MRI sequences of the LV for quantitative analysis, In 4th IEEE International Conference on Image Processing and its Applications, The Netherlands, pp. 393-396, 1992.

[212] Fleagle, S. R., Thedens, D. R., Ehrhardt, J. C., Scholz, T. D. and Skorton, D. J., Automated Segmentation of LV Borders from Spin-Echo MRI: Experimental and Clinical Feasibility Studies, Investigative Radiology, Vol. 26, No. 4, pp. 295-303, 1991.

[213] Szekely, G., Lelemen, A., Brechbuhler, C. and Greig, G., Segmentation of 2-D and 3-D objects from MRI volume data using constrained elastic deformation of flexible Fourier surface models, Jour. of Medical Image Analysis, Vol. 1, No. 1, pp. 19-34, 1996.

[214] Clarysse, P., Poupon, F., Barbier, B. and Magnin, I. E., 3-D Boundary Extraction of the Left Ventricule by a Deformable Model with A-Priori Information, Proc. of the IEEE International Conference in Image Processing, Vol. 2, IEEE Signal Processing Soc., pp. 492-495, 1995.

[215] Bardinet, E., Cohen, L. D., Ayache, N., Analyzing the deformation of the LV of the heart with a parametric deformation model, Research Report 2797, INRIA, Sophia-Antipolis, France, 1996.

[216] Bardinet, E., Cohen, L. D., Ayache, N., Tracking and motion analysis of the left ventricle with deformable superquadratics, Medical Image Analysis, Vol. 1, No. 2, pp. 129-149, 1996.

[217] Ayache, N., Medical Computer Vision, Virtual Reality and Robotics, Image and Vision Computing, Vol. 13, No. 4, pp. 295-313, May 1995.

[218] Staib, L. H. and Sinusas, A., Cardiac SPECT Restoration using MR-based Support Constraints, Proceedings of the IEEE International Conference on Image Processing, IEEE Press, Los Alamitos, CA, pp. 480-483, 1995.

[219] Nastar, C. and Ayache, N., Fast Segmentation, Tracking and Analysis of Deformable Objects, Proc. of the Fourth International Conference on Computer Vision (ICCV), Berlin, Germany, pp. 275-279, 1993.

[220] Staib, L. H. and Duncan, J. S., Parameterically Deformable Contour Models, International Conference in Computer Vision, pp. 98-102, 1989.

[221] Miller, J. V., Breen, D. E., Lorensen, W. E. and O'Bara, R. M., Geometrically deformable models: A method for extracting closed geometric models from volume data, In Siggraph Proceedings of Computer Graphics, Vol. 25, No. 4, pp. 217-226. July 1991.

[222] Chen, C. W. and Huang, T. S., Modeling, Analysis and Visualization of Left Ventricle Shape and Motion by Hierarchical Decomposition, IEEE Trans. on Pattern Analysis and Machine Intelligence, Vol. 16, No. 4, pp. 342-356, 1994.

[223] Revankar, S. and Sher, D., Constrained Contouring in the Polar Coordinates, Proceedings of the IEEE Computer Vision and Pattern Recognition (CVPR), Aggarwal, J. K., Aloimonos, Y. and Bolle, R. M., pp. 688-689, June 1993.

[224] Wei, Wu., Boundary Estimation of Left Ventricle in Ultrasound Images, Masters Thesis, Department of Electrical Engineering, The University of Washington, Seattle, 1992.

[225] O'Donel, T., Gupta, A. and Boult, T. E., A Periodic Generalized Cylinder Model with Local Deformations for Tracking Closed Contours Exhibiting Repeating Motion, Proc. of the 12th IAPR International Conference on Pattern Recognition, Vol. 1, Jerusalem, Israel, International Association for Pattern Recognition, IEEE Computer Soc. Inf. Process. Assoc. Israel, pp. 397-402, 1994.

[226] Williams, D. J. and Shah, M., A fast algorithm for active contour and curvature estimation, Computer Vision, Graphics and Image Understanding, Vol. 55, No. 1, pp. 14-26, Jan. 1992.

[227] Cootes, T. F., Taylor, C. J., Cooper, D. H. and Graham, J., Active Shape Models: Their Training and Applications, Computer Vision and Image Understanding, Vol. 61, No. 1, pp. 38-59, Jan. 1995.

[228] McInerney, T. and Terzopoulous, D., A dynamic finite element surface model for segmentation and tracking in multidimensional medical images with application to cardiac 4-D image analysis, Computerized Medical Imaging and Graphics, Vol. 19, No. 1, pp. 69-83, Jan. 1995.

[229] McInerney, T. and Terzopoulous, D., Deformable Models in Medical Image Analysis: A Survey, Medical Image Analysis, Vol. 1, No. 2, pp. 91-108, 1996.

[230] Nielsen, P. M. F., Le Grice, I. J., Smaill, B. H. and Hunter, P. J., Mathematical model of geometry and fibrous structure of the heart, Am. J. of Physiology, Vol. 260, (4 Pt 2), pp. 1365-1378, April 1991.

[231] Nielsen, P. M. F., The Anatomy of the Heart: A finite element model, Ph.D. Thesis, University of Auckland, New Zealand, 1987.

[232] Zienkiewicz, O. C. and Morgan, K., Finite element and approximation, Wiley, New York, ISBN: 0-4719-8240-7, 1982.

[233] Samadani, R., Adaptive Snakes: Control of Damping and Material Parameters, Proceedings of SPIE - The International Society for Optical Engineering - Geometric method in computer vision, Vol. 1570, San Diego, CA, pp. 202-213, 1991.

[234] Lipson, P., Yuille, A. L., O'Keefe, D., Cavanaugh, J., Taffe, J. and Rosenthal, D., Deformable templates for feature extraction from medical images, In Faugeras, O., (ed), Computer Vision Proc. first European Conference in Computer Vision, Antibes, France, pp. 413-417, 1990.

[235] Sheehan, F.H., Haralick, R. M., Suri, J. S. and Shao, Y., Method for Determining the Contour of an In Vivo Organ Using Multiple Image Frames of the Organ, US Patent #: 5,734,739, March 31, 1998.

[236] Suri, J. S., Haralick, R. M. and Sheehan, F. H., Two Automatic Calibration Algorithms for Left Ventricle Boundary Estimation in X-ray Images, In Proc. of IEEE Int. Conf. of Engineering in Medicine and Biology (EMBS), Amsterdam, The Netherlands, ISBN: 90-9010005-9 (CD-ROM) SOE 9609001, pp. 1117-1119, 1996.

[237] Takeshita, T., Nozawa, S. and Kimura, F., On the Bias of Mahalanobis Distance Due to Limited Sample Size Effect, IEEE International Conference on Document Analysis and Recognition, pp. 171-174, 1993.

[238] Suri, J. S., Haralick, R.M. and Sheehan, F. H., Systematic Error Correction in Automatically Produced Boundaries in Low Contrast Ventriculograms, International Conference in Pattern Recognition, Vienna, Austria, Vol. IV, Track D, pp. 361-365, 1996.

[239] Brower, R. W., Evaluation of Pattern Recognition for the Apex of the Heart, Catheterization and Cardiovascular Diagnosis, Vol. 6, No. 2, pp. 145-157, 1980.

[240] Suri, J. S., Haralick, R. M. and Sheehan, F. H., Left Ventricle Longitudinal Axis Fitting and LV Apex Estimation Using a Robust Algorithm and its Performance: A Parametric Apex Model, Proc. of the International Conference in Image Processing, Santa Barbara, CA, Volume III, IEEE, ISBN: 0-8186-8183-7/97, pp. 118-121, 1997.

[241] Huber, P. J., Robust Estimation of a Location Parameter, Annals Math. Statis., Vol. 35, No. 1, pp. 73-101, Aug. 1964.

[242] Shao, Y., Automatic Detection of Left Ventricle Aorta Valve Location From an X-ray Image, Master Thesis, University of Washington, Aug. 1996.

[243] Zuniga, O. and Haralick, R.M., Integrated Directional Derivative Gradient Operator, IEEE Trans. on System, Man and Cybernetics, Vol. 17, No. 3, pp. 508-517, May/June 1987.

[244] Haralick, R. M. and Shapiro, L. G., Computer and Robot Vision, Addison-Wesley, Reading, Mass., Don Mills, Ont., ISSN: 0201108771 (v. 1) 0201569434 (v. 2), 1991.

[245] Sternberg, S. R., Grayscale Morphology, Computer Vision, Graphics, Image Processing, Vol. 35, No. 3, pp. 333-355, Sept. 1986.

[246] Suri, J. S., Haralick, R. M. and Sheehan, F. H., Effect of Edge Detection, Pixel Classification, Classification-Edge Fusion Over LV Calibration, A Two Stage Automatic System, Proceedings of the 10th Scandinavian Conference on Image Analysis (SCIA), Finland, Vol. 1, ISBN: 951-764-145-1, pp. 197-204, 1997.

[247] Suri, J. S., Haralick, R. M. and Sheehan, F. H., General Technique for Automatic Left Ventricle Boundary Validation: Relation Between Cardioangiograms and Observed Boundary Errors, Proceedings of Society for Computer Applications in Radiology (SCAR), Rochester, Minnesota, pp. 212-217, 1997.

[248] Zwehl, W., Levy, R., Garcia, E., Haendchen, R. V., Childs, W., Corday, S. R., and Meerbaum, S., Corday Validation of computerized edge detection algorithm for qualitative 2-D echocardiography, Circulation, Vol. 68, No. 5, pp. 1127-1135, Nov. 1983.

[249] Suri, J. S., Haralick, R. M. and Sheehan, F. H., Two Automatic Training-Based Forced Calibration Algorithms for Left Ventricle Boundary Estimation in Cardiac Images, Proc. of 19th International Conference of IEEE Engineering in Medicine and Biology (EMBS), Chicago, ISBN: 0-7803-4265-9 (CD-ROM) SOE 9710002, pp. 528-532, 1997.

[250] Suri, J. S., Haralick, R. M. and Sheehan, F. H., Automatic Quadratic Calibration for Correction of Pixel Classifier Boundaries to an Accuracy of 2.5 mm: An Application in X-Ray Heart Imaging, International Conference in Pattern Recognition, (ICPR) Brisbane, Australia, pp. 30-33, 1998.

[251] Kim, D. Y., Kim, J. J., Meer, P., Mintz, D. and Rosenfeld, A., Robust Computer Vision: A Least Median of Squares Based Approach, Technical Report, Center for Automation Research, University of Maryland, College Park, MD, 1989.

[252] Hampel, F. R., Ronchetti, E. M., Ronsseeuw, P. J. and Stahel, W. A., Robust Statistics - The Approach Based on Influence Functions, ISBN: 0-4718-2921-8, John Wiley and Sons, 1986.

[253] Holland, P. W. and Welsch, R. E., Robust Regression Using Iteratively Reweighted Least Squares, Communication Statistics, Vol. 6, No. 9, pp. 813-828, Aug, 1977.

[254] Hill, R. W. and Holland, P. W., Two Robust Alternatives to Least Squares Regression, Jour. of American Statistical Association, Vol. 72, pp. 828-833, Dec. 1977.

[255] Sampson, P. D., Bookstien, F. L., Sheehan, F. H. and Bolson, E., Eigenshape Analysis of Left Ventricular Outlines from Contrast Ventriculograms, In Marcus, L. F., Corti, M., Loy, A., Naylor, G. J. P. and Slice, D. E. (eds.), Advances in Morphometrics, NATO Advance Study Institute, Advance Plenum Press, pp. 211-233, 1996.

[256] Press, W. H., Flannery, B. P., Teukolsky, S. A. and Vetterling, W. T., Numerical Recipes in C, Cambridge University Press, 1988.

[257] Sampson, P. D., Fitting Conic Sections to Very Scattered Data: An Iterative Refinement of the Bookstein Algorithm, Computer Graphics and Image Processing, Vol. 18, No. 1, pp. 97-108, 1982.

[258] Suri, J. S. and Haralick, R. M., Coupled Constrained Calibration, Intelligent Systems Laboratory, Tech. Internal Report, University of Washington, Seattle, 1996.

[259] Geman, S., Geman, D., Graffigne, C. and Dong, P., Boundary detection by constrained optimization, IEEE Trans. on Pattern Analysis and Machine Intelligence, Vol. 12, No. 7, pp. 609-627, 1990.

[260] Chiou, G. I. and Hwang, J. N., A Neural Network Based Stochastic Active Contour Model (NNS-SNAKE) for Contour Finding of Distinct Features, IEEE Trans. in Image Proc., Vol. 4, No. 10, pp. 1407-1416, Oct. 1985.

[261] Tseng, Y.-H., Hwang, J.-N. and Sheehan, F. H., 3-D heart border delineation and motion estimation using ultrasound transthoracic images for assisted heart diseases diagnoses. Proceedings, International Conference on Image Processing, Los Alamitos, CA, IEEE Comput. Soc., Vol. 3, pp. 543-546, 1997.

[262] Tseng, Y. H., Hwang, J. N., Sheehan, F. H., 3-D Heart Modeling and Motion Estimation Based On Continuous Distance Transform Neural Networks And Affine Transform, VLSIVideo, Vol. 18, No. 3, pp. 207-218. 9806, April 1998.

[263] Chen, T., Lin, W. C. and Chen, C. T., Artificial neural networks for 3-D motion analysis - part I: rigid motion - part II: nonrigid motion, IEEE Trans. Neural Networks, Vol. 6, No. 6, pp. 1386-1393, pp. 1394-1401, (with T. Chen and C.-T. Chen), Nov. 1995,

[264] Suri, J. S., Active Contour Vs. Learning: Computer Vision Techniques in CT, MR and Xray Cardiac Imaging, Proceedings of The Fifth International Conference in Pattern Recognition and Information Processing, ISBN: 83-87362-16-6, pp. 273-277, 1999.

[265] Huang, T. S., Modeling, analysis and visualization of nonrigid object motion, International Conference on Pattern Recognition (ICPR), pp. 361-364, June 1990.

[266] Griffith, R. L., Grant, C. and Kaufman, H., An Algorithm for Locating the Aortic Valve and the Apex in Left Ventricular Angiocardiograms, IEEE Trans. on Biomedical Engineering, Vol. 21, No. 5, pp. 345-349, 1974.

[267] Suri, J. S. and Haralick, R. M., Integrated Directional Derivative Approach for Left Ventricle Apex Estimation: Tech. Report #: ISL-TR-96-05, Intelligent Systems Lab., Univ. of Washington, Seattle, 1996.

[268] Bardeen, C. R., Determination of the size of the heart by means of the Xrays, Am. J. of Anat., Vol. 23, pp. 423-487, 1918.

[269] Dodge, H. T., Sandler, H., Ballew, D. W. and Lord, J. D., The Use of Biplane Angiocardiology for the Measurement of Left Ventricular Volume in Man, The American Heart Jour., Vol. 41, pp. 762-776, Nov. 1960.

[270] Dodge, H. T., Sandler, H., Baxley, W. A. and Hawley, R. R., Usefulness and Limitations of Radiographic Method for Determining Left Ventricular Volume, The American Jour. of Cardiology (AJC), Vol. 18, pp. 10-23, July 1966.

[271] Marcus, M. L and Schuette, M. H., An Automated Method for the Measurement of Ventricular Volume, Circulation, Vol. 45, No. 1, pp. 65-76, Jan. 1972.

[272] Chapman, C. B., Baker, O. and Mitchell, J. H., Experiences with Cineflurographics Method for Measuring Ventricular Volume, Vol. 18, No. 1, pp. 25-30, July 1966.

[273] Jouan, A., Analysis of Sequence of Cardiac Contours by Fourier Descriptors for Plane Closed Curves, IEEE Trans. on Med. Imag., Vol. 6, No. 2, pp. 176-180, June 1987.

[274] Lewis, R. P. and Sandler, H., Relationships between changes in left ventricular dimensions and ejection fraction in Man, Circulation, Vol. 44, pp. 548-557, 1971.

[275] Kim, H. C., Min, B. G., Lee, M. M., Lee, Y. W. and Han, M. C., Estimation of local cardiac wall deformation and regional wall stress from biplane coronary cine angiogram, IEEE Tran. On Biomedical Engineering, Vol. 32, No. 7, pp. 503-512, July 1985.

[276] Wynne, J., Greeen, L. H., Mann, T., Levin, D. and Grossman, W., Estimation of Left Ventricular Volumes in Man from Biplane Cineangiograms Filmed in Oblique Projections, The American Jour. of Cardiology, Vol. 41, No. 4, pp. 726-732, April, 1978.

[277] Lehmkuhl, H., Machnig, Th., Eicker, B., Karth, K., Reynen, K. and Bachmann, K., Digital Subtraction Angiography: Feasibility of Densitometric Evaluation of Left Ventricular Volumes and Comparison to Measurements Obtained by the Monoplane Area-Length-Method, In Proc. of Computers in Cardiology, IEEE Press, pp. 29-32, 1993.

[278] Papapietro, S. E., Smith, R. L., Hood, W. P., Russell, R. O., Rackley, C. R. and Rogers, W. J., An optimal method for angiographic definition and quantification of regional left ventricular contraction, In Proc. of Computers in Cardiology, IEEE Press, pp. 294-295, 1978.

[279] Rickards, A., Seabra-Gomes, R. and Thurston, P., The assessment of regional abnormalities of the left ventricle by angiography, European Journal of Cardiology, Vol. 5, No. 2, pp. 167-182, 1977.

[280] Klausner, S. C., Blair, T. J., Bulawa, W. F., Jeppson, G. M., Jensen, R. L. and Clayton, P. D., Quantitative Analysis of Segmental Wall Motion Throughout Systole and Diastole in the Normal Human Left Ventricle, Circulation, Vol. 65, No. 3, pp. 580-590, March 1982.

[281] Gibson, D. G., Prewitt, T. A. and Brown, D. J., Analysis of left ventricle wall movement during isovolumic relaxation and its relation to coronary artery disease, Jour. of Heart Br., Vol. 38, pp. 1010-1019, 1976.

[282] Suri, J. S., Error measurement tools for cardiac projection images, International Conference in Applications of Pattern Recognition (ICAPR), Plymouth, England, Nov. 23-25, pp. 125-134, 1998.

[283] Sandler, H., Dimensional Analysis of the Heart - A Review, The American Jour. of the Medical Sciences, Vol. 260, pp. 56-70, July 1970.

[284] Hoffman, E. A. and Ritman, E. L., Shape and dimension of cardiac chambers: Importance of CT section thickness and orientation, Radiology, Vol. 155, No. 3, pp. 739-744, 1985.

[285] Hoffman, E. A. and Ritman, E. L., Invariant total heart volume in the intact thorax, Am. J. Physiol. Heart Circ. Physiol., Vol. 249, (4 Pt 2), pp. H883-H890, 1985.

[286] Hoffman, E. A., Ehman, R. L., Sinak, L. J., Felmlee, J. P., Chandrasekaran, K., Julsrud, P. R. and Ritman, E. L., Law of constant heart volume in humans: A non invasive assessment via X-ray CT, MRI and echo, Jour. of American College. Cardiology, Vol. 9, No. 2, 38A, 1987.

[287] Hoffman, E.A. and Ritman, E.L., Intra Cardiac Cycle constancy of total heart volume, Dynamic Cardiovascular Imaging, Vol. 1, pp. 199-205, 1988.

[288] Sinak, L. J., Hoffman, E. A., Julsrud, R. R., Mair, D. D., Seward, J. B., Hagler, D. J., Harris, L. D., Robb, R. A. and Ritman, E. L., Dynamic spatial reconstructor: Investigating congenital heart diseases in four dimensions, Cardiovascular Intervent. Radiology, Vol. 7, No. 3-4, pp. 124-137, 1984.

[289] Apicella, A., Wood, C. H., NessAiver, M., Measurement of Ventricle Volumes with Cardiac MRI, US Patent #: 5,273,040, Dec 28, 1993.

[290] Gould, K. L. and Kennedy, J. W., Analysis of wall dynamics and directional components of left ventricular contraction, The American Jour. of Cardiology, Vol. 38, No. 3, pp. 322-331, 1976.

[291] Bolson, E. L., Kilman, S., Sheehan, F. H. and Dodge, H. T., Left ventricular segmental wall motion - a new method using local direction information, In Proc. of Computers in Cardiology, IEEE Press, pp. 245-248, 1980.

[292] Sheehan, F. H., Stewart, D. K., Dodge, H. T., Mitten, S., Bolson, E. L. and Brown, B. G., Variability in the measurement of regional left ventricular wall motion from contrast angiograms, Circulation, Vol. 68, No. 3, pp. 550-559, 1983.

[293] Sheehan, F. H., Mathey, D. G., Schofer, J., Becher, H., Wygant, J. and Bolson, E. L., Measurement of Region Right Ventricular Wall Motion From Biplane Contrast Angiograms Using the Centerline Method, In Proc. of Computers in Cardiology, IEEE Press, pp. 149-152, 1991.

[294] Yang, P., Otto, C. M. and Sheehan, F. H., Effect of normalization in reducing variability in regional wall thickening, Jour. Of American Soc. Of Echocardiography (JASE), Vol. 10. No. 3, pp. 197-204, April 1997.

[295] Mancini, G. B. J., LeFree, M. T. and Vogel, R. A., Curvature analysis of normal ventriculograms: Fundamental Framework for the assessment of shape changes in man, In Proc. of Computers in Cardiology, IEEE Press, pp. 141-144, 1985.

[296] Dumesnil, J. G., Shoucri, R. M., Laurenceau, J. L. and Turcot, J., A Mathematical Model of the Dynamic Geometry of the Intact Left Ventricle and Its Application to Clinical Data, Circulation, Vol. 59, No. 5, pp. 1024-1034, May 1979.

[297] Dumesnil, J. G. and Shouchri, R. M., Quantitative relationships between LV ejection fraction and wall thickening and Geometry, The American Physiological Society, pp. 48-54, 1991.

[298] Beier, J., Joerke, T., Lempert, S., Wellnhofer, E., Oswald, H. and Fleck, E., A Comparison of Seven Different Volumetry Methods of Left and Right Ventricle Using Post-mortem Phantoms, In Proc. of Computers in Cardiology, IEEE Press, pp. 33-36, 1993.

[299] Santos, B. S., Ferreira, C. and Riberiro, V. G., A comparison of two models for quantification in LV function, In Proc. of Computers in Cardiology, IEEE Press, pp. 99-100, 1994.

[300] Duncan, J. S., Lee, F. A., Smeulders, A. W. M. and Zaret, B. L., A Bending Energy Model for Measurement of Cardiac Shape Deformity, IEEE Trans. on Med. Imag., Vol. 10, No. 3, pp. 307-320, 1991.

[301] Amini, A. A. and Duncan, J. S., Bending and stretching models for LV wall motion analysis from curves and surfaces, Image and Vision Computing, Vol. 10, No. 6, pp. 418-430, 1992.

[302] Duncan, J. S., Owen, R., Anandan, P., Staib, L., McCauley, T., Salazar, A. and Lee, F., Shape-based Tracking of Left Ventricle Wall Motion, In Proc. of Information Processing in Medical Imaging, pp. 41-44, 1991.

[303] Owen, R. L., Staib, L. H., Anandan, P. and Duncan, J. S., Measurement of Left Ventricular Wall Motion from Contour Shape Deformation Information Processing in Medical Imaging, Progress in Clinical and Biological Research, Wiley-Liss, Inc., New York, Vol. 363, pp. 541-556, 1989.

[304] Sheehan, F. H., Bolson, E. L. and Jin, H., Determining cardiac wall thickness by imaging and three dimensional modeling, University of Washington, Seattle, US Patent #: 5,601,084, Feb. 11, 1997.

[305] Clary, G. J., Pizer, S. M. and Fritsch, D. S., Left Ventricular Wall Motion Tracking via Deformable Shape Loci, In Proc. of Computers in Cardiology, IEEE Press, pp. 271-276, 1997.

[306] Fritsch, D. S., Pizer, S. M., Yu, L., Johnson, V. and Chaney, E. L., Segmentation of Medical Image Objects Using Deformable Shape Loci, Image Processing in Medical Imaging (IPMI), pp. 127-140, 1996.

[307] McEachen II, J. C., Nehorai, A. and Duncan, J. S., Estimating Cardiac Motion from Image Sequences Using Recursive Comb Filtering, Proc. of the IEEE International Conference in Image Processing, IEEE Signal Processing Soc., Vol. 2, pp. 496-499, Oct. 1995.

[308] McEachen II, J. C. and Duncan, J. S., A Constrained Analytic Solution for Tracking Non-Rigid Motion of the Left Ventricle, IEEE 18th Annual Northeast Bioengineering Conference, Univ. of Rhode Island, pp. 137-138, March 1992.

[309] Horn, B. K. P. and Schunk, B. G., Determining the optical flow, Artificial Intelligence, Vol. 17, pp. 185-203, 1981.

[310] Spiesberger, W. and Tasto, M., Processing of medical image sequence, in Image Sequence Analysis, Huang, T. S. (ed.) Springer Verlag, Berlin, Germany, Chapter 7, pp. 381-429, 1981.

[311] Nagel, H. H., Analysis techniques for image sequences, in Proc. of 4th International Joint Conference on Pattern Recognition, Kyoto, Japan, pp. 186-211, 1978.

[312] Mailloux, G. E., Bleau, A., Bertrand, M. and Petitclerc, R., Computer analysis of heart motion from two dimensional echocardiograms, IEEE Trans. on Biomedical Engineering, BME-34, No. 5, pp. 356-364, 1987.

[313] Song, S. M. and Leahy, R. M., Computation of 3-D velocity fields from 3-D cine CT images of a human heart, IEEE Trans. on Med. Imaging, Vol. 10, No. 3, pp. 295-306, 1991.

[314] Srikantan, G., Sher, D. and Newberger, E., Efficient Extraction of Local Myocardial Motion with Optical Flow and a Resolution Hierarchy, Proceedings of SPIE - The International Society for Optical Engineering, Vol. 1459, pp. 258-267, 1991.

[315] Gutierrez, M. A., Moura, L., Melo, C. P. and Alens, N., Computing Optical Flow in Cardiac Images for 3-D Motion Analysis, In Proc. of Computers in Cardiology, IEEE Press, pp. 37-40, 1993.

[316] Suri, J. S. and Haralick, R. M., Computing the gradient flow for LV apex computation, GIPSY command - An image processing package at Intelligence Systems Lab., University of Washington, Seattle, 1992.

[317] Von Land, C. D., Rao, S. R. and Reiber, J. H. C., Development of an improved centerline wall motion model, In Proc. of Computers in Cardiology, IEEE Press, pp. 687-690, 1990.

[318] Buller, V. G. M., van der Geest, R. J., Kool, M. D. and Reiber, J. H. C., Accurate three-dimensional wall thickness measurement from multi-slice short-axis MR imaging, In Proc. of Computers in Cardiology, IEEE Press, pp. 245-248, 1995.

[319] van der Geest, R. J., de Roos, A., van der Wall, E. E. and Reiber, J. H. C., Quantitative analysis of cardiovascular MR images, Int. J. Card. Im., Vol. 13, No. 3, pp. 247-258, 1997.

[320] Fleagle, S. R., Thedens, D. R., Stanford, W., Pettigrew, R.I., Richek, N. and Skorton, D. J., Multicenter trial for automated border detection in Cardiac MR imaging, Jour. of Magnetic Resonance Imaging, Vol. 4, No. 2, pp. 409-415, 1993.

[321] Suh, D. Y., Eisner, R. L., Mersereau, R. M. and Pettigrew, R. I., Knowledge-based system for boundary detection of 4-D cardiac MR image sequences, IEEE Tran. on Med. Imag., Vol. 12, No. 1, pp. 65-72, 1993.

[322] Suri, J. S., Two Dimensional Fast MR Brain Segmentation Using a Region-Based Level Set Approach, Int. Journal of Engineering in Medicine and Biology, Vol. 20, No. 4, pp. 84-95, 2001.

[323] Zavaljevski, A., Dhawan, A. P., Gaskil, M., Ball, W. and Johnson, J. D., Multi-level adaptive segmentation of multi-parameter MR brain images. Comput. Med. Imag. Graph, Vol. 24, No. 2, pp. 87-98, Mar-April 2000.

[324] Barra, V. and Boire, J. Y., Tissue segmentation on MR images of the brain by possibilistic clustering on a 3-D wavelet representation, J. Magn. Reson. Imag., Vol. 11, No. 3, pp. 267-78, 2000.

[325] Salle, F. Di., Formisano, E., Linden, D. E. J., Goebel, R., Bonavita, S., Pepino, A., Smaltino, F. and Tedeschi, G., Exploring brain function with Magnetic Resonance Imaging, European Journal of Radiology, Vol. 30, No. 2, pp. 84-94, 1999.

[326] Kiebel, S. J., Goebel, R. and Friston, K. J., Anatomically Informed Basis Functions, NeuroImage, Vol. 11, (6 Part 1), pp. 656-667, Jun. 2000.

[327] Zeng, X., Staib, L. H., Schultz, R. T. and Duncan, J. S., Segmentation and measurement of the cortex from 3-D MR images using coupled-surfaces propagation, IEEE Trans. on Med. Imag., Vol. 18, No. 10, pp. 927-37, Oct. 1999.

[328] Fischl, B., Sereno, M. I. and Dale, A. M., Cortical Surface-Based Analysis, I. Segmentation and Surface Reconstruction, NeuroImage, Vol. 9, No. 2, pp. 179-194, 1999.

[329] Linden, D., Kallenbach, U., Heinecke, A., Singer, W., Goebel, R., The myth of upright vision, a psycophysical and functional imaging study of adaptation to inverting spectacles, Perception, Vol. 28, No. 4, pp. 469-482, 1999.

[330] Stokking, R., Integrated Visualization of Functional and Anatomical Brain Images, Ph.D. Thesis, Utrecht University Hospital, Utrecht, The Netherlands, 1998.

[331] Smith, A. D. C., The Folding of the Human Brain, Ph.D. Thesis, University of London, London, UK, 1999.

[332] Hurdal, M. K., Mathematical and Computer Modelling of the Human Brain With Reference to Cortical Magnification and Dipole Source Localisation in the Visual Cortex, Ph.D. Thesis, Queensland University of Technology, School of Mathematical Sciences, Brisbane, Queensland, Australia, 1999.

[333] ter Haar, R., Zuiderveld, K. J., van Waes, P. F. G. M., van Walsum, T., van der Weijden, R., Weickert, J., Stokking, R., Wink, O., Kalitzin, S., Maintz, T., Zonneveld, F. and Viergever, M. A., Advances in 3-D diagnostic radiology, J. of Anatomy, Vol. 193, No. 3, pp. 363-371, 1998.

[334] Hashemi, R. H. and Bradley, Jr., W. G., MRI: The Basics, Lippincott, Williams and Wilkins, Baltimore, ISBN: 0-6831-8240-4, 1997.

[335] Haacke, E. M., Brown, R. W., Thompson, M. R. and Venkatesan, R., Magnetic Resonance Imaging: Physical Principles and Sequence Design, J. Wiley and Sons, New York, ISBN: 0-471-35128-8, 1999.

[336] Cohen, M. S. and Weiskopf, R. M., Ultra-fast Imaging, Magnetic Resonance in Medicine, Vol. 9, No. 1, pp. 1-37, 1991.

[337] Arnold, D., Riess, G., Mathews, P., Collins, D., Francis, G. and Antel, J., Quantification of disease load and progression in multiple sclerosis by means of proton MR spectroscopy. In proceedings of SMRM, 11th annual meeting, Berlin, Society SMRM, p. 1911, 1992.

[338] Vaidyanathan, M., Clarke, L. P., Hall, L. O., Heidtman, C., Velthuizen, R., Gosche, K., Phuphanich, S., Wagner, H., Greenburg, H. and Silbiger, M. L., Monitoring brain tumor response to therapy Using MRI segmentation, Magnetic Resonance Imaging, Vol. 15, No. 3, pp. 323-334, 1997.

[339] Clarke, L. P., Velthuizen, R. P., Clark, M., Gaviria, G., Hall, L., Goldgof, D., Murtagh, R., Phuphanich, S. and Brem, S., MRI Measurement of Brain Tumor Response: Comparison of Visual Metric and Automatic Segmentation, Magnetic Resonance Imaging, Vol. 16, No. 3, pp. 271-279, Apr. 1998.

[340] Höhne, K. H. and Hanson, W., Interactive 3-D Segmentation of MRI and CT Volumes Using Mathematical Operations, J. Comput. Assist. Tomogr., Vol. 16, No. 2, pp. 285-294, 1992.

[341] Galloway, R. L., Maciunas, R. J. and Edwards, C. A., Interactive Image Guided Neurosurgery, IEEE Trans. on Biomedical Engineering, Vol. 39, No. 12, pp. 1126-1231, Dec. 1992.

[342] Kikinis, R., Shenton, M. E., Ferig, G., Martin, J., Anderson, D., Metcalf, C., Gutman, R. G., McCarley, R. W., Lorensen, W., Cline, H. and Jolesz, F. A., Routine quantitative analysis of brain and cerebrospinal fluid spaces with MR imaging, J. of Magn. Reso. Imaging, Vol. 2, No. 6, pp. 619-629, 1992.

[343] Gerig, G., Martin, J., Kikinis, R., Kubler, O., Shenton, M. and Jolesz, F. A., Unsupervised tissue type segmentation of 3-D dual MR head data, Image and Vision Computing, Vol. 10, No. 6, pp. 349-360, 1992.

[344] Griffin, L. D., The Intrinsic Geometry of the Cerebral Cortex, Journal of Theoretical Biology, Vol. 166, No. 3, pp. 261-273, 1994.

[345] England, M. A. and Wakely, J., A Colour Atlas of the Brain and Spinal Cord. An Introduction to Normal Neuroanatomy, Wolfe Publishing, London, ISBN: 0-7234-1696-6, 1991.

[346] Fischbach, G. D., Mind and brain, Scientific American, Vol. 267, No. 3, pp. 48-57, Sept. 1992.

[347] Hofman, M. A., Size and shape of the cerebral cortex in mammals I. The cortical surface, Brain Behav. Evol., Vol. 27, No. 1, pp. 28-40, 1985.

[348] Hofman, M. A., On the evolution and geometry of the brain in mammals, Prog. Neurobiol, Vol. 32, No. 2, pp. 137-158, 1989.

[349] Todd, P. H., A geometric model for the cortical folding pattern of simple folded brains, J. Theor. Biol., Vol. 97, No. 3, pp. 529-538, 1982.

[350] Prothero, J. W. and Sundesten, J. W., Folding of the cerebral cortex, A scaling model, Brain Behav. Evol., Vol. 24, No. 2-3, pp. 152-167, 1984.

[351] Horowitz, A. L., MRI physics for radiologists: a visual approach, Springer-Verlag, New York, ISBN: 0-3879-4372-2, 1995.

[352] Vaughn, Jr., T. J., Radio frequency volume coils for imaging and spectroscopy, US Patent #: 5,886,596, March 23, 1999 and Radio frequency volume coils for imaging and spectroscopy, US Patent #: 5,557,247, Sept. 17, 1996.

[353] Srinivasan, R., Radio-Frequency Coil and Method for Resonance Imaging/Analysis, US Patent #: 5,777,474, Jul. 7, 1998.

[354] Narayana, P. N., Brey, W. W., Kulkarni, M. V. and Sievenpiper, C. L., Compensation for surface coil sensitivity variation in magnetic resonance imaging, Magn. Resonance Imaging, Vol. 6, No. 3, pp. 271-274, 1988.

[355] Angenent, S., Haker, S., Tennenbaum, A. and Kikinis, R., On the Laplace-Beltrami Operator and Brain Surface Flattening, IEEE Trans. on Med. Imag., Vol. 18, No. 8, pp. 700-711, 1999.

[356] Van Essen, D. C. and Drury, H. A., Structural and functional analyses of human cerebral cortex using a surface-based atlas, J. Neuroscience, Vol. 17, No. 18, pp. 7079-7102, Sept. 1997.

[357] Kaufman, A., 3-D Volume Visualization, Advances in Computer Graphics VI, Garcia, G. and Herman, I. (eds.), Springer-Verlag, Berlin, ISBN:0-3875-3455-5, pp. 175-203, 1991.

[358] Kelly, P., Kall, B. and Goerss, S., Stereotactic CT scanning for biopsy for intracranial lesion and function neurosurgery, Applied NeuroPhysiology, Vol. 46, No. 1-4, pp. 193-199, 1983.

[359] Schad, L. R., Boesecke, R., Schlegel, W., Hartmann, G. H., Sturm, V., Strauss, L. G. and Lerenz, W. J., 3-D image correlation of CT, MR and PET studies in radiotheraphy., Treatment planning of brain tumors, Journal of Computer Assisted Tomography, Vol. 11, No. 6, pp. 948-954, 1987.

[360] Peters, T. M., Hentri, C. J., Pike, G. B., Clark, J. A., Collins, D. L. and Olivier, A., Integration of stereoscopic DSA with 3-D image reconstruction for stereotactic planning, Stereotactic planning, Stereotatic and function Neurosurgery, Vol. 54-55, pp. 471-476, 1990.

[361] Ayache, N., Cinquin, P., Cohen, I., Cohen, L., Leitner, F. and Monga, O., Segmentation of complex 3-D medical object: A challenge and a requirement for computer assisted surgery planning and performance, in Computer Integrated Surgery, Taylor, R., Lavallée, S., Burdea, G., Moesges, et. R., (eds), Computer integrated surgery, technology and clinical applications, pp. 59-74, MIT Press, 1996.

[362] Vemuri, B. C., Guo, Y., Lai, S. H. and Leonard, C. M., Fast numerical algorithms for fitting multiresolution hybrid shape models to brain MRI, Med. Image Anal., Vol. 1, No. 4, pp. 343-362, Sept. 1997.

[363] Kikinis, R., Gleason, P. L., Moriarty, T. M., Moore, M. R., Alexander, E., Stieg, P. E., Matsumae, M., Lorensen, W. E., Cline, H. E., Black, P. and Jolesz, F. A., Computer assisted interactive three-dimensional planning for neurosurgical procedures, Neurosurgery, Vol. 38, No. 4, pp. 640-651, April 1996.

[364] Jolesz, F. A., Kikinis, R., Cline, H. E. and Lorensen, W. E, The use of computerized image processing for neurosurgical planning, In Astrocytomas: diagnosis, treatment and biology, Black, P. McL, Schoene, W., Lampson, L., (eds), Blackwell Scientific, Boston, pp. 50-56, 1993.

[365] Maciunas, R. J., Fitzpatrick, J. M., Gadamsetty, S. and Maurer, Jr., C. R., A universal method for geometric correction of magnetic resonance images for stereotactic neurosurgery, Stereotactic Funct. Neurosurg., Vol. 66, No. 1-3, pp. 137-140, 1996.

[366] Kosugi, Y., Watanabe, E., Goto, J., Watanabe, T., Yoshimoto, S., Takakura, K. and Ikebe, J., An articulated neuro-surgical navigation system using MRI and CT images, IEEE Trans. on Biomedical Engineering, Vol. 35, No. 2, pp. 147-152, 1999.

[367] Lemieux, L., Hagemann, G., Krakow, K. and Woermann, F. G., Fast, Automatic Segmentation of the Brain in T1-weighted Volume Magnetic Resonance Image Data, Proceedings of SPIE - The International Society for Optical Engineering, Image Processing, Hanson, K. (ed.), Vol. 3661, pp. 152-160, 1999.

[368] Jaaski, Y. J., Klien, F. and Kubler, O., Fast direct display of volume data for medical diagnosis, CVGIP, Graphical Models and Image Processing, Vol. 53, No. 1, pp. 7-18, 1991.

[369] Suri, J. S. and Bernstien, R., 2-D and 3-D Display of Aneurysms from Magnetic Resonance Angiographic Data, 6th International Conference in Computer Assisted Radiology, pp. 666-672, 1992.

[370] Suri, J. S., Kathuria, C. and Bernstien, R., Segmentation of Aneurymns and its 3-D Display from MRA Data Sets., Proceedings of SPIE - The International Society for Optical Engineering, Vol. 1771, pp. 58-66, 1992.

[371] Schiemann, T., Bomans, M., Tiede, U. and Höhne, K. H., Interactive 3-D segmentation, Proc. Visual Biomed. Comput., Vol. 1808, pp. 376-383, 1992.

[372] Saiviroonporm, P., Robatino, A., Zahajszky, J., Kikinis, R. and Jolesz, F. A., Real-Time Interactive 3-D Segmentation, Acad. Radiol., Vol. 5, No. 1, pp. 49-56, Jan. 1998.

[373] Zeng, X., Staib, L. H., Schultz, R. T. and Duncan, J. S., Segmentation and measurement of the cortex from 3-D MR images, Medical Image Computing and Computer-Assisted Intervention (MICCAI), pp. 519-530, 1998.

[374] Henri, C. J., Pike, G. B., Collins, D. L. and Peters, T. M., Three-dimensional display of cortical anatomy and vasculature: Magnetic Resonance Angiography versus Multimodality Integration, Journal of Digital Imaging, Vol. 4, No. 1, pp. 21-27, 1991.

[375] Pelizzari, C., Chen, G., Spelbring, D., Weichselbaum, R. and Chen, C., Accurate 3-D registration of CT, PET and/or MRI Images of Brain, Journal of Computer Assisted Tomography, Vol. 13, No. 1, pp. 20-26, 1989.

[376] Stokking, R., Zuiderveld, K. J., Hilleke, E., Pol, Hulshoff, van Rijk, P. P. and Viergever, M. A., Normal Fusion for 3-D Integrated Visualization of SPECT and MR Brain Images, The Journal of Nuclear Medicine, Vol. 32, No. 4, pp. 627-629, April 1997.

[377] Cuisenaire, O., Thiran, J-P., Macq, B., Michel, C., Volder, A. D. and Marques, F., Automatic Registration of 3-D MR Images with a Computerized Brain Atlas, Proceedings of SPIE - The International Society for Optical Engineering, Vol. 2710, pp. 438-448, 1996.

[378] Alpert, N. M., Bradshaw, J. F., Kennedy, D. and Correia, J. A., The principle axes transformation - A method for image registration, J. Nucl. Med., Vol. 31, No. 10, pp. 1717-1722, 1992.

[379] Neelin, P., Crossman, J., Hawkes, D. J., Ma, U. and Evans A. C., Validation of an MRI/PET landmark registration method using 3-D simulated PET images and point simulations, Comput., Med. Imaging Graph, Vol. 17, No. (4/5), pp. 351-356, 1993.

[380] Collins, D. L., Neelin, P., Peters, T. M. and Evans, A. C., Automatic 3-D intersubject registration of MR volumetric data in standardized Talairach space, J. Computer Assisted Tomography, Vol. 18, No. 2, pp. 192-205, 1994.

[381] Lemieux, L., Wieshmann, U. C., Moran, N. F., Fish, D. R. and Shorvon, S. D., The detection and significance of subtle changes in mixed-signal brain lesions by serial MRI scan matching and spatial normalization. Med. Image Anal., Vol. 2, No. 3, pp. 227-242, Sept. 1998.

[382] Hajnal, J. V., Saeed, N., Oatridge, A., Williams, E. J., Young, I. R. and Bydder, G. M., Detection of subtle brain changes using sub-voxel registration and subtraction of brain images, Journal of Computer Assisted Tomography, Vol. 19, No. 5, pp. 677-691, 1995.

[383] Grimson, W. E. L., Ettinger, G. J., Kapur, T., Leventon, M. E., Wells III, W. M. and Kikinis, R., Utilizing segmented MRI data in Image Guided Surgery, Inter. Journal of Pattern Recognition and Artificial Intelligence, Vol. 11, No. 8, pp. 1367-97, Feb. 1998.

[384] Höhne, K. H., Bomans, M., Pommert, A., Riemer, M., Tiede, U. and Wiebecke, G., Rendering Tomographics Volume Data: Adequacy and Methods for Different Modalities and Organs, In 3-D imaging in medicine: algorithms, systems, applications, Höhne, K. H., Fuchs, H. and Pizer, S. M., (eds) Springer-Verlag, Berlin, ISBN: 0-540-2663-3, 1990.

[385] Tiede, U., Höhne, K. H., Bomans, M., Pommert, A., Riemer, M. and Wiebecke, G., Investigation of Medical 3-D Rendering Algorithms, Computer Graphics and Applications (CGA), Vol. 10, No. 2, pp. 41-53, 1990

[386] Johnston, B., Atkins, M. S., Mackiewich, B. and Anderson, M., Segmentation of multiple sclerosis lesions in intensity corrected multispectral MRI, IEEE Trans. on Med. Imag., Vol. 15, No. 2, pp. 154-169, Apr. 1996.

[387] Wagner, M., Fuchs, M., Wishmann, H. A., Ottenberg, K. and Dossel, O., Cortex Segmentation from 3-D MR Images for MEG Reconstructions, In Baumgartner, C and Deecke, L., Biomagnetism: Fundamental Research and Clinical Applications, Series: Studies in Applied Electromagnetics and Mechanics, IOS Press in collaboration with Elsevier Science; Tokyo:Ohmsa, ISBN: 9-0519-9233-5, pp. 433-438, 1995.

[388] Dale, A. M. and Sereno, M. I., Improved localization of cortical activity by combining EEG and MEG with MRI Cortical Surface Reconstruction, A Linear Approach, Journal of Cognitive Neuroscience, Vol. 5, No. 2, pp. 162-176, 1993.

[389] Brant-Zawadski, M., MR imaging of the brain, Radiology, Vol. 166, No. 1, pp. 1-10, 1988.

[390] Drayer, B. P., Imaging of the aging brain, Parts I and II, Radiology, Vol. 166, No. 3, pp. 785-806, 1988.

[391] Tanabe, J., Amend, D., Schuff, N., Di Sclafani, V., Ezekeil, F., Norman, D., Fein, G. and Weiner, M. W., Tissue segmentation of the brain in Alzheimer's disease, Am. Journal of Neuroradiology Vol. 18, No. 1, pp. 115-123, Jan. 1997.

[392] Woermann, F. G., Free, S. L., Koepp, M. J., Sisodiya, S. M. and Duncan, J. S., Abnormal cerebral structure in juvenile myoclonic epilepsy demonstrated with voxel-based analysis of MRI, Brain, Vol. 122, No. 11, pp. 2101-2107, 1999.

[393] Zubenko, G. S., Cullivan, P., Nelson, J. P., Belle, S. H., Huff, F. J. and Wolf, G. L., Brain imaging abnormalities in mental disorders of late life, Arch. Neurol., Vol. 47, No. 10, pp. 1107-1111, 1990.

[394] Lawrie, S. M. and Abukmeil, S. S., Brain abnormality in schizophrenia, A systematic and quantitative review of volumetric magnetic resonance imaging studies, British Journal of Psychiatry, Vol. 172, pp. 110-120, Feb. 1998.

[395] Velthuizen, R. P., Hall, L. O. and Clarke, L. P., Feature Extraction for MRI Segmentation, J. Neuroimaging, Vol. 9, No. 2, pp. 85-90, 1999.

[396] DeCarli, C. and Horwitz, B., Method for Quantification of Brain Volumes From MRI, US Patent #: 5,262,945, Nov. 16, 1993.

[397] Wright, I. C., Mc Guire, P. K., Poline, J. B., Travere, J. M., Murray, R. M. and Firth, C. D., A voxel-based method for the statistical analysis of gray and white matter density applied to schizophrenia, NeuroImage, Vol. 2, No. 4, pp. 244-252, 1995.

[398] Carswell, H., Functional MR techniques reveal the brain at work, Diagn. Imaging (San Francisco), Vol. 14, No. 12, pp. 86-92, Dec. 1992.

[399] Golay, X., Kollias, S., Stoll, G., Meier, D. and Valavanis, A., A New Correlation-Based Fuzzy Logic Clustering Algorithm for fMRI, Magnetic Resonance in Medicine, Vol. 40, No. 2, pp. 249-260, 1998.

[400] Lotze, M., Erb, M., Flor, H., Huelsmann, E., Godde, B. and Grodd, W., fMRI Evaluation of Somatotopic Representation in Human Primary Motor Cortex, NeuroImage, Vol. 11. No. 5, pp. 473-481, May 2000.

[401] Goldszal, A. F., Davatzikos, C., Yamazaki, Y., Solomon, J., Zhang, Y., Dagher, A. and Bryan, R. N., An image processing system for functional-structural correlational analysis of fMRI/MR brain images, NeuroImage, Vol. 9, No. 6, S151, 1999.

[402] Dawant, B. M., Zijdenbos, A. P. and Margolin, R. A., Correction of intensity variations in MR images for computer added tissue classification, IEEE Trans. on Med. Imag., Vol. 12, No. 4, pp. 770-781, 1993.

[403] Meyer, C. R., Bland, P. H. and Pipe, J., Retrospective correction of intensity inhomogeneities in MRI, IEEE Trans. on Med. Imag., Vol. 14, No. 1, pp. 36-41, 1995.

[404] Guillemaud, R. and Brady, M., Estimating the bias field of MR images, IEEE Trans. on Med. Imag., Vol. 16, pp. 238-251, 1997.

[405] Sled, J. G., Zijdenbos, A. P. and Evans, A. C., A non-parametric method for automatic correction of intensity nonuniformity in MRI data, IEEE Trans. on Med. Imag., Vol. 17, No. 1, pp. 87-97, Feb. 1998.

[406] Lai, Shang-Hong and Fang, M., A new variational shape-from-orientation approach to correcting intensity inhomogeneities in magnetic resonance images, Jour. of Medical Image Analysis, Vol. 3, No. 4, pp. 409-424, 1999.

[407] Nyul, L. G. and Udupa, J. K., On standardizing the MR image intensity scale, Magn. Reson. Med., Vol. 42, No. 6, pp. 1072-81, Dec. 1999.

[408] Kumar, A., Welti, D. and Ernst, R. R., NMR Fourier Zeugmatography, J. Magn. Reson., Vol. 18, pp. 69-83, 1975.

[409] Tootell, R. B. H. and Taylor, J. B., Anatomical Evidence for MT/V5 and Additional Cortical Visual Areas in Man, Cereb. Cortex, Vol. 1, No. 1, pp. 39-55, Jan./Feb. 1995.

[410] Tootell, R. B. H., Hadjikhani, N. K., Mendola, J. D., Marrett, S. and Dale, A. M., From retinotopy to recognition: fMRI in human visual cortex, Trends in Cognitive Sciences, Vol. 2, No. 5, pp. 174-183, 1998.

[411] Goualher, G. L., Barillot, C. and Bizais, Y., Modeling cortical sulci using active ribbons, International Journal of Pattern Recognition and Artificial Intelligence (IJPRAI), Vol. 11, No. 8, pp. 1295-1315, 1997.

[412] Goualher, G. L., Collins, D. L., Barillot, C. and Evans, A. C., Automatic identification of cortical sulci using a 3-D probabilistic atlas, Proceedings of Medical Image Computing and Computer Assisted Interventions (MICCAI), pp. 509-518, 1998.

[413]   Saeed, N., Hajnal, J. V. and Oatridge, A., Automated brain segmentation from single slice, multi-slice, or whole-volume MR scans using prior knowledge, Jour. Computer Assisted Tomography, Vol. 21, pp. 192-201, 1997.

[414]   Iwaoka, H., Hirata, T. and Matsuura, H., Optimal pulse sequence for MRI-computing accurate T1, T2 and proton density images, IEEE Trans. on Med. Imag., Vol. 6, No. 4, pp. 360-369, 1987.

[415]   Filippi, M., Rocca, M. A., Wiessmann M., Mennea S., Cercignani, M., Yousry, T. A., Sormani, M. P. and Comi, G., A comparison of MR imaging with fast-FLAIR, HASTE-FLAIR and EPI-FLAIR sequences in the assessment of patients with multiple sclerosis, Magn. Reson. Imaging, Vol. 17, No. 8, pp. 105-10, 1999.

[416]   Martin, J., Pentland, A. and Kikinis, R., Shape analysis of brain structures using physical and experimental modes, Proc. of computer vision and pattern recognition (CVPR), pp. 725-755, 1994.

[417]   Lundervold, A., Duta, N., Taxt, T. and Jain, A. K., Model-guided Segmentation of Corpus Callosum in MR images, Proceedings of CVPR, Vol. 1, pp. 231-237, 1999.

[418]   Weis, S., Kimbacher, M., Wenger, E. and Neuhold, A., Morphometric analysis of the corpus callosum using MRI: Correlation of measurements with aging in healthy individuals, Am. Journal of Neuroradiology, Vol. 14, No. 3, pp. 637-645, 1993.

[419]   Ghanei, A., Solitanian-Zadeh, H. and Windham, J. P., Segmentation of the hippocampus from brain MRI using deformable contours, Computerized Medical Imaging and Graphics (CMIG), Vol. 22, No. 3, pp. 203-216, May-Jun 1998.

[420]   Cowell, P. A., Allen, L. S., Kertesz, A., Zalatimo, N. S. and Denenberg, B. H., Human corpus callosum, A stable mathematical model of regional neuroanatomy, Brain and Cognition, Vol. 25, No. 1, pp. 52-66, 1994.

[421]   Worth, A. J., Makris, N., Caviness, V. S. and Kennedy, D. N., Neuroanatomical Segmentation in MRI: Technological Objectives, International Journal of Pattern Recognition and Artificial Intelligence, Vol. 11, No. 8, pp. 1161-1187, 1997.

[422]   Hill, A., Cootes, T. F. and Taylor, C. J., A Generic System for Image Interpretation Using Flexible Templates, Proc. British Machine Vision Conference (BMVC), pp. 276-285, 1992.

[423]   Crespo-Facorro B., Kim, J., Andreasen, N. C., Spinks R O'Leary, D. S., Bockholt, H. J., Harris, G. and Magnotta, V. A., Cerebral cortex: a topographic segmentation method using magnetic resonance imaging, Psychiatry Res., Vol. 100, No. 2, pp. 97-126, Dec. 2000.

[424]   Kikinis, R., Shenton, M., Jolesz, F., Gerig, G., Martin, J., Anderson, M., Metcalf, D., Guttmann, C., Mc Carley, R. W., Lorensen, W. and Cline, H., Routine Quantitative Analysis of Brain and CFS with MR Imaging, J. of Mag. Resonance in Medicine, Vol. 2, No. 6, pp. 619-629, 1992.

[425] Rusinek, H., deLeon, M. J., George, A. E., Stylopoulos, L. A., Chandra, R., Smith, G., Rand, T., Mourino, M. and Kowalski, H., Alzheimer's disease: Measuring loss of cerebral gray matter with MR imaging, Radiology, Vol. 178, No. 1, pp. 109-114, 1991.

[426] Johnston, B., Atkins, M. S., Mackiewich, B. and Anderson, M., Segmentation of multiple sclerosis lesions in intensity corrected multispectral MRI, IEEE Trans. on Med. Imag., Vol. 14, No. 2, pp. 154-169, 1996.

[427] Jones, E. G. and Peters, A., Cerebral Cortex, Vol. 8B, Comparative Structure and Evolution of Cerebral Cortex, Part II, Plenum Press, NY and London, ISBN: 0-306-43653-3, 1990.

[428] Hendelman, W. J., Student's Atlas of Neuroanatomy, W. B. Saunders, ISBN: 0-7216-5428-2, 1994.

[429] Rademacher, J., Caviness, V. S. and Steinmetz, H., Topographical Variation of the Human Primary Cortices: Implications for Neuroimaging, Brain Mapping and Neurobiology, Cerebral Cortex, Vol. 3, No. 4, pp. 313-329, July 1993.

[430] Menhardt, W. and Schmidt, K-H., Computer Vision on MRI, Pattern Recognition Letters, Vol. 8, No. 2, pp. 73-85, 1988.

[431] Clarke, L. P., Velthuizen, R. P., Camacho, M. A., Heine, J. J., Vaidyanathan, M., Hall, L. O., Thatcher, R. W. and Silbiger, M. L., Review of MRI Segmentation: Methods and Applications, Magn. Reso. Imaging, Vol. 13, No. 3, pp. 343-368, 1995.

[432] Binford, T. O., Survey of Model-Based Image Analysis Systems, Inter. Journal of Robotics Research, Vol. 1, No. 1, pp. 18-64, 1982.

[433] Pal, N. R. and Pal, S. K., A review on image segmentation techniques, Pattern Recognition, Vol. 26, No. 9, pp. 1277-1294, 1993.

[434] Kong, T. and Rosenfield, A., Digital Topology: Introduction and Survey, Computer Vision, Graphics and Image Processing, Vol. 48, No. 3, pp. 357-393, Dec. 1989.

[435] Saeed, N., Magnetic Resonance image segmentation using pattern recognition and applied to image registration and quantification, NMR in Biomedicine, Vol. 11, No. 4-5, pp. 157-167, 1998.

[436] Barillot, C., Gibaud, B., Lis, O., Luo, L. M., Bouliou, A., LeCerten, G., Collorec, R. and Coatrieux, J. L., Computer Graphics in Medicine: A Survey. CRC Critical Reviews in Biomedical Engineering, Vol. 15, No. 4, pp. 269-307, 1988.

[437] Barillot, C., Surface and Volume Rendering Techniques To Display 3-D Data, An Overview of Basic Principles Shows Advances in Display Techniques, IEEE Engineering in Medicine and Biology, Vol. 12, No. 1, pp. 111-119, 1993.

[438] Zucker, S. W., Region growing: Childhood and Adolescence, Computer Graphics and Image Processing (CGIP), Vol. 5, No. 3, pp. 382-399, 1976.

[439] Adams, R. and Bischof, L., Seeded region growing, IEEE Trans. on Pattern Analysis and Machine Intelligence, Vol. 16, No. 6, pp. 641-647, 1994.

[440] Justice, R. K., Stokely, E. M., Strobel, J. S., Ideker, R. E. and Smith, W. M., Medical image segmentation using 3-D seeded region growing, Proceedings of SPIE - The International Society for Optical Engineering, Vol. 3034, pp. 900-910, 1997.

[441] Liu, A., Pizer, S., Eberly, D., Morse, B., Rosenman, J., Chaney, E., Bullitt, E. and Carrasco, V., Volume registration using the 3-D core: Proceedings of SPIE - The International Society for Optical Engineering, Vol. 2359, pp. 217-226, 1994.

[442] Talairach, J., Szikla, G., Tournoux, P., Prosalentis, A. and Bornas-Ferrier, M., Atlas d'Anatomie Stiriotaxique du Tilenciphale, Masson, ISBN: 0-8657-7293-2 (Thieme Medical Publishers), 1967.

[443] Talairach, J. and Tournoux, P., Co-planar Stereotactic Atlas of the Human Brain, 3-D Proportional System, An Approach to Cerebral Imaging, Georg Thieme Verlag, Stuttgart, 1988.

[444] Bohm, C., Grertz, T. and Thurfjell, L., The role of anatomic information in quantifying functional neuroimaging data, Journal of Neural Transmission (Suppl.), Vol. 37, pp. 67-78, 1992.

[445] Seitz, R., Bohm, C., Greitz, T., Roland, P. and Eriksson, L., Blomqvist, B., Rosenqvist, B. and Nordell, B., Accuracy and precision of the computerized brain Atlas programme for localization and quantification in PET, J. Cereb. Blood Flow Metab., Vol. 10, No. 4, pp. 443-457, 1990.

[446] Evans, A. C., Marrett, S., Torrescorzo, J., Ku, S. and Collins, L., MRI-PET correlation in the 3-D using a VOI atlas, J. Cereb. Blood Flow Metab., Vol. 11, No. 2, pp. A69-78, 1991.

[447] Bajcsy, R. and Kosvacis, S., Multiresolution elastic matching, Computer Vision, Graphics and Image Processing, Vol. 46, No. 1, pp. 1-21, 1989.

[448] Van Essen, D. C. and Drury, H. A., Structural and functional analyses of human cerebral cortex using a surface-based atlas, Journal of Neuroscience, Vol. 17, No. 18, pp. 7079-7102, Sept. 1997.

[449] Collins, D. L., Holmes, C. J., Peters, T. M. and Evans, A. C., Automatic 3-D model-based neuroanatomical segmentation, Human Brain Mapping, Vol. 3, No. 3, pp. 190-208, 1995.

[450] Gibaud, B., Garlatti, S., Barillot, C. and Faure, E., Computerised Brain Atlases vs. Decision Support Systems: A Methodological Approach, Artificial Intelligence in Medicine, Vol. 14, No. 1, pp. 83-100, Jan. 1998.

[451] Sandor, S. and Leahy, R., Surface-based labelling of cortical anatomy using a deformable atlas, IEEE Trans. on Med. Imag., Vol. 16, No. 1, pp. 41-54, Feb. 1997.

[452] Sandor, S. R., Atlas-Guided Deformable Models for Automatic Labelling of MR Brain Images, Ph.D. Thesis, University of Southern California, Los Angeles, CA, 1994.

[453] Ferrant, M., Cuisenaire, O. and Macq Benoit, M., Multi object segmentation of brain structures in 3-D MRI using a Computerized Atlas, Proceedings of SPIE - The Inter. Society for Optical Engineering, Medical Imaging, Vol. 3661, pp. 986-995, 1999.

[454] Lim, K. O. and Pfefferbaum, A., Segmentation of MR brain images into cerebrospinal fluid spaces, white and gray matter, J. of Computer Assisted Tomography (JCAT), Vol. 13, No. 4, pp. 588-593, 1989.

[455] Harris, G. J., Barta, P. E., Pengk, L. W., Lee, S., Brettschneider, P. D., Shah, A., Henderer, J. D., Schlaepfer, T. E. and Pearlson, G. D., MR volume segmentation of gray matter and white matter using manual thresholding: dependence on image brightness, Am. J. of Neuro Radiology (AJNR), Vol. 15, No. 2, pp. 225-230, Feb. 1994.

[456] Falcao, A. X., Uudpa, J. K., Samarasekera, S., Sharma, S., Hirsch, B. E. and Lotufo, R. D. A., User-Steered Image Segmentation Paradigms: Live Wire and Live Lane, Graphical Models and Image Processing, Vol. 60, No. 4, pp. 233-260, 1998.

[457] Geman, S. and Geman, D., Stochastic Relaxation, Gibbs' Distribution and the Bayesian Restoration of Images, IEEE Trans. on Pattern Analysis and Machine Intelligence, Vol. 6, No. 6, pp. 721-741, 1984.

[458] Wells III, W. M., Grimson, W. E. L., Kikinis, R. and Jolesz, F. A., Adaptive Segmentation of MRI Data, IEEE Trans. on Med. Imag., Vol. 15, No. 4, pp. 429-442, Aug. 1992.

[459] Gerig, G., Kubler, O. and Jolesz, F. A., Nonlinear anisotropic filtering of MRI data, IEEE Trans. on Med. Imag., Vol. 11, No. 2, pp. 221-232, 1992.

[460] Joshi, M., Cui, J., Doolittle, K., Joshi, S., Van Essen, D., Wang, L. and Miller, M. I., Brain segmentation and the generation of cortical surfaces, NeuroImage, Vol. 9, No. 5, pp. 461-476, 1999.

[461] Dempster, A. D., Laird, N. M. and Rubin, D. B., Maximum likelihood from incomplete data via the EM algorithm, J. R. Stat. Soc., Vol. 39, No. 1, pp. 1-37, 1977.

[462] Kao, Yi-Hsuan, Sorenson, J. A., Bahn, M. M., and Winkler, S. S., Dual-Echo MRI segmentation using vector decomposition and probability technique: A two tissue model, Magnetic Resonance in Medicine, Vol. 32, No. 3, pp. 342-357, 1994.

[463] Kapur, T., Model based three dimensional Medical Image Segmentation, Ph.D. Thesis, Artificial Intelligence Laboratory, Massachusetts Institute of Technology, Cambridge, MA, May 1999.

[464] Li, S., Markov Random Field Modeling in Computer Vision, Springer Verlag, New York Berlin Heidelberg Tokyo, p. 264, ISBN: 0-387-70145-1, 1995.

[465] Held, K., Rota Kopps, E., Krause, B., Wells, W., Kikinis, R. and Muller-Gartner, H., Markov random field segmentation of brain MR images, IEEE Trans. on Med. Imag., Vol. 16, No. 6, pp. 878-887, 1998.

[466] Bezdek, J. C, Hall, L. O., Review of MR image segmentation techniques using pattern recognition, Medical Physics, Vol. 20, No. 4, pp. 1033-1048, March 1993.

[467] Hall, L. O. and Bensaid, A. M., A comparison of neural networks and fuzzy clustering techniques in segmenting MRI of the brain, IEEE Trans. in Neural Networks, Vol. 3, No. 5, pp. 672-682, Sept. 1992.

[468] Pham, D. L., Prince, J. L., Dagher, A. P. and Xu, C., An Automated Technique for Statistical Characterization of Brain Tissues in Magnetic Resonance Imaging, International Journal of Pattern Recognition and Artificial Intelligence, Vol. 11, No. 8, pp. 1189-1211, 1997.

[469] Pham, D. L. and Prince, J. L., An Adaptive Fuzzy C-Means Algorithm for Image Segmentation in the Presence of Intensity Inhomogeneities, Pattern Recognition Letters, Vol. 20, No. 1, pp. 57-68, 1999.

[470] Pham, D. L. and Prince, J. L., Adaptive Fuzzy Segmentation of Magnetic Resonance Images, IEEE Trans. on Med. Imag., Vol. 18, No. 9, pp. 737-752, 1999.

[471] Ostergaard, L.R. and Larsen, Ole Vilhelm, Applying Voting to Segmentation of MR Images, In Amin, A., Dori, D., Freeman, H. and Pudil, P. (eds), Advances in Pattern Recognition, Springer Berlin Heidelberg New York, Lecture notes in computer science, Vol. 1451, pp. 795-804, 1998.

[472] Duda, R. O. and Hart, P. E., Pattern Classification and Scene Analysis, John Wiley and Sons, NY, ISBN: 0-4712-2361-1, 1973.

[473] Rosenfeld, A. and Kak, A., Digital Picture Processing, Academic Press, Inc., NY, ISBN: 0-12597-301-2, 1982.

[474] Jain, A. K., Murty, M. N. and Flynn, P. J., Data Clustering: A Review, ACM Computing Surveys, Vol. 31, No. 3, pp. 264-323, Sept. 1999.

[475] Kandel, A., Fuzzy Techniques in Pattern Recognition, Wiley Interscience, NY, ISBN: 0-4710-9136-7, 1982.

[476] Acton, P. D., Pilowsky, L. S., Kung, H. F. and Ell, P. J., Automatic segmentation of dynamic neuroreceptor single-photon emission tomography images using fuzzy clustering, Eur. J Nucl. Med., Vol. 26, No. 6, pp. 581-90, 1999.

[477] Serra, J., Image analysis and mathematical morphology, Academic Press, Inc., London, UK, ISBN: 0-1263-7240-3, 0126372411 (v. 2), 1982.

[478] Sternberg, S. R., Grayscale Morphology, Computer Vision, Graphics, Image Processing, Vol. 35, No. 3, pp. 333-355, Sept. 1986.

[479] Bomans, M., Höhne, K.-H., Tiede, U. and Martin, R., 3-D Segmentation of MR Images of the Head for 3-D Display, IEEE Trans. on Med. Imag., Vol. 19, No. 2, pp. 177-37, 1990.

[480] Hildreth, E. C., The Detection of Intensity Changes by Computer and Biological Vision Systems, Computer Vision, Graphics and Image Processing, Vol. 22, No. 1, pp. 1-27, April 1983.

[481] Höhne, K. H., Bomans, M., Tiede, U. and Riemer, M., Display of multiple 3-D objects using the generalized voxel model., Prod. of Conf.

Med. Imaging, II, Proceedings of SPIE - The International Society for Optical Engineering, Vol. 914, pp. 850-854, 1988.

[482] Suri, J. S., Kumar, S. and Chou, Yu-Yu, Studying Cytology of the Uterine Cervix on Win.98/NT Platform Using Imaging Techniques: A Carcinoma-Situ and Cancerous Cell Detection and Scoring, Proceedings of the First Meeting of Engineering in Medicine and Biology, Atlanta, GA, Vol. 2, p. 1133, 1999.

[483] Robert, L. and Malandain, G., Fast Binary Image Processing Using Binary Decision Diagrams, Computer Vision and Image Understanding, Vol. 72, No. 1, pp. 1-9, Oct. 1998.

[484] Malandain, G., Bertrand, G. and Ayache, N., Topological segmentation of discrete surfaces, Int. Journal of Computer Vision, Vol. 10, No. 2, pp. 183-197, 1993.

[485] Bertrand, G., Everat, J. C. and Couprie, M., Image segmentation through operators based upon topology, Journal of Electronic Imaging, Vol. 6, No. 4, pp. 395-405, 1997.

[486] Lemieux, L., Hagemann, G., Krakow, K. and Woermann, F. G., Fast, Accurate and Reproducible Automatic Segmentation of the Brain in T1-weighted Volume Magnetic Resonance Image Data, Magnetic Resonance in Medicine, Vol. 42, No. 1, pp. 127-135, 1999.

[487] Sandor, S. and Leahy, R., A 3-D morphological algorithm for automated labelling of the cortex in magnetic resonance images, In AAAI Spring Symposium Applications of Computer Vision in Medical Image Processing, Palo Alto, CA, March 1994.

[488] Sckolowska, E. and Newell, J. A., Multilayered image representation structure and application in recognition of parts of brain anatomy, Patt. Recog. Lett., Vol. 4, No. 4, pp. 223-230, 1986.

[489] Sckolowska, E. and Newell, J. A., Recognition of the anatomy using a symbolic structural model of a CT image of the brain, Proceedings of the Second International Conference on Image Processing and Applications (ICIPA), pp. 233-237, 1986.

[490] Sckolowska, E., Newell, J. A. and Raya S. P., Low-level segmentation of 3-D magnetic resonance images: A rule based system, IEEE Trans. on Med. Imaging, Vol. 9, No. 1, pp. 327-337, 1990.

[491] Sonka, M., Tadikonda, S. K. and Collins, S. M., Knowledge based interpretation of MR brain images, IEEE Trans. on Med. Imag., Vol. 15, No. 4, pp. 443-452, 1996.

[492] Dhawan, A. P. and Juvvadi, S., Knowledge-based analysis and understanding of medical images, Comput. Methods Programs Biomed, Vol. 33, No. 4, pp. 221-39, 1990.

[493] Dhawan, A. P. and Arata, L., Knowledge-Based Multi-Modality Three-Dimensional Analysis of the Brain, Am. J. Physiol. Imaging, Vol. 7, No. 3/4, pp. 210-219, 1992.

[494] Clark, M., Knowledge-Guided Processing of Magnetic Resonance Images of the Brain, Ph.D. Thesis, Department of Computer Science and Engineering, University of South Florida, Tampa, 2000.

[495] Suri, J. S. and Tsai, J.-P., Expert System for low level segmentation of microscopic images of human embryos, in Proceedings of the World Congress of Expert Systems, Orlando, FL, pp. 308-313, 1991.

[496] Suri, J. S. and Tsai, J.-P., Knowledge-Based Analysis of Computer Tomography of Human Chest, in Proceedings of the World Congress of Expert Systems, Orlando, FL, pp. 2671-2678, 1991.

[497] Haralick, R. M. and Shanmugan K., Textural Features for Image Classification, IEEE Trans. on Syst., Man and Cybernetics, Vol. 3, No. 6, pp. 141-152, 1973.

[498] Peleg, S. H., Naor, J., Hartley, R. and Aunir, D., Multiple Resolution Texture Analysis and Classification, IEEE Trans. on Pattern Analysis and Machine Intelligence, Vol. 6, No. 4, pp. 518-523, July 1984.

[499] Cross, G. R. and Jain, A. K., Markov Random Field Texture Models, IEEE Trans. on Pattern Analysis and Machine Intelligence, Vol. 5, No. 1, pp. 25-39, 1983.

[500] Lachmann, F. and Barillot, C., Brain tissue classification from MRI data by means of texture analysis, Medical Imaging VI: Image Processing, Proceedings of SPIE - The International Society for Optical Engineering, Medical Imaging, Vol. 1652, pp. 72-83, 1992.

[501] Eklundh, J. O., Yamamoto, H. and Rosenfeld, A., A relaxation method for multispectral pixel classification, IEEE Trans. on Pattern Analysis and Machine Intelligence, Vol. 2, No. 1, pp. 72-75, Jan. 1980.

[502] Ehricke, H. H., Problems and Approaches for Tissue Segmentation in 3-D MR Imaging, Proceedings of SPIE - The International Society for Optical Engineering, Medical Imaging, Image Processing, Vol. 1233, pp. 128-137, 1990.

[503] Reddick, W. E., Glass, J. O., Cook, E. N., Elkin T. D. and Deaton, R. J., Automated Segmentation and Classification of Multispectral MRI of Brain Using Artifical Neural Networks, IEEE Trans. on Med. Imag., Vol. 16, No. 6, pp. 911-918, Dec. 1997.

[504] Clark, J. W., Neural network modelling, Phys. Med. Biol. Vol. 36, No. 10, pp. 1259-317, Oct. 1991.

[505] Wang, Y., Adah, T., Kung, S. and Szabo, Z., Quantification and segmentation of brain tissues from MR images: a probabilistic neural network approach, IEEE Trans. on Image Processing, Vol. 7, No. 8, pp. 1165-1181, 1998.

[506] Chiou, G. I. and Hwang, J.-N., A Neural Network Based Stochastic Active Contour Model (NNS-SNAKE) for Contour Finding of Distinct Features, IEEE Trans. on Image Proc., Vol. 4, No. 10, pp. 1407-1416, Oct. 1985.

[507] Koster, A. S. E., Linking Models for Multiscale Image Segmentation, Ph.D. Thesis, Utrecht University, Utrecht, The Netherlands, 1995.

[508] Vinken, K. L., Probabilistic multiscale image segmentation by the Hyperstack, Ph.D. Thesis, Utrecht University, Utrecht, The Netherlands, 1995.

[509] Niessen, W. J., Multiscale Medical Image Analysis, Ph.D. Thesis, Image Sciences Institute, Utrecht University, Utrecht, The Netherlands, 1997.

[510] Koster, A. S. E., Vincken, K. L., De Graff, C. N., Zander, O. C. and Viergever, M. A., Heuristis linking models in multiscale image segmentation, Computer Vision and Image Understanding, Vol. 65, No. 3, pp. 382-402, 1997.

[511] Vincken, K. L., Koster, A. S. E. and Viergever, M. A., Probabilistic multiscale image segmentation, IEEE Trans. on Pattern Analysis and Machine Intelligence, Vol. 2, No. 19, pp. 109-120, 1997.

[512] Niessen, W., Romeny, B. and Viergever, M. A., Geodesic Deformable Models for Medical Image Analysis, IEEE Trans. on Med. Imag., Vol. 17, No. 4, pp. 634-641, Aug. 1998.

[513] Niessen, W., Vincken, K. L., Weickert, J., Romeny, B. M. Ter Haar and Viergever, M. A., Multiscale Segmentation of Three-Dimensional MR Brain Images, Vol. 31, No. 2/3, pp. 185-202, 1999.

[514] Teo, P. C., Shapiro, G. and Wandell, B. A., Creating Connected Representations of Cortical Gray Matter for Functional MRI Visualization, IEEE Trans. on Med. Imag., Vol. 16, No. 6, pp. 852-863, 1997.

[515] Cline, H. E., Dumoulin, C. L., Hart, H. R., Lorensen, W. E. and Ludke, S., 3-D reconstruction of the brain from MRI using a Connectivity Algorithm, Magnetic Resonance in Medicine, Vol. 5, No. 5, pp. 345-352, 1987.

[516] Canny, J., A computational approach to edge detection, IEEE Trans. on Pat. Anal. and Mach. Int., Vol. 8, No. 6, pp. 679-698, 1986.

[517] Monga, O., Deriche, R., Malandain G. and Cocquerez, J. P., Recursive filtering and edge tracking: two primary tools for 3-D edge detection, Image and Vision Computing, Vol. 4, No. 9, pp. 203-214, Aug. 1991.

[518] Deriche, R., Recursively Implementing the Gaussian and Its Derivatives, Srinivasan, V., Ong, S. H., Ang, Y. H. (eds.), Proc. Second Int. Singapore Conf. on Image Proc., Singapore, pp. 263-267, 1992.

[519] Kennedy, D. N., Filipeck, P. A. and Caviness, V. S., Anatomic Segmentation and volumetric calculations in Nuclear MR imaging, IEEE Trans. on Med. Imag., Vol. 8, No. 1, pp. 1-7, 1989.

[520] Djuric, P. M. and Fwu, Jong-Kae, Boundary detection in noisy vector fields, In Proceedings of SPIE - The International Society for Optical Engineering, Medical Imaging, Image Processing, Vol. 2434, Loew, M. H. (ed.), pp. 730-741, 1995.

[521] Xuan, J., Adali, T. and Wang, Y., Segmentation of MR brain image: Integrating region growing and edge detection, Proceedings of the IEEE International Conference On Image Processing, Washington, DC, Vol. 3, pp. 544-547, 1995.

[522] Zuniga, O. and Haralick, R. M., Integrated Directional Derivative Gradient Operator, IEEE Trans. on System, Man and Cybernetics (SMC), Vol. 17, No. 3, pp. 508-517, May/June 1987.

[523] Wikins, K. and Terzopolous, D., Snakes: Active Contour Models, International Jour. of Computer Vision, Vol. 1, No. 4, pp. 321-331, 1988.

[524] Atkins, M. S. and Mackiewich, B. T., Fully automatic segmentation of the brain in MRI, IEEE Trans. on Med. Imag., Vol. 17, No. 1, pp. 98-107, Feb. 1998.

[525] Gang, X., Segawa, E. and Tsuji, S., Robust active contours with insensitive parameters, Pattern Recognition, Vol. 27, No. 7, pp. 879-884, 1994.

[526] Ranganath, S., Analysis of the effects of snake parameters on contour extraction, Proceedings of the 2nd International Conference on Automation, Robotics, Computer Vision (CARCV), Singapore, pp. CCV 4.5.1-CV 4.5.5, 1992.

[527] Amini, A., Tehrani, S. and Weymouth,T., Using dynamic programming for minimizing the energy of active contours in the presence of hard constraints, in Proceedings Second Int. Conf. Computer Vision (ICCV), Tarpon Springs, FL, pp. 95-99, 1988.

[528] Nastar, C. and Ayache, N., Fast Segmentation, Tracking and Analysis of Deformable Objects, Proceedings of the Fourth International Conference on Computer Vision (ICCV), Berlin, Germany, pp. 275-279, 1993.

[529] Staib, L. H. and Duncan, J. S., Parametrically Deformable Contour Models, Proceedings of Int. Conference in Computer Vision (ICCV), pp. 98-102, 1989.

[530] Ip, Horace H. S. and Shen, D., An affine invariant active contour model (AI-snake) for model-based segmentation, Image and Vision Computing, Vol. 16, No. 2, pp. 135-146, 1998.

[531] Duta, N. and Sonka, M., Segmentation and Interpretation of MR brain images: an improved active shape model, IEEE Trans. on Med. Imag., Vol. 17, No. 6, pp. 1049-1062, 1998.

[532] Lipson, P., Yuille, A. L., O'Keefe, D., Cavanaugh, J., Taffe, J. and Rosenthal, D., Deformable templates for feature extraction from medical images, In Faugeras, O. (ed.), Computer Vision Proc. First European Conference in Computer Vision, France, pp. 413-417, 1990.

[533] Menet, S., Saint-Marc, P. and Medioni, G., Active contour models: overview, implementation and applications, Proceedings of the IEEE International Conference on Systems, Man and Cybernetics Conference Proceedings, Vol. 929, pp. 194-199, 1990.

[534] Perona, P. and Malik, J., Scale space and edge detection using anisotropic diffusion, IEEE Trans. on Pattern Analysis and Machine Intelligence, Vol. 12, No. 7, pp. 629-639, Apr. 1990.

[535] Sethian, J. A., An Analysis of Flame Propagation, Ph.D. Thesis, Department of Mathematics, University of California, Berkeley, CA, 1982.

[536] Osher, S. and Sethian, J., Fronts propagating with curvature-dependent speed: algorithms based on Hamiltons-Jacobi formulations, J. Comput. Physics, Vol. 79, No. 1, pp. 12-49, 1988.

[537] Rouy, E. and Tourin, A., A viscosity solutions approach to shape-from-shading, SIAM J. of Numerical Analysis, Vol. 23, No. 3, pp. 867-884, 1992.

[538] Caselles, V., Catte, F., Coll, T. and Dibos, F., A geometric model for active contours, Numerische Mathematik, Vol. 66, pp. 1-31, 1993.

[539] Chopp, D. L., Computing Minimal Surfaces via Level Set Curvature Flow, Journal of Comput. Physics, Vol. 106, No. 1, pp. 77-91, 1993.

[540] Caselles, V., Kimmel, R. and Shapiro, G., Geodesic active contours, Int. Journal of Computer Vision (IJCV), Vol. 22, No. 1, pp. 61-79, 1997.

[541] Malladi, R., Sethian, J. A. and Vemuri, B. C., Shape Modeling with Front Propagation, IEEE Trans. on Pattern Analysis and Machine Intelligence, Vol. 17, No. 2, pp. 158-175, Feb. 1995.

[542] Cao, S. and Greenhalgh, S., Finite-difference solution of the eikonal equation using an efficient, First-arrival, wavefront tracking scheme, Geophysics, Vol. 59, No. 4, pp. 632-643, April 1994.

[543] Chen, S., Merriman, B., Osher, S. and Smereka, P., A Simple Level Set Method for Solving Stefan Problems, Journal of Comput. Physics, Vol. 135, No. 1, pp. 8-29, 1997.

[544] Adalsteinsson, D. and Sethian, J. A., The fast construction of extension velocities in level set methods, J. Compu. Phys., Vol. 148, No. 1, pp. 2-22, 1999.

[545] Kichenassamy, S., Kumar, A., Olver, P., Tannenbaum, A. and Yezzi, A., Conformal curvatures flows: from phase transitions to active vision, Arch. Rational Mech. Anal., Vol. 134, No. 3, pp. 275-301, 1996.

[546] Yezzi, A., Kichenassamy, S., Kumar, A., Olver, P. and Tannenbaum, A., A geometric snake model for segmentation of medical imagery, IEEE Trans. on Med. Imag., Vol. 16, No. 2, pp. 199-209, 1997.

[547] Siddiqui, K., Lauriere, Y. B., Tannenbaum, A. and Zucker, S. W., Area and length minimizing flows for shape segmentation, IEEE Trans. on Image Proc., Vol. 7, No. 3, pp. 433-443, 1998.

[548] Sethian, J. A., Level Set Methods and Fast Marching Methods: Evolving Interfaces in computational geometry, fluid mechanics, Computer Vision and Material Science (2nd ed.), Cambridge University Press, Cambridge, UK, ISBN: 0-521-64204-3, 1999.

[549] Sethian, J. A., Three-dimensional seismic imaging of complex velocity structures, US Patent #: 6,018,499, Jan. 25, 2000.

[550] Suri, J. S., Haralick, R. M. and Sheehan, F. H., Greedy Algorithm for Error Correction in Automatically Produced Boundaries from Low Contrast Ventriculograms, Pattern Analysis and Applications (PAA), Vol. 3, No. 1, pp. 39-60, Jan. 2000.

[551] Berger, M. J., Local Adaptive Mesh Refinement, Journal of Computational Physics, Vol. 82, No. 1, pp. 64-84, 1989.

[552] Sethian, J. A., Curvature Flow and Entropy Conditions Applied to Grid Generation, J. Computational Physics, Vol. 115, No. 2, pp. 440-454, 1994.

[553] Tababai, A. J. and Mitchell, O. R., Edge location to subpixel values in digital imagery, IEEE Trans. on Pattern Analysis and Machine Intelligence, Vol. 6, No. 2, pp. 188-201, March 1984.

[554] Huertas, A. and Medioni, G., Detection of intensity changes with subpixel accuracy using Laplacian-gaussian masks, IEEE Trans. on Pattern Analysis and Machine Intelligence, Vol. 8, No. 5, pp. 651-664, Sept. 1986.

[555] Gao, J., Kosaka, A. and Kak, A. C., A deformable model for human organ extraction, Proceedings IEEE International Conference on Image Processing (ICIP), Vol. 3, pp. 323-327, Chicago, 1998.

[556] Schroeder, W. J., Zarge, J. A. and Lorensen, W. E., Decimation of Triangle Meshes, Computer Graphics, Vol. 26, No. 4, pp. 65-169, 1987.

[557] Boissonnat, J. D., Shape Reconstruction from Planar Cross-Sections, Computer Vision, Graphics and Image Processing (CVGIP), Vol. 44, No. 1, pp. 1-29, 1988.

[558] Geiger, B., Construction et utilisation des modhles d'organes en vue de l'assistance au diagnostic et aux interventions chirurgicales, Ph.D. Thesis, Universiti Sophia Antipolis, France, 1993.

[559] Carman, G. J., Drury, H. A. and Van Essen, D. C., Computational Method for Reconstructing and Unfolding the Cerebral Cortex, Cerebral Cortex, Vol. 5, No. 6, pp. 506-517, Dec. 1995.

[560] Suri, J. S., Brain cavity reconstruction from MRI serial-cross sections, MS Thesis, University of Illinois, Chicago, 1990.

[561] Tatsumi, H., Takaoki, E., Omura, K. and Fujito, H., A new method of 3-D reconstruction from serial section by computer graphics using meta-balls: Reconstruction of Hepatoskeletal System formed by Ito Cells in the Cod Liver, Comput. Biomed. Res., Vol. 23, No. 1, pp. 37-45, Feb. 1990.

[562] MacDonald, D., Avis, D. and Evans, A. E., Proximity constraints in deformable models for cortical surface identification, Proceedings of the First International Conference on Medical Image Computing and Computer-Assisted Intervention (MICCAI), pp. 650-659, 1998.

[563] MacDonald, D., Avis, D. and Evans, A. E., Multiple surface identification and matching in Magnetic Resonance images, Proceedings of SPIE - The International Society for Optical Engineering, Bellingham, WA, Vol. 2359, pp. 160-169, 1994.

[564] MacDonald, D., Kabani, N., Avis, D. and Evans, A. C., Automated 3-D Extraction of Inner and Outer Surfaces of Cerebral Cortex from MRI, NeuroImage, Vol. 12, No. 3, pp. 340-356, 2000.

[565] Davatzikos, C. A. and Prince, J. L., An active contour model for mapping the cortex, IEEE Trans. on Med. Imag., Vol. 14, No. 1, pp. 65-80, 1995.

[566] Davatzikos, C. A. and Bryan, R. N., Using a deformable surface model to obtain a shape representation of cortex, IEEE Trans. on Med. Imag., Vol. 15, No. 6, pp. 785-795, 1996.

[567] Vaillant, M. and Davatzikos, C., Finding parametric representations of the cortical sulci using an active contour model, Medical Image Analysis, Vol. 1, No. 4, pp. 295-315, Sept. 1997.

[568] McInerney, T. and Terzopoulos, D., Topology adaptive deformable surfaces for medical image volume segmentation, IEEE Trans. on Med. Imag., Vol. 18, No. 10, pp. 840-850, Oct. 1999.

[569] McInerney, T. and Terzopoulos, D., Topologically Adaptable Snakes, 5th International Conference in Computer Vision (ICCV), pp. 840-845, 1995.

[570] McInerney, T. and Terzopoulos, D., Medical Image Segmentation Using Topologically Adaptable Surfaces, In: Troccaz, J., Grimson, E. and Mösges, R. (eds) CVRMed-MRCAS'97, Springer Berlin Heidelberg New York, ISBN 3-540-62734-0, Lecture notes in computer science, Vol. 1205, pp. 23-32, 1997.

[571] Terzopoulos, D., Witkin, A. and Kass, M., Constraints on deformable models: Recovering 3-D shape and nonrigid motion, Artificial Intelligence, Vol. 36, No. 1, pp. 91-123, 1988.

[572] Cohen, I., Cohen, L. and Ayache, N., Using deformable surfaces to segment 3-D images and inter-differential structures, CVGIP: Image Understanding, Vol. 56, No. 2, pp. 242-263, Sept. 1992.

[573] Fischl, B., Sereno, M. I. and Dale, A. M., Cortical Surface-Based Analysis II. Inflation, Flattening and a Surface-Based Coordinate System, Neuro Image, Vol. 9, No. 2, pp. 195-207, 1999.

[574] Malladi, R. and Sethian, J. A., An O (N log N) algorithm for shape modeling, Applied Mathematics, Proc. Natl. Acad. Sci (PNAS), USA, Vol. 93, No. 18, pp. 9389-9392, Sept. 1996.

[575] Malladi, R. and Sethian, J. A., A real-time algorithm for medical shape recovery, International Conference on Computer Vision (ICCV), pp. 304-310, 1998.

[576] Suri, J. S., Singh, S., Laxminarayan, S., Zeng, X., Reden, L., Fast Shape Recovery Algorithms Using Level Sets in 2-D/3-D Medical Imagery: A Review, Revised and Submitted to International Journal, 2001.

[577] Schiemann, T., Bomans, M., Tiede, U. and Höhne, K. H., Interactive 3-D Segmentation, in Robb, R. A. (ed.), Visualization in Biomedical Computing II, Proceedings SPIE 1808, pp. 376-383, 1992.

[578] Schiemann, T., Nuthmann, J., Tiede, U. and Höhne, K. H., Segmentation of the Visible Human for High Quality Volume Based Visualization, in Höhne, K. H. and Kikinis, R. (eds), Visualization in Biomedical Computing, Proceedings VBC, Vol. 1131 of Lecture Notes in Computer Science, Springer-Verlag, Berlin, pp. 13-22, 1996.

[579] Schiemann, T., Tiede, U. and Höhne, K. H., Segmentation of the Visible Human for High Quality Volume Based Visualization, Med. Image Anal. (MIA), Vol. 1, No. 4, pp. 263-270, 1997.

[580] Lorensen, W. E. and Cline, H., Marching Cubes: A High Resolution 3-D Surface Construction Algorithm, ACM Computer Graphics, Proceedings of Siggraph, Vol. 21, No. 4, pp. 163-169, July 1987.

[581] Cline, H. E., Lorensen, W. E. and Ludke, S., Two algorithms for the three-dimensional reconstruction of tomograms, Med. Phys., Vol. 15, No. 3, pp. 320-327, 1988.

[582] Shu, R., Zhou, C. and Kankanhalli, M. S., Adaptive Marching Cubes, The Visual Computer, Vol. 11, No. 4, pp. 202-217, 1995.

[583] Guéziec, A. and Hummel, R., Exploiting triangulated surface extraction using tetrahedral decomposition, IEEE Trans. on Visual and Comp. Graphics, Vol. 1, No. 4, pp. 328-342, 1995.

[584] Guéziec, A., Surface simplification inside a tolerance volume, IBM Research Report RC-20440, 1996.

[585] Montani, C., Scateni, R. and Scopigno, R., Discretized marching cubes, In Bergeron, R. D., and Kaufman, A. E., (eds), Proceedings of Visualization, IEEE Computer Society Press, pp. 281-287, 1994.

[586] Sarah, F. and Gibson, F., Constrained elastic surface nets: Generating smooth surfaces from binary segmented data. In Proceedings Medical Image Computing and Artificial Intelligence (MICCAI), M.I.T., pp. 888-898, 1998.

[587] Van-Gelder, A. and Wilhems, J., Topological considerations in isosurface generation, ACM Trans. Graph., Vol. 13, No. 3, pp. 337-375, 1994.

[588] Leventon, M. E., Grimson, W. Eric L. and Faugeras, O., Statistical Shape Influence in Geodesic Active Contours, Proceedings of the Computer Vision and Pattern Recognition (CVPR), Vol. 1, pp. 316-323, 2000.

[589] Suri, J. S., Liu, K., Singh, S., Laxminarayana, S., Reden, L., Shape Recovery Algorithms Using Level Sets in 2-D/3-D Medical Imagery: A State-of-the-Art Review, Accepted for Publication in International Journal of IEEE Trans. in Information Technology in Biomedicine, 2001.

[590] Lorigo, L. M., Grimson, W. Eric L., Faugeras, O., Keriven, R., Kikinis, R., Nabavi, A. and Westin, Carl-Fredrick, Two Geodesic Active Contours for the Segmentation of Tubular Structures, In Proc. of the Computer Vision and Pattern Recognition (CVPR), pp. 444-451, 2000.

[591] Yezzi, A., Tsai, A. and Willsky, A., A statistical approach to snakes for bimodal and trimodal imagery, In Proc. of Int'l Conf. Comp. Vision (ICCV), pp. 898-903, 1999.

[592] Guo, Y. and Vemuri, B., Hybrid geometric active models for shape recovery in medical images, In Proc. of Int'l Conf. Inf. Proc. in Med. Imaging (IPMI), pp. 112-125, Springer-Verlag, 1999.

[593] Zhu, S. C. and Yuille, A., Region competition: Unifying snakes, region growing, and Bayes/MDL for multiband image segmentation, IEEE Trans. on Pattern Anal. Machine Intell., Vol. 18, No. 9, pp. 884-900, 1996.

[594] Kapur, T., Brain Segmentation, M.S. Thesis, Artificial Intelligence Lab., Massachusetts Institute of Technology, Cambridge, MA, 1995.

[595] Kapur, T., Grimson, W. E. L., Wells III, W. M. and Kikinis, R., Segmentation of brain tissue from Magnetic Resonance Images, Medical Image Analysis, Vol. 1, No. 2, pp. 109-127, 1996.

[596] Kapur, T., Model based three dimensional Medical Image Segmentation, Ph.D. Thesis, Artificial Intelligence Laboratory, Massachusetts Institute of Technology, Cambridge, MA, May 1999.

[597] Ivins, J. and Porrill, J., Statistical Snakes: active region models, Proceedings of the 5th British Machine Vision Conference Proceedings, Vol. 2, pp. 377-386, 1994.

[598] Porrill, J. and Ivins, J., A Semi-Automatic Tool For 3-D Medical Image Analysis Using Active Contour Models, Medical Informatics, Vol. 19, No. 1, pp. 81-90, 1994.

[599] Poon, C. S. and Braun, M., Image segmentation by a deformable contour model incorporating region analysis, Physics, Medicine and Biology (PMB), Vol. 42, No. 9, pp. 1833-1841, 1997.

[600] Ronfard, R., Region-Based Strategies for Active Contour Models, International Journal of Computer Vision, Vol. 13, No. 2, pp. 229-251, 1994.

[601] Land, E. H., The retinex theory of color vision, Scientific American, Vol. 237, No. 6, pp. 108-129, 1977.

[602] Cohen, L., On active contour models and balloons, Computer Vision, Graphics and Image Processing: Image Understanding, Vol. 53, No. 2, pp. 211-218, March 1991.

[603] Prince, J. L. and Xu, C., A New External Force Model for Snakes, in Proc. of the Int. Conference in Computer Vision and Pattern Reco. (CVPR), pp. 66-71, 1997.

[604] Xu, C. and Prince, J. L., Generalized gradient vector flow external forces for active contours, Int. Journal of Signal Processing, Vol. 71, No. 2, pp. 131-139, 1998.

[605] Xu, C., Pham, D. L. and Prince, J. L., Finding the Brain Cortex Using Fuzzy Segmentation, Isosurfaces and Deformable Surface Models, Proceedings of the XVth International Conference on Information Processing in Medical Imaging (IPMI), pp. 399-404, 1997.

[606] Xu, C., Pham, D. L., Rettmann, M. E., Yu, D. N. and Prince, J. L., Reconstruction of the Human Cerebral Cortex from Magnetic Resonance Images, IEEE Trans. on Med. Imag., Vol. 18, No. 6, pp. 467-480, 1999.

[607] Xu, C., Pham, D. L., Rettmann, M. E., Yu, D. N. and Prince, J. L., Reconstruction of the Central Layer of the Human Cerebral Cortex from MR images, in Proceedings of the First International Conference on Medical Image Computing and Computer Assisted Interventions (MICCAI), pp. 482-488, 1998.

[608] Xu, C., Rettman, M. E., Yu, D. N., Pham, D. L. and Prince, J. L., A Spherical Map for Cortical Geometry, 4th International Conference on

Functional Mapping of the Human Brain, Montreal, Quebec, Canada, NeuroImage, Vol. 7, No. 4, pp. 734, 1998.

[609] Mangin, J. F., Frouin, V., Bloch, I., Rigis, J. and Lopez-Krahe, J., From 3-D Magnetic Resonance Images to structural representations of the cortex topography using topology preserving deformation, J. Math. Imag. Vision, Vol. 5, No. 4, pp. 297-318, 1999.

[610] Angenent, S., Haker, S., Tannenbaum, A. and Kikinis, R, Conformal Geometry and brain flattening, Proceedings of Medical Image Computing and Computer-Assisted Intervention (MICCAI), pp. 271-278, 1999.

[611] Angenent, S., Haker, S., Tannenbaum, A. and Kikinis, R., On the Laplace-Beltrami Operator and Brain Surface Flattening, IEEE Trans. on Med Imaging, Vol. 19, No. 7, pp. 665-670, 2000.

[612] Haker, S., Angenent, S., Tannenbaum, A. and Kikinis, R., Nondistorting flattening maps and the 3-D visualization of colon CT images, IEEE Trans. on Med Imaging, Vol. 19, No. 7, pp. 665-670, 2000.

[613] Xu, C., On the relationship between the parametric and geometric active contours, Internal Technical Report, Department of Electrical and Computer Engineering, Johns Hopkins University, Baltimore, MD, 1999.

[614] Suri, J. S., Leaking Prevention in Fast Level Sets Using Fuzzy Models: An Application in MR Brain, Inter. Conference in Information Technology in Biomedicine, pp. 220-226, 2000.

[615] Suri, J. S., White Matter/Gray Matter Boundary Segmentation Using Geometric Snakes: A Fuzzy Deformable Model, To appear in Int. conference in Application in Pattern Recognition (ICAPR), Rio de Janeiro, Brazil, March 11-14, 2001.

[616] Zeng, X., Volumetric Layer Segmentation Using a Generic Shape Constraint with Applications to Cortical Shape Analysis, Ph.D. Thesis, Department of Electrical Engineering, Yale University, New Haven, CT, May 2000.

[617] Gomes, J. and Faugeras, O., Reconciling Distance Functions and Level Sets, Tech Report, INRIA, April 1999; also in Journal of Visual Communication and Image Representation, Vol. 11, No. 2, pp. 209-223, 2000.

[618] Le Goualher, G., Procyk, E., Collins, L., Venegopal, R., Barillot C. and Evans, A., Automated extraction and variability analysis of sulcal neuroanatomy, IEEE Trans. on Med. Imag., Vol. 18, No. 3, pp. 206-217, March 1999.

[619] Baillard, C., Hellier, P. and Barillot, C., Segmentation of 3-D Brain Structures Using Level Sets, Research Report 1291, IRISA, Rennes Cedex, France, 16 pages, Jan. 2000.

[620] Baillard, C., Hellier, P. and Barillot, C., Cooperation between level set techniques and dense 3d registration for the segmentation of brain structures, In Int. Conference on Pattern Recognition, Vol. 1, pp. 991-994, 2000.

[621] Baillard, C., Barillot, C. and Bouthemy, P., Robust Adaptive Segmentation of 3-D Medical Images with Level Sets, Research Report 1369, IRISA, Rennes Cedex, France, 26 pages, Nov. 2000.

[622] Suri, J. S., Haralick, R. M. and Sheehan, F. H., General Technique for Automatic Left Ventricle Boundary Validation: Relation Between Cardioangiograms and Observed Boundary Errors, In Proc. of Society for Computer Applications in Radiology (SCAR), Rochester, Minnesota, pp. 212-217, 1997.

[623] Aboutanous, G. B. and Dawant, B. M., Automatic Brain Segmentation and Validation: Image-based versus Atlas-based Deformable Model, Proceedings of SPIE - The Inter. Society for Optical Engineering, Vol. 3034, pp. 299-310, 1997.

[624] Vannier, M. W., Pjlgram, T. K., Speidel, C. M., Neumann, L. R., Rickman, D. L. and Schertz, L. D., Validation of MRI Multispectral Tissue Classification, Computerized Medical Imaging and Graphics, Vol. 15, No. 4, pp. 217-223, 1991.

[625] Zwehl, W., Levy, R., Garcia, E., Haendchen, R. V., Childs, W., Corday, S. R. and Meerbaum, S., Validation of computerized edge detection algorithm for qualitative 2-D echocardiography, Circulation, Vol. 68, No. 5, pp. 1127-1135, Nov. 1983.

[626] Yu, D., Xu, C., Rettmann, M. E., Pham, D. L. and Prince, J. L., Quantitative Validation of a Deformable Cortical Surface Model, Proceedings of SPIE Medical Imaging, Kenneth M. Hanson (ed.), Vol. 3979, pp. 1593-1604, 2000.

[627] Kohn, M. I., Tanna, N. K., Herman, G. T., Resnick, S. M., Mozley, P. D., Gur, R. E., Alavi, A., Zimmerman, R. A. and Gur, R. C., Analysis of brain and CSF volumes with MR imaging; part I. methods, reliability and validation, Radiology, Vol. 178, No. 1, pp. 123-130, 1991.

[628] Grabowski, T. J., Frank, R. J., Szmuski, N. R., Brown, C. K. and Damasio, H., Validation of Partial Tissue Segmentation of Single-Channel Magnetic Resonance Images of the Brain, Vol. 12, No. 6, pp. 640-656, Dec. 2000.

[629] Ayache, N., Cinquin, P., Cohen, I., Cohen, L., Leitner, F. and Monga, O., Segmentation of Complex 3-D Medical Objects: A Challenge and Requirement for Computer-Assisted Surgery Planning and Performance, In Taylor, R. H., Lavallée, Burdea, G. C. and Mösges, R. (eds): Computer-integrated surgery: technology and clinical applications, The MIT Press, pp. 59-74, 1996.

[630] Haacke, E. M. and Liang, Zhi-Pei, Challenges of Imaging Structure and Function with MRI, IEEE Engineering in Medicine and Biology, Vol. 19, No. 5, pp. 55-62, Sept./Oct. 2000.

[631] Turner, R. and Ordidge, R. J., Technical Challenges of Function MRI, IEEE Engineering in Medicine and Biology, Vol. 19, No. 5, pp. 42-52, Sept./Oct. 2000.

[632] Kaufman, A., Trends in Volume Visualization and Volume Graphics, Scientific Visualization: Advances and Challenges, Rosenblum, L., *et al.* (eds.), Academic Press, Inc., London, pp. 3-19, ISBN: 0-1222-7742-2, 1994.

[633] Vokurka, E. A., Thacker, N. A. and Jackson, A., A fast model independent method for automatic correction of intensity nonuniformity in MRI data, J. Magn. Reson. Imaging, Vol. 10, No. 4, pp. 550-62, Oct. 1999.

[634] Herlin, I. L., Nguyen, C. and Graffigne, C., A deformable region model using Stochastic processes applied to echocardiographic images, Proceedings of CVPR, Urbana, IL, IEEE Computer Society, pp. 534-539, 1992.

[635] Neuenschwander, W., Fua, P., Szekely, G. and Kubblier, O., Initializing Snakes, in Proc. IEEE Conference in Computer Vision and Pattern Reco. (CVPR), pp. 658-663, 1994.

[636] Kimia, B. B., Tannenbaum, A. R. and Zucker, S. W., Shapes, shocks and deformations, I: The components of shape and the reaction-diffusion space, International Journal of Computer Vision (IJCV), Vol. 15, No. 3, pp. 189-224, 1995.

[637] Siddiqi, K. Tresness, K. J. and Kimia, B. B., Parts of visual form: Ecological and psychophysical aspects, Perception, Vol. 25, No. 4, pp. 399-424, 1996.

[638] Stoll, P., Tek, H. and Kimia, B. B., Shocks from images: Propagation of orientation elements, In Proc. of Computer Vision and Pattern Recognition (CVPR), Puerto Rico, IEEE Computer Society Press, pp. 839-845, 1997.

[639] Tek, H. and Kimia, B. B., Deformable bubbles in the reaction-diffusion space, in Proc. of the 5th Int. Conference in Computer Vision (ICCV), Cambridge, Massachusetts, pp. 156-162, 1995.

[640] Volker, R. and Roland, P., MR method for the reduction of motion artifacts and device for carrying out the method, US Patent #: 5,933,006, Aug. 3, 1999.

[641] Malandain, G. and Fernandez-Vidal, F., Euclidean Skeletons, Image and Vision Computing (IVC), Vol. 16, No. 5, pp. 317-327, April 1998.

[642] Ballester, M. A., Gonzlez, Z. A. and Brady, J. M., Combined Statistical and Geometrical 3-D Segmentation and Measurement of Brain Structures, Proc. IEEE Workshop on Biomedical Image Analysis, Santa Barbara, CA, IEEE Computer Society, pp. 499-508, 1998.

[643] González, M. A., Ballester, A. Z. and Brady, J. M., Measurement of Brain Structures based on Statistical and Geometrical 3-D Segmentation, In Proc. of Medical Image Computing and Computer-Assisted Intervention (MICCAI), Lecture Notes in Computer Science, Springer Verlag, 1998.

[644] Xu, C., Pham, D. L. and Prince, J. L., Medical Image Segmentation Using Deformable Models, In SPIE Handbook of Medical Imaging (Vol.

2): Medical Image Processing and Analysis, Sonka, M., Fitzpatrick, J. M., (eds.), ISBN 0-8184-3622-4, 2000.

[645] Suri, J. S., Modeling Segmentation Issues Via Partial Differential Equations, Level Sets, and Geometric Deformable Models: A Revisit, In Preparation for Inter. Journal, 2001.

[646] Rettmann, M. E., Xu, C., Pham, D. L. and Prince, J. L., Automated segmentation of sulcal regions, In Proc. of Medical Image Computing and Computer-Assisted Intervention (MICCAI), pp. 158-167, 1999.

[647] Rettmann, M. E., Han, X. and Prince, J. L., Watersheds on Cortical Surface for Automated Sulcal Segmentation, Proc. of IEEE/SIAM workshop on Mathematical Morphology and Biomedical Image Analysis (MMBIA), pp. 20-27, 2000.

[648] Lohmann, G. and Cramon, D. Y. von, Sulcal basins and sulcal strings as new concepts for describing the human cortical topography, In IEEE Workshop on Biomedical Image Analysis (BIA), pp. 24-33, 1998.

[649] Lohmann, G. and Cramon, D. Y. von, Automatic labelling of the human cortical surface using sulcal basins, Medical Image Analysis, Vol. 4, No. 3, pp. 179-88, Sept. 2000.

[650] Liang, J., McInerney, T. and Terzopoulos, D., Interactive Medical Image Segmentation with United Snakes, In Proceedings of 2nd International Conference on Medical Image Computing and Computer Assisted Interventions (MICCAI), Cambridge, England, Lecture Notes in Computer Science, Vol. 1679, ISBN: 3-540-66503-X, pp. 116-127, Sept. 1999.

[651] Liang, J., McInerney, T. and Terzopoulos, D., United Snakes (Towards a More Perfect Union of Active Contour Techniques), in IEEE Seventh International Conference on Computer Vision, Kerkyra, Greece, 1999.

[652] Paragios, N. and Deriche, R., Geodesic Active Regions: A New Paradigm to Deal with Frame Partition Problems in Computer Vision, Journal of Visual Communication and Image Representation, Special Issue on Partial Differential Equations in Image Processing, Computer Vision and Computer Graphics, Dec. 2000.

[653] "http://www.bic.mni.mcgill.ca/", McConnell Brain Imaging Center, Montreal Neurological Institute, McGill University, Canada.

[654] Ibsrcma, "http://neuro-www.mgh.harvard.edu/cma/ibsr", The Internet Brain Segmentation Repository, Center for Morphometric Analysis, Massachusetts General Hospital, Boston, MA.

[655] Jolesz, F. A., Image-guided Procedures and the Operating Room of the Future, Radiology, Vol. 204, No. 3, pp. 601-612, May 1997.

[656] Jolesz, F. A. and Kikinis, R., The vision of image-guided computerized surgery: the high-tech operating room. In Taylor, R. H., Lavalle, S., Burdea, G. C. (eds.), Computerized Integrated Surgery, M.I.T Press, Cambridge, Mass., pp. 717-721, 1994.

[657] Mumford, D. and Shah, J., Optimal approximations by piece-wise smooth functions and associated variational problems, Communications on Pure and Applied Mathematics, Vol. 42, No. 5, pp. 577-68, 1989.

[658] Woermann, F. G., Free, S. L., Koepp, M. J., Sisodiya, S. M. and Duncan, J. S., Abnormal cerebral structure in juvenile myoclonic epilepsy demonstrated with voxel-based analysis of MRI, Brain, Vol. 122 (Pt 11), pp. 2101-2108, Nov. 1999.

[659] Zelaya, F., Flood, N., Chalk, J. B., Wang, D., Doddrell, D. M., Strugnell, W., Benson, M., Ostergaard, L., Semple, J. and Eagle, S., An evaluation of the time dependence of the anisotropy of the water diffusion tensor in acute human ischemia, Magn. Reson. Imag., Vol. 17, No. 3, pp. 331-348, Apr. 1999.

[660] Harris, G., Andreasen, N. C., Cizadlo, T., Bailey, J. M., Bockholt, H. J., Magnotta, V. A. and Arndt, S., Improving tissue classification in MRI: a three-dimensional multispectral discriminant analysis method with automated training class selection, J Comput. Assist. Tomogr., Vol. 23, No. 1, pp. 144-54, Jan. 1999.

[661] Johnston, B., Atkins, M. S. and Booth, K. S., Three-dimensional partial volume brain tissue segmentation of multispectral Magnetic Resonance Images using stochastic relaxation, Proceedings of SPIE - The International Society for Optical Engineering, In Dougherty, E. R. (ed.), Non-Linear Image Processing VI, Vol. 2180, pp. 268-279, 1994.

[662] Snell, J. W., Merickel, M. B., Ortega, J. M., Goble, J. C., Brookeman, J. R. and Kassell, N. F., Segmentation of the brain from 3-D MRI using a hierarchical active surface template, Proceedings of SPIE - The International Society for Optical Engineering, Vol. 2167, pp. 2-9, 1994.

[663] Alexander, M. E., Baumgartner, R., Summers, A. R., Windischberger, C., Klarhoefer, M., Moser, E. and Somorjai, R. L., A wavelet-based method for improving signal-to-noise ratio and contrast in MR images, Magn. Reson. Imag., Vol. 18, No. 2, pp. 169-80, 2000.

[664] Makoto, N. and Takashi, M., Edge Preserving Smoothing, Computer Graphics and Image Processing (CGIP), Vol. 9, No. 4, pp. 394-407, 1979.

[665] Yousry, T. A., Schimd, U. D., Alkadhi, H., Schmidt, D., Peraud, A., Buettner, A. and Winkler, P., Localization of the motor hand area to a knob on the precentral gyrus, a new landmark, Brain, Vol. 120, No. 1, pp. 141-157, 1997.

[666] Bentum, M. J., Lichtenbelt, B. B. A. and Malzbender, T., Analysis of Gradient Estimators in Volume Rendering, IEEE Trans. on Visualization and Computer Graphics, Vol. 2, No. 3, pp. 242-254, Sept. 1996.

[667] Lichtenbelt, B., Crane, R. and Naqvi, S., Introduction to Volume Rendering, Hewlett-Packard Company, ISBN: 0-13-861683-3, Hewlett-Packard Professional Books, Prentice Hall, 1998.

[668] Kaufman, A., Bakalash, R., Cohen, D. and Yagel, R., Architecture for Volume Rendering - A Survey, IEEE Engineering in Medicine and Biology, pp. 18-23, Dec. 1990.

[669] Levoy, M., Display of Surfaces from Volume Data, IEEE Computer Graphics and Applications (CGA), Vol. 5, No. 3, pp. 29-37, May 1988.

[670] Levoy, M., A Hybrid Ray Tracer from Rendering Polygon and Volume Data, IEEE Computer Graphics and Applications, Vol. 10, No. 2, pp. 33-40, March 1990.

[671] Levoy, M., Volume Rendering Using the Fourier Projection Slice Theorem, In Proceedings of Graphics Interface, Canadian Information Processing Society, pp. 61-69, 1992.

[672] Koo, Yun-Mo, Choel, Hi and Shin, Y. G., Object order template based approach for stereoscopic volume rendering, J. of Visualization and Computer Animation, Vol. 10, No. 3, pp. 133-142, 1999.

[673] Lacroute, P. and Levoy, M., Fast Volume Rendering Using a Shear-Warp Factorization of the Viewing Transformation, Computer Graphics, Vol. 28, No. 4, pp. 451-458, Aug. 1994.

[674] Guo, B., A Multiscale Model for Structure-Based Volume Rendering, IEEE Trans. on Visualization and Computer Graphics, Vol. 1, No. 4, pp. 291-301, Dec. 1995

[675] Udupa, J. K., Hung, H.-M. and Chuang, K.-S., Surface and Volume rendering in Three-Dimensional Imaging: A comparison, J. Digital Imaging, Vol. 4, No. 3, pp. 159-168, 1991.

[676] Heckbert, P. S., Survey of texture mapping, IEEE Computer Graphics and Applications, Vol. 6, No. 11, pp. 56-67, 1986.

[677] Heckbert, P. S., Fundamentals of Texture Mapping and Image Warping, Master's Thesis, Dept. of Electrical and Computer Science, Univ. of California, Berkeley, June 1989.

[678] Bier, E. A. and Sloan, K. R., Two part texture mappings, IEEE Computer Graphics and Applications, Vol. 6, No. 9, pp. 40-53, 1986.

[679] Hughes, T., The finite element method, Prentice Hall, Englewood Cliffs, NJ, ISBN: 0-486-411-818, 1987.

[680] Friston, K. J., Jezzard, P. and Turner, R., Analysis of function MRI time series, Human Brain Mapping, Vol. 2, pp. 69-78, 1994.

[681] Friston, K. J., Frith, C. D., Turner R. and Frackowiak, R. S. J., Characterizing evoked hemodynamics with fMRI, NeuroImage, Vol. 2, No. 2, pp. 157-165, 1995.

[682] Friston, K. J., Holmes, A. P., Poline, J-B., Grasby, P. J., Willams, S. C. R., Frackowiak, R. S. and Turner, R., Analysis of fMRI time series revisted, NeuroImage, Vol. 2, No. 1, pp. 45-53, 1995.

[683] Belliveau, J. W., Kennedy, D. and McKinstry, R. C., Functional mapping of the human visual cortex by MRI, Science, Vol. 254, pp. 716-719, 1991.

[684] Raichle, M. E., Behind the scenes of functional brain imaging: a historical and physiological perspective, Proc. Natl. Acad. Sci., Vol. 95, No. 3, pp. 765-772, 1998.

[685] Friston, K. J., Imaging cognitive anatomy, Trends in Cognitive Sciences, Vol. 1, No. 1, pp. 21-27, April 1997.

[686] Kim, S. G. and Ugurbil, K., Functional Magnetic Resonance Imaging of the Human Brain, J. Neurosci. Methods, Vol. 74, No. 2, pp. 229-243, 1997.

[687] Woods, R. P., Cherry, S. R. and Mazziotta, J. C., Rapid Automated algorithm for aligning and reslicing PET images, Journal of Computer Assisted Tomography, Vol. 16, No. 4, pp. 620-633, 1992.

[688] Friston, K. J., Ashburner J., Frith, J. D., Poline, J. B., Heather J. D. and Frackowiak R. S. J., Spatial registration and normalization of images, Human Brain Mapping, Vol. 3, No. 3, pp. 165-189, 1995.

[689] Friston, K. J., Williams, S., Howard, R. Frackowiak, R. S. and Turner, R., Movement-related effects in fMRI time-series, Magn. Reson. Med., Vol. 35, No. 3, pp. 346-55, Mar. 1996.

[690] Biswal, B. B and Hyde, J. S., Contour-Based registration technique to differentiate between task-activated and head motion-induced signal variations in fMRI, Magn. Reson. Med. (MRM), Vol. 38, No. 3, pp. 470-476, 1997.

[691] Goebel, R., Linden, D. E. J., Lanfermann, H., Zanella, F. E. and Singer, W., Functional imaging of mirror and inverse reading reveals separate coactivated networks for oculomotion and spatial transformations, Neuroreport, Vol. 9, No. 4, pp. 713-719, 1998.

[692] Poldrack, R. A., Desmond, J. E., Glover, G. H. and Gabrieli, J. D. E., The neural basis of visual skill learning: An fMRI study of mirror reading, Cerebral Cortex, Vol. 8, No. 1, pp. 1-10, 1998.

[693] Goebel R., Khorram-Sefat D., Muckli, L., Hacker H. and Singer W., The constructive nature of vision: direct evidence from fMRI studies of apparent motion and motion imagery, Eur. Jour. of Neuroscience, Vol. 10, No. 5, pp. 1563-1573, 1998.

[694] Kulynych, J. J., Vladar, J. and Jones, D. W., Superior temporal gyrus volume in schizophernia: a study using MRI morphometry assisted by surface rendering, Am. Journal of Psychiatry, Vol. 153, No. 1, pp. 50-56, 1996.

[695] Goebel, R. and Singer, W., Cortical surface-based statistical analysis of fMRI data, Human Brain Mapping, Vol. 9, No. 2, p. 64, 1999.

[696] Drury, H. A., Van Essen, D. C., Corbetta, M. and Snyder, A. Z., Surface-based analyses of the human cerebral cortex. In Brain Warping, Toga, A., *et al.* (eds.), Academic Press, Inc., pp. 337-363, 1999.

[697] Drury, D., Van Essen, D., Anderson C., Lee C., Coogan T. and Lewis J., Computerized mapping of the cerebral cortex: A multiresolution flattening method and surface-based coordinate system, J. Cognitive Neurosci., Vol. 8, No. 1, pp. 1-28, 1996.

[698] Van Essen, D. C., Drury, H. A., Joshi, S. and Miller, M. I., Functional and structural mapping of human cerebral cortex: Solutions are in the surfaces, Proc. Natl. Acad. Sci. (PNAS), Vol. 95, No. 3, pp. 788-795, 1997.

[699] Gabrieli, J. D. E., Poldrack, R. A. and Desmond, J. E., The role of the left prefrontal cortex in language and memory, Proc. Natl. Acad. Sci. (PNAS), Vol. 95, No. 3, pp. 906-913, 1998.

[700] Friedman, L., Kenny, J. T. and Wise, A. L., Brain activation during silent word generation evaluated with fMRI, Brain Language, Vol. 64, No. 2, pp. 231-256, Sept. 1998.

[701] Fiez, J. A. and Petersen, S. E., Neuroimging studies of word reading, Proc. Natl Acad Sci, Vol. 95, No. 3, pp. 914-921, 1998.

[702] Neville, H. J., Bavelier, D., Corina, D., Rauschecker, J., Karni, A., Lalwani, A., Braun, A., Clark, V., Jezzard, P. and Turner, R., Cerebral organization for language in deaf and hearing subjects: biological constraints and effect of experience, Proc. Natl Acad Sci (PNAS), Vol. 95, No. 3, pp. 922-929, 1998.

[703] Schlosser, M. J., Aoyagi, N., Fulbright, R. K., Gore, J. C. and McCarthy, G., Functional MRI studies of auditory comprehension, Human Brain Mapping, Vol. 6, No. 1, pp. 1-13, 1998.

[704] Hykin, J., Moore, R., Clare, S., Baker, P., Johnson, I., Bowtell, R., Mansfield, P. and Gowland, P., Fetal brain activity demonstrated by functional MRI, Research Letters, The Lancet, Vol. 354, pp. 645-646, Aug. 21, 1999.

[705] Wakai, R. T., Leuthold, A. C. and Martin, C. B., Fetal auditory evoked responses detected by magnetoencephalopathy, Am. J. Obstet. Gynecol., Vol. 174, No. 5, pp. 1484-1486, 1996.

[706] Francis, S., Rolls, E. T., Bowtell, R., McGlone, F., O'Doherty, J., Browing, A., Clare, S. and Smith, E., The representation of pleasant touch in the brain and its relationship with taste and olfactory areas, Neuroreport, Vol. 10, pp. 453-459, 1999.

[707] Chee, M. W., O'Craven, K. M., Bergida, R., Rosen, B. R. and Saoy, R. L., Auditory and visual word processing studied with fMRI, Human Brain Mapping, Vol. 7, No. 1, pp. 15-28, 1999.

[708] Howard, R. J., ffytche, D. H., Barnes, J., McKeefry, D., Ha, Y., Woodruff, P. W., Bullmore, E. T., Simmons, A., Williams, S. C., David, A. S. and Brammer, M., The functional anatomy of imaging and perceiving color, Neuroreport, Vol. 9, No. 6, pp. 1019-1023, 1998.

[709] Beason-Held, L. L., Purpura, K. P., Krasuski, J. S., Maisog, J. M., Daly, E. M., Mangot, D. J., Desmond, R. E., Optican, L. M., Schapiro, M. B. and VanMeter, J. W., Cortical regions involved in visual texture perception: a fMRI study, Brain Res. Cogn. Brain. Res., Vol. 7, No. 2, pp. 111-118, Oct. 1998.

[710] Rao, S. M., Bandettini, P. A., Binder, J. R., Bobholz, J. A., Hammeke, T. A., Stein, E. A., Hyde, J. S., Relationship between finger movements

rate and functional MR signal change in human primary motor cortex, J. Cereb. Blood Flow Metab., Vol. 16, No. 6, pp. 1250-1254, 1996.

[711] Schlaug, G., Sanes, J. N., Thangaraj, V., Darby, D. G., Jäncke, L., Edelman, R. R. and Warach, S., Cerebral activation covaries with movement rate, Neuroreport, Vol. 7, No. 4, 879-883, 1996.

[712] Stokking, R., van Isselt, H., van Rijk, P., de Klerk, J., Huiskens, T., Mertens, I., Buskens, E. and Viergever, M. A., Integrated Visualization of Functional and Anatomic Brain Data: A Validation Study, Journal of Nuclear Medicine, Vol. 40, No. 2, pp 311-316, Feb. 1999

[713] Jernigan, T. L., Salmon, D. P., Butters, N. and Hesserlink, J. R., Cerebral structure on MRI, part II: Specific changes in Alzheimer's and Huntington's diseases, Biological Psychiatry, Vol. 29, No. 1, pp. 68-81, 1991.

[714] Stone, L. A., Albert, P. S. and Smith, M. E., Changes in the amount of diseased white matter over time in patients with relapsing-remitting multiple sclerosis, Neurology, Vol. 45, No. 10, pp. 1808-1814, 1995.

[715] Tanabe, J., Amend, D., Schuff, N., Di Sclafani, V., Ezekeil, F., Norman, D., Fein, G. and Weiner, M. W., Tissue segmentation of the brain in Alzheimer's disease, American Journal of Neuroradiology, Vol. 18, No. 1, pp. 115-123, 1997.

[716] Dastidar, P., Heinonen, T., Vahvelainen, T., Elovaara, I. and Eskola, H., Computerized volumetric analysis of lesions in multiple sclerosis using new semi-automatic segmentation software, Medical Biology Engineering Computation, Vol. 37, No. 1, pp. 104-107, 1999.

[717] Filippi, M., Mastronardo, G., Rocca, M. A., Pereira, C. and Comi, G., Quantitative volumetric analysis of brain magnetic resonance imaging from patients with multiple sclerosis, Journal of Neurological Science, Vol. 158, No. 2, pp. 148-153, 1998.

[718] Vaidyanathan, M., Clarke, L. P., Hall, L. O., Heidtman, C., Velthuizen, R., Gosche, K., Phuphanich, S.,Wagner, H., Greenberg, H. and Silbiger, M. L., Monitoring brain tumor response to therapy using MRI segmentation, Magnetic Resonance Imaging, Vol. 15, No. 3, pp. 323-334, 1997.

[719] Dickson, S., Thomas, B. T. and Godddard, P., Using neural networks to automatically detect brain tumors in MR, International Journal of Neural Systems, Vol. 8, No. 1, pp. 91-99, 1997.

[720] Kikinis, R., Guttmann, C. R., Metcalf, D., Wells, W. M., Ettinger, G. J., Weiner, H. L. and Jolesz, F. A., Quantitative follow-up of patients with multiple sclerosis using MRI: technical aspects, Journal of Magnetic Resonance Imaging, Vol. 9, No. 4, pp. 519-530, 1999.

[721] Udupa, J. K., Three dimensional visualization and analysis methodologies: a current prospective, Radiographics, Vol. 19, No. 3, pp. 783-806, 1999.

[722] Guttman, C. R., Kikinis, R., Anderson, M. C., Jakab, M., Warfield, S. K., Killiany, R. J., Weiner, H. L. and Jolesz, F. A., Quantitative

follow-up of patients with multiple sclerosis using MRI: Reproducibility, Journal of Magnetic Resonance Imaging, Vol. 9, No. 4, pp. 509-518, 1999.

[723] O'Riordan, J. I., Gawne Cain, M., Cloes, A., Wang, L., Compston, D. A., Toffs, P. and Mileer, D. H., T1 hypointense lesion load in secondary progressive multiple sclerosis: a comparison of pre versus post contrast loads and of manual versus semi automated threshold techniques for lesion segmentation. Multiple Sclerosis, Vol. 4, No. 5, pp. 408-412, 1998.

[724] Molyneux, P. D., Wang, L., Lai, M.,Tofts, P. S., Mosley, I. F. and Miller, D. H., Quantitative techniques for lesion load measurement in multiple sclerosis: an assessment of the global threshold technique after non uniformity and histogram matching corrections, European Journal of Neurology, Vol. 5, No. 1, pp. 55-60, 1998.

[725] Vinitski, S., Gonzalez, C. F., Knobler, R., Andrews, D., Iwanaga, T. and Curtis, M., Fast tissue segmentation based on a 4-D feature map in characterization of intracranial lesions, Journal of Magnetic Resonance Imaging, Vol. 9, No. 6, pp. 768-776, 1999.

[726] Magnotta, V. A., Heckel, D., Andreasen, N. C., Cizadlo, T., Corson, P. W., Ehrhardt, J. C. and Yuh, W. T., Measurement of brain structures with artificial neural networks: two and three-dimensional applications, Radiology, Vol. 211, No. 3, pp. 781-790, 1999.

[727] Joshi, M., Cui, J., Doolittle, K., Joshi, S., Van Essen, D., Wang L. and Miller, M. I., Brain segmentation and the generation of cortical surfaces, NeuroImage, Vol. 9, No. 5, pp. 461-76, 1999.

[728] Karayiannis, N. B. and Pai, P. I., Segmentation of magnetic resonance images using fuzzy algorithms for learning vector quantization, IEEE Trans. on Med. Imag., Vol. 18, No. 2, pp. 172-180, 1999.

[729] Velthuizen, R. P., Hall, L. O. and Clarke, L. P., Feature extraction of MRI segmentation. Journal of Neuroimaging, Vol. 9, No. 2, pp. 85-90, 1999.

[730] Shareef, N., Wang, D. L. and Yagel, R., Segmentation of medical images using LEGION, IEEE Trans. on Med. Imag., Vol. 18, No. 1, pp. 74-91, 1999.

[731] Harris, G., Andreasen, N. C., Cazadlo, T., Bailey, J. M., Bockholt, H. J., Magnotta, V. A. and Arndt, S., Improving tissue classification in MRI: a three-dimensional multispectral discriminant analysis method with automated training class selection, Journal of Computer Assisted Tomography, Vol. 23, No. 1, pp. 144-154, 1999.

[732] Dale, A. M., Fischl, B. and Sereno, M. I., Cortical surface-based analysis. I. Segmentation and surface reconstruction, NeuroImage, Vol. 9, No. 2, pp. 179-194, 1999.

[733] Pachai, C., Zhu, Y. M., Grimaud, J., Hermier, M., Dromigny-Badin, A., Boudraa, A., Gimenez, G., Confavreux, C. and Froment, J. C., A pyramidal approach for automatic segmentation of multiple sclerosis lesions in brain MRI, Computer and Medical Imaging Graphics, Vol. 22, No. 5, pp. 399-408, 1998.

[734] van Waesberghe, J. H., van Buchem, M. A., Fillipi, M., Castelijns, J. A., Rocca, M. A., van der Boom, R., Polman, C. H. and Barkhof, F., MR outcome parameters in multiple sclerosis: comparison of surface-based thresholding segmentation and magnetization transfer ratio histographic analysis in relation to disability (a preliminary note), American Journal of Neuroradiology, Vol. 19, No. 10, pp. 1857-1862, 1998.

[735] Manousakas, I. N., Undrill, P. E., Cameron, G. G. and Redpath, T. W., Split-and-merge segmentation of magnetic resonance medial images: performance evaluation and extension to three dimensions, Computers in Biomedical Research, Vol. 31, No. 6, pp. 393-412, 1998.

[736] Glass, J. O. and Reddick, W. E., Hybrid artificial neural network segmentation and classification of dynamic contrast-enhanced MR imaging (DEMRI) of osteosarcoma, Magnetic Resonance Imaging, Vol. 16, No. 9, pp. 1075-1083, 1998.

[737] Lee, C., Huh, S., Ketter, T. A. and Unser, M. Unsupervised connectivity-based thresholding segmentation of midsagittal brain MR images, Computers in Biology and Medicine, Vol. 28, No. 3, pp. 309-338, 1998.

[738] Heinonen, T., Dastidar, P., Kauppinen, P., Malmivuo, J. and Eskola, H., Semi-automatic tool for segmentation and volumetric analysis of medical images, Medicine Biology Engineering and Computers, Vol. 36, No. 3, pp. 291-296, 1998.

[739] Clark, M. C., Hall, L. O., Goldgof, D. B., Velthuizen, R., Murtagh, F. R. and Silbiger, M. S., Automatic tumor segmentation using knowledge based techniques, IEEE Trans. on Med. Imag., Vol. 17, No. 2, pp. 187-201, 1998.

[740] Atkins, M. S. and Mackiewich, B. T., Fully automatic segmentation of the brain in MRI, IEEE Trans. on Med. Imag., Vol. 17, No. 1, pp. 98-107, 1998.

[741] Bedell, B. J. and Narayana, P. A., Automatic segmentation of gadolinium-enhanced multiple sclerosis lesions, Magnetic Resonance in Medicine, Vol. 39, No. 6, pp. 935-940, 1998.

[742] Mohamed, F. B., Vinitski, S., Faro, S. H., Gonzalez, C. F., Mack, J. and Iwanaga, T., Optimization of tissue segmentation of brain MR images based on multispectral 3-D feature maps, Magnetic Resonance Imaging, Vol. 17, No. 3, pp. 403-409, 1999.

[743] Burghart, C. R., Perozzoli, A. and Rembold, U., Knowledge based segmentation, Studies in Health Technology Information, Vol. 50, pp. 353-354, 1998.

[744] Summers, P. E., Bhalerao, A. H. and Hawkes, D. J., Multiresolution, model-based segmentation of MR angiograms, J. Magnetic Resonance Imaging, Vol. 7, No. 6, pp. 950-957, 1997.

[745] Alfano, B., Brunetti, A., Covelli, E. M.,Quarantelli, M., Panico, M. R., Ciarmiello, A. and Salvatore, M., Unsupervised, automated segmentation of the normal brain using a multispectral relaxometric magnetic

resonance approach, Magnetic Resonance in Medicine, Vol. 37, No. 1, pp. 84-93, 1997.

[746] Jackson, E. F., Narayana, P. A. and Falconer, J. C., Reproducibility of nonparametric feature map segmentation for determination of normal intracranial volumes with MR imaging data, J. of Magnetic Resonance Imaging, Vol. 4, No. 5, pp. 692-700, 1994.

[747] Clarke, L. P., Velthuizen, R. P., Phuphanich, S., Schellenberg, J. D., Arrington, J. A. and Silbiger, M., MRI: stability of three supervised segmentation techniques, Magnetic Resonance Imaging, Vol. 11, No. 1, pp. 95-106, 1993.

[748] Bedell, B. J., Narayana, P. A., Wolinsky, J. S., A dual approach for minimizing false lesion classification on magnetic resonance images, Magnetic Resonance in Medicine, Vol. 37, No. 1, pp. 94-112, 1997.

[749] Stoll, E., Stern, C., Stucki, P. and Wildermuth, S., A new filtering algorithm for medical magnetic resonance and computer tomography images, Journal of Digital Imaging, Vol. 12, No. 1, pp. 23-28, 1999.

[750] Harris, G. J., Barta, P. E., Peng, L. W., Lee, S., Brettschneider, Shah, A., Henderer, J. D., Schlaepfer, T. E. and Pearlson, G. D., MR volume segmentation of gray matter and white matter using manual threshold: dependence on image brightness, American Journal of Neuroradiology, Vol. 15, No. 2, pp. 225-230, 1994.

[751] Narayana, P. A. and Borthakur, A., Effect of radio frequency inhomogeneity correction on reproducibility of intra-cranial volumes using MR image data, Magnetic Resonance in Medicine, Vol. 33, No. 3, pp. 396-400, 1995.

[752] Bedell, B. J. and Narayana, P. A., Automatic removal of extrameningial tissues from MR images of human brain, Journal of Magnetic Resonance Imaging, Vol. 6, No. 6, pp. 939-943, 1996.

[753] Rovaris, M., Rocca, M. A., Sormani, M. P., Comi, G. and Filippi, M., Reproducibility of brain MRI lesion volume measurements in multiple sclerosis using a local thresholding technique: effects of formal operator training, European Journal of Neurology, Vol. 41, No. 4, pp. 226-230, 1999.

[754] Filippi, M., Horsfield, M. A., Hajnal, J. V., Narayana, P. A., Udupa,J. K., Yousary, T. A., Zijdenbos, A., Quantitative assessment of magnetic resonance imaging lesion load in multiple sclerosis, Journal of Neurology, Neurosurgery and Psychiatry, Vol. 64 (suppl.), pp. S88-S93, 1998.

[755] Bedell, B. J., Narayana, P. A. and Johnston, D. A., Three-dimensional MR image registration of the human brain, Magnetic Resonance in Medicine, Vol. 35, No. 3, pp. 384-390, 1996.

[756] Hummel, R. A. and Zucker, S. W., On the foundations of relaxation labeling processes, IEEE Trans. on Pattern Analysis and Machine Intelligence, Vol. 5, No. 3, pp. 267-287, 1983.

[757] Rosenfeld, A., Hummel, R. A. and Zucker, S. W., Scene labeling by relaxation operations, IEEE Trans. on Sys., Man and Cyber., Vol. SMC-6, No. 6, pp 420-433, 1976.

[758] Titterington, D. M., Smith, A. F. M. and Makov, U. E., Statistical Analysis of Finite Mixture Distributions, ISBN: 0-4719-0763-4, Wiley, Chichester, UK, 1985.

[759] Dempster, A. P., Laird, N. M. and Rubin, D. B., Maximum likelihood from incomplete data, J. Roy. Stat. Soc., Vol. 39, No. 1, pp. 1-38, 1977.

[760] Liang, Z., Jaszczak, R. J. and Coleman, R. E., Parameter estimation of finite mixtures using the EM algorithm and information criteria with application to medical image processing, IEEE Trans. on Nucl. Sci., Vol. 39, No. 4, pp. 1126-1133, 1992.

[761] Liang, Z., MacFall, J. R. and Harrington, D. P., Parameter estimation and tissue segmentation from multispectral MR images, IEEE Trans. on Med. Imag., Vol. 13, No. 3, pp. 441-449, 1994.

[762] Redner, R. A. and Walker, H. F., Mixture densities, maximum likelihood and the EM algorithm, SIAM Review, Vol. 26, pp. 195-239, 1984.

[763] Santago, P. and Gage, H. D., Statistical models of partial volume effect, IEEE Trans. on Imag. Proc., Vol. 4, No. 11, pp. 1531-1540, 1995.

[764] Sclove, S. L., Application of the conditional population-mixture model to image segmentation, IEEE Trans. on Pattern Analysis and Machine Intelligence, Vol. 5, No. 4, pp. 428-433, 1983.

[765] Titterington, D. M., Some recent research in the analysis of mixture distributions, Statistics, Vol. 21, pp. 619-641, 1990.

[766] Sanjay-Gopal, S. and Hebert, T. J., Bayesian pixel classification using spatially variant finite mixtures and the generalized EM algorithm, IEEE Trans. on Image Proc., Vol. 7, No. 7, pp. 1014-1028, 1998.

[767] Berger, J. O., Statistical Decision Theory and Bayesian Analysis, ISBN: 3-5409-6098-8, Springer-Verlag, New York, 1980.

[768] Chellappa, R. and Jain, A. K., Markov Random Fields: Theory and Applications, ISBN: 0-1217-0608-7, Academic, New York, 1993.

[769] Hebert, T. and Leahy, R., A generalized EM algorithm for 3-D Bayesian reconstruction from Poisson data using Gibbs' priors, IEEE Trans. on Med. Imag., Vol. 8, No 2, pp. 194-202, 1989.

[770] Luenberger, D. G., Linear and Nonlinear Programming, ISBN 0-2011-57940-2, Addison-Wesley, Reading, Massachusetts, 1984.

[771] Galatsanos, N. P. and Katsaggelos, A. K., Methods for choosing the regularization parameter and estimating the noise variance in image restoration and their relation, IEEE Trans. on Imag. Proc., Vol. 1, No. 3, pp. 322-336, 1992.

[772] Hilgers, J. W., A note on estimating the optimal regularization parameter, SIAM J. Numer. Anal., Vol. 17, No. 3, pp. 472-473, 1980.

[773] Johnson, V. E., Wong, W. H., Hu, X. and Chen, C. T., Image restoration using Gibbs' priors: boundary modeling, treatment of blurring and selection of hyperparameter, IEEE Trans. on Pattern Analysis and Machine Intelligence, Vol. 13, No. 5, pp. 413-425, 1992.

[774] Thompson, A. M., Brown, J. C., Kay, J. W. and Titterington, D. M., A study of methods of choosing the smoothing parameter in image restoration by regularization, IEEE Trans. on Pattern Analysis and Machine Intelligence, Vol. 13, pp. 326-339, 1991.

[775] Raff, U. and Newmann, F. D., Automated lesion detection and lesion quantification in MR images using auto-associative memory, Medical Physics, Vol. 19, No. 1, pp. 71-79, 1992.

[776] Johnston, B., Atkins, M. S., Mackiewich, B. and Anderson, M., Segmentation of multiple sclerosis lesions in intensity corrected multispectral MRI, IEEE Trans. on Med. Imag., Vol. 15, No. 2, pp. 154-169, 1996.

[777] Rusinek, H., de Leon, M. J., George, A. E., Styopoulos, L. A., Chandra, R., Smith, G., Rand, T., Mourino, M. and Kowalski, H., Alzheimer's disease: measuring loss of cerebral gray matter with MR imaging, Radiology, Vol. 178, No. 1, pp. 109-114, 1999.

[778] Schuff, N., Vermathen, P., Maudsley, A. A. and Weiner, M. W., Proton magnetic resonance spectroscopic imaging in neurodegenerative diseases, Current Science, Vol. 76, No. 6, pp. 800-807, 1999.

[779] Mackay, S., Meyerhoff, D. J., Constans, J. M., Norman, D., Fein, G. and Weiner, M. W., Regional gray and white matter metabolite differences in subjects with AD with subcortical ischemic vascular dementia and elderly controls with 1H magnetic resonance spectroscopic imaging, Archives in Neurology, Vol. 53, No. 2, pp. 167-174, 1996.

[780] Soher, B. J., Young, K., Govindraju, V. and Maudsley, A. A., Automated spectral analysis III: Application to in vivo proton MR spectroscopy and spectroscopic imaging, Magnetic Resonance in Medicine, Vol. 40, No. 6, pp. 822-831, 1998.

[781] Nagatomo, Y., Wick, M., Prielmeier, F. and Frahm, J., Dynamic monitoring of cerebral metabolites during and after transient global ischemia in rats by quantitative proton NMR spectroscopy in-vivo, NMR in Biomedicine, Vol. 8, No. 6, pp. 265-270, 1995.

[782] Rooney, W. D., Goodkin, D. E., Schuff, N., Meyerhoff, D. J., Norman, D. and Weiner, M. W., 1H MRSI of normal appearing white matter in multiple sclerosis, Multiple Sclerosis, Vol. 3, No. 4, pp. 231-217, 1997.

[783] Arnold, D. L., Matthews, P. M., Francis, G. S., O'Connor J. and Antel, J. P., Proton Magnetic Resonance Spectroscopic Imaging for metabolic characterization of demyelinating plaques, Annals Neurology, Vol. 31, No. 3, pp. 235-241, 1992.

[784] Hennig, J., Theil, T. and Speck, O., Improved sensitivity to overlapping multiplet signals in in-vivo proton spectroscopy using multiecho volume selective(CPRESS) experiment, Magnetic Resonance in Medicine, Vol. 37, No. 6, pp. 816-820, 1997.

[785] Pouwels, P. J. and Frahm, J., Regional metabolite concentrations in human brain as determined by quantitative localized proton MRS, Magnetic Resonance in Medicine, Vol. 39, No. 1, pp. 53-60, 1998.

[786] Sarchielli, P., Presciutti, O., Pelliccioli, R., Tarducci, R., Gobbi, G., Chiarini, P., Alberti, A., Vicinanza, F. and Gallai, V., Absolute quantification of brain metabolites by proton magnetic resonance spectroscopy in normal appearing white matter of multiple sclerosis patients, Brain, Vol. 122, No. 3, pp. 513-521, 1999.

[787] Narayana, P. A., Doyle, T. J., Lai, D. and Wolinsky, J. S., Serial proton magnetic resonance spectroscopic imaging, contrast-enhanced magnetic resonance imaging and quantitative lesion volumetry in multiple sclerosis, Annals in Neurology, Vol. 43, No. 1, pp. 56-71, 1998.

[788] Doyle, T. J., Pathak, R., Wolinsky, J. S. and Narayana, P. A., Automated Proton Spectroscopic Image Processing, Journal of Magnetic Resonance Series B, Vol. 106, No. 1, pp. 58-63, 1995.

[789] Samarasekera, S., Udupa, J. K., Yukio, M., Wei, L. and Grossman, R. I., A new computer-assisted method for the quantification of enhancing lesions in multiple sclerosis, Journal of Computer Assisted Tomography, Vol. 21, No. 1, pp. 145-151, 1997.

[790] Gawne-Cain, M. L., O'Riordan, J. I., Coles, A., Newell, B., Thompson, A. J. and Miller, D. H., MRI lesion volume measurement in multiple sclerosis and its correlation with disability: a comparison of fast fluid attenuated inversion recovery (FLAIR) and spin echo sequences, Journal of Neurology and Neurosurgery Psychiatry, Vol. 64, No. 2, pp. 197-203, 1998.

[791] Rovaris, M., Rocca, M. A., Capra, R., Prandini, F., Martinelli, V., Comi, G. and Filippi, M., A comparison between the sensitivities of 3-mm and 5-mm thick serial brain MRI for detecting lesion volume changes in patients with multiple sclerosis, Journal of Neuroimaging, Vol. 8, No. 3, pp. 144-147, 1998.

[792] Jackson, E. F., Narayana, P. A. and Falconer, J. C., Reproducibility of non-parametric feature map segmentation for determination of normal human intracranial volumes with MR imaging data, Journal of Magnetic Resonance Imaging, Vol. 4, No. 5, pp. 692-700, Sept. 1994.

[793] MacKay, S., Ezekiel, F., Di Sclafani, V., Meyerhoff, D. J., Gerson, J., Norman, D., Fein, G. and Weiner, M. W., Alzheimer's disease and subcortical ischemic vascular dementia: evaluation by combining MR imaging segmentation and H-1 MR spectroscopic imaging, Radiology, Vol. 198, No. 2, pp. 537-545, 1998.

[794] Saunders, D. E., Howe, F. A., van den Boogaart, A., Griffiths, J. R. and Brown, M. M., Discrimination of metabolite from lipid and macromolecule resonances in cerebral infarction in humans using short echo proton spectroscopy, Journal of Magnetic Resonance Imaging, Vol. 7, No. 6, pp. 1116-1121, 1997.

[795] Frahm, J., Bruhn, H., Hanicke, W., Merbolt, K. D., Mursch, K. and Markakis, E., Localized proton NMR spectroscopy of brain tumors using short-echo time STEAM sequences, Journal of Computer Assisted Tomography, Vol. 15, No. 6, pp. 915-922, 1991.

[796] Nelson, S. J., Nalbandian, A. B., Proctor, D. B. and Vigneron, D. B., Registration of images from sequential MR studies of the brain, Journal of Magnetic Resonance, Vol. 4, No. 6, pp. 877-883, 1994.

[797] Maudsley, A. A., Wu, Z., Meyerhoff, D. J. and Weiner, M. W., Automated processing for 1H spectroscopic imaging using water reference deconvolution, Magnetic Resonance in Medicine, Vol. 31, No. 6, pp. 589-595, 1994.

[798] Young, K., Govindraju, V., Soher, B. J. and Maudsley, A. A., Automated spectral analysis I. Formation of a priori information by spectral simulation, Magnetic Resonance in Medicine, Vol. 40, No. 6, pp. 812-815, Dec. 1998.

[799] Young, K., Soher, B. J. and Maudsley, A. A., Automated spectral analysis II: application of wavelet shrinkage for characterization of non-parametrized signals, Magnetic Resonance in Medicine, Vol. 40, No. 6, pp. 816-821, 1998.

[800] Pouwels, P. J. and Frahm, J., Differential distribution of NAA and NAAG in human brain as determined by quantitative localized proton MRS, NMR in Biomedicine, Vol. 10, No. 2, pp. 73-78, 1997.

[801] Matthews, P. M., Pioro, E., Narayanan, S., De Stefano, N., Fu, L., Francis, G., Antel, J., Wolfson, C. and Arnold, D. L., Assessment of lesion pathology in multiple sclerosis using quantitative MRI morphometry and magnetic resonance spectroscopy, Brain, Vol. 119, No. 3, pp. 715-722, 1996.

[802] Gutowski, N. J., Newcombe, J. and Cuzner, M. L., Tenascin-R and C in multiple sclerosis lesions: relevance to extracellular matrix remodelling, Neuropathology and Applied Neurobiology, Vol. 25, No. 3, pp. 207-214, 1999.

[803] Trapp, B. D., Peterson, J., Ransohoff, R. M., Rudick, R., Mork. S. and Bo, L., Axial transection in the lesions of multiple sclerosis, New England Journal of Medicine, Vol. 29, No. 5, pp. 278-85, 1998.

[804] Gehrmann, J., Banati, R. B., Cuzner, M. L., Kreutzberg, G. W. and Newcombe, J., Amyloid precursor protein (APP) expression in multiple sclerosis lesions, Glia, Vol. 15, No. 2, pp. 141-51, 1995.

[805] McManus, C., Berman, J. W., Brett, F. M., Staunton, H., Farrell, M. and Brosnan, C. F., MCP-1, MCP-2 and MCP-3 expression in multiple sclerosis lesions: an immunohistochemical and in situ hybridization study, Journal of Neuroimmunology, Vol. 86, No. 1, pp. 20-29, 1998.

[806] Aquino, D. A., Capello, E., Weisstein, J., Sanders, V., Lopez, C., Tourtellotte, W. W., Brosnan, C. F., Raine, C. S. and Norton, W. T., Multiple sclerosis: altered expression of 70- and 27-kDa heat shock proteins in lesions and myelin, Journal of Neuropathology Experimental Neurology, Vol. 56, No. 6, pp. 664-72, 1997.

[807] Li, W., Quigley, L., Yao, D. L., Hudson, L. D., Brenner, M., Zhang, B. J., Brocke, S., Mc Farland, H. F. and Webster, H. D., Chronic relapsing experimental autoimmune encephalomyelitis: effects of insulin-like

growth factor-I treatment on clinical deficits, lesion severity, glial responses and blood brain barrier defects, Journal of Neuropathology Experimental Neurology, Vol. 57, No. 5, pp. 426-38, 1998.

[808] Constans, J. M., Meyerhoff, D. J., Gerson, J., Mackay, S., Norman, D., Fein, G. and Weiner, M. W., H-1 MR spectroscopic imaging of white matter signal hyperintensities: Alzheimer's disease and ischemic vascular dementia, Radiology, Vol. 198, No. 2, pp. 537-545, 1996.

[809] Pan, J. W., Hetherington, H. P., Vaughan, J. T., Mitchell, G., Pohost, G. M. and Whitaker, J. N., Evaluation of multiple sclerosis by 1-H spectroscopic imaging at 4.1 T, Magnetic Resonance in Medicine, Vol. 36, No. 1, pp. 72-77, 1996.

[810] Hirsch, J. A., Lenkinski, R. E. and Grossman, R. I., MR spectroscopy in the evaluation of enhancing lesions in the brain in multiple sclerosis, American Journal of Neuroradiology, Vol. 17, No. 10, pp. 1829-1836, 1996.

[811] De Stefano, N., Federico, A. and Arnold, D. L., Proton magnetic resonance spectroscopy in brain white matter disorders, Italian Journal of Neurological Science, Vol. 18, No. 6, pp. 331-339, 1997.

[812] Filippi, M., Rocca, M. A., Horsfield, M. A., Rovaris, M., Pereira, C., Yousry, T. A., Colombo, B. and Comi, G., Increased spatial resolution using a three-dimensional T1-weighted gradient-echo MR sequence results in greater hypointense lesion volumes in multiple sclerosis, American Journal of Neuroradiology, Vol. 19, No. 2, pp. 235-238, 1998.

[813] Filippi, M., Horsfield, M. A., Ader, H. J., Barkhof, F., Bruzzi, P., Evans, A., Frank, J. A. and Grossman, R. I., Guidelines for using quantitative measures of brain magnetic resonance imaging abnormalities in monitoring the treatment of multiple sclerosis, Annals in Neurology, Vol. 43, No. 4, pp. 499-506, 1998.

[814] Miller, D. H., Grossman, R. I., Reingold, S. C. and McFarland, H. F., The role of magnetic resonance techniques in understanding and managing multiple sclerosis, Brain, Vol. 121, No. 1, pp. 3-24, 1998.

[815] Filippi, M., Rovaris, M., Sormani, M. P., Horsfield, M. A., Rocca, M. A., Capra, R., Prandini, F. and Comi, G., Intraobserver and interobserver variability in measuring changes in lesion volume on serial brain MR images in multiple sclerosis, American Journal of Neuroradiology, Vol. 19, No. 4, pp. 685-687, 1998.

[816] Erickson, B. J. and Avula, R. T., An algorithm for automatic segmentation and classification of magnetic resonance brain images, Journal Digital Imaging, Vol. 11, No. 2, pp. 74-82, 1998.

[817] Zijdeenbos, A. P. and Dawant, B. M., Brain segmentation and white matter lesion detection in MR images, Critical Reviews in Biomedical Engineering, Vol. 22, No. 5-6, pp. 401-465, 1994.

[818] Filippi, M., Horsfield, M. A., Hajnal, J. V., Narayana, P. A., Udupa, J. K., Yousry, T. A. and Zijdenbos, A., Quantitative assessment of magnetic resonance imaging lesion load in multiple sclerosis, Journal

of Neurology and Neurosurgery Psychiatry, Vol. 64, No. 1, pp. 88-93, 1998.

[819] Michaelis, T., Helms, G. and Frahm, J., Metabolic alterations in brain autopsies: proton NMR identification of free glycerol, NMR in Biomedicine, Vol. 9, No. 3, pp. 121-124, 1996.

[820] Filippi, M., Mastronardo, G., Rocca, M. A., Capra, R., Gasperini, C., Rovaris, M., Bastianello, S. and Comi, G., Detecting new lesion formation in Multiple Sclerosis: The relative contributions of monthly dual-echo and T1-weighted scans after triple-dose gadolinium, European Neurology, Vol. 40, No. 3, pp. 146-150, 1998.

[821] Malladi, R. and Sethian, J. A., A Unified Approach to Noise Removal, Image-Enhancement and Shape Recovery, IEEE Trans. on Image Processing, Vol. 5, No. 11, pp. 1554-1568, Nov. 1996.

[822] Rouy, E. and Tourin, A., A viscosity solutions approach to shape-from-shading, SIAM J. of Numerical Analysis, Vol. 23, No. 3, pp. 867-884, 1992.

[823] Sethian, J.A., A fast marching level set method for monotonically advancing fronts, Proc. Natl. Acad. Science, Applied Mathematics, Vol. 93, No. 4, pp. 1591-1595, Feb. 1996.

[824] Adalsteinsson, D. and Sethian, J. A., The fast construction of extension velocities in level set methods, J. Computational Physics, Vol. 148, No. 1, pp. 2-22, 1999.

[825] Sedgewick, R., Algorithms in C, Fundamentals, data structures, sorting, searching, Addison-Wesley, ISBN: 0-2013-1452-5, (v. 1), 1998.

[826] Suri, J. S., Singh, S. and Reden, L., Computer Vision and Pattern Recognition Techniques for 2-D and 3-D MR Cerebral Cortical Segmentation: A State-of-the-Art Review, Accepted for Publication in Journal of Pattern Analysis and Applications, Vol. 4, No. 3, Sept. 2001.

[827] Astley, S. M., Taylor, C. J., Boggis, C. R. M., Asbury, D. L. and Wilson, M., Cue generation and combination for mammographic screening, in Brogan, Carr and Gale (eds), Visual Search II, Taylor and Francis, London, 1993.

[828] Belhomme, P., Elmoataz, A., Herlin, P. and Bloyet, D., Generalized region growing operator with optimal scanning: application to segmentation of breast cancer images, Journal of Microscopy, Vol. 186, No. 1, pp. 41-50, 1997.

[829] Besag, J. E., On the statistical analysis of dirty pictures, Journal of Royal Statistical Society, Series B, Vol. 48, No. 3, pp. 259-302, 1986.

[830] Betal, D., Roberts, N., Whitehouse, G. H., Segmentation and numerical analysis of microcalcifications using mathematical morphology, The British Journal of Radiology, Vol. 70, No. 837, pp. 903-917, 1997.

[831] Bishop, C., Neural networks for pattern recognition, Clarendon Press, New York, ISBN: 0-1985-3849-9, 1997.

[832]   Blom, J., Topological and geometrical aspects of image structure, Ph.D dissertation, Utrecht University, Utrecht, Holland, 1992.

[833]   Bovis, K. J. and Singh, S., Enhancement techniques evaluation using quantitative measures on digital mammograms, Proc. 5th International Workshop on Digital Mammography (IWDM), Toronto, June 11-14, 2000 (to appear).

[834]   Bovis, K. J. and Singh, S., Detection of Masses in Mammograms Using Texture Measures, Proc. 15th International Conference on Pattern Recognition, Barcelona, IEEE Press, Vol. 2, pp. 267-270, 2000.

[835]   Byng, J. W., Yaffe, M. J., Lockwood, G. A., Little, L. E., Tritchler, D. L. and Boyd, N. F., Automated analysis of mammographic densities and breast carcinoma risk, Cancer, Vol. 80, No. 1, pp. 66-74, 1997.

[836]   Cardenosa, G., Breast imaging companion, Lippincott-Raven, ISBN: 0-3975-1778-5, Philadelphia, 1997.

[837]   Cayley, A., On contour and slope lines, London, Edinburgh, Dublin, Philosph. Mag. J. Sci., Vol. 18, pp. 264-268, Oct. 1859.

[838]   Chalana, V. and Kim, Y., A methodology for evaluation of boundary detection algorithms on medical images, IEEE Trans. on Med. Imaging, Vol. 16, No 5, pp. 642-652, 1997.

[839]   Chan, H. P., Wei, D., Helvie, M. A., Sahiner, B., Adler, D. D., Goodsitt, M. M. and Petrick, N., Computer-aided classification of mammographic masses and normal tissue: linear discriminant analysis in texture feature space, Phys. Med. Biol., Vol. 40, No. 5, pp. 857-876, 1995.

[840]   Chan, H. P., Lo, S. C. B., Sahiner, B., Lam, K. L. and Helvie, M. A., Computer-aided detection of mammographic microcalcifications: pattern recognition with an artificial neural network, Medical Physics, Vol. 22, pp. 1555-1567, 1995.

[841]   Chan, H. P., Sahiner, B., Lam, K. L., Petrick, N., Helvie, M. A., Goodsitt M. M. and Adler, D. D., Computerized analysis of mammographic microcalcifications in morphological and texture feature space, Medical Physics, Vol. 25, No. 10, pp. 2007-2019, 1998.

[842]   Chandrasekhar, R., Systematic segmentation of mammograms, Ph.D. Thesis, Electrical and Electronic Engineering Department, University of Western Australia, Perth, Australia, 1996.

[843]   Chandrasekhar, R. and Attikiouzel, Y., A simple method for automatically locating the nipple on mammograms, IEEE Trans. on Med. Imag., Vol. 16, No. 5, pp. 483-494, 1997.

[844]   Chang, Y. L. and Li, X., Adaptive image region growing, IEEE Trans. on Image Processing, Vol. 3, No. 6, pp. 868-872, 1994.

[845]   Collins, S. H., Terrain parameters directly from the digital terrain model, Canadian Survey, Vol. 29, No. 5, pp. 507-518, 1975.

[846]   Conners, R. W. and Harlow, C. A., Toward a structural textural analyser based on statistical methods, Computer Graphics and Image Processing, Vol. 12, pp. 224-256, 1980.

[847] Egan, R. L., Breast imaging: diagnosis and morphology of breast diseases, ISBN: 0-7216-2320-4, W. B. Saunders, Philadelphia, 1988.

[848] Pauwels, E. J. and Frederix, G., Finding salient regions in images, Computer Vision and Image Understanding, Vol. 75, No. 1/2, pp. 73-85, 1999.

[849] Frigui, H. and Krishnapuram, R., A robust competitive clustering algorithm with applications in computer vision, IEEE Trans. on Pattern Analysis and Machine Intelligence, Vol. 21, No. 5, pp. 450-465, 1999.

[850] Gamagami, P., Atlas of mammography: new early signs in breast cancer, ISBN: 0-8654-2481-0, Blackwell Science, Cambridge, Massachusetts, 1996.

[851] Gauch, J. M., Image segmentation and analysis via multiscale watershed hierarchies, IEEE Trans. on Image Processing, Vol. 8, No. 1, pp. 69-79, 1999.

[852] Gonzalez, R. C. and Woods, R. E., Digital image processing, ISBN: 0-2015-0803-6, Addison Wesley, New York, 1993.

[853] Griffin, L. D., Colchester, A. F. C. and Robinson, G. P., Scale and segmentation of gray-level images using maximum gradient paths, Proc. Information processing in Medical Imaging Conference, Wye, UK, pp. 256-272, 1991.

[854] Goddard, C. C., Filbert, F. J., Needham, G. and Deans, H. E., Routine receiver operating characteristic analysis in mammography as a measure of radiologists' performance, The British Journal of Radiology, Vol. 71, No. 850, pp. 1012-1017, 1998.

[855] Goodsitt, M. M., Chan, H. P., Liu, B., Guru, S. V., Morton, A. R., Keshavmurthy, S. and Petrick, N., Classification of compressed breast shapes for the design of equalisation filters in x-ray mammography, Medical Physics, Vol. 25, No. 6, pp. 937-947, 1998.

[856] Gupta, R. and Undrill, P. E., The use of texture analysis to delineate suspicious masses in mammography, Physics Medicine and Biology, Vol. 40, No. 5, pp. 835-855, 1995.

[857] Hair, J. F., Anderson, R. E., Tatham, R. L. and Black, W. C., Multivariate data analysis, 5th ed., ISBN: 0-1389-4858-5, Prentice Hall, New Jersey, 1998.

[858] Hansen, M. W. and Higgins, W. E., Relaxation methods for supervised image segmentation, IEEE Trans. on Pattern Analysis and Machine Intelligence, Vol. 19, No. 9, pp. 949-962, 1997.

[859] Haralick, R. M., Shanmugam, K. and Dinstein, I., Textural features for image classification, IEEE Trans. on System, Man and Cybernetics, Vol. 3, No. 6, pp. 610-621, 1973.

[860] Haus, A. G., Screen-Film Processing Systems and Quality Control in Mammography, Kodak Health Sciences Monograph Based on a Lecture Presented at the Symposium on the Physics of Clinical Mammography Sponsored by the American College of Radiology, St Louis, 1990.

[861] Heywang-Köbrunner, S. H., Shreer, I. and Dershaw, D. D., Diagnostic breast imaging - Mammography, sonography, magnetic resonance imaging and interventional procedures, Thieme, Stuttgart, 1997.

[862] Heath, M. D. and Bowyer, K. W., The digital database for screening mammography, Proc. International Workshop on Digital Mammography (IWDM), Toronto, 2000. http://marathon.csee.usf.edu/Mammography/Database.html.

[863] Highnam, R., Brady, M. and Shepstone, B., A representation for mammographic image processing, Medical Image Analysis, Vol. 1, No. 1, pp. 1-18, 1996.

[864] Highnam, R. and Brady, M., Mammographic image analysis: computational imaging and vision, Computational Imaging and Vision, Vol. 14, Kluwer Academic Publishers, 1999.

[865] Hong, T. H., Dyer, C. R. and Rosenfeld, A., Texture primitive extraction using an edge based approach, IEEE Trans. on Systems, Man and Cybernetics, Vol. 10, No. 10, pp. 659-675, 1980.

[866] Hoover, A., Paptisle, C. J., Jiang, X., Flynn, P. J., Bunke, H., Goldof, D. B., Bowyer, K., Eggert, D. W., Fitzgibbon, A. and Fisher, R. B., An experimental comparison of range image segmentation algorithms, IEEE Trans. on Pattern Analysis and Machine Intelligence, Vol. 18, No. 7, pp. 673-689, 1996.

[867] Ibrahim, N., Fujita, H., Hara, T. and Endo, T., Automated detection of clustered microcalcifications on mammograms: CAD system application to MIAS database, Phys. Med. Biol., Vol. 42, No. 12, pp. 2577-2589, 1997.

[868] Illingworth, J. and Kittler, J., A survey of Hough transform, Computer Vision, Graphics and Image Processing, Vol. 44, No. 1, pp. 87-116, 1988.

[869] Jain, A. K. and Dubes, R. C., Algorithms for clustering data, ISBN: 0-1302-2278-x, Prentice Hall, Englewood Cliffs, N.J., 1988.

[870] Jain, A. K., Duin, R. P. W. and Mao, J., Statistical pattern recognition: a review, IEEE Trans. on Pattern Analysis and Machine Intelligence, Vol. 22, No. 1, pp. 4-37, 2000.

[871] Jain, R., Kasturi, R. and Schunck, B., Machine vision, McGraw-Hill International Editions, Singapore, 1995.

[872] Kallergi, M., Carney, G. M. and Gaviria, J., Evaluating the performance of detection algorithms in digital mammography, Medical Physics, Vol. 26, No. 2, pp. 267-275, 1999.

[873] Karssemeijer, N., Stochastic model for automated detection of calcifications in digital mammograms, Image and Vision Computing, Vol. 10, No. 6, pp. 369-375, 1992.

[874] Karssemeijer, N., Detection of stellate distortions in mammograms using scale space operators, Proc. IPMI 95, Kluwer, pp. 335-346, 1995.

[875] Karssemeijer, N. and te Brake, G., Combining single view features and asymmetry for detection of mass lesions, Proc. 4th International Workshop on Digital Mammography, pp. 95-102, Nijmegen, The Netherlands, 1998.

[876] Kegelmeyer, W. P., Pruneda, J. M., Bourland, P. D., Hillis, A., Riggs, M. W. and Nipper, M. L., Computer-aided mammographic screening for spiculated lesions, Radiology, Vol. 191, No. 2, pp. 331-337, 1994.

[877] Kim, J. K. and Park, H. W., Statistical texture features for detection of microcalcifications in digitised mammograms, IEEE Trans. in Med. Imag., Vol. 18, No. 3, pp. 231-238, 1999.

[878] Kitchen, L. and Rosenfeld, A., Edge evaluation using local edge coherence, IEEE Trans. on Systems, Man and Cybernetics, Vol. 11, No. 9, pp. 597-605, 1981.

[879] Klette, R. and Zamperoni, P., Handbook of image processing operators, John Wiley, Chichester, UK, ISBN: 0-4719-5642-2, 1996.

[880] Kobatake, H., Murakami, M., Takeo, H. and Nawano, S., Computerised detection of malignant tumors on digital mammograms, IEEE Trans. on Med. Imag., Vol. 18, No. 5, pp. 369-378, 1999.

[881] Kopans, D., Breast imaging (2nd ed.), ISBN: 0-3975-1302-X, Lippincott-Raven, Philadelphia, 1998.

[882] Kupinski, M. A. and Giger, M. L., Automated seeded lesion segmentation on digital mammograms, IEEE Trans. on Med. Imag., Vol. 17, No. 4, pp. 511-517, 1998.

[883] Lau, T. and Bischof, W. F., Automated detection of breast tumors using the asymmetry approach, Computers and Biomedical research, Vol. 24, No. 3, pp. 273-295, 1991.

[884] Laws, K. I., Textured image segmentation, Ph.D. Thesis, Dept. of Electrical Engineering, University of Southern California, Los Angles, Jan. 1980.

[885] Li, L., Qian, W. and Clarke, L. P., Digital mammography: computer assisted diagnosis method for mass detection with multi-orientation and multiresolution wavelet transforms, Academic Radiology, Vol. 4, No. 11, pp. 724-731, 1997.

[886] Mandlebrot, B. B., The fractal geometry of nature, ISBN: 0-7167-1186-9, Freeman, New York, 1982.

[887] Marks, D., Dozier, J. and Frew, J., Automated basin delineation from digital elevation data, Geoprocessing, Vol. 2, pp. 299-311, 1984.

[888] Masek, M., Attikiouzel, Y. and deSilva, C. J. S., Automatic removal of high intensity labels and noise from mammograms, Proc. International Workshop on Digital Mammography (IWDM), Toronto, 2000.

[889] Maxwell, J. C., On hills and dales, London, Edinburgh, Dublin, Philosph. Mag. J. Sci., 4th series, Vol. 40, pp. 421-425, Oct. 1859.

[890] Mehnert, A. and Jackway, P., An improved seeded region growing algorithm, Pattern Recognition Letters, Vol. 18, No. 10, pp. 1065-1071, 1997.

[891] Mendez, A. J., Tahoces, P. G., Lado, M. J., Souto, M. and Vidal, J. J., Computer aided diagnosis: texture features to discriminate between malignant masses and normal breast tissue in digitised mammograms, Computer Assisted Radiology and Surgery, 11th International Symposium and Exhibition (CAR), pp. 342-346, 1997.

[892] Mendez, A. J., Tahoces, P. G., Lado, M. J., Souto, M. and Vidal, J. J., Computer aided diagnosis: automatic detection of malignant masses in digitised mammograms, Medical Physics, Vol. 25, No. 6, pp. 957-964, 1998.

[893] Metz, C. E., Basic principles of ROC analysis, Seminars in Nuclear Medicine, Vol. 8, No. 4, pp. 283-298, 1978.

[894] Miller, P. and Astley, S., Classification of breast tissue by texture analysis, Image and Vision Computing, Vol. 10, No. 5, pp. 277-283, 1992.

[895] Ng, S. L. and Bischof, W. F., Automated detection and classification of breast tumours, Computers and Biomedical Research, Vol. 25, No. 3, pp. 218-237, 1992.

[896] Pal, S. K. and Majumder, D. D., Fuzzy mathematical approaches to pattern recognition, ISBN: 0-4702-7463-8, Wiley, New York, 1986.

[897] Parr, T., Zwiggelaar, R., Astley, S., Boggis, C. and Taylor, C., Comparison of methods for combining evidence for stellate lesions, Proc. 4th International Workshop on Digital Mammography, Nijmegen, The Netherlands, pp. 71-78, June 1998.

[898] Petrick, N., Chan, H. P., Wei, D., Sahiner, B., Helvie, M. A. and Adler, D. D., Automated detection of breast masses using adaptive contrast enhancement and texture classification, Medical Physics, Vol. 23, No. 10, pp. 1685-1696, 1996.

[899] Petrick, N., Chan, H. P., Sahiner, B. and Wei, D., An adaptive density-weighted contrast enhancement filter for mammographic breast mass detection, IEEE Trans. on Med. Imag., Vol. 15, No. 1, pp. 59-67, 1996.

[900] Petrick, N., Chan, H. P., Sahiner, B. and Helvie, M. A., Combined adaptive enhancement and region-growing segmentation of breast masses on digitized mammograms, Medical Physics, Vol. 26, No. 8, pp. 1642-1654, 1999.

[901] Pohlman, S., Powell, K. A., Obuchowsky, N. A., Chilocote, W. A. and Grundfest-Broniatowski, S., Quantitative classification of breast tumours in digitized mammograms, Medical Physics, Vol. 23, No. 8, pp. 1337-1345, 1996.

[902] Polakowski, W. E., Cournoyer, D. E., Rogers, S. K., Desimio, M. P., Ruck, D. W., Hoffmeister, J. W. and Raines, R. A., Computer-aided breast cancer detection and diagnosis of masses using difference of Gaussians and derivative-based feature saliency, IEEE Trans. on Med. Imag., Vol. 16, No. 6, pp. 811-819, 1997.

[903] Pratt, W. K., Digital image processing, John Wiley, New York, 1991.

[904] Puecker, T. K. and Douglas, D. H., Detection of surface specific points by local parallel processing of discrete terrain elevation data, Computer, Vision, Graphics and Image Processing, Vol. 4, pp. 375-387, 1975.

[905] Qian, W., Li, L. and Clarke, L. P., Image feature extraction for mass detection in digital mammography: influence of wavelet analysis, Medical Physics, Vol. 26, No. 3, pp. 402-408, 1999.

[906] Rao, R. M. and Bopardikar, A. S., Wavelet transforms, ISBN: 0-2016-3463-5, Addison Wesley, Reading, Massachusetts, 1998.

[907] Rangayyan, R. M., El-Faramawy, N. M., Leo Desautels, J. E. and Alim, O. A., Measures of acutance and shape for classification of breast tumors, IEEE Trans. on Med. Imag., Vol. 16, No. 6, pp. 799-810, 1997.

[908] Rangayyan, R. M., Shen, L., Shen, Y., Desautels, J. E. L., Bryant, H., Terry, T. J., Horeczko, N. and Rose, M. S,, Improvement of sensitivity of breast cancer diagnosis with adaptive neighbourhood contrast enhancement of mammograms, IEEE Trans. on Information Technology in Biomedicine, Vol. 1, No. 3, pp. 161-169, 1997.

[909] Revol, C. and Jourlin, M., A new minimum variance region growing algorithm for image segmentation, Pattern Recognition Letters, Vol. 18, No. 3, pp. 249-258, 1997.

[910] Roberts, S., Parametric and non-parameteric unsupervised cluster analysis, Pattern Recognition, Vol. 30, No. 2, pp. 261-272, 1997.

[911] Rosenfeld, A., Image Analysis and Computer Vision, Computer Vision and Image Understanding, Vol. 78, No. 2, pp. 222-302, 2000.

[912] Sahiner, B., Chan, H. P., Wei, D., Petrick, N., Helvie, M. A., Adler, D. D. and Goodsitt, M. M., Image feature selection by a genetic algorithm: application to classification of mass and normal breast tissue, Medical Physics, Vol. 23, No. 10, pp. 1671-1683, 1996.

[913] Sahiner, B., Chan, H. P., Petrick, N., Wei, D., Helvie, M. A., Adler, D. D. and Goodsitt, M. M., Classification of mass on normal breast tissue: A convolution neural network classifier with spatial domain and texture features, IEEE Trans. on Med. Imag., Vol. 15, No. 5, pp. 598-610, 1996.

[914] Sahiner, B., Chan, H. P., Petrick, N., Helvie, M. A. and Goodsitt, M. M., Computerized characterization of masses on mammograms: The rubber band straightening transform and texture analysis, Medical Physics, Vol. 25, No. 4, pp. 516-526, 1998.

[915] Sahoo, P. K., Soltani, S. and Wong, A. K. C., A survey of thresholding techniques, Computer Vision, Graphics and Image Processing, Vol. 41, No. 2, pp. 233-260, Feb. 1988.

[916] Singh, S. and Al-Mansoori, R., Identification of region of interest in digital mammograms, Journal of Intelligent Systems, Vol. 10, No. 2, pp. 183-210, 2000.

[917] Sonka, M., Hlavac, V. and Boyle, R., Image processing, analysis and machine vision, ISBN: 0-5349-5393-X, PWS Publishing, New York, 1999.

[918] Spiesberger, W., Mammogram inspection by computer, IEEE Trans. on Biomedical Engineering, Vol. 26, pp. 213-219, 1979.

[919] Suckling, J., Parker, J., Dance, D., Astley, S., Hutt, I., Boggis, C., Ricketts, I., Stamatakis, E., Cerneaz, N., Kok, S., Taylor, P., Betal, D. and Savage, J., The mammographic images analysis society digital mammogram database, Exerpta Medica, International Congress Series, Vol. 1069, pp. 375-378, 1994. http://www.wiau.man.ac.uk/services/MIAS/MIAScom.html.

[920] Taylor, P., Hajnal, S., Dilhuydy, M-H. and Barreau, B., Measuring image texture to separate difficult from easy mammograms, The British Journal of Radiology, Vol. 67, pp. 456-463, 1994.

[921] te Brake, G. M., Karssemeijer, N. and Hendriks, J., Automated detection of breast carcinomas not detected in a screening program, Radiology, Vol. 207, No. 2, pp. 465-471, 1998.

[922] Theodoridis, S. and Koutroumbas, K., Pattern Recognition, ISBN: 0-1268-6140-4, Academic Press, San Diego, 1999.

[923] Vincent, L. and Soille, P., Watershed in digital spaces: an efficient algorithm based on immersion simulations, IEEE Trans. on Pattern Analysis and Machine Intelligence, Vol. 13, No. 6, pp. 583-598, 1991.

[924] Umbaugh, S. E., Computer vision and image processing, ISBN: 0-1326-4599-8, Prentice Hall, Upper Saddle River, 1998.

[925] Wang, T. C. and Karayiannis, N. B., Detection of microcalcifications in digital mammograms using wavelets, IEEE Trans. on Med. Imaging, Vol. 17, No. 4, pp. 498-509, 1998.

[926] Wei, D., Chan, H. P., Petrick, N., Shahiner, B., Helvie, M. A., Adler, D. D. and Goodsitt, M. M., False-positive reduction technique for detection of masses on digital mammograms: Global and local multiresolution texture analysis, Medical Physics, Vol. 24, No. 6, pp. 903-914, 1997.

[927] Weszka, J., Dyer, C. and Rosenfeld, A., A comparative study of texture measures for terrain classification, IEEE Trans. on Systems, Man and Cybernetics, Vol. 6, No. 4, pp. 269-285, 1976.

[928] Winsberg, F., Elkin, M., Macy, J., Bordaz, V. and Weymouth, W., Detection of radiographic abnormalities in mammograms by means of optimal scanning and computer analysis, Radiology, Vol. 89, pp. 211-215, 1967.

[929] Wirth, M. A., Choi, C. and Jennings, A., A nonrigid-body approach to matching mammograms, Proceedings of The Institute of Electrical Engineers Conference on Image Processing, Vol. 465, pp. 484-488, 1999.

[930] Wolberg, W. H., Benign breast disease and breast cancer tutorial, Http://www.surgery.wisc.edu/wolberg, 2000.

[931] Yin, F. F., Giger, M. L., Vyborny, C. J., Doi, K. and Schmidt, R., Comparison of bilateral-subtraction and single-image processing techniques in the computerised detection of mammographic masses, Investigative Radiology, Vol. 28, No. 6, pp. 473-481, 1993.

[932] Zadeh, L. A, Fuzzy logic and its applications, Academic Press, New York, 1965.

[933] Zahid, N., Limouri, M. and Essaid, A., A new cluster-validity for fuzzy clustering, Pattern Recognition, Vol. 32, No. 7, pp. 1089-1097, 1999.

[934] Zhang, Y. J. and Gerbrands, J. J., Comparison of thresholding techniques using synthetic images and ultimate measurement accuracy, Proc. of 11th International Conference on Pattern Recognition, Vol. 3, pp. 209-213, 1992.

[935] Zhang, Y. J. and Gerbrands, J. J., Objective and quantitative segmentation evaluation and comparison, Signal Processing, Vol. 39, No. 1-2, pp. 43-54, 1994.

[936] Zhang, Y. J., A survey on evaluation methods for image segmentation, Pattern Recognition, Vol. 29, No. 8, pp. 1335-1346, 1996.

[937] Zhang, Y. J., Evaluation and comparison of different segmentation algorithms, Pattern Recognition Letters, Vol. 18, pp. 963-974, 1997.

[938] Zwiggelaar, R., Schumm, J. E. and Taylor, C. J., The detection of abnormal masses in mammograms, Proc. Medical Image Understanding Workshop, pp. 65-68, Oxford, 1997.

[939] Zwiggelaar, R., Anatomical classification of linear structures in mammograms, Proc. Medical Image Understanding Workshop, pp. 201-204, Oxford, 1997.

[940] Zwiggelaar, R., Parr, T. C., Boggis, C. R. M., Astley, S. M. and Taylor, C. J., Statistical modelling of lines and structures in mammograms, Proc. Medical Imaging, Newport Beach, CA, Vol. 3034, pp. 510-521, 1997.

[941] Zwiggelaar, R., Astley, S. and Taylor, C., Detecting the central mass of a speculated lesion using scale-orientation signatures, Proc. 4th International Workshop on Digital Mammography, pp. 63-70, Nijmegen, Holland, 1998.

[942] Zwiggelaar, R., Parr, T. C., Schumm, J. E., Hutt, I. W., Taylor, C. J., Astley, S. M. and Boggis, C. R. M., Model-based detection of spiculated lesions in mammograms, Medical Image Analysis, Vol. 3, No. 1, pp. 39-63, 1999.

[943] Antani, S., Kasturi, R. and Jain, R., Pattern Recognition Methods in Image and Video Databases: Past, Present and Future, In: Amin, A. *et al.* (eds), Advances in Pattern Recognition, Springer, Lecture Notes in Comp. Science, Vol. 1451, pp. 31-53, 1998.

[944] Banks, P., Chan, J., Cleary, M., Delsol, G., De Wolf- Peeters, C., Gatter, K., Grogan, T., Harris, N., Isaacson, P., Jaffe, E., Mason, D., Pileri, S., Ralfkiaer, E., Stein, H. and Warnke, R., Mantle Cell Lymphoma: A Proposal for Unification of Morphologic, Immunologic and Molecular Data, Am. J. Surg. Pathology, Vol. 16, No. 7, pp. 637-640, 1992.

[945]   Bauman, I., Nenninger, R., Harms, H., Zwierzina, H., Wilms, K., Feller, A. C., Meulen, V. T. and Muller-Hermelink, H. K., Image Analysis Detects Lineage-Specific Morphologic Markers in Leukemic Blast Cells, Am. J. Clin. Pathol., Vol. 105, No. 1, pp. 23-30, 1995.

[946]   Campo, E. and Jaffe, E., Mantle Cell Lymphoma, Arch. Pathol. Lab. Med., Vol. 120, No. 1, pp. 12-14, 1996.

[947]   Chan, J., Banks, B. M., *et al.*, A Revised European-American Classification of Lymphoid Neoplasms Proposed by the International Lymphoma Study Group, Am. J. Clin. Pathol., Vol. 103, No. 5, pp. 543-560, 1995.

[948]   Cheng, Y., Mean shift, mode seeking and clustering, IEEE Trans. on Pattern Anal. Machine Intell., Vol. 17, No. 8, pp. 790-799, 1995.

[949]   Cho, K. and Meer, P., Image Segmentation from Consensus Information, Comp. Vis. and Image Understanding, Vol. 68, No. 1, pp. 72-89, 1997.

[950]   Comaniciu, D., Foran, D. and Meer, P., Shape-Based Image Indexing and Retrieval for Diagnostic Pathology, Proc. Int'l Conf. on Pattern Recognition, Brisbane, Australia, pp. 902-904, 1998.

[951]   Comaniciu, D., Meer, P., Foran, D. and Medl, A., Bimodal System for Interactive Indexing and Retrieval of Pathology Images, IEEE Workshop on Applications of Comp. Vis., Princeton, New Jersey, pp. 76-81, 1998.

[952]   Comaniciu, D. and Meer, P., Distribution Free Decomposition of Multivariate Data, Pattern Analysis and Applications, Vol. 2, No. 1, pp. 22-30, 1999.

[953]   Comaniciu, D. and Meer, P., Mean Shift Analysis and Applications, IEEE Int'l Conf. Comp. Vis., Kerkyra, Greece, pp. 1197-1203, 1999.

[954]   Comaniciu, D., Meer, P., Xu, K. and Tyler, D., Retrieval Performance Improvement through Low Rank Corrections, IEEE Workshop on Content-Based Access of Image and Video Lib., Fort Collins, Colorado, pp. 50-54, 1999.

[955]   Comaniciu, D., Georgescu, B., Meer, P., Chen, W. and Foran, D., Decision Support System for Multiuser Remote Microscopy in Telepathology, IEEE Symposium on Computer-Based Medical Systems, Stamford, Connecticut, pp. 150-155, 1999.

[956]   Comaniciu, D., Meer, P. and Foran, D., Image Guided Decision Support System for Pathology, Machine Vision and Applications, Vol. 11, No. 4, pp. 213-224, 2000.

[957]   Cox, I. J., Miller, M. L., Minka, T. P. and Yianilos, P. N., An Optimized Interaction Strategy for Bayesian Relevance Feedback, IEEE Conf. on Comp. Vis. and Pattern Recognition, Santa Barbara, California, pp. 553-558, 1998.

[958]   Das, M., Riseman, E. M. and Draper, B. A., FOCUS: Searching for Multi-colored Objects in a Diverse Image Database, IEEE Conf. on Comp. Vis. and Pattern Recognition, San Juan, Puerto Rico, pp. 756-761, 1997.

[959] Efron, B. and Tibshirani, R., An Introduction to the Bootstrap, ISBN: 0-4120-4231-2, Chapman & Hall, New York, 1993.

[960] Flickner, M., Sawhney, H., Niblack, W., Ashley, J., Huang, Q., Dom, B., Gorkani, M., Hafner, J., Lee, D., Petkovic, D., Steele, D. and Yanker, P., Query by Image and Video Content: The QBIC System, Computer, Vol. 9, No. 9, pp. 23-31, 1995.

[961] Fukunaga, K. and Hostetler, L.D., The Estimation of the Gradient of a Density Function, with Applications in Pattern Recognition, IEEE Trans. on Info. Theory, Vol. IT-21, No. 1, pp. 32-40, 1975.

[962] Fukunaga, K., Introduction to Statistical Pattern Recognition (2nd ed.), ISBN: 0-1226-9851-7, Computer science and scientific computing series, Academic Press, Boston, 1990.

[963] Kauppinen, H., Seppanen, T. and Pietikainen, M., An Experimental Comparison of Autoregressive and Fourier-Based Descriptors in 2-D Shape Classification, IEEE Trans. on Pattern Analysis Machine Intell., Vol. 17, No. 2, pp. 201-207, 1995.

[964] Kittler, J., Hatef, M., Duin, R. P. W. and Matas, J., On Combining Classifiers, IEEE Trans. on Pattern Analysis Machine Intell., Vol. 20, No. 3, pp. 226-238, 1998.

[965] Kuhl, F. P. and Giardina, C.R., Elliptic Fourier Features of a Closed Contour, Comp. Graphics Image Process., Vol. 18, No. 3, pp. 236-258, 1982.

[966] Liu, F. and Picard, R. W., Periodicity, Directionality and Randomness: World Features for Image Modeling and Retrieval, IEEE Trans. on Pattern Analysis Machine Intell., Vol. 18, No. 7, 722-733, 1996.

[967] Liu, Y. and Dellaert, F., A Classification Based Similarity Metric for 3-D Image Retrieval, IEEE Conf. on Comp. Vis. and Pattern Recognition, Santa Barbara, California, pp. 800-805, 1998.

[968] Ma, W. Y. and Manjunath, B.S., NETRA: A Toolbox for Navigating Large Image Databases, IEEE Int'l Conf. Image Process., Santa Barbara, California, Vol. 1, pp. 568-571, 1997.

[969] Mao, J. and Jain, A. K., Texture Classification and Segmentation using Multiresolution Simultaneous Autoregressive Models, Pattern Recognition, Vol. 25, No. 2, pp. 173-188, 1992.

[970] Moghaddam, B. and Pentland, A., Probabilistic Visual Learning for Object Representation, IEEE Trans. on Pattern Analysis Machine Intell., Vol. 19, No. 7, pp. 696-710, 1997.

[971] Nastar, C., Mitschke, M. and Meihac, C., Efficient Query Refinement for Image Retrieval, IEEE Conf. on Comp. Vis. and Pattern Recognition, Santa Barbara, California, pp. 547-552, 1998.

[972] Ortega, M., Rui, Y., Chakrabarti, K., Mehrotra, S. and Huang, T.S., Supporting Similarity Queries in MARS, ACM Multimedia, Seattle, Washington, pp. 403-413, 1997.

[973] Pentland, A., Picard, R.W. and Sclaroff, S., Photobook: Content-based manipulation of image databases, Int'l. J. of Comp. Vis., Vol. 18, No. 3, pp. 233-254, 1996.

[974] Persoon, E., and Fu, K. S., Shape Discrimination using Fourier Descriptors, IEEE Trans. on Systems, Man and Cybern., Vol. 7, No. 3, pp. 170-179, 1977.

[975] Petrakis, E. G. M. and Faloutsos, C., Similarity Searching in Large Databases, IEEE Trans. on Knowledge and Data Engn., Vol. 9, No. 3, pp. 435-447, 1997.

[976] Picard, R. W., Kabir, T., Liu, F., Real-time Recognition with the Entire Brodatz Texture Database, IEEE Conf. on Comp. Vis. and Pattern Recognition (CVPR), New York, pp. 638-639, 1993.

[977] Popat, K. and Picard, R. W., Cluster-Based Probability Model and Its Application to Image and Texture Processing, IEEE Trans. on Image Process., Vol. 6, No. 2, pp. 268-284, 1997.

[978] Press, W. H., Teukolsky, S. A., Vetterling, W. T. and Flannery, B. P., Numerical Recipes in C (2nd ed.), ISBN 0-521-43108-5, Cambridge University Press, Cambridge, 1992.

[979] Rui, Y., She, A.C. and Huang,T.S., A Modified Fourier Descriptor for Shape Matching in MARS, In: Chang SK (ed) Image Databases and Multimedia Search, Series of Software Engn. and Knowledge Engn., Vol. 8, World Scientific Publishing, Singapore, pp. 165-180, 1998.

[980] Sedgewick, R., Algorithms in C++, Addison-Wesley, New York, 1992.

[981] Sharma, R., Pavlovic, V. I. and Huang, T. S., Toward Multimodal Human-Computer Interface, Proceedings of the IEEE, Vol. 86, No. 5, pp. 853-869, 1998.

[982] Tagare, H. D., Jaffe, C. C. and Duncan, J., Medical Image Databases: A Content-based Retrieval Approach, J. Am. Medical Inform. Assoc., Vol. 4, No. 3, pp. 184-198, 1997.

[983] Trucco, E. and Verri, A., Introductory Techniques for 3-D Computer Vision, Prentice Hall, NJ, ISBN: 0-1326-1108-2, 1998.

[984] Wyszecki, G. and Stiles, W. S., Color Science: Concepts and Methods, Quantitative Data and Formulae (2nd ed.), Wiley, New York, 1982.

[985] Bamber, J. C., Speckle Reduction, in Wells, P. N. T., Advances in ultrasound techniques and instrumentation, Churchill Livingstone Inc. New York, NY, USA, pp. 55-67, 1993.

[986] Harris, R. A. and Wells, P. N. T., Ultimate limits in ultrasound image resolution, in Wells, P. N. T., Advances in ultrasound techniques and instrumentation, Churchill Livingstone Inc., New York, pp. 55-67, 1993.

[987] Harris, R. A., Follett, D. H., Halliwell, M. and Wells, P. N. T., Ultimate limits in ultrasound image resolution, Ultrasound in Med. Biol, Vol. 17, No. 6, pp. 547-558, 1991.

[988] Belliveau, J. W., Kennedy, D. N., McKinstry, R. C., Buchbinder, B. R., Weisskoff, R. M., Cohen, M. S., Vevea, J. M., Brady, T. J. and Rosen, B. R., Functional mapping of the human visual cortex by magnetic resonance imaging, Science, Vol. 254, No. 5032, pp. 716-719, 1991.

[989] Orrison, Jr., W. W., Lewin, D. J., Sanders, J. A., Hartshorne, M. F., Functional Brain Imaging, Mosby Publishers, ISBN 0-8151-6509-9, 1999.

[990] Pauling, L. and Coryell, C. D., The Magnetic Properties and Structure of Hemoglobin, Oxyhemoglobin and Carbonmonoxyhemoglobin, Proc. Natl. Acad. Sci., USA, Vol. 22, No. 3, pp. 210-216, 1936.

[991] Ogawa, S., Lee, T. M., Nayak, A. S. and Glynn, P., Oxygenation-sensitive contrast in magnetic resonance image of rodent brain at high magnetic fields, Magnetic Resonance in Medicine, Vol. 14, No. 1, pp. 68-78, 1990.

[992] Turner, R., Le Bihan, D., Monen, C. T. W., Despres, D., Frank, J., Echo-planar time course MRI of cat brain oxygenation changes, Magnetic Resonance in Medicine, Vol. 22, No. 1, pp. 159-166, Nov. 1991.

[993] Kwong, K. K., Belliveau, J. W., Chesler, D. A., Goldberg, I. E., Weisskoff, R. M., Poncelet, B. P., Kennedy, D. N., Hoppel, B. E., Cohen, M. S., Turner, R., Cheng H-M., Brady, T. J. and Rosen, B. R., Dynamic magnetic resonance imaging of human brain activity during primary sensory stimulation, Proc. Natl. Acad. Sci., USA, Vol. 89, No. 12, pp. 5675-5679, 1992.

[994] Fox, P. T., Raichle, M. E., Focal physiological uncoupling of cerebral blood flow and oxidative metabolism during somatosensory stimulation in human subjects, Proc. Natl. Acad. Sci., USA, Vol. 83, No. 4, pp. 1104-1144, 1986.

[995] Penfield, W., The evidence for a cerebral vascular mechanism in epilepsy, Ann. Intern. Med., Vol. 7, No. 3, pp. 303-310, 1933.

[996] Fisel, C. R., Ackerman, J. L., Buzton, R. B., Garrido, L., Belliveau, J. W., Rosen, B. R. and Brady, T. J., MR contrast due to microscopically heterogeneous magnetic susceptibility: Numerical simulations and applications to cerebral physiology, Magnetic Resonance in Medicine, Vol. 17, No. 2, pp. 336-347, 1991.

[997] Turner, R., Jezzard, P., Wen, H., Kwong, K. K., Le Bihan, D., Zeffiro, T., Balaban, R. S. and Balaban, R. S., Functional mapping of the human visual cortex at 4 and 1.5 Tesla using deoxygenation contrast EPI, Magnetic Resonance in Medicine, Vol. 29, No. 2, pp. 277-281, 1993.

[998] Chatfield, C. and Collins, A., Introduction to Multivariate Analysis, Chapman and Hall, London, ISBN: 0-4121-6040-4, 1980.

[999] Ogawa, S., Menon, R. S., Tank, D. W., Kim, S. G., Merkle, H., Ellerman, J. M. and Ugurbil, K., Functional brain mapping by blood oxygenation level-dependent contrast magnetic resonance imaging. A comparison of signal characteristics with a biophysical model, Biophysics Journal, Vol. 64, No. 3, pp. 803-812, 1993.

[1000] Weisskoff, R. M., Zuo, C. S., Boxerman, J. L. and Rosen, B. R., Microscopic susceptibility variation and transverse relaxation: Theory and experiment, Magnetic Resonance in Medicine, Vol. 31, No. 6, pp. 601-610, 1994.

[1001] Kennan, R. P., Zhong, J. and Gore, J. C., Intravascular susceptibility contrast mechanisms in tissues, Magnetic Resonance in Medicine, Vol. 31, No. 1, pp. 9-21, 1994.

[1002] Boxerman, J. L., Bandettini, P. A., Kwong, K. K., Baker, J. R., Davis, T. L., Rosen, B. R. and Weisskoff, R. M., The intravascular contribution to fMRI signal change: Monte Carlo modeling and diffusion-weighted studies *in-vivo*, Magnetic Resonance in Medicine, Vol. 34, No. 1, pp. 4-10, 1995.

[1003] Menon, R. S., Hu, X., Adriany, G., Andersen, P., Ogawa, S. and Ugurbil, K., BOLD based functional MRI at 4 Tesla includes a capillary bed contribution: echo-planar imaging correlates with previous optical imaging using intrinsic signals, Magnetic Resonance in Medicine, Vol. 33, No. 3, pp. 453-459, 1995.

Index

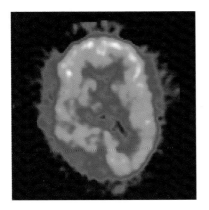 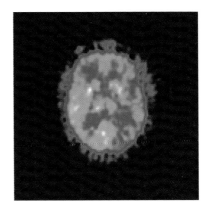

Plate 1: Sample PET images (courtesy of Keith A. Johnson, Harvard Medical School, Boston, source: The Whole Brain Atlas).

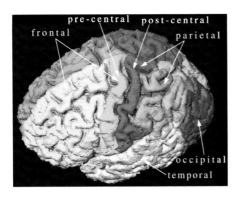 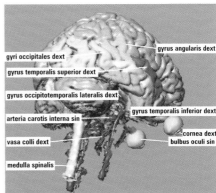

Plate 2: **Left**: Labeling of the cerebral lobes and regions in 3-D from the posterior end (courtesy of Xioalan Zeng, R2 Technology, Inc., Los Altos, CA). **Right**: Labeling of the cortex in 3-D from the posterior end (reproduced with permission from [340]. © Lippencott, Williams and Wilkins 1992). Both images are computer-generated. The algorithms used are discussed in Sub-sections 4.5.4 and 4.3.4.2.

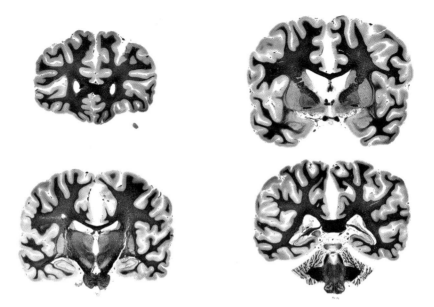

Plate 3: Specimen showing the brain sections (courtesy of John I. Johnson, Neuroscience Program, Michigan State University, source: //www.brainmuseum.org). Four sections of the human brain. The darker region is the WM and the area around it is the GM.

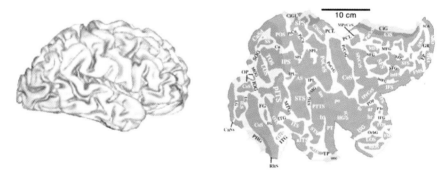

Plate 4: Flattening of the cerebral cortex using Van Essen's method (reproduced with permission from [356]. © 1997 Society for Neuroscience).

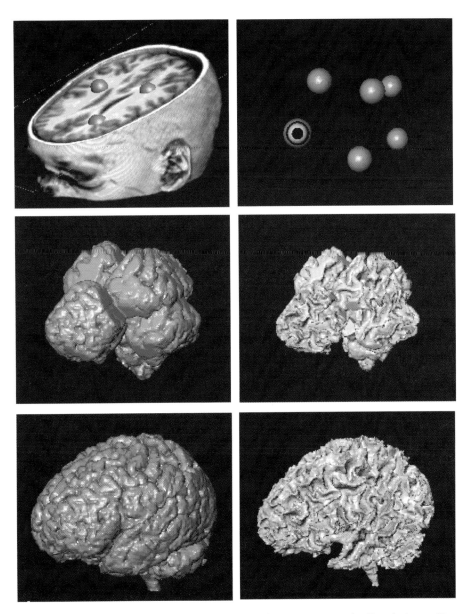

Plate 5: Propagation of the outer (pink) and inner (yellow) bounding surfaces. **Top Left**: embedded sphere sets as initializations shown in unedited 3-D MR brain volume. **Top Right**: outer (pink) and inner (yellow) bounding spheres. **Middle Left**: intermediate step in GM surface propagation. **Middle Right**: intermediate step in WM surface propagation. **Bottom Left**: final result of the segmented GM/CSF surface. **Bottom Right**: final result of the segmented WM/GM surface (© 1999 IEEE. Reprinted with permission from [327]).

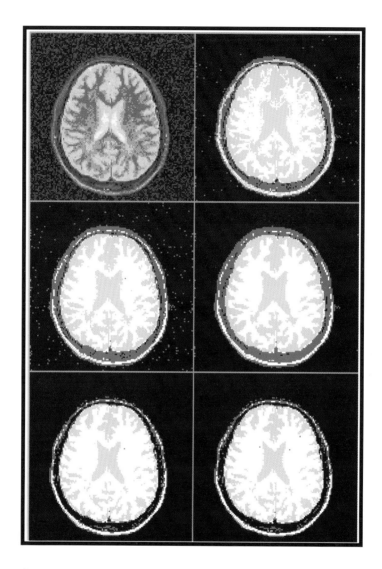

Plate 6: Segmentation of an MRI image: an MRI T_2-weighted image (top left), segmentation using the EM-CMM algorithm (top right), segmentation using the ML-SVMM algorithm (middle left), segmentation using the MAP-SVMM algorithm using $b = 1$ (middle right), segmentation using the MAP-SVMM algorithm using $b = 10$ (bottom left), and segmentation using the MAP-SVMM algorithm using $b = 1000$ (bottom right).

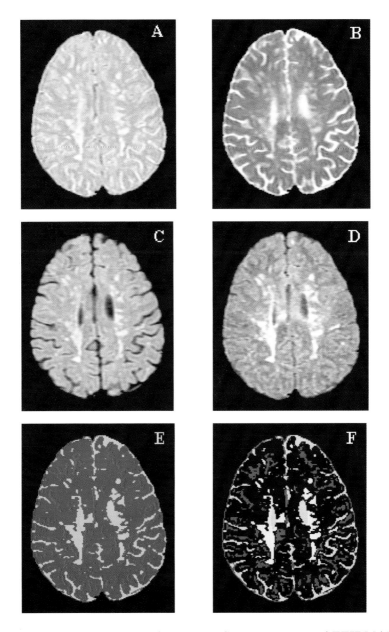

Plate 7: An axial MR image from an MS patient using AFFIRMATIVE pulse sequence: **Top Left**: using early-echo FSE. **Top Right**: using late-echo FSE. **Middle Left**: using early-echo FLAIR/MTC. **Middle Right**: using late-echo FLAIR/MTC. **Bottom Left** and **Bottom Right**: segmented results shown. Pink colored White Matter, gray colored Gray Matter, blue colored CSF, yellow colored MS lesions. Note that the MRIAP program minimizes false lesion classification by the use of FSE and flow information from FSE, FLAIR/MTC and flow images (MRSI data courtsey of the MR Lab., University of Texas Medical School, Houston, TX).

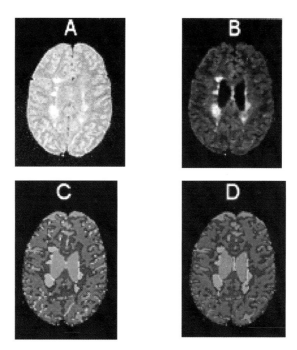

Plate 8: **Top Left**: unsegmented image acquired after early echo FSE (labeled A). **Top Right**: unsegmented late echo FLAIR/MTC (labeled B). **Bottom Left**: segmented FSE image (labeled C). **Bottom Right**: segmented FLAIR/MTC image (labeled D) (MRI data courtesy of the MR Lab., University of Texas Medical School, Houston, TX).

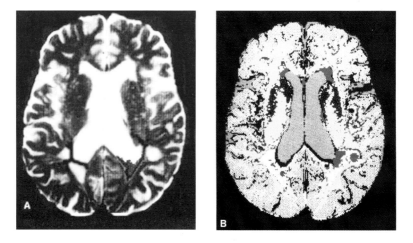

Plate 9: Feature map classification method. T_2-weighted image of MS patient showing lesions (bright areas) in the periventricular region (A). Segmented image-based Multi-spectral 3-D feature map showing two lesions in red (T_1-weighted component) and pink (T_2-weighted and proton density component) colors from the same patient (reproduced by permission of John Wiley & Sons Inc. from [725]. © 1999).

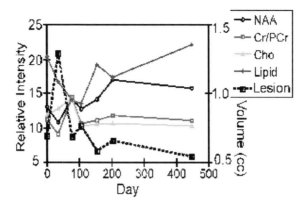

Plate 10: Time dependent temporal lipid and other metabolite concentration variations in an acute lesion rich area shown with different curves. This figure shows the relative intensity of metabolites against water as an internal reference and lesion volume. Note the time dependent metabolite normalization except for lipids. The lipid concentration remained higher when the lesion volume reached a maximum (courtesy of P. A. Narayana, University of Texas Medical School, Houston, TX).

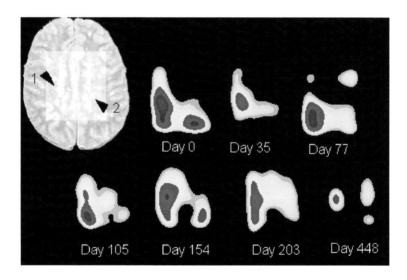

Plate 11: A spectroscopic VOI highlighted on 3 mm thick collapsed (left most) image with arrow heads occurs on enhancing lesion sites. Temporal changes in lipids in the enhancing lesions in different scan sessions are shown. Note, initially a slow increase was seen and then normalization of lipids occurred after 30 weeks (reproduced by permission of John Wiley & Sons Inc. from [787]. © 1998).

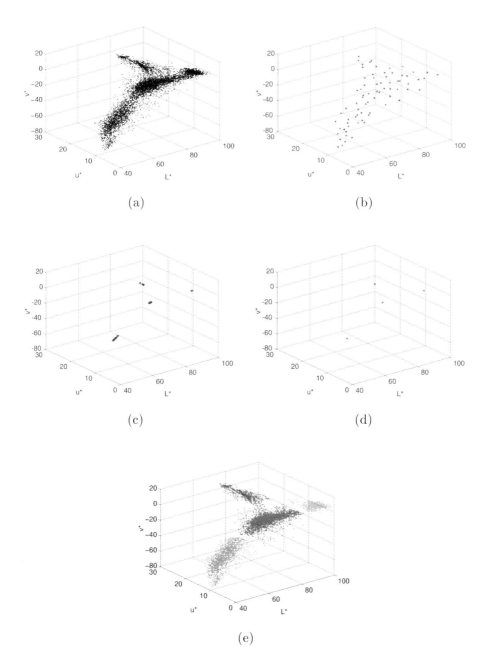

Plate 12: (a) Color vectors. (b) Sample set. (c) Cluster center candidates. (d) Cluster centers. (e) Delineated clusters. The color vectors are randomly sampled yielding the sample set which converges to cluster center candidates from which the cluster centers are extracted.